Travellers' Health
How to stay healthy abroad

Editor's Health Warning

We've done our best to make sure that the information in this book is accurate and up-to-date at time of going to press. You can find updates and further information on our web-site at **www.travellers-health.info**

Advice from books — and from websites — has its limitations, however, and can never take account of your own individual needs and circumstances. Advice offered here is not intended to be a substitute for skilled medical care, when such care is available.

Travellers' Health
How to stay healthy abroad

Fourth Edition

Devised and edited by
Dr Richard Dawood

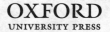

OXFORD
UNIVERSITY PRESS

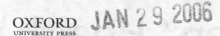

OXFORD

UNIVERSITY PRESS

Oxford University Press, Great Clarendon Street, Oxford OX2 6DP

Oxford University Press is a department of the University of Oxford.
It furthers the University's objective of excellence in research, scholarship,
and education by publishing world-wide in

Oxford New York

Auckland Bangkok Buenos Aires
Cape Town Chennai Dar es Salaam Delhi Hong Kong Istanbul
Karachi Kolkata Kuala Lumpur Madrid Melbourne Mexico City Mumbai
Nairobi São Paulo Shanghai Taipei Tokyo Toronto

and an associated company in Berlin

Oxford is a registered trade mark of Oxford University Press
in the UK and in certain other countries

Published in the United States
by Oxford University Press Inc., New York

Library of Congress Cataloging in Publication Data
Travellers' health: how to stay healthy abroad/ devised and edited by Richard
Dawood.– 4th ed.
Includes bibliographical references and index.
1. Travel–Health aspects. 2. Tropical medicine. I. Dawood, Richard M.
RA783.5.T68 2002 613.6'8–dc21 2001053129
ISBN 0 19 262947 6 (pbk. : alk. paper)
10 9 8 7 6 5 4 3 2 1

Typeset by EXPO Holdings, Malaysia
Printed in Great Britain
on acid-free paper by Biddles Ltd, Guildford & King's Lynn

To Gillian, Jamie, Harry and Archie

Foreword

Travellers' Health is an essential part of going abroad. You can never know too much about health hazards out on the road, and Richard Dawood has assembled a star cast of experts to reassure and terrify at the same time. This rich and authoritative latest edition should be taken at least once a day, before, during and after travelling.

London   Michael Palin
March 2002

Preface to the fourth edition

Since the first edition of this book was published in 1986, the global travel industry has more than doubled in size — a growth matched by much greater interest in travellers' health. The concept of travel medicine as a unified field encompassing many disciplines has become widely acknowledged: travel medicine is now a distinct medical specialty in its own right. There is a thriving International Society of Travel Medicine, that has brought together experts and practitioners from all over the world; and there are many regional and local organizations and professional associations devoted to the same cause. International bodies such as the WHO, and national health departments in many countries, are increasingly aware of travel-related health risks and the importance of reducing them. But there is still no room for complacency.

Consider, for example, the current global burden of poverty and ill-health* - now increasing, not receding:

- Number of people with no access to safe drinking water: 1100 million (according to one assessment, no fewer than half the world's hospital beds are occupied by people suffering from 'diseases they drank')
- Number of people with no access to adequate sanitation: 2400 million
- Number of malnourished children in developing countries: 149 million
- Number of people killed by water related diseases each year: 5 million
- Number of people living on less than $1 per day — the official yardstick of poverty: 1200 million
- Number of children dying each year from vaccine-preventable diseases: 2 million
- Number of African children living with HIV: 1.1 million

Travel to developing countries is one of the fastest growing sectors in the travel industry: it can bring economic growth, and can be a force for good: but travellers need to be alert, informed, and well-prepared, if they are to minimize risks to their own health that can sometimes be substantial.

Diseases that seemed to be in decline, just two decades ago, are now back with a vengeance. In the 1980s, I had to struggle to find a clinician with first-hand knowledge of diphtheria to contribute a chapter on that subject for this book's first edition: the only experts were in semi-retirement; during the Nineties, a huge epidemic in the former Soviet Union put diphtheria back on the global agenda. Other diseases that then seemed barely to merit attention included TB, HIV and anthrax. Yellow fever has reappeared in South American cities for the first time in forty years. Ebola, hantavirus, Nipah, variant CJD at least thirty new, emerging or re-emerging infecting organisms have appeared during the past 30 years, and the problem is getting worse. Even smallpox has resurfaced as a possible concern.

Improving our systems for surveillance and response is a high priority. We rely heavily on the expertise of the World Health Organization and the US government's Centers for Disease Control and Prevention (CDC). In the UK, tropical medicine resources and expertise suffered a tragic decline during the Eighties and Nineties. What seemed a quaint relic of an embarrassing colonial past, proved a soft target for cuts in government spending. Tropical expertise within the British Army also declined — as vividly evidenced by the high toll of malaria in British troops posted to Sierra Leone during 2000. Belatedly, there's a new government initiative to improve the situation (Getting ahead of the Curve — see Further reading.

The most common travel-related illnesses are more mundane: two fifths of all international travellers suffer from travellers' diarrhoea; most often a minor inconvenience, endured in silence, it can easily become a miserable experience, disrupting travel plans, causing expense, and occasionally resulting in hospitalization and prolonged illness. Some travellers have come to regard diarrhoea as inevitable or acceptable — the norm; it is not. It is interesting, though, that the likelihood of developing travellers' diarrhoea has not diminished in 40 years; despite the huge growth in our awareness of health issues that are closer to home, large numbers of travellers are still not getting the information they need to stay healthy, or are not putting it into practice. Another 'mundane' problem is on the increase: sexually transmitted diseases — especially among young people: the 'safe sex' messages of the 1980s and 1990s have been diluted or forgotten: in the UK, the prevalence of gonorrhoea has risen sharply, while syphilis is for the first time now back at post-World War II levels.

Since the last edition of this book, many new travel health issues have come to the fore. Not least among them is the problem of flight-related deep vein thrombosis (DVT), considered in greater detail elsewhere in this book. Like most 'new' issues, this is in fact an old one that we have had good cause to cover before. There are those in the airline industry who insist that the problem is due purely to immobility — having nothing to do with inadequate leg room, or the cramped conditions that prevail in the economy class cabin, or any other factors that are a feature of long-haul air travel; and that DVT is therefore not the airlines' problem. But the recent finding that as many as ten per cent of long-haul air travellers suffer from symptomless blood clots gives new grounds for concern, and new urgency to the more detailed research that is now under way. Similar concerns apply to other aspects of in-flight health: the airline industry has done little to lay to rest passenger concerns about cabin air quality, or to combat the growing problem of 'air rage' and its causes. In a recent instance of the latter, the acquittal of an American rock star has exposed a dangerous legal loophole: he successfully blamed his violent rampage through the First Class cabin of a British Airways jet on an interaction between alcohol and a commonly-used sleeping tablet, thereby avoiding liability for his actions.

The relentless spread of drug-resistant malaria continues to leave havoc in its wake, sometimes in unexpected ways. One consequence of its spread is the near uselessness, in some parts of the world, of the previously trusted antimalarial drug combination, chloroquine and Paludrine. Medicines that are non-toxic, and that are therefore considered to have limited potential for causing harm, are increasingly being made available to the public without the need for a doctor's prescription: in the UK, this is true for chloroquine and Paludrine, which are currently the only antimalarial drugs on pharmacy sale. In the UK, there are numerous examples on record of people suffering severe or fatal malaria as a direct consequence of purchasing chloroquine and Paludrine at a pharmacy, bypassing the opportunity for skilled medical advice. One recent case includes a woman in her fifties, who lost both legs from complications of severe malaria, following a trip to the Gambia, having sought advice at her local pharmacy. Chloroquine and Paludrine cause harm by giving inadequate protection, and in my own view their pharmacy sale is an unacceptable anomaly.

One welcome addition to our antimalarial armoury is atovaquone + proguanil (Malarone) — which was licensed in Norway in 1997, in the USA in 2000, and in the UK and the rest of Europe in 2001. The first new antimalarial drug in almost a decade, Malarone combines a high degree of effectiveness with a low rate of side effects, though at higher cost than its predecessors. There are new drugs and vaccines against other travel-related ills that are now at advanced stage of development. They, like Malarone, are the product of a massive and sustained research effort: it is increasingly clear that they, too, will cost us more. Healthcare costs are a controversial issue in most parts of the world, perhaps nowhere more so than at present in the UK, where most healthcare is funded from general taxation. But should the taxpayer bear the cost of more, better vaccines and medicines, offering improved protection and greater peace of mind, for business and leisure travellers alike? Should travellers' health, now or in the future, be funded from the same purse as neonatal intensive care, accident and emergency medicine, or cancer research? Like health insurance, the costs of travel medicine should be part of the costs of travel, though in the UK, cost issues are a nettle that we have not yet fully grasped.

Pharmaceutical costs have spawned a shadowy trade in counterfeit and adulterated vaccines and medicines that pose a real and serious hazard to local people and travellers in many parts of the world. One of my patients recently acquired hepatitis A ten months after receiving a supposed hepatitis A vaccine in the Ukraine (p. 556). The dangers of fakes are an important reason why travellers should receive their vaccines in the safety of their home environment, and should travel with their own supply of medicines like antimalarials or antibiotics, rather than attempting to buy them abroad in an effort to save costs.

Vaccination against polio has been remarkably successful, and a global campaign has eliminated the disease from many parts of the world: the next two years will show whether or not the efforts can be sustained and followed through to successful global eradication. But polio has a sting in its tail: the virus used in the oral vaccine may persist in the environment, and is capable of reverting to a more virulent, disease-producing form: we may not yet have seen the last of it.

The terrorist attacks on New York of September 11th 2001 and their aftermath have had profound effects upon travel, upon the travel industry and upon travel medicine. Some of these are considered elsewhere in this book, but it is noteworthy that they have not been exclusively negative. For example, the anthrax attacks triggered a massive research initiative into ways of combating anthrax toxin: within a matter of weeks, X-ray crystallography studies of its structure revealed an innate vulnerability — an 'Achilles' heel' — a previously unknown target for development of new drugs against this ancient scourge. Similarly, the fear that stocks of smallpox virus might have fallen into the hands of bioterrorists has triggered the accelerated development of new smallpox vaccines, as well as a new, tailor-made oral drug against smallpox. If only the same research effort and resources could be mobilized and channelled against some of the other tropical and infectious diseases that claim a heavy toll. In the post September 11th era, perhaps there will be broader acceptance that 'an infectious disease in one country is the concern of all' (p. 602).

What health risks should travellers know about? Which travellers are at highest risk? A recent study suggests our traditional approach may be seriously flawed. Of cases of hepatitis A in travellers from Canada, only seven per cent occurred in people whose destination, manner or style of travel fell into a category of 'high risk.' Further analysis revealed that if every high-risk traveller had been vaccinated against hepatitis A, the overall toll would have been cut by *just seven per cent*. Health precautions for travel need to be applied and understood much more widely if they are to have an impact — they are for everyone, not just those at 'high risk'.

This book has been thoroughly updated and revised. It has its own website, at www.travellers-health.info. Wherever you are bound, I hope you will find it both thought-provoking and helpful.

London   R.M.D.
April 2002

*See also Taipale et al., *War or Health* – Further reading

From the Preface to previous editions

From the moment they leave the security of their accustomed environment, travellers are at risk. Hazards arise not just from strange diseases they encounter on their travels, but from other factors too: home comforts such as a safe water supply, sanitation and public hygiene controls, legal safety standards for motor vehicles and road maintenance, to give just a few examples, may not seem very inspiring, and are easily taken for granted when they are present, but simply do not exist in many popular travel destinations. Environmental factors such as arduous conditions, adverse climate, and high altitude may constitute a hazard; and so may travellers' own behaviour while away — on holiday, free from the restraints of the daily routine, and determined to have a good time with scant regard for the consequences.

When illness or injury occurs abroad, travellers are again at a disadvantage — from inability to communicate with a doctor on account of language or cultural difficulties, inability to find a doctor owing to ignorance of the local medical system, inability perhaps to pay for skilled care in a sudden emergency. They may be a complete absence of skilled medical care, or of medical facilities of a standard acceptable to travellers from technologically sophisticated countries.

When symptoms of an illness acquired abroad do not appear until *after* return home (up to a year later, for example, in certain cases of malaria) a final hazard becomes apparent: the symptoms may be unfamiliar, may pass unrecognized, and the correct diagnosis may not be considered until it is too late.

This book offers neither an exhaustive catalogue of obscure tropical diseases nor a course of training in first aid; it *is* an anthology of invited, *specialist* opinion on a wide range of problems of concern to travellers; concern, either because a genuine hazard exists that travellers should know about, and should take precautions to avoid, or because a disease or hazard which in fact constitutes no real threat has been the potential source of unwarranted anxiety.

It is a popular misconception that exotic infections pose the principal danger to travellers' health. While this book presents detailed information and advice about disease hazards and their prevention, other, no less important hazards have not been neglected. Accidents, for example, are the single most frequent cause of death in travellers abroad, causing 25 times as many deaths as infectious diseases. Some accidents and disasters are indeed indiscriminate, and raise issues of safety and security that concern all of us. Most accidents involving travellers, however, like the majority of travellers' health problems, are in fact preventable or under a considerable degree of individual control. People worry increasingly about the dangers of blood transfusion and other forms of medical treatment abroad; prevention of accidents is the most effective way of reducing these risks as well.

Travel may have other unexpected implications for health, not traditionally encompassed by Travel Medicine: an unwanted pregnancy, the possible consequence of failure of absorption of the Pill during a severe bout of traveller's diarrhoea, can ruin the memory of a holiday no less surely than a tropical disease.

The scope of this book largely reflects the range of problems which I have come across during my own travel — often without having been able to deal with them to my own satisfaction at the time — and many subjects discussed here have not previously been given detailed attention in books for travellers. A specialist view is presented on each topic, because the range of subjects considered extends beyond the first-hand experience and expertise of any one individual, and because when travellers are most in need of information or advice about health, they need advice that they can trust and depend on, not myth that has simply been handed on.

Like the rest of medicine, however, travellers' health is not an exact science, and consensus is lacking on many crucial issues. A recent survey found visitors from different countries to the same part of East Africa following no fewer than *eighty* different antimalarial regimes (but an alarming 30% of the visitors were taking no precautions at all). Some of the problems raised in this book have no satisfactory solution, or have solutions that remain a matter of opinion or the subject of debate. Readers will therefore detect differences of opinion between contributors to this book, or may disagree with their conclusions, and we hope that this will stimulate and encourage further debate.

In general, the quality of advice on health matters customarily given to travellers has not been good: adequate pre-travel information and advice are the exception rather than the rule — or this book would not be necessary.

Doctors in developed countries receive minimal training in, and remain largely unfamiliar with, hazards outside their own environment. In a report on the deaths of seven travellers who succumbed to acute mountain sickness while trekking in the Himalayas, Dr John Dickinson pointed out that three of the seven who died were themselves doctors. As Dr Dickinson explains on p. 224, all of those deaths could readily have been avoided. And enough doctors were stricken with diarrhoea on a recent British Medical Association Congress in Egypt, to make headline news at home. Worse still, a third of the doctors attending a gastroenterology convention in Mexico were also stricken.

Deaths still occur in developed countries from malaria, and occur in previously fit, healthy young travellers; initial symptoms are all too easily confused with influenza and deterioration is often rapid without prompt treatment. In the past decade, some 50 000 cases of malaria have occurred in travellers entering Europe. Each year, there are now more than 2000 cases of malaria in travellers entering the UK, and around 1000 cases in travellers entering the USA — for both countries, these figures have trebled over the past ten years. Most of the travellers either did not seek or receive appropriate advice, or did not follow it; many of them, however, knew about the dangers, but simply could not be bothered with precautions. The number of people coming home with malaria rises steadily every year.

Doctors tend to be poor educators; we have depressingly little to show for our efforts to educate the general public on even such a clear-cut issue as the effects of cigarette smoking on health. How much more difficult, then, is it for doctors to provide large numbers of departing travellers with detailed information and effective advice for their trip when the usual forum for doing so is a single, hurried consultation, just before departure. There are limits to what can be achieved in or should be expected from a medical consultation under the best of circumstances, even when the doctor is well-motivated and well-informed about the subject, and the traveller is receptive, has a perfect memory, and is good at doing what he or she is told.

What kind of advice should travellers receive? A list of rules and instructions given without explanation or justifications carries the implication that travellers are incapable of understanding the principles involved, are not interested, or do not 'need' to know. It is hardly surprising that advice offered on such condescending terms is seldom followed for long.

The best advice is not a list of do's and don'ts, but is based on information, a clear, rational explanation from which a conclusion is obvious. Information is a powerful weapon, and I believe that travellers should have the opportunity to choose for themselves how much they 'want' or 'need' to know; to an extent, this book is a personal statement of the kind of information I believe should be readily available to anyone interested.

Throughout this book, we have studiously avoided giving blanket advice to consult a doctor without stating the reason for doing so. 'Consult your doctor' is a useful formula to enable advice-givers to evade difficult issues, but is a particularly unhelpful one when it relates to a problem which may arise abroad. It is not easy to find a doctor in a remote place, or to communicate with one in an alien land. Merely finding a doctor does not guarantee that correct advice or treatment will be given. Some 85% of the world's population have never seen a doctor, and never will; advice for travellers must take account of the fact that travellers to many parts of the world will be in the same position.

Advice from doctors, travel agents, embassies, or immunization centres too often goes no further than to provide details of statutory vaccination certificate entry requirements. Few legal requirements now remain, and they are generally no more than public health measures, designed to protect countries from imported disease; they should not be confused with, and are no substitute for, clear advice and instruction on staying healthy abroad. All those who dispense 'advice' which is in fact limited to information about statutory requirements have a responsibility to make it clear that additional precautions are almost always necessary for personal protection. Such further precautions need to be spelt out in detail: advice to 'take care with food hygiene' is practically meaningless to anyone who has never given serious thought to the problems of travelling or living in an environment where total absence of 'basic' sanitary measures is the norm; there is growing public awareness of food safety and hygiene issues, however, which can only help for the future.

In the time since this book first appeared, there has been undoubted growth in interest and awareness of the health problems of travel, and it would be gratifying to think that this book might have made even a small contribution to the process. One group has patently failed to make any large scale contribution, however: the travel industry still views health information for travel as bad for business, or not its concern, a few travel agents appear to see farther than the commission on their next sale. They argue that, since they are not doctors, it is not their responsibility to dispense health advice; but they belittle the problems instead of pointing out the need for advice and directing travellers to suitable sources.

> 'I cannot for the life of me understand the logic in your telling readers about the pollution problem in Rio de Janeiro. Somehow it seems a very self-destructive tack for a publication supposed to encourage, not discourage, world travel. You are doing both your readers and your advertisers a disservice.'
> New York advertising agency executive for VARIG,
> writing to withdraw all further advertising
> from Condé Nast *Traveler* magazine.
>
> 'We rejoice in the enrichments of travel, but our aim is to give readers the fullest information, frankly and fairly. They know it's a big world, where sometimes it's sunny and sometimes it rains. Isn't travel just as likely to be discouraged when it begins in illusion and ends in frustration and disappointment?'
> Harold Evans, Founding Editor,
> Condé Nast *Traveler* magazine, New York

An American survey showed that only 28% of travellers to malarial areas had received any kind of notification from their travel agent that malaria might be a possible hazard. A British victim of malaria, which was acquired on a holiday in the Gambia, was actually told by the travel agent who made the booking that there was no malaria in the Gambia. A Dutch survey showed that travellers who had used travel agents as their sole source of advice were in fact at even greater risk than those who had not troubled to seek advice from any source. There are cases on record where elderly people have been booked on tours to Peru, without any warning about the dangers of high altitude, and have died as a result. One-third of British travel brochures make no reference to health whatsoever, according to another recent survey, while only 10% give any useful specific health information.

More problems for travellers means more work for consular officials, who now receive a record number of requests for assistance. In 1988, in an attempt to reduce the burden, the British Government made repeated requests to the Association of British Travel Agents to include information leaflets with tickets. These requests were turned down.

There have been well-substantiated reports in the British Press of injured and sick tourists, in many resorts, being taken for treatment not to the nearest or most suitable hospital, but to the one that pays the largest commission to the local representative of the tour company. London's *Sunday Times* identified a number of representatives who had received 'backhanders'. In most cases this is against company policy, and the newspaper reports resulted in staff dismissals; however, travel companies appear to be doing little to stamp out what is still believed to be a widespread practice. Journalists from the *Sunday Times*, posing as tour representatives were easily able to discover the going rates of commission paid by local hospital doctors, ambulance services, and even undertakers. In many resorts, representatives also receive commissions from companies that hire mopeds and motorcycles to tourists — that cause many of the injuries in the first place.

Tour companies are in a position to influence, monitor, and enforce hygiene and safety standards in hotels and resorts; the opportunity to do so is currently being ignored, even though many companies are fully aware of the hazards. Instead, travellers face shabby attempts to disclaim legal liability for the consequences, thinly concealed in the fine print of the brochures.

There are occasional praiseworthy exceptions: some of the best immunization centres anywhere in the world are owned and operated by travel companies, such as the British Airways Clinics, and the Thomas Cook unit in London. Most of the travel trade has far to go, however, to the extent that those who care about travellers' health still cannot regard them as partners with shared objectives. New European legislation may shortly be introduced to formalize liability of travel agents and tour operators for the information they provide. Meanwhile, judge your travel agent by the extent of visible concern for your health and safety.

If the foregoing gives a rather gloomy view of the state of affairs confronting today's traveller — for whom it is tempting, though incorrect, to assume that advances in medical technology at home have been matched by like progress in combating disease abroad — it is because gloom is justified. Close to *half* of all international travellers experience some kind of adverse effect upon their health as a result of their trip. The majority of problems are inevitably minor ones; but Britons now take over 25 million trips abroad every year, Americans take almost 40 million trips, and more than a million Americans now travel by air every day. The scale on which international travel is now taking place lends perspective to the problem (see also p. 8).

Travellers' health has been a neglected corner of medicine for too long, but more attention from doctors and anyone else can only be a partial solution; ultimately travellers have to look after themselves, and this book aims to give them the power to do so. In this book, the problems have been addressed by experts. It is my fervent hope, and has been my sole purpose in initiating and presenting this project, that travellers will take note of its conclusions.

R.M.D.

Contents

Appendices

List of contributors

Professor Michael Barer
Professor of Clinical Microbiology, Department of Microbiology and Immunolgy, University of Leicester, Leicester, UK

Professor Christopher Bartlett
Visiting Professor at University College London and London School of Hygiene and Tropical Medicine, London, UK

Dr Buddha Basnyat
Medical Director, Nepal International Clinic, Nepal; Medical Director, Himalaya Rescue Association; Professor of Clinical Physiology, Institute of Medicine in Katmandu, Nepal; Consultant in Medicine, Patan Hospital, Nepal

Dr Laura Bedford
Médécins sans Frontières, Herat, Afghanistan

Dr Ron Behrens
Consultant in Tropical and Travel Medicine, Hospital for Tropical Diseases, London, UK; Senior Lecturer, London School of Hygiene and Tropical Medicine, London, UK

Dr Alan Benson
Visiting Consultant, RAF Centre for Aviation Medicine, Henlow, UK

Dr Delia B. Bethel
Specialist Registrar in Paediatrics, John Radcliffe Hospital, Oxford, UK

Dr Herbert A. Brant
Formerly Professor of Clinical Obstetrics and Gynaecology at University College Hospital, London

Dr Ian F. Burgess
Director, Medical Entomology Centre, Cambridge University, Cambridge, UK

Nicholas Cameron MC
Research and Risk Management Consultant, AKE Ltd., UK

Dr Elphis Christopher
Consultant in Family Planning and Reproductive Care, Haringey NHS Trust, London, UK

Dr Jonathan H. Cossar
General Practitioner; Primary Care Consultant Advisor, Scottish Centre for Infection and Environmental Health, Glasgow, UK

Dr George Cowan
Medical Director, UK Joint Committee on Higher Medical Training; Past President, Royal Society of Tropical Medicine and Hygiene; formerly Consultant Physician, British Army

Professor Christopher Curtis
Department of Medical Parasitology, London School of Hygiene and Tropical Medicine, London, UK

Dr Robert N. Davidson
Consultant Physician, Department of Infectious Diseases & Tropical Medicine, Northwick Park Hospital, Harrow, UK

Dr Peter Davies
Consultant Respiratory Physician, Cardiothoracic Centre and Aintree University Hospital, Liverpool, UK

Andrew Dawood
Specialist in Prosthodontics, Dental Clinic, 45 Winepole Street, London, UK

Dr Richard Dawood
Specialist in Travel Medicine and Medical Director, Fleet Street Clinic, London

Dr Carol Dow
Chief Medical Adviser, Foreign and Commonwealth Office, London, UK

Dr Elizabeth Driver
Medical Consultant and Partner, Arnold and Porter, London, UK; Honorary Clinical Lecturer, University College & Middlesex School of Medicine, London, UK; Consultant, Medical Research Council Toxiology Unit, Carshalton, UK

Dr D. Peter Drotman
Senior Medical Officer, National Center for Infectious Diseases, Centers for Disease Control and Prevention, Atlanta, US

Ms Paula Dudley
Podiatrist, The Fleet Street Clinic, London, UK

Dr Jules Eden
Director, E-med, London UK

Professor Jean Emberlin
Director, National Pollen Research Unit, University College, Worcester, UK

Dr Richard Fairhurst
Director, Accident and Emergency Department, Chorley District Hospital, Chorley, UK; Medical Director, Lancashire Ambulance Service; Medical Director, NHS Direct North West Coast, UK

Mr Timothy ffytche
Consultant Ophthalmologist, Moorfields Eye Hospital; Consultant Ophthalmologist, Hospital for Tropical Diseases, London, UK

Dr Susan Fisher-Hoch
Virologist and Medical Epidemiologist, School of Public Health, University of Texas, Houston, USA

Ms Agnes Fletcher
Parliamentary Affairs Manager, Disability Rights Commission, London, UK

Dr Hemda Garelick
Principal Lecturer in Environmental Microbiology, Middlesex University, London, UK

Dr Larry Goodyer
Lecturer in Clinical Pharmacy, King's College London, London, UK

Paul Goodyer
Managing Director, Nomad Travellers Store and Medical Centre, London, UK

Professor Brian M. Greenwood
Professor of Tropical Medicine, Clinical Research Unit, London School of Hygiene and Tropical Medicine, London, UK

Dr Richard Harding
Consultant in Biomechanics and Injury Causation, Biodynamic Research Corporation, San Antonio, Texas, USA; formerly Consultant in Aviation Medicine, RAF Centre for Aviation Medicine, Farnborough, UK

Professor John Hawk
Consultant Dermatologist, St John's Dermatology Centre, St Thomas' Hospital, London, UK; Head of the Photobiology Unit, St Thomas' Hospital, London, UK

Mr Basil Helal
Consultant Orthopaedic Surgeon, The London Hospital and the Royal National Orthopaedic Hospital, London, UK

Dr David L. Heymann
Executive Director, Communicable Diseases, World Health Organisation, Geneva, Switzerland

Dr Chris Johnson
Consultant Anaesthetist, Southmead Hospital, Bristol, UK

Dr Jonathan E. Kaplan
Medical Epidemiologist, Centers for Disease Control and Prevention, Atlanta, USA; Attending Physician, Veterans Affairs Medical Center, Atlanta, USA

Dr Arnold F. Kaufmann
Expert Consultant, Emergency Preparedness and Response Branch, Centers for Disease Control and Prevention, Atlanta, USA

Andreas King
Director, SERM, London, UK; Formerly Assistant Editor of *Water & Waste Treatment Journal*

Dr Richard Knight
Associate Specialist in General Medicine, Royal Sussex County Hospital, Brighton, UK; Formely Professor of Parasitology, Department of Medical Microbiology, University of Nairobi, Kenya

Dr Gil Lea
Consultant, Travel Health Sections, Communicable Disease Surveillance Centre, Public Health Laboratory Service, Colindale, UK

Roger Lewis†
Formerly Research specialist in international drug traffic; formerly Visiting Professor, National Research Council — IERROSS, Salerno, Italy

Dr Diana N. J. Lockwood
Consultant Leprologist, Hospital for Tropical Diseases, London, UK; Senior Lecturer, London School of Hygiene and Tropical Medecine, London, UK

Dr Iain B. McIntosh
General Practitioner, Stirling, Scotland, UK

Dr Martin Mitcheson
Former Clinical Director, South West Regional Drug Advisory Service, Bristol, UK

Dr John Naponick
Medical Administrator, Department of Health and Hospitals, Office of Public Health, Alexandria, Louisiana, USA

Dr Nebojša Nikolić
Lecturer, Faculty of Maritime Studies, Rijeka College of Maritime Studies, Rijeka, Croatia

Professor Geoffrey Pasvol
Professor of Infection and Tropical Medicine, the Lister Unit, Imperial College School of Medicine, Northwick Park and St Mark's Hospital, Harrow, Middlesex, UK

Dr John Paul
Consultant Medical Microbiologist and Director, Brighton Public Health Laboratory, Brighton, UK

Dr Michael Phelan
Consultant Psychiatrist and Honorary Senior Lecturer, Charing Cross Hospital, London, UK

Dr Ernst Philipp
Consultant Physician, Centre for Health in Employment and the Environment, Department of Occupational Health & Safety, Bristol Royal Infirmary, Bristol, UK

Dr Robin Philipp
Occupational Physician and Director, Centre for Health in Employment and the Environment, Department of Occupational Health & Safety, Bristol Royal Infirmary, Bristol, UK

Ms Ellen Poage
Registered Nurse and Health Educator, Fort Myers, Florida, USA

Professor Daniel Reid
Honorary Professor, University of Glasgow, UK; Visiting Professor, University of Strathclyde, UK; Formerly Director, Scottish Centre for Infection and Environmental Health, Glasgow, UK

Surgeon-Commander Simon Ridout
Formerly Principal Medical Officer, Royal Naval Air Station, Culdrose, UK

Dr C. J. Schofield
London School of Hygiene and Tropical Medicine, London, UK

Professor Gordon Seward
Emeritus Professor, Oral and Maxillo-Facial Surgery, University of London, London, UK

Ms Jean Sinclair,
Public Health Specialist and Marine Biologist, Medical Trainer, the Voluntary Service Overseas, UK

Dr David Smith†
Former Senior Lecturer in Clinical Tropical Medicine, Liverpool School of Tropical Medicine, Liverpool, UK

Dr Alastair Smith
President, International & Maritime Health Consultants inc.; independent consultant to the cruise and maritime industry; formerly Vice President and Medical Director, P&O and Princess Cruises

Dr David Snashall
Senior Lecturer in Occupational Medicine, Guy's and St Thomas' Hospitals, London, UK; Occupational Physician and Chief Medical Adviser to the British Foreign and Commonwealth Office and Department for International Development

Dr Tom Solomon
Lecturer in Neurology and Honorary Lecturer in Medical Microbiology and Tropical Medicine, University of Liverpool, Liverpool, UK

Dr S. Bertel Squire
Senior Lecturer in Clinical and Tropical Medicine and Consultant Physician, Division of Tropical Medicine, Liverpool School of Tropical Medicine, Liverpool, UK

Dr Rollin Stott
Senior Medical Officer (Research), Defence Research Agency, Centre for Human Sciences, Department of Aeromedicine and Neuroscience, Farnborough, UK

Dr David Swerdlow
Medical Epidemiologist, Centers for Disease Control and Prevention, Atlanta, USA

Colonel (retired) Michael J. G. Thomas
Clinical Director, the Blood Care Foundation, UK

Pamela Thorne
Research Psychologist, Centre for Health in Employment and the Environment, Department of Occupational Health and Safety, Bristol Royal Infirmary, Bristol, UK

Dr C. Louise Thwaites
Research Registrar, University of Oxford Wellcome Trust Clinical Research Unit, Ho Chi Min City, Vietnam

Dr Francisco Vega-López
Consultant Dermatologist, University College London Hospitals NHS Trust, London, UK

Professor David Warrell
Professor of Tropical Medicine and Infectious Diseases and Founding Director of the Centre of Tropical Medicine, University of Oxford, Oxford, UK; Honorary Clinical Director, Alistair Reid Venom Research Unit, Liverpool School of Tropical Medicine, Liverpool, UK; Consultant to the World Health Organisation, the Royal Geographical Society, the British Army, and the Medical Research Council

Dr Tony Waterston
Honorary Senior Clinical Lecturer in Child Health, University of Newcastle, Newcastle-upon-Tyne, UK

Dr Peter Watkins
Honorary Consultant Physician, King's College Hospital, London, UK

Dr Mary E. Wilson
Associate Professor of Medicine, Harvard Medical School, Cambridge, Massachusetts, USA; Associate Professor of Population and International Health, Harvard School of Public Health, Cambridge, Massachusetts, USA; Chief of Infectious Diseases and Director, Travel Resource Center, Mount Auburn Hospital, Cambridge, Massachusetts, USA

Dr David M. Wright
Consultant Microbiologist and Reader in Medical Microbiology, Department of Medical Microbiology, Imperial College, London, UK

Professor Arie J. Zuckerman
Dean and Director of the World Health Organisation Collaborating Centre for Reference and Research on Viral Diseases, Royal Free and University College Medical School, London, UK

Dr Jane N. Zuckerman
Director, Academic Centre for Travel Medicine and Vaccines, The Royal Free Travel Health Centre, Royal Free and University College Medical School, London, UK

Acknowledgements

I should like to record the debt that this book owes to contributors to previous UK and US editions, and to others who have given expert advice on specific points over the years. These have included: Andrew Agle, John Becher, Dr Norman Begg, Lt. Col John Dickinson, Dr Herbert DuPont, Dr Christopher Ellis, Mr Peter Fison, Dr William Foege, Dr Anthony Hall, Dr Donald Hopkins, Barbara Hornby, Dr Robert Horsburgh, Dr Peter Janke, Dr Jay Keystone, Edward Lee, Dr Hans Lobel, Professor Denis Mitchison, Air Commodore Anthony Nicholson, Dr Peter Oliver, Peta Pascoe, Dr John Pettit, Nancy Piet Pelon, Dr Thomas Quan, Dr Sonia Richards, Dr Simon Ridout, Rod Robinson, Dr George Schmid, Dr Stan Schwartz, Dr Bonita Stanton, Professor Robert Steffen, Gary Stoller, Aaron Sugarman, Dr Theodore Tsai, Dr Mary Warrell, Louise Weiss, Dr Philip Welsby, Dr Martin Wolfe, and Dr George Wyatt.

Of the past contributors, sadly Col. Jim Adam, Dr Stanley Browne, Dr David Haddock, and Dr Clinton Manson-Bahr are deceased, and Roger Lewis and Dr David Smith died before this edition was published.

This project owes much to the assistance and goodwill of many: they include a large number of colleagues, friends and erstwhile travelling companions who have contributed to my own knowledge of travel medicine; and too many people to name individually who have provided advice and practical help with this project since work began on the first edition of this book in the early 1980s.

For this edition, it is a pleasure to welcome many new contributors, and to acknowledge the role of many who have been involved in this project from its start: I thank all of the contributors for their wisdom, patience and participation, and for sharing their expertise. The drawings of insects are by Amanda Callaghan, and the drawings of snakes and other venomous creatures are by Professor David Warrell.

Special thanks also to: Sophie Chadwick and all my colleagues at the Fleet Street Clinic; Harold Evans; Thomas J. Wallace and my colleagues at Condé Nast *Traveler* in New York; Graham Boynton and colleagues at the Daily Telegraph; Anna and Barry Giles; and Alison Langton, Susan Harrison, Kate Martin and the many others at Oxford University Press who have worked tirelessly on this project over the years.

About using this book

- This book contains more information than other health books for travellers: is all this information really necessary? For example, all most travellers really *need* to know about rabies is that it is a serious disease, spread by animal bites. If you are unlucky enough to be bitten abroad, however, as I have been, your life may suddenly depend upon having detailed information you would probably not want to carry in your head: how to treat the bite, what kind of vaccine to insist on, and what to do. It is not always possible to predict what will happen when you travel, and health information based on 'just a few tips' to follow won't always help you. The main objective of this book is to draw together all the health information you might need, direct from the experts who really know. You may not want to read all of it in advance, and you may choose not to follow all of the precautions we suggest, but having the information available at least allows *you* to make that choice

- This book is mainly about prevention, so to get the most from it you should become familiar with it before you travel. It will also help you deal with problems that occur while you are travelling, though diagnosis of infectious diseases may be difficult even with skilled medical care and laboratory facilities

- Don't be put off by the names of strange diseases you have not come across before, or by some of the more technical information we provide You do not have to know everything, and the important practical points are summarized at the end of each chapter, but I believe it is important for us to try to give you the background information on which our advice is based

- *If you are travelling only within North America, northern Europe, and Australasia,* most of the infectious and parasitic diseases referred to in the first half of this book will not be a significant hazard. All travellers should be immunized against tetanus (p. 100), however, and the sections on diarrhoea (p. 17), rabies (p. 217), and Chapter 5 on diseases spread by insects (p. 130) may also be relevant to you. There is much more to the subject of health problems in travellers than infectious diseases, as you will see from the second half of the book

- If you are travelling elsewhere, especially to *Africa, Asia, or Latin America,* the sections on diseases of poor hygiene and diseases spread by insects will be particularly important. An indication of the geographical distribution of specific diseases is summarized in Appendix 3

- Remember that accidents are the commonest cause of death in travellers, and that most accidents are preventable (p. 290); malaria is the most serious tropical disease hazard that travellers are likely to come across (p. 130); hepatitis A is common and serious, but is preventable with a safe and effective vaccine (p. 55); diarrhoea and sunburn are the two 'minor' problems that most often interfere with travel plans, and they too are preventable

- Depending on the nature of your trip, the risk of other diseases is probably small anyway, but simple precautions can often dramatically reduce or eliminate the risks altogether; this book is for travellers whose health abroad is too important to be left to chance

- There's no substitute for understanding the basics, when it comes to protecting your health abroad. But for additional information, and to keep you up-to-date with news of outbreaks and other developments, you can find a detailed listing of specialist sources and websites in Appendix 8. Links to all of these sites can be found on the book's own web-site at **www.travellers-health.info**

Introduction

Staying healthy abroad: why and how

Prevention is the only strategy for staying healthy abroad that any traveller can afford to trust. Personal health precautions really work, and the time you invest in understanding and applying them will be amply rewarded.

Dr Richard Dawood devised this project and is the editor of this book. He has travelled in more than 80 countries around the world — and has survived.

Staying healthy abroad is not a question of luck and is too important to be left to chance. Knowledge is power: the purpose of this book is to give you the information you need to *prevent* health problems when you travel, before they occur.

Why prevention?

Of all the hazards and infectious diseases to which travellers are exposed abroad, some are lethal, many are dangerous, and several have long-term effects on health and well-being; some, also, may be passed on to family, friends, and contacts on return home.

The majority of health problems in travellers, however troublesome at the time, tend to be relatively minor in their long-term implications: this is just as well, given the large numbers of travellers who experience illness abroad, but goes some way towards explaining the meagre attention that such problems have generally received.

A problem does not have to be serious, however, to have a devastating effect upon the success or enjoyment of a trip. An undignified bout of diarrhoea can be all it takes to mar an eagerly awaited holiday, force a major change of travel plans, or abort a vital business trip.

Health problems in travellers are common. The risks are not decreasing, and we are all susceptible. Health care abroad is costly, travel is expensive, our leisure time is precious and some business travellers have much at stake; if for no other reason than the most mercenary ones, prevention is a strategy for health that no traveller can afford to neglect.

Prevention: who is responsible?

Can travel health issues be legislated away? Many of the world's most interesting travel destinations are developing countries with limited resources and unreliable infrastructure: on matters of health, local legislation is largely meaningless.

By contrast, in more developed countries, extensive health and safety legislation is now the norm, and travellers can and do benefit. Lower your guard at your peril, however: there are still serious lapses. Recent examples of problems at European resorts and destinations include major shortcomings in swimming pool safety at hotels, outbreaks of legionnaires' disease, frequent contamination of ice and ice machines, and cases of food poisoning and diarrhoea — including one of the UK's largest outbreaks of *Giardia* (58 laboratory-confirmed cases imported in 1997, traced to a single hotel in Greece). In 1998, 120 British holidaymakers came down with salmonellosis at a hotel in Mallorca. Dangers and health risks can't just be made to disappear by decree.

The travel industry can and must do more. As the aftermath of the September 11th terrorist attacks on New York vividly demonstrated, however, the industry is perilously vulnerable to economic circumstances and to our changing travel habits. We need the travel industry to be strong enough to be *able* to do more! Good practices need to be universally applied, particularly at hotels and resorts that are under the virtual control of operators from Western countries, or that use their name (such as hotels belonging to international chains, even though they may be locally owned and run): good fire safety, food hygiene, pool safety and vehicle safety, for example, ought to be the norm wherever western tour operators regularly send their clients. So should adequate information about health risks — something that European Union directives now provide for. Too often, however, litigation after failure proves to offer a more potent incentive to good practice than a proactive, industry-led approach to health promotion.

The point I want to make is that, whatever your government, your tour operator, your airline, your travel agent (or indeed your employer, secretary or travelling companion) may or may not do for you, responsibility for your health abroad ultimately rests with only one person: YOU.

Devising a strategy

Do not delegate responsibility for your health abroad to anyone else, however busy or preoccupied you may be with more pressing preparations for your trip; take personal charge. Business travellers are consistently at fault in this regard. Many people are surprised to discover that business travellers are often less well informed about health than the average package tourist! Even when they have made efforts in the past to find out about health precautions, they tend not to update their knowledge, and all to easily become complacent about the risks.

Intelligence, good health, and an extensive general knowledge do not absolve you from the need to obtain careful advice and up-to-date information about the health risks of travel that apply to your particular circumstances and travel plans, from a reliable source. This book will help you do that. Even if you are well-informed about health issues that apply to your home environment, you must never assume that this will help you abroad: many of the precautions that are necessary for travel are not logical or intuitive.

Remember that not all doctors are equally able to provide the information you need, and many will probably not provide more than a part of it unless you ask specifically about each point that concerns you. 'Most physicians are remarkably ill-informed about health risks abroad and appropriate protective measures', according to one senior US public health official. Recent surveys of local health departments and specialized travel clinics in the USA found significant variation in the reliability of the advice on offer, even from supposedly knowledgeable sources. Periodic surveys of travel advice from British General Practitioners have yielded similarly depressing results, though the situation is undoubtedly improving as a result of increasing interest in travel medicine as a medical specialty. Doctors are *not* the sole source of reliable health advice: nurses and other staff at immunization centres, travel clinics and university health centres frequently have considerable experience and more time to talk to you. Listen carefully to them. It helps to develop a good relationship with a local, specialist travel clinic that you can turn to for all your travel health requirements.

Specific prevention measures

Immunization offers protection from several important diseases, and should not be neglected (see pp. 553–67). Vaccines against hepatitis A were an important development, and although more expensive, have now largely succeeded in replacing the unpopular gamma-globulin injection. Current typhoid vaccines have fewer side effects than their predecessor. The only remaining formal vaccination certificate requirements for travel relate to yellow fever. There's an increasing trend towards 'combined' vaccines — diphtheria and tetanus, hepatitis A and B, and hepatitis A and typhoid are examples of travel vaccines that are now commonly given in a single injection. Many vaccines also now offer the prospect of long-term protection.

And among current issues in travel medicine is whether rabies vaccine should be used more often for prevention, given the scarcity of immune globulin for treatment (p. 229) — all travellers to developing countries should now consider carefully whether they might benefit from protection.

Be aware of the pitfalls, however. Vaccination *regulations* are generally designed to protect countries rather than travellers, and not all individuals to whom you may turn for advice are able to make this important distinction. Regulations and *recommendations* for each country in the world are liable to change from time to time, and so should be confirmed before departure (see Appendix 1).

Immunizations don't work if they have not been given or are allowed to lapse, and their timing requires thought; not all of them offer 100 per cent protection. For frequent travellers, a strategy of continuous protection is an attractive option that offers many advantages over the conventional 'trip-by-trip' approach.

Keep in mind that only a small minority of disease risks can be prevented by immunization: no traveller who has undergone even a full course of immunization should ever be allowed to assume that no further precautions will be necessary.

Prevention (prophylaxis) with drugs is an essential protective measure for travellers to malarial areas (see pp. 130–50) — malaria is a potential killer that should never be underestimated. Drug resistance is now widespread, and growing: it limits the usefulness of trusted remedies, and looms ahead for every new drug we have so far come up with. Chloroquine, once the most widely used preventive drug, is effective on its own in only a limited number of destinations; it is now so ineffective in parts of Africa that some countries have banned its commercial importation. Reports of side effects have contributed to a decline in popularity of mefloquine (Lariam), introduced in the early Nineties (and also to a rise in travel-related cases of malaria); it is doubtful whether all these reports were justified, and problems with using Lariam now seem much less common. Perhaps that is because we are better at using it, but in any event it remains an important and effective drug under appropriate circumstances. Doxycycline, a tetracycline antibiotic, is now more widely used, though it too is not free from side effects. The most important new addition to our armoury is atovaquone/proguanil (Malarone), which is highly effective, has a very low rate of side effects, and unlike other drugs can be discontinued just seven days after leaving a malarial area.

Anti-malarial drugs are never enough on their own, however, and measures to avoid mosquito bites remain of the utmost importance.

Drug treatment can sometimes also be used to prevent certain diarrhoeal diseases, and this may be an appropriate option in special circumstances; but the issue is a controversial one (see pp. 37–8); the desired results are more likely to be achieved by careful precautions with food, water, and hygiene.

Preventing individual diseases by taking medication may seem an attractive concept, but unfortunately this is not a precaution on which travellers can rely.

General precautions

In most cases, each disease of concern to the traveller does not have its own, unique, specific preventive measure. There is, after all, a limit to the number of possible ways in which diseases can spread. Whether you are in Kathmandu, Kabul, or Corfu, and whether the problem you are trying to avoid is amoebic dysentery, giardiasis or plain old travellers' diarrhoea, the principles of food hygiene are just the same. And anti-insect precautions, assiduously followed, will protect you from dengue fever in the Caribbean just as surely as from filariasis in West Africa and unpleasant diseases in many other countries around the world.

Although detailed information about a large number of diseases appears in this book, and the list of hazards may at first glance appear frightening, the important point to realize is that prevention is not only feasible in virtually every case, but is usually not difficult; it follows logical principles that relate directly to how the disease is spread. The mode of spread holds the key to prevention of each disease, but this book presents further details as well — to add interest, to provide perspective, and to give purpose to precautions that might otherwise seem obscure or not really necessary.

Because some preventive measures are common to many diseases, a degree of overlap between chapters in a book of this type is inevitable. I make no apology for this repetition which serves to emphasize their importance.

Food hygiene One of my favourite surveys of visitors to East Africa found that only 2 per cent of them were taking adequate dietary precautions. Are dietary precautions a lost cause? Unfortunately, nothing less than a process of education or re-education in the fundamental principles of hygienic food preparation will protect travellers to most countries outside northern Europe, North America, or Australasia. Appetite is a poor guide to food safety, and food should never be assumed to be safe unless you know that it has been freshly and thoroughly cooked (heat sterilized) — in the case of meat, until no red colour remains. Let this rule guide your choice from even the most tempting menu. Satisfy yourself that today's lunch is not yesterday's evening meal, re-heated and re-arranged. Intricate delicacies that have received much handling during preparation, and cold platters left out in the open, are highly likely to have been contaminated. Prawns, oysters, and other seafood feed by filtering the water around them; they are rapidly able to accumulate dangerous levels of bacteria and viruses, and only 4 per cent of shellfish-growing areas in the Mediterranean now produce seafood that is fit to eat. Shellfish should be boiled vigorously for at least 10 minutes, or preferably avoided altogether. Even within the USA, public health officials estimate that the risk of gastrointestinal illnesses is 18 000 greater from eating shellfish than from eating fish. Fruit and vegetables need careful preparation — they should be freshly cooked or freshly peeled. In Western countries, we have become so used to thinking of foods such as salad vegetables as 'healthy' that many of the necessary precautions are frankly counter-intuitive.

Observing food precautions means that you won't always be able to eat what you want or what is on offer when you are hungry. The principles of food hygiene are of crucial importance to travellers, and are discussed again at length in the next chapter and elsewhere throughout the book (see also Appendix 5).

Expensive hotels Many travellers draw comfort from the fact that they will be staying in multi-starred or 'luxurious' establishments, but these offer no firm guarantee of safety from diseases of poor hygiene: it is a grave error to assume that the food they serve must automatically be safe, or to allow yourself a false sense of security. One serious outbreak of amoebic dysentery and amoebic liver abscesses in a group of Italian tourists was traced to raw vegetables served on ice at a luxury hotel in Phuket. Surveys have repeatedly found appalling examples of poor hygiene standards and contaminated food in hotel kitchens at popular European resorts; the UK consumer publication *Holiday Which?* has repeatedly concluded that a hotel's star rating bears little relation to the standard of food hygiene in its kitchen. I have myself seen junior, migrant waiters at a top Paris hotel use their breath to polish plates and glasses. If in doubt about local hygiene standards, have a look at the kitchen yourself, and check for flies; do you see any food left lying around exposed? Flies cannot discriminate between the plate of a wealthy tourist and any of their other preferred habitats. African flies carry African diseases, and you can acquire dysentery from the foot of a single fly. (Avoiding flies can sometimes be hard: in Africa's Rift Valley, 'fly counts' in a typical home reach 30 000–40 000 per 24-hour period.)

Low budget travellers are not necessarily at greater risk of illness than travellers who only stay in luxury hotels. Whether you eat in a street market or anywhere else, you can rely on the same principles of food hygiene to protect you. Do you enjoy eating bread fresh from the oven, food that you have selected and watched cooking, and fresh fruit, peeled carefully yourself? (I always travel with a small spoon and a sharp knife for just this purpose). Food like this is easy to find and is cheap, appetizing, and almost always safe to eat.

Clean hands It is all very well to wash your hands before a meal, but if you then proceed to wipe your hands on a filthy towel that has been contaminated by others, and then touch a grubby bathroom door handle, you are literally asking for trouble. In developing countries, regard your hands as an 'unclean' surface, and avoid eating food that you have handled directly.

Water safety and purification are discussed in detail on pp. 78–83. In most countries outside northern Europe, North America, and Australia, water from the public drinking supply is likely to be just a very dilute solution of sewage, and should be regarded as such unless known to be safe.

Ice is only as pure as the water from which it is made (p. 71). But even when the water supply is safe, chilling happens to be an excellent way of preserving bacteria and viruses. Ice machines readily become contaminated: it takes a careful programme of maintenance and de-contamination to ensure their continuing safety — even, for example, in the supposedly hygienic setting of British hospitals, where such programmes are understood and in place, but where a recent survey found 75% of hospital ice machines to be visibly dirty and most to be heavily contaminated. In an investigation by *Holiday Which?* into ice from randomly selected resorts in France, the UK, Portugal, and Spain, the most disgusting example of faecal contamination was found in ice cubes from a luxury hotel in Biarritz: 19 out of 69 samples from bars and cafés were 'dubious' and 26 were harmful. The situation in developing countries is generally much worse.

Hospitality is a dangerous pitfall for the unwary. It takes diplomacy and determination to refuse food prepared (unhygienically) by someone who has clearly gone to great lengths in order to please an honoured visitor. This can be an extremely delicate problem in rural areas in developing countries, where food is anyway scarce. My personal advice is not to relax your standards of food hygiene under any circumstances; plead illness, use any excuse, and if necessary, even permit the food to be put on your plate and toy with it, but *do not eat food you consider to be suspect*. The possible embarrassment of such a situation, and reluctance to offend one's host (genuine offence is rarely taken), must be balanced against the risk of illness that may ruin your trip or put you out of action for several days.

Insects transmit a multitude of diseases, not all of which can be prevented individually, and their bites can be a painful nuisance. With the relentless spread of drug-resistant malaria, personal protection from insects has become even more important. A notable advance is the use of bed nets impregnated with insecticide, which have proved to be over 30 times more effective than untreated nets, and in places where they have been introduced on a wide scale, the incidence of malaria has fallen considerably. Such methods are discussed in depth on pp. 207–16. Travellers to some infected areas can expect to be bitten by malaria-bearing mosquitoes at least once a day.

Sex Sex abroad has always been a risky business, but the penalties are now higher. In the UK, heterosexual sex is now the commonest route of spread of HIV. And of the 1746 cases of HIV infection in heterosexuals reported during 2000, 1371 infections (79 per cent) originated abroad, making this by far the most important source of imported, lethal infection. Estimates of HIV infection rates in many countries are of dubious accuracy, and as Dr Peter Drotman explains elsewhere in this book, they are not a reliable basis for decisions about countries where sex might be 'safe.' As far as the risks of HIV are concerned, where you go is less important than what you do when you get there.

It has been estimated that there are in excess of two million prostitutes in Thailand alone, most of whom have had 5000 sexual partners by the age of nineteen: and that one-third of male visitors to Thailand have sex with prostitutes, more than 70 per cent of whom are thought to be infected with sexually transmitted diseases at any one time. In some parts of the country, in excess of 70 per cent of prostitutes are believed to be HIV positive.

Sun Since people from cooler climates have been travelling to sunny places in ever greater numbers, the incidence of skin cancer has risen significantly: the incidence of melanoma, the most serious form, is now rising in many countries by around 7 per cent each year — a higher rate than for any other cancer. Skin cancers are now known to be related not just to long-term exposure to ultraviolet light, but also with acute episodes of sunburn. (Did you know that lying in the sun could also be a significant source of extra calories? One estimate is that it adds about 300 calories per hour per 100 pounds of body weight, to your body's total energy intake!)

Exposure to ultraviolet light also causes cataract formation and retinal damage: protect your eyes with good quality sunglasses that filter out the harmful rays.

The environment holds many hazards, including heat, cold, the effects of high altitude, the bites of wild animals, and accidents — the biggest hazard of all. A large part of this book is devoted to such subjects, and it is often the simplest precautions that are most important. For example, if you have children and you rent a car abroad, remember that child seats cut their risk of dying in a car crash by 70 per cent. And according to a recent analysis of 100 000 accidents, the risk of dying in the front seat in a car crash is five times higher when passengers in the back are not wearing seat belts. If you are planning to use a moped or motorcycle, your risk of injury is at least 40 times greater than if you use a car. A bicycle helmet reduces the risk of head injury by 70 per cent. These dangers don't just mysteriously vanish when you go abroad, and in fact may be amplified by reduced access to good emergency care.

Many accidents abroad relate to alcohol (at least 20 per cent of drownings, for example). Remember that drinks may not come in standard measures, or even in standard strengths. Many countries have lower blood alcohol limits for drivers, and in many countries there is also a high likelihood of being tested. Pedestrians involved in accidents are also likely to be tested. The penalties are generally high. Travel insurance policies often exclude cover for accidents, injuries and losses that take place while under the influence of alcohol.

And when exploring 'the environment', don't drink and hike! Half of the 100 deaths that occurred in a study of outdoor accidents (such as drownings and falling off cliffs) were related to alcohol.

Remember to travel unobtrusively, be discreet with your possessions, and avoid flourishing large sums of money in poor areas: as the late Dr. Alistair Reid, an expert on hazards from wild animals, once pointed out, the greatest animal danger to travellers is man.

Health in the air

Deep vein thrombosis (DVT) is attracting much attention, and so are other issues relating to in-flight health (p. 258). It is now clear that travellers can do much to reduce their own risk of DVT, and some of the necessary precautions are considered in greater detail on pp. 257–9.

Safety and security

Issues surrounding personal security are discussed in detail on p. 304. Especially since the September 11th terrorist attacks, hazards from security breaches loom large in people's minds, but there are many other ways that safety and security can be compromised, that are under direct individual control. Local people, and local police and military, may easily misinterpret hobbies such as planespotting, as 12 British and two Dutch travellers to Greece in 2001 recently discovered to their cost; your inability to explain what you are doing in the local language can make matters worse. Apart from other considerations, health and hygiene conditions in overseas prisons can be extremely dangerous. Photography also has its dangers: it is amazing how many people find themselves tempted to take pictures of 'No Photography' signs in countries where such matters are taken extremely seriously. I once spent most of a day negotiating for the release of a distinguished American oral surgeon, arrested in Tamanrasset for doing just this; and was arrested myself, elsewhere in Africa, for photographing a billboard about malaria.

Illness abroad

When prevention fails or the unavoidable occurs, coping with illness abroad and, if necessary, getting yourself or someone else home again quickly, demands resourcefulness and judgement. It helps if a doctor can be found, and knowledge of the local language is a valuable asset. Often, though, self-help is everything. A carefully constructed personal medical kit can be a valuable aid (p. 573).

Medical treatment abroad may itself be dangerous. Public awareness of HIV has helped draw attention to some of the hazards: screened and unscreened blood transfusions; non-sterile needles, syringes, and medical and dental instruments; acupuncture; and surgery may all spread the virus (see p. 468); hepatitis B is much more common however, and is spread by the same routes. There are numerous examples of travellers undergoing immunization in poor countries and subsequently developing hepatitis B. Not all medical attention is undertaken voluntarily. Have a car accident in Turkey, and you will almost certainly have to provide a blood sample for measurement of your blood alcohol level; the sterility of the needle that is used will probably depend on precisely where you are unfortunate enough to have your accident.

Other hazards include drugs and vaccines that may be ineffective or dangerous; in some poor countries, where the likelihood of being bitten by a dog, and the frequency of rabies, are both high, the locally produced rabies vaccine may be almost as dangerous as the disease itself. Doctors have reported nine deaths in Pakistan following post-exposure rabies vaccination attributed to fake or adulterated vaccines. As I write this, one of my patients is suffering from an acute infection with hepatitis A, having been 'vaccinated' against hepatitis A just a few months previously, in eastern Europe.

Medical skills and standards of practice also vary, and in particular, women should always make sure that a chaperone is present when they are examined. In some countries, there may be an over-enthusiasm for surgical treatment, and this is undoubtedly the case in many European ski resorts; other than in a desperate emergency — a situation that is usually self-evident — repatriation is usually possible prior to any surgery.

The most usual problems, however, are inadequacy of emergency services, and scarcity or inaccessibility of skilled medical facilities. Places with quite reasonable facilities for local people may not necessarily be capable of dealing with emergencies in foreigners, and this remains a problem at resorts — particularly island resorts — all over the world. Each year, there is a distressing toll of injuries in young tourists who are injured in moped accidents on islands that have no facilities, or only limited facilities, for neurosurgical care. On the relatively well-developed island of Crete, for example, visitors who are injured on the south side of the island face a three-hour ambulance journey to the main hospital. With head injuries in particular, survivability may well hinge on your proximity to medical care.

Adequate insurance may remove anxiety about expense and should provide for emergency repatriation if necessary, but it is also important to have enough cash available to cover immediate costs. A general awareness of the main, likely health risks will be invaluable. Specific advice for coping with individual diseases is given in each of the chapters on the main diseases.

In my view, *all* travellers to remote areas with limited medical facilities should also have a knowledge of basic first aid both for their own benefit and the benefit of others and should attend a course of instruction if necessary.

Coming home

The value of a post-tropical check-up is discussed in Appendix 7. All travellers should realize, however, that it is possible for symptoms of infectious diseases — especially malaria — not to appear until several weeks, or even longer, after return home. When symptoms do appear, their significance may not be recognized immediately: roughly half of all fatal malaria cases are initially misdiagnosed as flu. The worst place to be is a country that sees few cases: the death rate for travellers with malaria is 10 times higher in Japan than in the US. There are other pitfalls too: one vacationer died recently from appendicitis, misdiagnosed as travellers' diarrhoea. If illness does develop after a trip, make sure that your doctor understands that you have been travelling.

Attitude

A positive attitude to health and perception of one's health as a vital element in the success of a trip, rather than as an inconvenient obstacle to enjoyment, are powerful weapons indeed for any traveller.

And finally

The message of this book is not that you should worry about each and every disease or problem that is mentioned here, every time and wherever you travel; or, worse still, that you would be better off staying at home. It is simply this: by informing yourself of the nature of the hazards that travellers face and how these hazards can be overcome, you will learn healthy travel habits that will open new horizons and protect you wherever you go. You could, of course, learn them the hard way, as I have had to do on many of my own travels, in which case you need read no further . . .

Travellers' health: an overview

The unprecedented scale and speed of modern-day international travel means that ever-increasing numbers of travellers are exposed to unfamiliar infectious diseases and other hazards. Understanding the nature, size, and range of the problems can help the traveller minimize the risks from preventable illnesses.

Professor Daniel Reid is the former Director of the Scottish Centre for Infection and Environmental Health in Glasgow.
Dr Jonathan H. Cossar is a general practitioner and research associate at the Scottish Centre for Infection and Environmental Health.

Defining and monitoring the disease hazards that travellers face is a crucial step towards their prevention. Since 1973, the Scottish Centre for Infection and Environmental Health (SCIEH) has been conducting intensive epidemiological surveillance on the illnesses affecting returning travellers. This has helped to define the perspective of illnesses associated with travel, to evaluate the effectiveness of pre-travel health advice, and to develop a computerized database designed to give advice on suitable antimalarial drugs and appropriate immunizations for travellers (see TRAVAX, p. 671).

Introduction

Although there have been notable medical advances in combating disease risks, today's traveller is still vulnerable to health hazards on account of the very nature of travel itself. Travel exposes the individual to new cultural, psychological, physical, physiological, emotional, environmental, and microbiological experiences and challenges. The traveller's ability to adapt to, cope with, and survive these challenges is influenced by many variable factors including his or her pre-existing physical, mental, immunological, and medical status. Examples of travellers at higher risk are shown in Table 1.1.

Risk is further modified by personality, experience, and behaviour, which may each differ with age, gender, culture, race, social status, and education.

The final aspect of this challenge relates specifically to exposure to an unfamiliar environment with different climate, altitude, sunlight, hygiene, insects, pollution, safety, disease prevalence, and so on. For these reasons it is not surprising that health problems affecting the traveller have been recognized throughout history.

Table 1.1 Travellers at higher risk of infection

The young (less mature/exposed immune system)
The elderly (immunosenescence)
The pregnant (altered immunity/medication restrictions)
The less experienced (less adept at minimizing risks)
Those with pre-existing disease (immune system under stress)
The immunocompromised (less disease resistance)
The adventurer/backpacker (increased microbiological spectrum/dose)
The 'sex traveller' (high-risk behaviour with a high-risk population)

Historical background

Awareness of the dangers from infection imported by travellers is not new. It was in response to outbreaks of plague during the Middle Ages, following the arrival of ships from the East, that Venice and Rhodes introduced the first travel health regulations. On arrival, ships were kept at a distance and travellers detained in isolation for 40 days (*quaranta giorni*) before they were allowed to proceed to their final destination. First imposed by the Venetian Republic in 1377, this was the origin of the concept of quarantine, with other cities and countries following its example until some form of sanitary regulation became the general rule in many countries during the next five centuries.

There are numerous historical accounts of illness within various groups of mobile personnel who have been required to travel at different periods. Notable among these were people involved with military operations in colonial times and missionaries who lived and worked abroad.

The scale of the problem

The number of travellers crossing international boundaries has increased tremendously in recent years. National and international bodies such as the UK Central Statistical Office (CSO), the World Health Organization (WHO), the International Civil Aviation Organization (ICAO), and the World Tourism Organization (WTO) provide valuable statistics on the numbers involved.

Groups contributing to the growth in travel include tourists, business travellers, technical experts, pilgrims, migrant workers, refugees, immigrants, military personnel, political representatives, sporting participants and spectators, and the travel support services. Of particular significance has been the growth of the 'package tour' (although the proportion of holiday visits from the UK has now stabilized at around 55 per cent). In 1949, 26 million international tourists were recorded (Table 1.2) whereas by 2000 this had risen to 699 million. Between 1949 and 1999, there was a 50-fold increase in numbers of scheduled air passengers and a 32-fold increase in UK residents travelling abroad; the proportion of those travelling beyond Europe has increased 111-fold. International tourist arrivals in North America have also increased spectacularly, from 6 180 000 in 1950 to more than 80 million in 1995 (CSO, WTO, and ICAO figures). In 2000 the number of passengers carried worldwide on scheduled services was over 1.6 billion. Current annual expenditure on tourism is in excess of $500 billion.

Table 1.2 Growth in international travel

	1949	1960	1970 (Millions)	1980	1995	2000
Total no. of international tourists	26	69	160	285	565	699
Total no. of air travellers	31	106	386	748	1288	1647
Total visits abroad by UK residents	1.7	6	11.8	17.5	41.5	56.8

In former times, when sea voyages were the customary method of travelling long distances, the period spent at sea was nearly always longer than the incubation period of the most likely infections. This provided an effective safeguard for the inhabitants of the countries to which infected travellers were bound, and also gave a longer time to appreciate the significance of any symptoms that appeared during the return voyage.

Today, this mode of travel has become relatively much less common (although there has been a resurgence in the leisure cruise market). Moreover, with modern air transport the infected patient may well arrive home some days before the appearance of clinical signs of disease. Between 1948 and the present time, the fastest passenger aircraft cruising speed has risen from 340 miles per hour to 1356 miles per hour (in Concorde). Thus, with China but a jet flight away, a fresh epidemic strain of influenza can be imported to New York in a matter of 16 hours or to London in 14 hours.

Modern travel ensures that there are no countries in the world where human demographics and behaviour, technological and industrial practices, environmental change, international commerce, microbial adaptation, and changing priorities in public health can occur in isolation, without implications for potential transmission of infection by travellers.

Health risks

Logically enough, most travellers tend to think of travel health problems in terms of specific risks they might expect in a particular country or countries. However, the 'true' health risk reflects a complex relationship between the traveller, micro-organisms/hazards, and location/environment; it is not something that can be simply looked up in a reference book. The higher-risk regions include the tropics and subtropics of Africa, Asia, and Central and South America, but due to the wide and changing variations of climate, topography, sanitation, agricultural practices, and industrial development found not only within continents, but even within a single country, mapping infections geographically is complex and potentially misleading. In general terms, the greater the climatic and cultural contrast with the home country, the greater the risk.

Headlines may be made by 'newsworthy' imported infections such as the 2055 malaria notifications recorded for the UK in 1995 (54% due to *P. falciparum*) or the 78% of heterosexually acquired AIDS cases which were contracted abroad. However, it is only by epidemiological studies that the true perspective of the risks can be defined — for example, collaborative, multidisciplinary studies on the patterns of illness in over 14 000 returning travellers have been carried out at SCIEH since 1973 and, correlation of these results with those of other researchers around the world has helped to define the comparative risk of illness to travellers, as shown in Table 1.3.

Undoubtedly most illnesses encountered by travellers are simply not recorded, and this is especially the case with less serious (though still troublesome) afflictions such as gastrointestinal problems. Ongoing studies continue in a number of countries to determine the frequency and types of illness encountered by travellers, and to place these in perspective. Although much of the data are incomplete, and depends for their quality on such factors as the enthusiasm of the researcher, meaningful conclusions are still possible, and attack rates can be calculated for different health problems (Fig. 1.1).

Table 1.3 Profile of travellers at higher risk

Package holidaymakers
Inexperienced travellers
Travellers heading further south, particularly to northern Africa
Summer travellers
Younger age groups (specifically 20–29 years)
Smokers
Travellers with excessive alcohol intake and those involved in road traffic accidents

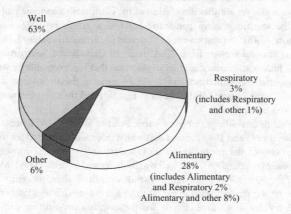

Well
63%

Respiratory
3%
(includes Respiratory
and other 1%)

Other
6%

Alimentary
28%
(includes Alimentary
and Respiratory 2%
Alimentary and other 8%)

Fig. 1.1 Reports of illness in 14 227 holidaymakers (1973–85).

The spectrum of health problems associated with travel

Relaxed attitudes and reduced inhibitions are natural elements of holiday enjoyment. The traveller may thus accept risks that would be avoided in everyday life, such as experimenting with unfamiliar food and drink or participating in hazardous sports. Alcohol may increase such behaviour, contribute to road traffic accidents, or lead to neglect of precautions against mosquito bites or of regular antimalarial prophylaxis and to acceptance of risk of exposure to sexually transmitted diseases. Narcotic drug abuse can have similar influences in addition to the risk of hepatitis B from intravenous drug injections.

Some illnesses may be induced by travel itself, such as motion sickness and upsets to the circadian rhythms; unaccustomed exercise or the effects of altitude may exacerbate pre-existing cardiovascular or respiratory problems. Exposure to unfamiliar infectious agents and the stress of altered climate and environment may also cause problems for the unwary traveller, and these may be compounded by the differing medical practices encountered overseas.

Some diseases less common in one country may be more prevalent in another, and this may lead to problems when travellers become complacent about immunization before travelling. For example, as a consequence of the social catharsis in the former USSR, collapse of the public health infrastructure which previously delivered a highly efficient immunization programme, allied to consumer suspicion of the efficacy of the vaccines and safety of the needles used, now means that population immunity has fallen below protective levels for some common pathogens. It is therefore not surprising that over 50 000 cases of diphtheria were reported in the newly independent states of the former Soviet Union during the mid-1990s (see p. 103). A disease that had previously been virtually eradicated has now re-emerged to threaten both the native population and visitors from abroad with inadequate immunity.

Cholera provides yet another illustration of the continually changing global pattern of illness; the seventh cholera pandemic reached a zenith in 1992, when WHO reported a total of 461 783 cases, with 8072 deaths (5291 in Africa alone). During 1992 there were confirmed reports from 20 African, 19 Central and South American, 15 Asian, and 7 European countries. Thus an infection that is preventable by simple basic hygiene and effective sanitation had again become a global scourge due to the appearance of different types of the cholera organism and the overwhelming ubiquity of tourism and travel.

With regard to fatal illness, a review carried out at SCIEH of 952 Scots who died abroad between 1973 and 1988 showed that whilst infection accounted for only a small proportion (4%) of the mortality, cardiovascular disease was the most frequently recorded cause of death (69%), followed by accidents and injuries (21%). Most deaths occurred in the 50 to 69-year age range (50%), with the highest mortality associated with cardiovascular illness (34%) in the 60 to 69 age range. This highlights the risks of a strenuous holiday in a warm climate for those with a pre-existing cardiovascular problem, especially in older travellers (p. 503).

The same review noted that the highest death rate from accidents and injuries (32%) occurred in the 20 to 29-year age group, with road traffic accidents the largest single contributor to this group of preventable deaths. It is alarming to note that, with motor registrations in China at a rate of 5 vehicles per 1000 population, the current Chinese road death rate is already at a level similar to that in the USA, which has 770 vehicle registrations per 1000 population. Motor registrations in China are now growing at the rate of 10 to 20% a year, and as developing countries open up to tourism, tourist deaths and injuries from road traffic accidents are bound to increase. Such data highlight the importance of ensuring that travellers understand what can be done to reduce the risks (see p. 291).

A final illustration of the crucial link between lifestyle and infection is HIV infection. In the words of a recent WHO report, 'casual sexual contacts are common among leisure travellers unaccompanied by their partner. This is most clear in the case of sex tourism'. Sexual fidelity and appropriate health education are the only sure ways to avoid sexually transmitted diseases and AIDS.

Travellers are, however, often vulnerable to events that are outside their direct control, as the terrorist attacks on New York in September 2001 sadly illustrate.

Environmental issues

Pioneer tourists or travellers, anxious to explore the most newly accessible areas in remote parts of the world, are often exposed to unfamiliar hazards. For example, in developing countries, city growth can lead to overcrowding, poor hygiene, inadequate sanitation, and contaminated drinking water. Not only does this result in high rates of infection in the shanty towns and *favelas* surrounding these cities, but also has the potential for spread to more immunologically vulnerable people who may be visiting and mixing with the local population.

The economic demands of burgeoning populations dictate major man-made environmental changes: reservoirs and dams for water storage and electricity generation; new roads driven through untouched forests; de-forestation and re-forestation. Such changes encourage 'aggressor' strains of flora, fauna, insects and micro-organisms, previously contained by a natural balance built up over thousands of years, to emerge. These have a dramatic impact upon the entire ecological infrastructure, with unforseeable consequences for the development and transmission of disease. This situation has obvious implications for newcomers to those areas particularly affected.

Responsibilities for the traveller

Effective public education and, ultimately, changes in behaviour by travellers themselves, stand to make the greatest contribution to reducing the rate of health problems in travel. Simple truisms such as 'there is a price to pay for the freedom to travel', 'if travellers don't pick up infections, they cannot pass them on', and 'immunizations and medications protect against only 5 to 10 per cent of the problems encountered by travellers, the rest relate to their personal behaviour', need to be communicated and understood. Basic educational messages about avoiding mosquito bites and malaria, personal hygiene, food handling, sexual behaviour, and drug abuse require continual reinforcement and need to be acted upon.

It is important for travellers to understand the impact of tourism upon local populations, and to appreciate its social and environmental costs. The detrimental effects to health and welfare of the rapid growth of tourism in poor countries include the accelerated consumption and overloading of resources (from land for building to sewage disposal facilities, food, and water supplies) and the disruption of local agricultural practices (with environmental damage and competition for resources). It has been estimated that up to 80% of the profits from tourism are returned to affluent, tourist-donor countries; all too often, the only beneficiaries in the local communities are relatively small numbers of temporary, low-paid, low-status workers.

Furthermore, host countries may realize too late that uncontrolled tourism not only fails to solve their foreign debt problems but extracts an unacceptable price in terms of the loss of native cultures, political instability, and the importation of foreign values and new diseases. Levels of pollution, disease, crime, violence, prostitution, and drug abuse can escalate, threatening the very tourists responsible for promoting these changes in the first place, as well as the native population, which may suffer yet further when the country loses popularity after being branded as 'unsafe'. Better understanding of such factors may ultimately encourage greater social responsibility.

Postscript

Though vulnerable to the impact of world events, international travel and tourism remain some of the world's fastest growing and financially lucrative industries. Throughout history, migration and travel — whether driven by commerce, necessity, warfare, or recreation — have been intimately associated with transmission of infection. The scale and speed of modern-day travel, and current changes in demographics, industry, the environment, and public health infrastructure mean that opportunities for microbial adaptation and global epidemic spread have never been greater.

It is clearly not possible to ensure that every tourist and traveller is counselled individually by a health care professional prior to travel — there are too many economic and practical constraints. It is therefore all the more important for individuals to take responsibility for their own personal health and welfare when travelling abroad. There is an educational opportunity to consider the rationale of socially responsible tourism e.g. exploring the concept that we all share a 'global village' and that the welfare of our fellow 'villager' is directly related to our own personal behaviour. With this insight the individual traveller is far more likely to effect the personal changes required to reduce the risks from preventable travel-related health problems, and to halt the other socially and environmentally destructive consequences of global tourism.

2 Diseases spread mainly by food, drink, and poor hygiene

Diarrhoea and intestinal infections

'Travel broadens the mind and loosens the bowels' — Sherwood Gorbach.

Millions of travellers, all over the world, have discovered for themselves how true this statement can be. However, travellers' diarrhoea is both preventable and readily treatable.

Dr Ron Behrens is the only NHS consultant in Travel and Tropical Medicine and is Director of the Travel Clinic of the Hospital for Tropical Diseases, London, and Senior Lecturer at the London School of Hygiene and Tropical Medicine, where he conducts research into ways of improving travellers' health. **Professor Michael Barer** is a medical microbiologist at the University of Leicester, where he teaches and conducts research on infections of the gastrointestinal tract.

- If you already have diarrhoea and want help, turn to '**What to do about diarrhoea**' on p. 29.
- If you want quick, simple advice on how to avoid getting diarrhoea in the first place, turn to '**Prevention**' on p. 37, '*How diarrhoeal diseases are spread*' (p. 19) and Appendix 5.
- If you want to understand why these measures may or may not work, read on!

No fewer than two-thirds of all international travellers suffer from diarrhoea abroad. Travellers' diarrhoea is not merely a trivial inconvenience: some 13 per cent of sufferers are confined to bed, and a further 40 per cent are forced to change their itinerary.

What are the risks?

Any kind of travel increases the likelihood of developing diarrhoea, and the level of risk is influenced by two main factors: where you come from, and where you are going.

As far as the risk of diarrhoea is concerned, the world can be broadly divided into three regions:

- **High risk:** Latin America, Africa, southern Asia

- **Low risk:** United States, Canada, northwestern Europe, Australia, New Zealand, and Japan
- **Intermediate risk:** northern Mediterranean, China, eastern Europe, and the former Soviet Union

When a person from a low risk region travels to a high risk region, the likelihood of developing a diarrhoeal illness is about 40 per cent. When the same individual travels to an intermediate risk area, the rate of illness is approximately 10 per cent. For a traveller who goes from one low risk region to another, the risk is between two and five per cent — higher than the rate of illness in people who resist the urge to travel and just stay at home. Naturally, the longer the trip, the more likely it is that illness will occur.

The two to five per cent background rate of diarrhoea among low risk travellers arises from many factors, including: the stress of travel itself; the fact that many more meals are eaten at restaurants or prepared by others, with greater opportunity for contamination than when food is prepared at home; increased alcohol consumption; and the presence of poorly-absorbed salts and other non-infective diarrhoea-producing substances found in local, unfamiliar food and water sources.

The rate of diarrhoea when a person from a high risk region travels to either another high risk region or to a lower risk region is probably about the same two to five per cent background rate. This reduced susceptibility, compared with travellers from low risk areas, is a further indication that the infectious organisms that cause illness are widespread throughout the developing world.

Certain types of traveller are at higher risk, and therefore need to take much more careful precautions if they wish to avoid illness:

- Travellers who are elderly, or very young
- Travellers living under conditions of reduced hygiene, in close contact with the local community
- Travellers who have little or no opportunity to choose for themselves what food and drink they consume
- Travellers with an important underlying disease including: diabetes mellitus requiring insulin, heart disease requiring regular medication, chronic liver disease, and acquired immune deficiency syndrome (AIDS)
- Travellers taking medication to reduce gastric acid secretion — especially potent drugs like PPIs (proton pump inhibitors e.g. omeprazole).

Diarrhoea: not just a problem for travellers

As far as most healthy western travellers are concerned, a diarrhoeal episode is uncomfortable, at worst debilitating, and may last for up to a few weeks. But for malnourished children in the developing world, diarrhoeal illnesses are life-threatening: at a rough estimate, there are around 1.3 billion episodes, leading to death in at least five million children around the world each year; the true figure may be much higher than this.

The principal cause of death is severe dehydration, and administration of fluids is a simple measure that can prevent death. In addition to appalling mortality rates,

diarrhoeal diseases contribute substantially to chronic ill health, increased susceptibility to other diseases, and poor economic performance in countries where they are
uncontrolled. Addressing such problems is, not surprisingly, one of the World Health
Organization's most pressing concerns.

How diarrhoeal diseases are spread: the cornerstone of prevention

Most cases of travellers' diarrhoea are caused by micro-organisms that either damage
the gut or interfere with the normal mechanisms that control water flow across the gut
wall. Many different micro-organisms including bacteria, viruses, and protozoa may
be responsible. Fortunately, at least for the purposes of this chapter, all the agents of
major concern to adult travellers are transmitted in the same manner: you must
actually swallow contaminated material to contract the disease.

This has two important practical consequences. First, you should identify and take
pains to avoid food, drink, or anything else you might swallow that has a high risk of
being contaminated. Second, you should ensure that you do not touch the food you
eat, or (if you must use your fingers) that your hands are scrupulously clean and as dry
as possible (if necessary, use clean paper tissues or napkins to handle food while
eating); plates and cutlery should also be clean and dry.

If your appetite is at its strongest when confronted with mysterious, aromatic, alien
delicacies, then you have a simple choice: either to accept the risks involved in
satisfying your gastronomic curiosity, or to establish whether or not the food is safe,
and to choose something else if it isn't.

Food poisoning is by no means uncommon, even in developed countries such as the
UK. In most outbreaks, investigation usually reveals that a breakdown in
recommended food preparation or storage practices is responsible.

Thus, even in a country where organisms that cause diarrhoea are not common in
the environment and virtually never contaminate the water supply, the diseases they
cause remain inadequately controlled despite widely disseminated knowledge of
hygienic catering practices.

Unfortunately, the micro-organisms responsible for diarrhoeal disease do not mark
their presence in the food they contaminate by making it look or smell rotten. Instead,
the reverse may occasionally be true, since organisms that cause food spoilage can
prevent the growth of diarrhoea-causing organisms. In practice, well-cooked food,
that is to say food whose temperature has exceeded the boiling point of water for at
least 15 minutes, is nearly always safe.

If not eaten straight away, cooked food should be protected from possible sources of
contamination, and refrigerated immediately. This period is often where contamination
occurs. Contact by hands, flies, cutlery, or the cutting board onto which uncooked food is
placed leads to contamination. Small numbers of surviving bacteria may grow at
phenomenal rates if left in a slowly cooling medium (i.e. recently cooked food). In
addition, room temperature in tropical countries is much closer to that required for
optimal bacterial growth, so safe storage times without refrigeration are much shorter.

Bacteria of the type relevant to this discussion may divide once every 20 minutes: a
single bacterial cell weighing one millionth of a gram could (under optimum

conditions) divide enough times in 24 hours for its offspring to weigh around four million kilograms — or about the weight of a small ship. Clearly bacterial growth of this magnitude could never occur, but these figures serve to illustrate that even minimally contaminated food that has been stored at tropical room temperatures for brief periods cannot be considered safe.

Specific food hazards

Bacteria need moisture to survive, and so dry foods (e.g. breads) are safer than those that are moist (e.g. salads, sauces). Other factors include the acid content of the item (citrus is generally safe because of its citric and ascorbic acid content), and salt or sugar content — syrups and jams, for example, should also be safe.

The following foods can be particularly risky:

Shellfish and seafood

These have been the source of many outbreaks of food-borne disease. In many instances this is a consequence of their mode of feeding, which involves filtration of large volumes of seawater, predisposing them to the accumulation of microorganisms like vibrios, *Plesiomonas*, *Aeromonas*, and hepatitis viruses. This is a problem only where seawater is contaminated, but in many parts of the world it is usual for untreated human excreta to be deposited close to areas where shellfish are collected. With poor handling or storage, they may also become contaminated after harvesting.

Vegetables, salads, and fruit

The use of human faeces as fertilizer (night soil) — a practice widespread in the tropics — makes salads and uncooked fresh vegetables risky unless they have been carefully washed with clean water. Even where night soil is not used, salads and fresh fruit are still quite common sources of infection because they frequently become contaminated during transit, storage, or preparation.

In contrast, travellers to remoter areas who peel fruit themselves without contaminating the contents and eat the fruit immediately are at little risk of infection from this source.

Rice

Freshly cooked rice is also generally safe. However, it is common practice in many restaurants and communities for the leftovers to be reheated at the next meal. *Bacillus cereus*, a bacterium that often contaminates rice even in the UK, is able to survive the initial cooking process by producing heat-resistant spores. Left to their own devices in the interval between meals, these spores germinate and the subsequent bacterial growth converts the surrounding rice into a deadly emetic cocktail, lying in wait for the unwary consumer. It is now known that, by this stage, the emetic toxin is so robust that even pressure-cooking will not destroy it.

Drinks

Water purification is dealt with in detail in Chapter 3. However, as has already been suggested in relation to salads, water contamination is not a matter that can be ignored: ice, ices, and anything else prepared locally from suspect water supplies should be considered contaminated, since freezing will kill only a fraction of any organisms present. Remember, that even the most stylish breaststrokers swallow small quantities of water while swimming.

Milk products

Unpasteurized milk (and ice cream or yoghurt made from it) should always be avoided. Diarrhoeal diseases are rarely contracted in this way, but other diseases such as brucellosis and tuberculosis are a real problem in some regions. Listeriosis is a disease that has received much recent publicity and has also been linked to certain dairy products.

Brucellosis and listeriosis

Brucellosis is a bacterial disease acquired from animals. It occurs with varying but moderate frequency in most areas of the world outside northern Europe, Australia, New Zealand, the United States, and Canada. This disease has non-specific symptoms characterized by fever, headache, profuse sweating, chills, weight loss, depression, joint pains, and generalized aching.

For the traveller, risk of infection arises from eating unpasteurized dairy products, particularly goat cheese. Every year a number of cases are reported in recent travellers to southern Europe, Africa, the Middle East, and South America. Most cases respond to several weeks' treatment with a combination of antibiotics. However, delay in diagnosis and initiation of appropriate therapy may lead to prolonged disability. Because the time interval between consuming the contaminated food item and onset of illness is typically a month or more, the important diagnostic clue of having eaten cheese or other unpasteurized dairy product may have been forgotten. The lengthy incubation period combined with the non-specific symptoms of brucellosis are important factors contributing to the frequent delays in diagnosis that often occur.

In addition to brucellosis, a variety of other infections can be acquired from eating goat cheese in areas where pasteurization is not the norm. Bacterial infections are most common and include **bovine tuberculosis, listeriosis, salmonellosis**, and a variety of diarrhoeal agents. Listeriosis presents a particular hazard for pregnant women (see p. 488). The mother may have no symptoms, or may have a mild febrile illness; but the mother's infection may result in fetal infection. This can lead to miscarriage, stillbirth, or meningitis and septicaemia in the newborn.

Eggs

The importance of eggs as a possible source of salmonella infections has received extensive attention in the UK, but it is a problem in many countries where intensive farming methods are used, including the USA. Salmonella infections predominate in growing chickens and are much less frequent in the egg-laying population. Where individual eggs have been tested the infection rate is no greater than 1 in 1000 eggs. There is no evidence to suggest that travellers are at greater risk of acquiring egg-associated salmonellosis at present. In fact it is possible that less intensive egg production methods that do not involve large flocks and battery conditions are less likely to produce contaminated eggs. The greatest risk is related to bulk catering where large numbers of pooled eggs are used. Uncooked or lightly cooked eggs, and foods made with them, such as mayonnaise, sauces, mousses, milk shakes, ice cream, and sandwiches, are frequently incriminated. Thorough cooking kills the organisms.

Alcohol

Due caution should also be taken with alcoholic drinks, which should not be assumed to be self-sterilizing. Furthermore, excessive alcohol intake may itself cause diarrhoea by an irritant action. Alcohol within a drink has a dehydrating effect, and reduces the amount of water actually available for rehydration. For these reasons, alcoholic drinks are not recommended as a source of water intake in hot countries.

Food from buffets

People eat more buffet food when they travel. The food looks appealing, and it is a way to try many local dishes. However, buffet foods are often the highest risk items, and should usually be avoided. If it is absolutely essential to eat food from a buffet, and it is not possible to have something prepared freshly for you, the principles of food safety discussed in this chapter should be followed closely. If there is a flame under any of the items and the food is steaming, choose food from directly over the flame: this is more likely to be at a safe temperature.

Aeroplane food

Food served on aeroplanes can be a source of intestinal infection. This is not surprising considering the large number of meals prepared, the frequent flight delays that occur, and the time in the air before some meals are served. Aeroplane meals on flights originating in tropical or semitropical developing countries are even more likely to be contaminated: take careful precautions, or better still, don't eat it.

Cruise ships

Food and water can be considered safe on most cruise ships, and the greatest risk usually arises when consuming meals on shore excursions during the cruise, which is when food precautions are particularly important. Precautions should also be followed carefully if there is any suspicion that food or water is being taken on board in a high-risk area.

Flies

Flies live with equal happiness on dung and on food. If you allow flies to walk on your food and then you eat it, for all practical purposes you are eating excrement. Flies are important vectors in the 'faecal–oral' transmission of infection. Avoid buffets and cold food that have not been protected with fly screens.

Hands

Micro-organisms sticking to your hands easily contaminate food if you are careless. A conscious effort not to bring your hands up to your mouth unless they are clean is therefore worthwhile. Proper hand drying after washing is an equally important part of the cleansing process.

Other modes of transmission

Several diarrhoea-causing organisms can be transmitted directly from person to person or from animals. However, in most cases transmission will involve swallowing contaminated material, so the precautions outlined above will remain effective. Transmission via fine droplets produced by coughing or sneezing is a possible route for the viral agents of diarrhoea. Rotaviruses and Norwalk-like viruses (previously called small round structured virus (SRSv)) may also be transmitted in this way, and remain largely uncontrolled world-wide. They are notorious for evading even the most careful cross-infection precautions in modern hospitals, and Norwalk-like virus has caused serious outbreaks on board cruise ships (p. 277).

Organisms responsible for travellers' diarrhoea

Identifying and understanding the organisms that cause diarrhoea are very important steps in developing rational treatments and control measures. The brief details given here are intended to help the reader understand the various patterns of infections and choose the right treatment. The organisms concerned differ greatly in their geographic distribution, as well as in the frequency and severity of the diseases they cause. The principal agents are listed in Fig. 2.1, and prominent causes of travellers' diarrhoea are described below. Details of treatment are given on pp. 29–35 and summarized in Fig. 2. 2.

Enterotoxigenic *Escherichia coli* (ETEC)

ETEC bacteria multiply in the small intestine and make toxins, which are responsible for most, if not all, of the symptoms. They are responsible for up to one third of cases of travellers' diarrhoea (as well as being a major cause of diarrhoea in local children, often resulting in life-threatening illness).

The toxins interact with cells called enterocytes situated on the lining of the small intestine and cause an uncontrolled activation of the mechanisms by which water is normally moved across the gut wall. The result is a dramatic net flow of salt and water into the gut.

The large intestine normally absorbs one or two litres of water passing down from the small intestine daily. It has a reserve absorbing capacity of a further two to three litres that must be exceeded before diarrhoea appears. Given that in severe cases several litres of fluids may be lost in the stools, the level of disturbance is impressive, to say the least.

ETEC diarrhoea is self-limiting and rarely lasts more than 48 hours.

Another type of *E. Coli* — *E. Coli* 0157:H7 — has been responsible for a number of outbreaks in the UK and the USA that have received much publicity, particularly on account of the kidney failure (haemolytic uraemic syndrome) that can sometimes be a complication in children. This type of *E. Coli* is seldom associated with travel.

Shigella

Organisms of the *Shigella* group, along with some strains of *E. coli* that don't produce the toxins mentioned above, are responsible for bacillary dysentery. *Shigella* organisms are responsible for up to 15 per cent of travellers' diarrhoea. It takes only 10 organisms to start an infection.

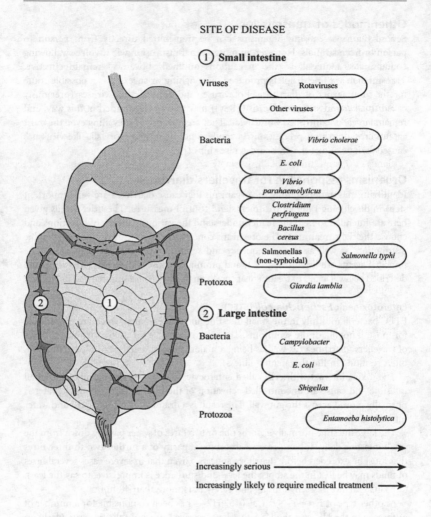

SITE OF DISEASE

① Small intestine

Viruses
- Rotaviruses
- Other viruses

Bacteria
- *Vibrio cholerae*
- *E. coli*
- *Vibrio parahaemolyticus*
- *Clostridium perfringens*
- *Bacillus cereus*
- Salmonellas (non-typhoidal) — *Salmonella typhi*

Protozoa
- *Giardia lamblia*

② Large intestine

Bacteria
- *Campylobacter*
- *E. coli*
- *Shigellas*

Protozoa
- *Entamoeba histolytica*

Increasingly serious ⟶

Increasingly likely to require medical treatment ⟶

Fig 2.1 The main infectious causes of diarrhoea

Shigellosis occurs characteristically in two phases: an initial feverish phase with profuse watery diarrhoea, leading to a prolonged illness with loose and frequent stools containing blood and mucus, whose passage may be associated with considerable pain. The initial phase is probably caused by the multiplication of bacteria in the small intestine. Their offspring travel down into the large intestine, where they invade the gut lining. This invasion causes a failure of the normal absorption process producing a small amount of bleeding and secretion of mucus by glands lining the bowel wall. The illness may be very unpleasant indeed, with delirium and dehydration in the early phase, particularly in children, while the prolonged phase may last up to a month.

Salmonellas (non-typhoid)

Salmonella infections (salmonellosis) may account for up to 10 per cent of cases of travellers' diarrhoea. They predominantly affect the lower end of the small intestine.

The organisms penetrate deeper than the shigellas and become localized in lymph glands of the intestinal wall. Surprisingly, they seem to produce less damage than the shigellas, and the disease is limited to a week of mild to moderate diarrhoea containing mucus but rarely any blood. An infection without any bowel symptoms, just fever and rigors or shivering with fever, is a common feature of salmonella infection.

Rotaviruses

Rotaviruses account for less than 1 per cent of cases. In contrast to the bacteria causing intestinal infections, only very small numbers of viral particles are required to initiate an illness, which is one of the reasons why they remain uncontrolled even in industrialized countries.

The tiny viral particles — less than 0.0001 mm in diameter — multiply within the small intestinal enterocytes, destroying their ability to absorb fluids and greatly reducing the levels of many digestive enzymes. Failure to absorb nutrients, which then pass into the large intestine, may further impair water absorption and diarrhoea may be severe, especially in children under the age of two. The mechanism of immunity to rotaviruses is unclear at present. Infections continue to occur in adult life but the resulting disease becomes milder.

Other viruses

Norwalk-like virus is a poorly understood virus that is extremely difficult to combat. It causes diarrhoea and vomiting and can spread rapidly, both by direct contact and by droplet spread; it is highly contagious and infection produces no lasting immunity. There is no vaccine. It can be a particular problem on cruise ships — total ship decontamination involves taking the ship out of service and cleaning every surface with chlorine bleach — an unpleasant, costly, and destructive process that is sometimes the only way to stamp out infection.

Giardia lamblia

This protozoon parasite occurs throughout the world (see p. 45) and is able to stick firmly to the wall of the small intestine. It probably accounts for less than 3 per cent of cases of travellers' diarrhoea, though it accounts for a much larger proportion of cases of diarrhoea persisting after return home.

In prolonged infections it destroys the inward projections of the gut (called villi), which are responsible for absorbing digested food. If untreated, this may lead to a state of malnutrition characterized by a number of vitamin deficiencies.

The early phase of the disease varies from a self-limiting mild condition to an extremely unpleasant profuse watery diarrhoea succeeded by a chronic phase with bulky, extremely foul-smelling, pale grey stools that indicate failure to absorb digested food. The second phase may persist at various levels of severity for months or even years.

Cryptosporidium

The increasing recognition of this organism (a distant relative of the malarial parasite) over the past 10 years as a cause of diarrhoeal disease is another reminder that although we know a great deal, we still don't know nearly enough.

Cryptosporidium is now known to be prominent as a cause of travellers' diarrhoea. The organism lives in the enterocytes of the small intestine and stimulates an outflow of water that normally lasts up to 10 days but that can persist for several weeks. None of the treatments described here apart from rehydration therapy can affect the course of cryptosporidiosis. Moreover, the organism is resistant to all chemical means of water decontamination available to the traveller (including iodine). The likely sources of cryptosporidiosis for the traveller include contaminated water supplies and faecal-oral transmission via food-handlers or close contact with an infected individual.

Boiled water and well-cooked food provide the only guarantees against this alarming 'new' hazard.

Cyclospora

A recently recognized organism causing persistent diarrhoea in travellers through Nepal and Peru, as well as a major outbreak in the USA that was linked to raspberries imported from Guatemala (contamination of water used for crop-spraying is believed to have been the cause).

Entamoeba histolytica

E. histolytica is another protozoan parasite, related to free-living amoebae so commonly studied in school biology classes. Like *Giardia* it is a relatively uncommon cause of travellers' diarrhoea, accounting for less than 3 per cent of cases. *E. histolytica* occurs in most tropical countries and may cause amoebic dysentery (see p. 47), a disease of the large intestine that is not dissimilar to the 'bacillary dysentery' mentioned above.

The active disease-producing stage of this organism's lifecycle, the 'trophozoites', invade the intestinal wall, causing bleeding and mucus production. Tissue destruction may be extensive and leads to ulcers in the large intestine. Trophozoites may spread to the liver (in about one in five cases) and occasionally (in about one in 1000 cases) produce liver abscesses. Spread to other parts of the body, notably the lungs and the brain, rarely occurs and usually has fatal consequences.

Bacillary and amoebic dysentery are very difficult to distinguish. The presence of blood or mucus in the stool always requires medical attention and if one cannot, by microscopic examination of the stool, separate the cause, medical advice on correct treatment should be sought.

Giardia and *Entamoeba* are discussed further in the next chapter.

Unidentified causes

In surveys attempting to establish the cause of diarrhoeal illness in almost any group of individuals, no clearly defined infecting agent may be found in over 60 per cent of cases. It seems likely that there are several as yet unidentified causative organisms involved.

Over the past 20 years, no fewer than five 'new' major infectious causes of diarrhoeal disease have been brought to light (rotavirus, *Campylobacter*, *Clostridium difficile*, *Cryptosporidium*, and *Cyclospora*) and we have no reason to suspect that the next 20 years will not bring similar discoveries.

Patterns of illness

The main patterns of illness that occur in travellers with intestinal infection are summarized in Table 2.1.

Table 2.1 Patterns of illness

Vomiting only:	This is most likely to be caused by toxins produced by bacteria such as *Staphylococcus aureus* and *Bacillus cereus*: vomiting typically occurs one to five hours after eating contaminated food.
Vomiting and diarrhoea (gastroenteritis):	This is usually due to a toxin (from *S. aureus* or *B. cereus*) or a virus (Norwalk virus or rotavirus); the incubation period and the absence or presence of fever are sometimes helpful in identifying the likely cause.
Watery diarrhoea:	More than half of people with travellers' diarrhoea have a non-specific syndrome of watery diarrhoea without excessive vomiting, fever, or blood or mucus in the stools. Between 3 and 40 unformed stools are passed over a three to five day period, often with abdominal cramps and pain. Cholera can cause an extreme form of this syndrome, with profound fluid loss (up to 3 litres per day) — see next chapter.
Diarrhoea with fever or blood (dysentery):	When fever or passage of bloody mucoid stools (dysentery) occur, the traveller usually has an infection caused by a bacterium that invades the intestinal lining and produces inflammation. Anti-microbial treatment is necessary. The two major causes of this syndrome in travellers are *Shigella* spp. and *Campylobacter jejuni*. Other less common causes are *Aeromonas* spp., *Vibrio parahemolyticus*, *Entamoeba histolytica* (see also p. 46) and noninfectious inflammatory bowel disease.
Persistent diarrhoea:	When diarrhoea lasts longer than two weeks it is usually due to: *Giardia*; lactose malabsorption; bacterial overgrowth syndrome; persistent infection by a bacterial agent; nonspecific injury pattern of the gut.
Typhoid fever:	The person with typhoid will have high fever, headache, abdominal pain and either constipation or diarrhoea.

Table 2.2 Types of bacterial food-poisoning

Causal agent	Incubation period	Symptoms	Comments
Salmonellas (non-typhoid)	6–72 hrs (usually 12–36 hrs)	Diarrhoea, abdominal pain, vomiting, and fever	See text
Clostridium perfringens	8–22 hrs (usually 12–18 hrs)	Diarrhoea, abdominal pain (vomiting is rare)	Toxin formed in small intestine
Staphylococcus aureus	1–7 hrs (usually 2–4 hrs)	Nausea, vomiting, abdominal pain, prostration, dehydration, low temperature, sometimes diarrhoea	Preformed toxin in the food (hence rapid onset)
Campylobacter	1–11 days (usually 2–5 days)	Abdominal pain, diarrhoea, sometimes with blood, fever	Similar to shigellosis; probably very common
Bacillus cereus	1–5 hrs or 8–16 hrs	Predominantly vomiting Predominantly diarrhoea	Preformed toxins made in small intestine
Vibrio parahaemolyticus	2–48 hrs (usually 12–24 hrs)	Abdominal pain, diarrhoea, sometimes nausea, vomiting, fever, and headaches	Toxins made in small intestine; classically caught from uncooked seafood

Enteropathogens

Several other agents of diarrhoeal disease (enteropathogens) are known to be important, although their exact significance to travellers is not established. They are all considered causes of 'food-poisoning', a rather loose term that denotes any acute illness attributable to recent consumption of food. Information regarding these is summarized in Table 2.2. They can to a certain extent be differentiated by the sufferer on the basis of the interval between eating contaminated food and the onset of the symptoms, and the nature of the symptoms themselves.

- There are many non-infectious causes of diarrhoea and blood in the stool (e.g. anxiety and haemorrhoids respectively). ***Blood in the stool always warrants investigation by a doctor.***
- Typhoid does not usually cause severe diarrhoea; fever is always present (see p. 448)

Two other enteropathogens that can cause a severe illness if not appropriately treated are those that cause typhoid and cholera.

Table 2.3   Non-infectious causes of diarrhoea

Agent	Incubation	Signs and Symptoms	Food
Ciguatera fish poisoning (ciguatera toxin)	2–6 hrs	Abdominal pain, nausea, vomiting, diarrhoea.	A variety of large reef fish, including grouper, red snapper, amberjack, and barracuda
Shellfish toxins (diarrhoeic, neurotoxic, amnesic)	30 mins– 2 hrs	Nausea, vomiting, diarrhoea, and abdominal pain accompanied by chills, headache, and fever	Shellfish, primarily mussels, oysters, scallops, and shellfish from Florida
Nitrite poisoning Pesticides (organo-phosphates) Mushroom toxin, Drugs, including proguanil and chloroquine			

Typhoid

The bacterium responsible for typhoid is called *Salmonella typhi*, and shows a pattern of invasion similar to that seen with the other salmonellas. However, after localizing in the lymph glands of the large intestine and terminal small intestine, there is further spread into the blood. Symptoms take around seven days to appear after exposure (but may range from 3 to 60 days) and include fever, headache, abdominal pain, constipation, and, less frequently, diarrhoea. Typhoid is a serious systemic illness and a fatal outcome is common without treatment.

Cholera

You probably wouldn't be able to distinguish cholera from any other cause of diarrhoea; the disease and its treatment are described in greater detail in the next chapter (See p. 40).

Non–infectious causes of diarrhoea

Some non–infectious causes of diarrhoea are listed in Table 2.3

What to do about diarrhoea

Practical help for diarrhoea starts with a description of stool quality and pattern of onset of symptoms.

A simple approach based on such descriptions is presented in Fig. 2.2. The various courses of action — oral rehydration, seeking medical advice, antibiotics, and antidiarrhoeal medicines — are discussed in further detail below.

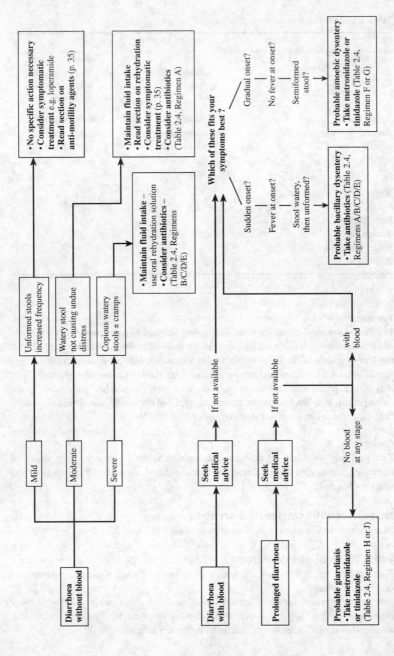

Fig 2.2 What to do about diarrhoea.

Four important points should be borne in mind when considering appropriate action:

1. Most cases of travellers' diarrhoea will resolve within 48 to 72 hours without any treatment.
2. Complications following diarrhoea are commoner in children, the elderly, or those with underlying medical problems.
3. Fluid replacement or rehydration by mouth is an effective, safe, and worthwhile part of treatment.
4. Diarrhoea containing blood or lasting more than four days warrants medical attention.

In the rare instances where travellers' diarrhoea is severe enough to be life threatening, it is adequate fluid replacement, not antibiotics, or antidiarrhoeal agents, that proves life saving.

Rehydration

Travellers' diarrhoea may cause dehydration even if mild. Sweating in hot climates leads to considerable body fluid losses. Fluid requirements are difficult to predict, but thirst is a reminder that the body needs fluid. Young children cannot communicate their thirst other than by crying or becoming drowsy, which makes them especially susceptible to dehydration.

Rehydration salts may be bought in a pharmacy as sachets containing a mixture of salt and glucose (e.g. Dioralyte or Electrolade) with instructions for use in water that is as clean as possible. Alternatively, using a plastic spoon designed to measure salt and sugar in the ratio of 1:8 to be made up in a glass of water is as effective — and is simpler and cheaper to make up. Otherwise, the proportions are as follows:

- 8 level or 4 heaped teaspoons of sugar (white, brown, or honey)
- plus 1/2 teaspoon of salt
- added to 1 litre of clean water.

Other carbohydrates produce the same effect as glucose or sucrose. These include 50 grams (10–15 teaspoons) per litre of powdered rice (and other cereals), which needs to be added to a small volume of boiling water before diluting to 1 litre. In some countries, rehydration solutions containing cereals may be available (e.g. Ceralyte).

Oral rehydration should be started early rather than later before judgement becomes impaired as the diarrhoea takes it toll and you weaken. Vomiting is often a major feature of dehydration: as you replace fluids vomiting will decrease. If necessary, regular small sips may be a better way of keeping the fluid down than taking large gulps, which may start further vomiting.

For healthy adults with mild to moderate attacks, an adequate intake of most non-alcoholic drinks will normally suffice. Rehydration fluids should always be prepared for infants.

When ministering to others, look for evidence of significant dehydration such as dry tongue, dark, concentrated, and smelly urine in small quantities, or no urine, and a weak, rapid pulse. If such evidence is found, particularly in children, the sufferer should be coerced to take as much rehydration solution as possible until he or she starts to pass urine of normal appearance and volume. A simple regimen for adults is to insist on a glass of oral rehydration solution for every bowel movement plus a further glass every hour.

For infants and children, careful fluid replacement is necessary. As a guide, 1.5 times the normal feed volume as rehydration solution while continuing the normal feed would be necessary. For children who are breast feeding, this should continue, with additional rehydration solution also provided although research has shown breast fed infants can obtain all they need from the breast alone. Anyone showing signs of dehydration would be well advised to seek immediate medical attention. As soon as someone you are caring for ceases to be able to drink, this should be treated as a medical emergency, and they should receive attention as soon as possible since intravenous rehydration may be necessary (see also pp. 497 and 578–9).

Antibiotics

- Most forms of diarrhoeal disease will resolve without the use of antibiotics.
- Antibiotics are of NO effect when the cause is a virus.

There are a number of fairly clear circumstances where antibiotics **are** needed for gut problems.

A doctor should prescribe any antibiotic treatment required. However, in an emergency the following regimens may be considered after consultation with Table 2.4 (p. 33):

Ciprofloxacin: There is considerable evidence for the efficacy of 'quinolones' — the antibiotic group that includes ciprofloxacin, norfloxacin, and ofloxacin. They are effective in the treatment of diarrhoea. They must not be used in children before puberty or in pregnant or breastfeeding women; and, because there have been occasional reports of dizziness and visual disturbance, you should find out how you react to ciprofloxacin before driving or operating machinery. Table 2.4 (regimens A and B) gives recommendations for the use of ciprofloxacin; the early administration of an antibiotic reduces the length and severity of symptoms. In many instances treatment can cut the expected duration of illness by half. Many different drug regimens have been evaluated, but the simplest is a single dose of ciprofloxacin taken at the first sign of diarrhoea. Drug resistance to quinolones can be a problem in some parts of the world, especially *Campylobacter* infections in Southeast Asia.

Azithromycin (Zithromax) is a possible alternative to these drugs, with the added advantage of being suitable for use in children. Drug-resistance is less widespread.

Metronidazole (Flagyl) is an effective and safe drug and can be used in the treatment of suspected amoebiasis and giardiasis. Minor side effects (compared with the illness you are treating) are fairly common and include: an unpleasant metallic taste, nausea, and a furry tongue. Unless you want a remarkably bad hangover you should not drink alcohol during treatment. The regimens for use of metronidazole for giardiasis are shown in Table 2.4 (regimens F and H). Tinidazole (Fasigyn) is an alternative that is simpler and slightly more pleasant to take.

Sulphamethoxazole with trimethoprim (Bactrim, Septrin). Once a common recommendation, this is now of limited use for the treatment of diarrhoea and bacillary dysentery (shigellosis). Resistance is widespread, and side effects (usually due

Table 2.4 Antibiotic regimens for treatment of various suspected causes of diarrhoea

Suspected cause	Regimen	Antibiotic	Age	Amount per dose	Doses per day and duration
Suspected bacillary dysentery (shigellosis), ETEC	A	Ciprofloxacin	Adult	500–750 mg	Single dose (may be sufficient in 80–90% of cases)
	B	Ciprofloxacin	Adult	500 mg	One dose twice a day for three days; opt for 3-day course in presence of fever blood.
Suspected bacillary dysentery (shigellosis), ETEC	C	Norfloxacin	Adult	400 mg	One dose twice a day for three days
	D	Ofloxacin	Adult	400 mg	One dose twice a day for three days
	E	Azithromycin	Adult	500 mg	Once daily for 3 days
			Child over 6 months (only with fever and bloody diarrhoea)	Initial dose: 10 mg per kg of body weight; thereafter 5 mg per kg	Once daily for 3 days
Suspected amoebiasis (see also p. 46)	F	Metronidazole (Flagyl)	Adult	750–800 mg	One dose three times per day for 5 days followed by diloxanide furoate (p. 46)
			8–12 yrs	400–500 mg	
			4–7 yrs	375–400 mg	
			2–3 yrs	200–120 mg	
			Under 2	80–120 mg	
	G	Tinidazole (Fasigyn)	Adult	2 g (4 tablets)	Daily for 5 days
			Child	50–60 mg per kilo of body weight	Daily for 3 days

Table 2.4 Antibiotic regimens for treatment of various suspected causes of diarrhoea (continued)

Suspected cause	Regimen	Antibiotic	Age	Amount per dose	Doses per day and duration
Suspected giardiasis	H	Metronidazole (Flagyl)	Adult	200–250 mg	One dose three times per day for 5 days
			8–12 yrs	200–250 mg	
			3–7 yrs	100–125 mg	
			Under 3	50–62 mg	
	I	Tinidazole (Fasigyn)	Adult	2 g (4 tablets)	Single dose, repeated once if necessary
			Child	50–75 mg per kg of body weight	
Suspected typhoid	J	Ciprofloxacin	Adult	500 mg	One dose twice a day for 14 days
	K	Chloramphenicol (Chloromycetin)	12 years - adult	500 mg – 1g	One dose four times per day
			8–12 years	250 mg	
			3–7 years	125 mg	

Notes:

1. Any antibiotic treatment should preferably be prescribed by a doctor. The above regimens are for emergency use only.

2. Use of the above regimens should be considered only after reading the accompanying text on antibiotics and consulting Fig 2.2.

3. For regimens F and H, the choice of doses given allows for different tablet sizes.

to the sulphamethoxazole component) can be a problem. Signs of toxicity are rashes, blood in the urine, and jaundice.

If, after starting ciprofloxacin for dysentery, there is no improvement after 36 hours, it is quite reasonable to take a course of metronidazole at the same time.

Drugs like ciprofloxacin are fairly effective in shortening diarrhoeal episodes in travellers. But for reasons to be discussed in the section on prevention, such treatment is not justified unless an important part of the trip will be ruined if the episode continues for too long.

New antibiotics New antibiotics are being developed to combat travellers' diarrhoea. These include Rifaximin, one of a new generation of antibiotics that is not absorbed and acts locally on the intestine.

Typhoid

Typhoid does not necessarily cause diarrhoea, and even if this does become a feature, it is seldom present early on. Typhoid often begins like a cold or flu with a headache, sore throat, and a gradually increasing fever. Signs of a serious infection are usually obvious, and the sufferer is confined to bed. A pulse of only 80 beats per minute or less, in the presence of an obviously high fever, makes typhoid a likely cause. The illness is more severe in the second week and the victim may become delirious.

Medical help should always be sought. In an emergency, antibiotic treatment with ciprofloxacin in the doses shown in Table 2.4 regimen J should be used.

Symptomatic treatment

'Anti-motility' agents

'Anti-motility' or antidiarrhoeal agents inhibit intestinal movement, and can reduce diarrhoea by 80 per cent. Their use is recommended mainly when sanitary arrangements are difficult (e.g. for long journeys) or to permit attendance at important meetings, and then limited to two to four doses. They should never be used when the sufferer has bloody diarrhoea or fever — they can make the illness worse. They can lead to constipation when used in excess.

With the above warnings in mind, the two antidiarrhoeal agents that might be considered are: loperamide hydrochloride (Imodium, Arret), and codeine phosphate. Dosages for adults are shown in Table 2.5.

Both drugs are chemically related to morphine, and may constitute a serious risk to children. The WHO advises that anti-secretory or binding agents should not be used in managing infants or children with diarrhoea, and these drugs should never be used in children below the age of 10 years.

There are very few circumstances where the administration of these drugs is absolutely necessary, but if you really feel obliged to use them, adhere closely to the regimens presented.

'Anti-secretory drugs'

The best known drug of this type is bismuth subsalicylate (Pepto-Bismol) — a widely used remedy in the USA; it can reduce diarrhoea by 50 per cent (p. 39). It should not be used in children.

Racecadotril (Hidrasec) is a newer drug that has a powerful effect on reducing water secretion into the gut. It is available in several countries, is considered to be safe and effective, and in trials has been widely used in children in combination with oral rehydration therapy. It is not likely to be made available in the UK or North America. However, it is part of a new generation of 'anti-secretory' drugs that represent a promising approach to reducing symptoms of diarrhoea in travellers, and trials on these drugs are continuing.

Adsorptive agents

Adsorbents such as attapulgite (Diasorb or Kaopectate) are very safe since they are not absorbed from the intestine, making them useful in children and pregnant women with travellers' diarrhoea. However, relapse is common as soon as treatment stops.

What to eat if you are ill

It is important to alter your diet during a bout of diarrhoea, because the intestine is injured by the infection and absorption of food is often impaired. Don't try to starve yourself! The gut needs energy for repair.

Table 2.5 Antidiarrhoeal agents

Drug	Age	Amount per dose	Doses per day
Loperamide hydrochloride (Imodium, Arret)	13–adult	2 mg	Two doses (4 mg) initially then one dose (2 mg) every four to six hours
	10–12 yrs	2 mg	One dose (2 mg) four times daily
Codeine phosphate	13–adult	30 mg	One dose up to four times daily
	10–12 yrs	15 mg	

With watery diarrhoea, take only liquids such as soups and broths and easily digestible foods such as saltine crackers. As stools assume some form and become soft, move on to foods like toast, potatoes, bananas, tortillas, and baked fish or chicken. Once stools become formed again, move back to a normal diet. Milk and dairy products should be avoided during the early stages of diarrhoea since lactose malabsorption may occur.

When to see a doctor

The major reasons for seeing a physician, either while travelling or on return home, include: temperature above 38°C; significant fever lasting longer than 48 hours;

When you've got to go...

Nothing adds to the misery and discomfort of a sudden attack of diarrhoea quite like the panic of discovering that there really is nowhere to go! On a long journey, away from a familiar environment, not speaking the language and not knowing what to ask for... Is there anything you can do when you really can't find a loo? That is the moment a basic understanding of the physics of diarrhoea can sometimes help.

Under normal circumstances, an average person produces about half a litre of gas every day that can only escape through the rectum. When the stool is solid, this presents no problem. A liquid stool, however, creates an impenetrable obstacle to its passage — as long as you remain in a vertical position.

Much of the discomfort and urgency associated with a bout of diarrhoea is due to exactly this: increasing bloating and distension of the rectum with gas, above a liquid stool.

The solution, if you can find somewhere to do it, is simply to lie on your side — preferably left side down: for anyone suffering from diarrhoea with cramps and gas, this is the position for maximal comfort.

RD

---

diarrhoea lasting longer than 4 days; severe diarrhoea with difficulty keeping up with fluid and salt replacement; and diarrhoea with blood.

Prevention

The most important preventive measures are outlined in the section on transmission, and the principal precautions necessary are summarized in Fig. 2.3, below.

Antibiotics are occasionally advocated for prevention and their use remains somewhat controversial. The main arguments against this practice are:

1. Some of the rare side effects of antibiotics are considerably worse than the diseases they may prevent.
2. Widespread consumption of antibiotics promotes the development of antibiotic-resistant bacteria. This may make other infections more difficult to treat.
3. Antibiotics make diagnosis difficult when infection does occur.

The main arguments in favour of the prophylactic use of antibiotics are:

1. Several regimens are known to be effective.
2. The personal cost of being out of action may outweigh the risks involved in taking antibiotics.

Our feeling is that antibiotics should be taken as a preventive **only** when important meetings or other plans are at risk, or when the traveller is already weakened from some long-standing illness (e.g. heart disease).

Travellers taking 'proton pump inhibitors' for gastric or duodenal ulcers to reduce gastric acidity may be at particular increased risk, and should consider taking antibiotics for prevention.

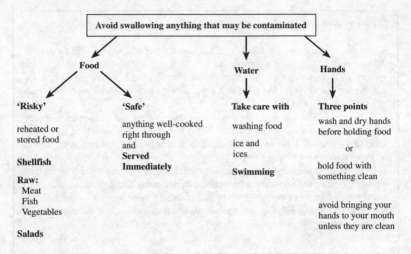

Fig 2.3 Preventing diarrhoea

The most suitable option for prevention is ciprofloxacin, in a dose of 500mg per day. Ciprofloxacin should not be used by children. The duration of antibiotic prophylaxis should not exceed two weeks.

Vaccination

Typhoid

Two vaccines are currently available against typhoid (see p. 561), and immunization against typhoid is recommended when travelling to areas where sanitation may be poor.

The injected Vi antigen vaccine causes very little reaction, and only a single dose is necessary. The oral typhoid vaccine is based ingeniously on freeze-dried bacteria that 'come to life' briefly in the small intestine and then 'commit suicide'.

All of the current typhoid vaccines have roughly the same effectiveness — around 50–90 per cent.

Cholera

Cholera vaccine is discussed on pp. 42 and 561.

Future vaccine developments

Vaccine initiatives are also being directed against many of the other agents important in diarrhoea, including ETEC, *Shigella*, *Campylobacter*, and rotavirus.

Other medicines for prevention

Bismuth subsalicylate (Pepto-bismol), taken in a dose of two tablets four times a day, with meals and at bedtime, for those with a trip lasting no more than three weeks, will prevent 65 per cent of the illnesses that would occur without prophylaxis. The only side effects of this approach are harmless blackening of stools and tongue; other salicylate-containing drugs should not be taken at the same time (notably aspirin), because this can lead to excessive salicylate blood levels. It is a popular option for travellers from the USA.

Lactobacilli are available in various preparations. These are bacteria originally from dairy products made into stable preparation. When taken, the concept is that the organisms displace the dangerous organisms and improve the symptoms. There is not much evidence to suggest they work either in treatment or in prevention of diarrhoea.

The traveller will find a host of tempting preparations offered to the current or potential sufferer in any local or foreign pharmacy. Many of these are useless, or actually damaging. For example, clioquinol (Entero-Vioform) is still a surprisingly popular remedy in some countries — despite being toxic and ineffective.

Persisting symptoms

Most diarrhoeal episodes in travellers last between 48 and 72 hours, but 10 per cent of people with travellers' diarrhoea have illnesses that last longer than a week, and 2 per cent have diarrhoea that lasts more than a month. In a small proportion of cases, the diarrhoea will last for 2 to 12 months.

In travellers with persistent diarrhoea, a different set of conditions is usually the cause — parasites like *Giardia*, for example; another common cause is lactose intolerance — reduced digestion and absorption of milk sugars following damage to the intestinal lining.

In a few unlucky individuals, post-infective diarrhoea syndrome may develop. When bowel symptoms do not return to normal after an acute attack, and irregular and frequent bowel movements are still occurring as long as three months later, but no infecting organisms are found on testing, this condition is the most likely cause. No major damage appears to occur. The symptoms are a nuisance, but invariably the condition resolves without specific treatment. Occasionally, changing diet or excluding dairy products produces some benefit.

Several other even rarer illnesses also became relatively more important in this context. These include tropical sprue, a poorly understood condition in which the normally sparsely populated small intestine contains large numbers of bacteria; and several of the parasitic worms dealt with on pp. 48–51. These illnesses are rarely life threatening but they are definitely sufficiently serious to warrant careful investigation.

Other, non-infective disorders, unrelated to travel other than by coincidence, may also cause diarrhoea, bleeding, and abdominal symptoms. Careful medical investigation is extremely important.

Summary of advice for travellers

• Most travellers' diarrhoea is the result of swallowing contaminated food, drink, or other material.

• The contaminating micro-organisms are rendered harmless by adequate cooking (temperatures above the boiling point of water, all the way through, for at least 15 minutes).

• Food remains safe only if eaten immediately after cooking or if sealed and refrigerated without delay.

• Precautions with food are summarized in Appendix 5.

• Diarrhoeal episodes are usually self-limiting, get better after one to three days, and require no specific treatment.

• When required, replacement of water losses is the first consideration of treatment, especially with children (p. 477).

• Guidelines for the place and use of antibiotics, anti-diarrhoeal medication, and other drugs are given on pp. 32–36.

• Diarrhoeal illnesses are not always avoidable.

Cholera

A new cholera strain appeared in Asia in 1992, and its impact is still being monitored. Meanwhile, cholera continues to cause outbreaks in parts of Africa, Asia, South America and the Pacific, particularly in relation to natural disasters, conflict, refugee camps, and conditions of poverty. In this setting, medical resources and knowledge failed to prevent 70 000 cases among Rwandan refugees living in Goma, a quarter of whom died. New vaccines, designed for such situations, are now available. The risk to travellers is extremely small.

Dr Ron Behrens is the only NHS consultant in Travel and Tropical Medicine and is Director of the Travel Clinic of the Hospital for Tropical Diseases, London, where he conducts research into ways of improving travellers' health.

Historical background

The anxiety and fear associated with the name cholera is usually out of all proportion to the severity of the disease in its modern context. The reason is clear: during the nineteenth century, cholera was a devastating illness, causing severe dehydration and death in most of those infected. The usual source of infection was the water supply, and large numbers of people were infected and killed.

The *Vibrio cholerae* bacteria that caused classic cholera (prior to 1961) were in fact slightly different from those that cause the disease today — and more dangerous. However, in 1992 a further new strain — the O139 'serotype' — was discovered in Bengal. The new mutant was recognized when it afflicted adults, a group that is normally relatively immune to cholera. The infection was in most ways similar to the original strains — causing a dramatic fluid loss, with vomiting and with litres of watery diarrhoea within hours of infection. If fluid replacement of 5–10 litres could not be provided rapidly, debility and death would ensue. It spread rapidly through Bangladesh, causing over 100 000 deaths in less than five months.

Throughout history, cholera has always tended to occur in pandemics (world-wide epidemics) lasting decades or longer.

The current (seventh) pandemic

The current pandemic started in Indonesia in 1961. It reached Latin America in 1992 (after an absence from the continent of more than a century) causing much panic but ultimately resulting in greatly improved hygiene and sanitation. However, cases in Asia have increased by 17% and large outbreaks continue to occur in West, Central, East, and southern Africa. There have also been outbreaks in Micronesia and Fiji. In 1999, WHO received official reports of cholera cases from 61 countries amounting to more than 250 000 confirmed cases with more than 10 000 deaths.

The strain of cholera involved is the El Tor 01 biotype; it is carried by humans via trade and commercial routes. It is much less virulent than classical cholera: after infection, severe diarrhoea develops in only 2–5 per cent of those infected, while over 75 per cent will have no symptoms at all.

To put the disease in its true perspective, even during an epidemic cholera accounts for less than 5 per cent of acute diarrhoeal cases in a poor community. Healthy carriers (people excreting the organism without symptoms) are an important catalyst to the spread of cholera, and remain infectious to others for more than five days after being infected.

Screening all migrants from infected areas would be highly impractical, and disease containment has never been effective in the past. Control of cholera epidemics is based on the following cardinal principles: isolate and treat patients until they are non-infectious, identify and treat their contacts, establish and enforce public hygiene measures such as protecting and treating drinking water, provide adequate sewage treatment and waste disposal, and secure uncontaminated food supplies. A main source of infection in the South American outbreaks was identified in the water storage pots kept by households. Contamination and spread of the bacteria occurred when householders scooped out water for personal use.

Legislation and control

In an effort to control the spread of cholera across international boundaries through travel, the World Health Organization introduced mandatory cholera vaccination in 1969. The intentions and scope of these regulations have on many occasions been over-interpreted and misapplied: measures such as placing aircraft passengers in quarantine, disinfecting mail, and prohibiting importation of tinned foodstuffs have been enforced at various times.

Control measures consisted mainly of checking immunization of travellers at borders, and reporting cases of cholera that did occur. Despite intensive surveillance, however, most countries could not prevent the spread of cholera across their borders — which was often carried by illegal immigrants via small, unsupervised ports.

International requirements for cholera immunization have had little impact on world-wide cholera spread and were formally abandoned in 1973. The WHO stopped publishing cholera vaccination certificates in 1989. The WHO, along with other organizations such as the Centers for Disease Control in the USA, does not now recommend cholera immunization for travellers, and states that immunization certificates should not be required of any traveller.

Cholera vaccination

The original injected cholera vaccine is now seldom used as it was found to protect only half of recipients, for a limited period. Serious reactions to cholera vaccine were occasionally reported, particularly when it was combined with typhoid vaccine; a more important drawback of cholera immunization was the false sense of security that it engendered.

How it is spread

The bacteria that cause the disease survive mainly in estuarine waters and semi-saline coastal lagoons; it has been suggested that certain kinds of algae act as an environmental reservoir.

Cholera is spread by contamination of food and water by faeces or raw sewage. Shellfish and seafood have been a major source of infection in South America, where ceviche — a dish that contains marinated uncooked fish — is a delicacy in many countries. Unwashed vegetables irrigated with contaminated water or untreated sewage are also a source.

Like all diarrhoeal illnesses, the likelihood of infection depends on the weakest link in the food and water hygiene chain. Even if water is decontaminated by boiling, or comes from a chlorinated source, contamination of ice cubes or of a slice of lemon placed in a glass will cause infection.

Children and people with blood group O are at greater risk of infection.

The illness

Diarrhoea caused by the El Tor strain is a mild illness, unlike the more profuse diarrhoea associated with classic cholera. Its onset is quite sudden, but in no way can it be differentiated from most other causes of travellers' diarrhoea. Vomiting is frequent and is thought to reflect dehydration; it improves as fluid replacement progresses.

Hospital management is not normally necessary unless sufficient oral fluid intake proves difficult, and intravenous rehydration is required. The illness lasts between three and five days and leaves no disability when properly treated.

Treatment

Oral antibiotics such as ciprofloxacin or erythromycin can reduce the length of infection and reduce fluid loss, if taken early in the illness.

The diarrhoea of cholera is no different from other types of travellers' diarrhoea, and its treatment with abundant quantities of oral rehydration solution is the simplest and most effective measure (see pp. 31–32). Since fluid loss is the most important complication of severe cholera, the development of effective oral rehydration therapy has completely disarmed the disease, reducing the death rate from over 80 per cent to less than 1 per cent.

Scientific research has established that the gut absorbs salt and water most rapidly and efficiently in the presence of a carbohydrate such as sugar or glucose. Rehydration fluids take advantage of this effect, and generally consist of glucose (or sucrose), salt, and water (the sugar can be replaced by a number of other carbohydrates such as powdered rice, potato, or wheat — the effect in the presence of salt is the same).

Cholera and the traveller

Cholera is a disease associated with slums and extreme poverty, and an absence of the most basic hygiene facilities and education. It is unusual for travellers to use water supplies or food from slum areas, and the risk of cholera in travellers is therefore low.

Until the epidemic of cholera in South America, the risk to travellers was less than 1 in a million. However more cases in travellers occurred as they received improperly prepared food and contaminated meals during travel to infected countries. In Europe, cases in immigrants and refugees are reported.

In 1999, six cases of cholera were imported into the USA, six into Western Europe, and five into Australia and New Zealand, with no deaths.

Future prospects for a vaccine

New vaccines against cholera and other diarrhoeal diseases are under trial. Using genetic manipulation techniques, cholera organisms that are 'sheep in wolf's clothing' have been created. One type uses killed bacteria, while another uses live organisms. What is unusual about these vaccines is that they are swallowed, so that immunity occurs in the intestine — at the natural site of infection. Protection against cholera with the killed bacteria oral vaccine was disappointingly low and short-lived in young children. (This vaccine uses a neutralized cholera toxin, which stimulates the intestine to produce antibodies to the toxin found in natural infection.) However, the combined vaccine has been shown to partially protect against diarrhoea caused by *Escherichia coli*, the bacteria responsible for most of travellers' diarrhoea, and it could be of considerable benefit to tropical travellers in the future.

The most promising vaccine is a mutant live cholera vaccine, *Vibrio cholera* CVD 103-HgR, which is drunk, infects the intestine, and secretes a deactivated replica toxin which does not cause diarrhoea but stimulates natural effective immunity. The vaccine organism is also handicapped so it cannot spread and infect others when it passes from the body. The vaccine has been shown to safe and it has been used in Switzerland.

CVD 103-HgR (Mutachol) — is licensed in Canada and is effective against cholera; that is, against serogroup O1 only. The vaccine is administered as a single dose and is approved for adults and children over 2 years of age.

Vaccination is not recommended for the prevention of cholera in the majority of travellers to endemic areas for the following reasons:
• the risk of acquiring cholera for travellers is generally low;
• the cost of the vaccine is relative high given the low risk of cholera infection.

However, travellers who may be at increased risk for acquiring cholera — for example, health professionals working in endemic areas, aid workers in refugee camps, travellers to remote cholera areas without access to safe water supplies — may wish to consider receiving the vaccine. Travellers should seek a detailed, individual risk assessment to determine their need for vaccination.

Summary of advice for travellers

• Current cholera outbreaks are a serious hazard to the local communities that are affected, but the risk to individual travellers is extremely small, and should not deter anyone from visiting affected regions.

• Cholera is spread by contaminated food and water; hygiene precautions are the most reliable way of avoiding risk.

• There are no official vaccination certificate requirements for travel to any country.

• Although the new cholera vaccines are not recommended by the WHO, they may provide worthwhile protection.

• Cholera is no longer the fearsome disease it once was, and is amenable to simple treatment.

Parasites from infected food and drink

Intestinal parasitic and protozoan infections are amongst the most common infections world-wide. The risk to travellers from these infections varies greatly according to geographic location visited, the food eaten, and local hygiene with respect to water and food.

Dr Richard Knight was a staff member at the London and Liverpool Schools of Tropical Medicine for 18 years. He has worked as physician, epidemiologist, and parasitologist in tropical countries for 17 years. He is now Associate Specialist in General Medicine, with a special interest in gastrointestinal disease, at the Royal Sussex County Hospital in Brighton, Sussex.

The mouth is a major portal of entry for human parasites. The infective stage may be ingested as microscopic protozoan cysts, worm eggs, or worm larvae that contaminate food or drink. Alternatively, food consumed may be tissue from an animal itself infected by a parasite such as *Toxoplasma* or a tapeworm; or fluke larvae from aquatic snail hosts may encyst in fish, crustaceans, or water plants.

Human parasites fall into two distinct groups: those that remain in the gut throughout most of their cycle in man — *resident intestinal parasites* (see Table 2.6); and those that leave the intestine soon after infection and disperse to other organs — *transient intestinal parasites* (see Table 2.7). The latter may manifest themselves as

Table 2.6 Resident intestinal parasites acquired from food and drink

	Location	Source of infection	Distribution
Protozoa			
Giardia	Small intestine	Cysts on food or in water	C
Cryptosporidium	Small intestine	Cysts on food or in water	C
Amoebiasis (*Entamoeba*)	Large intestine	Cysts on food or in water	PT
Helminths (worms)			
Herring worm (*Anisakis*)	Stomach and duodenum	Larval worm in fish	L
Roundworm (*Ascaris*)	Small intestine	Eggs on food	PT
Tapeworm (*Taenia*)	Small intestine	Larval cysts in meat	L
Intestinal flukes	Small intestine	Larval cysts in fish or on water plants	L
Abdominal angiostrongyliasis	Caecum	Larvae from molluscs on salads	L
Whipworm (*Trichuris*)	Large intestine	Eggs on food	PT

Key: C = cosmopolitan (worldwide); PT = pantropical (throughout the tropics); L = localized

disease weeks, months, or even years later. The number of potential parasite species transmitted in these ways exceeds 50, but some are rare or very local in their distribution; nevertheless, there is a significant chance that visitors might pick up one or more of them.

Travellers to rural areas, backpackers, and ecotourists are generally at greater risk, especially those who share in cultural experiences such as wedding or hunting feasts or local food specialities.

Table 2.7 Transient intestinal infections derived from food and drink

	Final location	Source of infection	Distribution
Protozoa			
Amoebiasis (*Entamoeba*)	Liver, rarely lung	Cysts on contaminated food or drink	PT
Toxoplasma	Most tissues including eye	Cysts in meat or from cat faeces	C
Helminths (worms)			
Trichinosis (*Trichinella*)	Muscle and elsewhere	Larval worm in meat	L
Cysticercosis (*Taenia solium*)	Brain, eye, and elsewhere	Eggs contaminate food	L
Hydatid (*Echinococcus*)	Liver, lung, and elsewhere	Eggs contaminate food and fingers	L
Liver flukes	Liver and biliary system	Larval cysts in fish or on vegetables	L
Lung flukes	Lung	Larval cysts in crayfish	L
Angiostrongylus cantonensis	Meninges of brain	Larvae from molluscs on salads	L
Toxocara	Liver, lung, eye, and brain	Eggs contaminate food and fingers	C

Key: C = cosmopolitan (worldwide); PT = pantropical (throughout the tropics); L = localized

Resident intestinal parasites

Some major symptoms and clinical features caused by the parasites listed in Table 2.6 are:

- Colicky abdominal pains — all species
- Upper abdominal pain, sometimes severe — *Ascaris, Anisakis*
- Simple diarrhoea — *Cryptosporidium*
- Diarrhoea with malabsorption (bulky, pale, offensive, and difficult to flush away) — *Giardia*
- Dysentery (diarrhoea with blood) — amoebiasis
- Worms seen in stool — *Ascaris*, tapeworms, threadworms
- Skin wheals (urticaria) and wheezing — *Ascaris*, intestinal flukes
- Itchy bottom — *Enterobius* and *Taenia saginata* (beef tapeworm)
- Retarded growth and malnutrition among children in heavily infected populations — *Ascaris, Trichuris*, and *Giardia*.

These infections are diagnosed by examining stool samples under the microscope and finding cysts, motile protozoa, eggs, or worms. Most can be effectively treated with antiparasitic drugs, and self-treatment is sometimes appropriate.

Protozoan infections

Giardasis

Giardia is a common cosmopolitan species. Most infections in the tropics are derived from infected children but animals, especially dogs, are also important; in Canadian ski resorts mountain beavers can contaminate water supplies. The parasite is pear shaped, flattened, and narrowed behind; it bears four pairs of flagellae. It adheres to the epithelial cells lining the gut by means of a sucking disc, affecting cell function with reduced absorption of nutrients, especially fats. Symptoms start within a few days with abdominal bloating; flatulence; poor appetite; and loose, pale, fatty stools. Morning diarrhoea is characteristic. The illness may subside spontaneously after a week or so but in some persons it is prolonged and debilitating.

Stool specimens show cysts or the swimming flagellate. Treatment is with metronidazole (400 mg, 3 times a day for 5 days) or tinidazole (2 g as a single dose). Self-treatment on clinical suspicion is justified. Some people have very persistent infections that are difficult to eradicate; they have a mild genetic immune defect. There is no relationship between this parasite and HIV.

Cryptosporidium and other small gut protozoa

Cryptosporidium is common and cosmopolitan; infection is often water borne. Farm animals are a common source, as are some domestic animals. The parasites invade epithelial cells and undergo repeated cycles of multiplication causing local damage and inflammation. The illness is often quite acute with watery diarrhoea, cramps, and fever; most infections are self-limiting after a week or so. Drug treatment is ineffective and usually not necessary.

Two related parasites are widespread but local. *Isospora* is reported especially from tropical Africa and the West Indies, while *Cyclospora* is common in Nepal and Latin America. Their life cycle is similar to *Cryptosporidium* — in fact all are biologically close to the malaria parasites. The illness they cause is often more severe than *Cryptosporidium,* more prolonged, and may resemble giardiasis with fatty stools. Both can be treated with co-trimoxazole (Septrin, Bactrim).

While the cysts of these three parasites are present in faecal specimens, they are commonly overlooked unless dried smears are fixed and specially stained. These infections are of major importance in persons with HIV, in whom they are the major secondary cause of the wasting, diarrhoeal, AIDS-related illness that is so common in tropical countries. Other gut protozoa called microspora cause similar problems in HIV patients but fortunately only transient diarrhoea in normal persons. These organisms are minute and require electron microscopy of gut biopsies to identify them; the commonest is *Enterocytozoon.*

Amoebiasis (amoebic dysentery)

Entamoeba histolytica once had a world-wide distribution but is now common only in the tropics, especially Southeast Asia, southern Africa, Mexico, and other parts of Latin America; Nepal has a bad reputation for this parasite. It is estimated to cause severe disease in 48 million people, killing 70 000 each year.

Swallowed cysts reach the large intestine. These 'hatch' to produce amoebae that live on the mucosal surface and usually invade it, resulting in ulcers that can severely damage the bowel wall. Invading amoebae are actively motile, killing host cells on contact and feeding on cell debris and red blood cells. Invading amoebae may enter local blood vessels and be carried to the liver to cause liver abscess (see below).

Symptoms start two weeks or sometimes a month or so after infection. Colicky pains and loose blood-stained stools may persist for weeks or even months, often with a relapsing course. Severe infections cause dysentery with bloody diarrhoea and, untreated, this may be a significant danger to life. More chronic infections can cause tumour-like masses called amoebomas.

Early diagnosis is essential and is best made by microscopic examination of fresh faeces or exudate taken from the rectal wall examined with a scope. Living invasive amoebae are actively motile and contain red blood cells. Finding amoebic cysts in stool specimens is of little value as they are indistinguishable from those of a harmless species called *Entamoeba dispar.* Even in the tropics this second species is much more common than *E. histolytica.* Travellers should beware of local laboratories that use unreliable methods and practitioners who offer unnecessary and sometimes toxic medications.

The standard course of treatment consists of metronidazole 750–800 mg, 3 times daily for 5 days, followed by diloxanide 500 mg 3 times daily for 10 days. Unless the second drug is given, relapses from persisting infection can occur. An alternative is metronidazole, taken alone for eight days, but this will give a lower rate of parasite elimination. There is a dilemma here for the traveller since amoebiasis is potentially dangerous and it is better to know whether one is really infected or not. Empirical treatment, even self-treatment, is sometimes justified, but when symptoms recur there will be the temptation to repeat it, when it is quite possible that the illness was not amoebiasis at all. Side-effects of metronidazole in short courses may be unpleasant but are unlikely to be serious; alcohol should not be taken. Tinidazole is an alternative to metronidazole; it has the advantage of being taken as single daily dose but is probably less effective.

Worm infections

Roundworm, whipworm, and threadworm infections
These are all common; they are nematode worms, whitish in colour, cylindrical in cross section, and pointed at both ends.

The **roundworm** (*Ascaris*) is usually about 30 cm in length and 4 mm in diameter. Infection occurs when eggs, usually on contaminated food and vegetables, are swallowed; after hatching in the intestine, larvae migrate through the lungs to be swallowed again and so back to the small intestine. Worms live free in the gut lumen and mature in about 9 weeks, when eggs appear in the faeces; they live for about a year. During the lung migration phase, wheezing and rashes can occur; later the main symptoms are colicky abdominal pains and loss of appetite. Worms may be passed per rectum. Illness is serious in heavily infected children, in whom bowel obstruction or migration into the bile and pancreatic duct may require surgical treatment. More than a billion people world-wide harbour this parasite, including perhaps one third of the population of Africa.

The **whipworm** (*Trichuris*) is much smaller, up to 4 cm in length. It lives in the lower colon and rectum, where it is attached to the mucosa by its narrower head end. There is no lung migration phase. Sources of infection are similar to *Ascaris*. Light infection may cause no symptoms but lower left abdominal pains and loose bowel habit with some blood can occur. Heavy infections in children can cause dysentery, constant straining at stool, and rectal prolapse.

Threadworms (*Enterobius*) are a familiar problem in children throughout the world. Despite some opinions to the contrary, they are common in the tropics and quite often picked up by travellers. The worms measure up to 1 cm and live in the large intestine; female worms migrate to the rectum and emerge from the anus at night to lay eggs on the skin. Allergic responses to the worm lead to scratching, and eggs are transferred to fingers, toys, food, furniture, and dust. Self-infection is common and prolongs the problem. Parents commonly notice worms in children's underpants or night attire. Children become irritable and sleep poorly.

Mebendazole is effective for all these infections, but is not recommended for children under 2 years. For *Ascaris* and *Trichuris*, 100 mg is given twice daily for 3 days. For threadworms a single 100 mg dose, repeated after 2 weeks is sufficient; this infection often spreads to close contacts and it is wise to treat all the family simultaneously to prevent reinfection. Piperazine should be used for children under 2 years with *Ascaris* or threadworm.

Tapeworms
Larval cysts of the beef tapeworm (*Taenia saginata*) occur in undercooked steak and beefburgers. The swallowed worm attaches to the gut wall, grows to maturity in 3 months, and may live many years; most are solitary. The worm is creamy white, flat, and segmented; it can reach 4 m in length. Mature segments containing eggs are shed

at the posterior end of the worm while new segments form at the narrow anterior end. Colicky pains and impaired or increased appetite are typical symptoms but many patients become aware of the problem when segments are seen in the stool, actively migrate through the anus, or are found in underpants. The life cycle of this parasite involves only humans and cattle; cattle become infected from eggs in human faeces.

Infection with the related pork tapeworm *(Taenia solium)* occurs when undercooked pig meat is eaten. Symptoms are similar except that worm segments are not motile and do not migrate through the anus. The importance of the pork tapeworm is that under conditions of poor hygiene, eggs can be swallowed by other people and can develop into cystic larval worms (as normally occurs when the eggs are swallowed by pigs). The result is a serious condition — cysticercosis (see below).

Several other tapeworms infect man including the fish tapeworm, found mainly in Canada, northern Europe, Scandinavia, and Russia; and the cosmopolitan dwarf tapeworm *(Hymenolepis)*, which requires no animal host in its cycle.

Tapeworm infections are treated with niclosamide, usually as a single dose before breakfast, and sometimes given with a laxative to help expel the worms.

Rarities

Symptoms caused by herring worm *(Anisakis)* occur within 24 hours of eating raw sea fish or squid containing the larval worm which burrows into the wall of the stomach or duodenum. There is upper abdominal pain and vomiting and emergency endoscopy may reveal the worm and enable its extraction. The worm occurs especially in the Pacific where whales and other cetaceans are the hosts for the adult worm; to infect man seafood must be eaten partly raw or lightly pickled. The Japanese delicacy sushi is particularly risky.

Intestinal flukes come in many sizes and include the giant *Fasciolopsis* of Southeast Asia acquired by eating water chestnuts, a local delicacy; other flukes are acquired from cysts in undercooked fish.

Abdominal angiostrongyliasis due to *Angiostrongylus costaricensis* was first described in Costa Rica in 1971. It is now recognized as being quite common, especially in children, in parts of Latin America and the Caribbean. Worms live in the arteries of the appendix area of the gut and set up local inflammation. The normal hosts are cotton rats and other rodents; transmission occurs via slugs that contain the larval stage. While humans are unlikely to eat slugs deliberately, their mucus trails containing larvae can easily contaminate salads and fallen fruit on the ground. Diagnosis is usually made at surgery for suspected appendicitis. There is no drug treatment.

Transient intestinal parasites

Major symptoms and clinical features of the parasites listed in Table 2.7 (p. 45) are:
* **Muscle pain and stiffness** — trichinosis
* **Raised blood eosinophil count** — most worm infections in tissue
* **Liver enlargement and pain** — liver flukes, amoebic liver abscess, hydatid cysts, *Toxocara*
* **Lung disease with cough and shortness of breath** — lung fluke, hydatid cyst
* **Fever and generalized illness** — amoebic liver abscess, toxoplasmosis, trichinosis

- **Allergic features** (wheals, facial swelling, and wheezing) — most worm parasites
- **Brain disease** with fits, meningitis, or brain tumour simulation — cysticercosis, *Angiostrongylus*, hydatid cyst, and toxoplasmosis
- **Eye disease** with visual impairment — *Toxoplasma, Toxocara*

The diagnosis may be difficult and require blood tests for specific antibody, imaging with ultrasound, and X-rays. Anti-parasitic drugs alone may not be sufficient and surgery may be necessary.

Amoebic liver abscess

This serious condition can occur during an attack of amoebic dysentery; but more commonly weeks or even years later. It presents with fever, rigors (shivers), and pain in the liver region, back, or right shoulder tip. The abscess contains dead liver tissue and can reach many centimetres in diameter. Untreated they enlarge progressively and rupture into adjacent structures. Ultrasound and antibody tests establish diagnosis. Metronidazole is used for treatment, but to prevent relapse, gut infection must be eliminated with diloxanide. Drainage of the abscess with a needle or surgery is sometimes needed.

Toxoplasmosis

Although the risk from cat boxes is well known, infection also follows eating undercooked meat containing tissue cysts. Hamburgers have a bad reputation and epidemic outbreaks can occur. A febrile illness with enlarged lymph nodes results and sometimes the retina is affected. Pregnant women are at special risk because the foetus may be infected. Latent infections can be reactivated in persons with late HIV infection. The resulting brain lesions can mimic a tumour; the retina may also be affected.

Trichinosis

Infection follows eating poorly cooked pig meat, but wild boar, bush pig, or even hippopotamus are other sources. Travellers may be tempted to partake in 'feasts'. After a short diarrhoeal illness patients develop generalized muscle pains, weakness, fever, prostration and swelling of the face and eyelids. The initial gut infection can be treated with mebendazole, if the cause is known, but once muscle is invaded by larval worms the steroid prednisolone must be used to control symptoms and limit damage to the heart.

Larval tapeworms causing cysticercosis and hydatid disease

In environments contaminated by human faeces of persons infected by the pork tapeworm, eggs may be ingested on food and man becomes an accidental intermediate host instead of the pig. Larval cysts, up to 2 cm, develop in any tissue but especially the brain, muscle, heart, or beneath the skin. Brain lesions can cause epilepsy or serious pressure effects. Drug treatment is available but difficult and surgery may be necessary. High-risk areas for travellers are Latin America (especially Mexico), central and southern Africa, and the Indian subcontinent.

Hydatid cysts are the larval cysts of the dog tapeworm *Echinococcus granulosus*. They may reach 10 cm or more in size and occur especially in the liver, lung, or brain.

Symptoms result from pressure or from leakage, leading to severe allergic reactions that may be fatal. Leakage may occur after trauma or during surgical procedures. Travellers are at risk especially in the Middle East, North and East Africa, and Latin America. Infection is derived from eggs in dog faeces that contaminate food and fingers; stroking infected dogs is a particular risk.

Fluke infections of liver and lung
Liver flukes cause painful liver enlargement and sometimes jaundice. Species of liver fluke occur in East and Southeast Asia and follow ingestion of pickled or undercooked fish. The sheep liver fluke *(Fasciola)* has a cosmopolitan distribution including Europe and South America. Infection follows ingestion of watercress and other water plants on which there are larval cysts.

Lung fluke infections occur in the Far East, South America, and West Africa and follow eating crayfish and other freshwater crustaceans. Larval flukes penetrate the gut, diaphragm, and lung to reach the bronchial airways, where pairs of worms live for many years. Symptoms include breathlessness, cough, and blood-stained sputum. Drug treatments for these fluke infections are available but some are rather toxic.

Eosinophilic meningitis due to **Angiostrongylus cantonensis**
This occurs in the Pacific area and follows ingestion of salads containing snails or their slime trails. The larval worm migrates to the meninges, where a chronic infection occurs; the diagnostic clue is numerous eosinophil cells in the cerebrospinal fluid and blood. The illness lasts several weeks and no specific treatment is yet available.

Toxocariasis
Infection rates for this dog roundworm are often high in the tropics and children are vulnerable to ingesting eggs from sand and soil contaminated by dog faeces. Heavy infections cause cough and wheezing or painful liver enlargement. A few children, even with light infections, develop retinal lesions that resemble eye tumours and epilepsy.

Summary of advice for travellers

- Understanding how parasites are transmitted is the key to reducing the risk.

- Particular hazards are contaminated water that has not been boiled or sterilized; undercooked meat, salads, and raw vegetables; fruit that cannot be peeled; cold drinks and cooked foods sold by street vendors.

- Self-treatment is appropriate for some protozoan and worm infections of the gut, and it may be helpful to take treatment medication as part of your medical kit.

- Seek medical advice on returning home if you develop symptoms or feel you have been at special risk. Tell your doctor where you have been and what you have eaten. Delays in diagnosis are often due to failure to take travel history into account.

- Keep in mind that stool samples often need a specialist laboratory for correct diagnosis and may need to be repeated a number of times before infection can be ruled out.

Poliomyelitis

As the result of a global immunization campaign, the final eradication of polio now seems close. For the time being, however, polio remains a risk in some parts of the world, and travellers should ensure that they don't miss out on protection.

Dr Tom Solomon has worked on polio and other central nervous system (CNS) infections in Vietnam and other parts of Southeast Asia since 1994. He continues to study CNS infections as a Lecturer in Neurology and Honorary Lecturer in Medical Microbiology and Tropical Medicine at the University of Liverpool.

The remarkable story of poliomyelitis encompasses some of the landmark achievements and successes of medical science in the twentieth century — in terms of diagnosis, prevention, and eradication.

Poliomyelitis (often known just as polio) has been around since antiquity. The earliest record of a withered, shortened leg with the characteristic appearances is an Egyptian stele of the eighteenth dynasty (1580–1350 BC). The name (derived from the Greek 'polio' meaning grey and 'myelos' meaning marrow or spinal cord) is descriptive of the pathological lesions that affect the grey matter in the anterior horn of the spinal cord, where lower motor nerves originate. The infectious nature of the disease was proved in the early 1900s by injecting spinal cord material from fatal polio cases into monkeys to reproduce the symptoms and the pathological lesions of the disease. The poliovirus was subsequently shown to be a small enterovirus (intestinal virus), transmitted between humans via the faeco-oral route, which occurs as three strains.

Before the late nineteenth century, polio was predominantly a sporadic disease that mostly affected children under five. Epidemiological evidence supports the idea that the virus was ubiquitous. Almost all under fives became infected, but in most there was no obvious illness, and they simply developed immunity; only the unlucky few developed the disease. Then, during the twentieth century, the disease pattern changed: it is speculated that because of improved hygiene, younger childen avoided infection, and large populations of uninfected and non-immune older children became vulnerable to infection, succumbing in mass epidemics.

Immunization

In the 1950s, two vaccines were produced. In the first (developed by Salk and others) formalin-inactivated (i.e. killed) poliovirus was injected into the skin; in the second (developed by Sabin and others) live virus which had been attenuated (i.e. changed to a mild form which does not cause disease) was used orally. There was a dramatic decline in polio epidemics in countries where the vaccines were used.

In 1988 the World Health Organization resolved to eradicate polio by the year 2000. Like smallpox before it, polio is a suitable target for global eradication (see also p. 601) because the virus is found only in humans (there is no animal reservoir to contend with), and cheap effective vaccines are available. The campaign consisted, in essence, of mass vaccination with the live oral polio vaccine and disease surveillance for clinically suspected cases of polio. Although there was initially some controversy, the campaign has undoubtedly been a success. By 1998 the Americas were free from polio, and transmission had been interrupted in the WHO Western Pacific Region (including China) and in the European Region (except for a small focus in southeast Turkey). A total of 5000 cases were reported in 1999, compared with more than 350 000 cases in 1988. Although cases were reported from 30 countries in 1999, these mostly came from one of three large foci of transmission: South Asia (India, Pakistan, and Afghanistan), West Africa (mainly Nigeria), and Central Africa (mainly Democratic Republic of Congo). Approximately 70% of remaining polio cases occur in India, but eradication from areas of conflict in Africa may ultimately prove to be the most difficult. For the latest update, visit the WHO web-site **www.who.int/vaccines-polio/**

When the WHO launched its campaign at the end of the 1980s there was controversy, particularly about the reliability of clinically diagnosed polio. It was argued that many cases attributed to the virus may not be polio, and that eradication would not have the dramatic impact on paralytic disease that was hoped for. To some extent this has been borne out. In many areas the number of children presenting with acute flaccid paralysis remains high, even after polio eradication. Attention is now focusing on other viral causes of acute flaccid paralysis: enteroviruses (such as enterovirus 71), respiratory viruses (such as adenovirus), and flaviviruses (such as Japanese encephalitis virus).

Clinical features

Infection with polioviruses can cause one of five clinical presentations: asymptomatic infection, 'abortive poliomyelitis' (a mild non-specific febrile illness), 'non-paralytic poliomyelitis' (essentially a viral meningitis syndrome), 'paralytic poliomyelitis' (which may be spinal or bulbar), or 'polio encephalitis' (which is rare). Of these, paralytic poliomyelitis affecting the spinal cord is the most frequently recognized syndrome. Typically the illness is biphasic: a couple of days of a non-specific fever is followed by a brief asymptomatic period before the central nervous system infection begins. This is heralded by more fever, headache, nausea, vomiting, neck stiffness, and limb paralysis. The paralysis is flaccid (floppy), progresses rapidly, and is usually asymmetrical, involving the legs more frequently than the arms. Paralysis is more likely in a limb that has been the site of an intramuscular injection or injury within 2–4 weeks before the onset of infection. There may be muscle pains early in the illness, and although these may be relieved by gentle exercise, this increases the severity of the paralysis that follows.

Recommendations for travellers

The oral polio vaccine is a mixture of live attenuated poliovirus types 1, 2, and 3, which can be given on a sugar lump. A booster dose is recommended for travellers to areas where polio is still endemic, unless they have received a dose within the previous 10 years. Individuals who have never been vaccinated should receive a primary immunization course of three doses at 1-month intervals. There is a very small risk (approximately one case per two million doses) of the vaccine reverting to a virulent form to cause poliomyelitis (vaccine-associated paralytic poliomyelitis) in a recipient or, via faeco-oral spread, to a household in contact with a recipient. However, this risk is greatly overshadowed by the risks of acquiring polio in endemic areas if you are not vaccinated. (See also p. 560.)

The vaccine should be delayed for those with a gastrointestinal upset (because of reduced absorption). It should not be given to those who have an immunodeficiency disorder or have a household contact with immunodeficiency, because they are more susceptible to vaccine-associated paralytic poliomyelitis. In these cases the inactivated vaccine should be given (three subcutaneous doses of 0.5 ml trivalent vaccine 1 month apart for primary immunization, or a single dose for a booster).

Interestingly, since polio has now been eradicated from the Americas, the only new cases reported in that region are vaccine-associated cases. The American Advisory Committee on Immunization Practices has therefore recently advised that for routine childhood vaccination in the USA inactivated polio vaccine should be used, rather than live vaccine. Whether the advice in the UK changes remains to be seen.

Summary of advice for travellers

- Polio remains a threat to travellers despite the success of the WHO polio eradication campaign.

- Travellers to endemic areas should receive a booster dose of oral polio vaccine (unless they have had one in the last 10 years) or a primary course (if they have never been vaccinated).

Viral hepatitis

Hepatitis is common in travellers to areas outside North America, northern Europe, and Australia, and may result in an unpleasant prolonged illness. All travellers should understand how the different types of hepatitis are spread.

Dr Jane N. Zuckerman is Head of the Academic Unit of Travel Medicine and Vaccines, Royal Free and University College Medical School, London.
Professor Arie J. Zuckerman is Dean and Director of the WHO Collaborating Centre for Reference and Research on Viral Diseases, Royal Free and University College Medical School, London.

Viral hepatitis is common throughout the world and is a major public health problem. At least six different viruses are capable of causing the infection, and the illnesses associated with each (which are all very similar) are as follows:

1. Hepatitis A, also known in the past as infectious hepatitis or epidemic jaundice
2. Hepatitis B, also known in the past as serum hepatitis
3. Hepatitis C, referred to in the past as non-A, non-B hepatitis
4. Hepatitis D (delta hepatitis)
5. Hepatitis E
6. Non-A, non-E hepatitis, which is caused by several different viruses (although, by definition, not by the viruses responsible for hepatitis A, B, C, D, E).

The viruses responsible for hepatitis A, B, C, D, and E have been 'characterized' (i.e. a great deal is known about their size, structure, and biology). Sensitive laboratory tests are available for detecting components of the viruses (viral antigens) and antibodies against the viruses in the blood or tissues of people who have been infected — and hence a diagnosis of infection can be made with precision.

The viruses responsible for some forms of non-A, non-E hepatitis have not, on the other hand, been fully characterized, and specific laboratory tests are not available for detecting them. The diagnosis of non-A, non-E hepatitis is thus made (as the name implies) in cases of hepatitis where hepatitis A, B, C, D, and E, and other viruses known to cause liver damage have been excluded.

The illness

The illness of all forms of hepatitis is similar, and results from acute inflammation of the liver. It is frequently heralded by symptoms such as fever, chills, headache, fatigue, generalized weakness, and aches and pains. A few days later, there is often loss of appetite, nausea, vomiting, right upper abdominal pain or tenderness, followed closely by dark urine, light-coloured faeces, and jaundice of the skin or the sclerae (outer coating of the eyeballs). Many infections, particularly in children, are without specific symptoms or without jaundice. In others, jaundice may be severe and prolonged; complete liver failure may occur, and the patient may lapse into a coma.

Hepatitis A

Hepatitis A is common in all parts of the world, but the exact incidence is difficult to estimate because of the high proportion of non-symptomatic cases and infections without jaundice. Surveys of antibody to hepatitis A have shown that while the prevalence of hepatitis A in industrialized countries (particularly North America, northern Europe, and Australia) is decreasing, the infection is virtually universal in most other regions, particularly in countries with warm climates.

Only one form of hepatitis A has been identified, and the antibody that develops against it persists for many years, frequently providing lifelong immunity.

The highest risk areas for hepatitis A include central and eastern Europe, the Mediterranean countries, the Middle East, and developing countries in Africa, Asia, and Central and South America.

How it is spread

Hepatitis A virus is spread by the faecal-oral route, usually by person-to-person contact, particularly in conditions of poor sanitation and overcrowding. Outbreaks result most frequently from faecal contamination of drinking water and food (although water-borne transmission is less often a factor in industrialized countries, or where the piped water supply has been adequately treated and chlorinated).

Food-borne outbreaks, which have become more important and frequent in developed countries, may be due to the shedding of the virus in the faeces of infected food handlers during the incubation period of the illness; the source of the outbreak can often be traced to cooking. Raw or inadequately cooked shellfish cultivated in sewage-contaminated tidal or coastal water, and raw vegetables grown in soil fertilized with untreated human faeces and excreta are associated with a high risk of infection with hepatitis A virus. Hepatitis A infection is frequently contracted by travellers from areas of low to areas of high prevalence. Hepatitis A virus is very rarely transmitted by blood transfusion or by inoculation.

The incubation period of the virus is between 3 and 5 weeks, with an average of 28 days.

Age incidence and seasonal patterns
All age groups are susceptible. The highest incidence is observed in children of school age, but in North America and in many countries in northern Europe most cases occur in adults, frequently after travel abroad. In temperate zones the characteristic seasonal trend is for an increase in incidence in the autumn and early winter months, falling progressively to a minimum in midsummer; but recently this seasonal trend has been lost in some countries. In many tropical countries, the peak of reported infection tends to occur during the rainy season with low incidence in the dry months.

Consequences of infection
The illness caused by hepatitis A is described above. Although the disease has a low mortality, patients may be incapacitated for many weeks. There is no evidence of persistence of infection with hepatitis A virus nor of progression to chronic liver disease.

Control
Control of the infection is difficult. Since faecal shedding of the virus and therefore infectivity is at its highest during the incubation period, strict isolation of cases is not a useful measure. Spread of infection is reduced by simple hygienic measures and the sanitary disposal of excreta.

Hepatitis A and the traveller
Protection against hepatitis A is strongly recommended for travellers who are not already immune (if necessary, this can be checked with a blood test) and who are travelling to endemic areas. One recent study demonstrated that the relative risk of contracting hepatitis A in unprotected travellers was 1 in 300 per month of travel in tourist/resort areas, increasing to a risk of 1 in 50 if the traveller is backpacking or trekking.

Several vaccines against hepatitis A are now licensed. Such vaccines represent a major step forward for travellers, eliminating the need for repeated doses of immunoglobulin. Amongst their many advantages, they are also considerably less painful, provide long-term immunity, and are safe. They do, however, need to be given at least 2 weeks in advance of travel for optimal protection.

Normal human immunoglobulin (gamma-globulin), if available, provides rapid protection but is a blood product and has been largely superseded by the new hepatitis A vaccines. Travellers who need rapid protection, but who also wish to be protected against hepatitis A in the longer term, may sometimes be given immunoglobulin, if available, and hepatitis A vaccine at the same time.

Apart from immunization, other preventive measures include strict personal hygiene, avoiding raw or inadequately cooked shellfish and raw vegetables, and not drinking untreated water or unpasteurized milk.

Hepatitis B

Like hepatitis A, hepatitis B occurs throughout the world. Its continued survival is ensured by the large number of individuals who are carriers of the virus, estimated to be at least 350 million world-wide. Hepatitis B can be spread either from carriers or from people with inapparent infection, or during the incubation period, illness, or early convalescence.

A person is defined as a carrier if hepatitis B surface antigen — a marker of the virus — persists in their circulation for more than 6 months following infection. A person may be a lifelong carrier and remain apparently healthy, although variable degrees of liver damage can occur.

The highest risk areas for hepatitis B include Southeast Asia, the People's Republic of China, the Pacific Islands, sub-Saharan Africa, and a number of countries in central Asia and South America. Note that in certain population groups the rates of infection are very high, especially among homosexual men, prostitutes, and drug addicts.

The prevalence of hepatitis B carriers varies from one region of the world to another. In North America, northern Europe, and Australia, 0.1% of the population are carriers (at least among blood donors); in central and eastern Europe, up to 5%; in southern Europe, countries bordering the Mediterranean, and parts of Central and South America, a higher frequency; and in parts of Africa, Asia, and the Pacific area, 20% or more of the apparently healthy population may be carriers.

The incidence of hepatitis B tends to be higher among adults living in urban communities and among those living in poor conditions. The infection may become established in closed institutions such as those for the mentally handicapped.

Certain groups of people — recipients of unscreened blood transfusions and blood products, health care and laboratory personnel, staff in institutions for the mentally handicapped, male homosexuals, prostitutes, and abusers of injectable drugs and narcotics — are at considerably increased risk of contracting hepatitis B. Travellers or expatriates belonging to any of these groups are at higher risk in countries where the carrier rate is high. The incidence of symptomatic and asymptomatic hepatitis B infection in long-term travellers, including expatriates, is 0.8–2.4 per 100 per month of travel. This figure falls up to 10 times lower in short-term travellers (travelling for less than one month) to endemic areas.

The incubation period is about 60–180 days.

How it is spread

Transmission of the infection may result from accidental inoculation with minute amounts of blood, which may occur during medical, surgical, or dental procedures; during immunization with inadequately sterilized syringes and needles; with sharing of needles during intravenous drug abuse; tattooing, ear piercing, and nose piercing;

acupuncture; and laboratory accidents and accidental inoculation with razors and similar objects that have been contaminated with blood.

However, hepatitis B is not spread exclusively by blood or blood products. Hepatitis B surface antigen and other markers of hepatitis B virus have been found in other body fluids such as saliva, menstrual and vaginal discharges, and seminal fluid, and these have been implicated as vehicles of transmission of the infection. In certain defined circumstances the virus may be infective by mouth, and there is much evidence for the transmission of hepatitis B by sexual contact. Persons who change sexual partners frequently are at high risk of hepatitis B.

In the tropics and in warm climates, additional factors may be important for the transmission of hepatitis B. These include traditional tattooing and scarification, blood-letting, ritual circumcision, and repeated biting by bloodsucking insects. Results of investigations into the role that biting insects play in the spread of hepatitis B are conflicting. Hepatitis B surface antigen has been detected in several species of mosquito and in bedbugs that have either been trapped in the wild or fed experimentally on infected blood, but no convincing evidence of multiplication of the virus in insects has been obtained. Mechanical transmission of the infection via an insect's biting parts is a theoretical possibility, but appears to be rare.

Hepatitis B also tends to occur within family groups, although the precise mechanism of intrafamilial spread is not known.

Transmission of hepatitis B virus from carrier mothers to their babies can occur around the time of birth and is an important factor in determining the prevalence of the infection in some regions, particularly in China and Southeast Asia.

The carrier state
Progression to the carrier state is more common in males, more likely to follow infections acquired in childhood than in adult life, and more likely to occur in people with natural or acquired immune deficiencies. The carrier state becomes established in approximately 5–10% of infected adults. In countries where hepatitis B infection is common the highest prevalence of surface antigen is found in children aged 4–8 years, with steadily declining rates among older age groups.

There is an urgent need to define the mechanisms that lead to the carrier state and to introduce methods of interruption of transmission. This is a complex and vexed issue, with considerable personal, social, and economic implications.

Consequences of infection
The symptoms and clinical manifestations of hepatitis B are similar to those of the other types of viral hepatitis. However, the picture is complicated by the carrier state and by chronic liver disease, which may follow the infection. Chronic liver disease may be severe and may progress to primary liver cancer. In many parts of the world primary liver cancer is one of the commonest human cancers, particularly in men.

Prevention and control
Immunization against hepatitis B can be carried out in two ways.

Passive immunization

This uses hepatitis B immunoglobulin (hepatitis B gamma-globulin), which contains antibody against hepatitis B. It is not used for prevention in travellers, but can offer protection after accidental exposure, such as when blood or other material containing hepatitis B surface antigen is inoculated, swallowed, or splashed in the eyes. Two doses administered 30 days apart are required: the first dose should preferably be administered within 48 hours, but not later than seven days following exposure. A course of active immunization should be started at the same time.

Active immunization

This uses a vaccine that contains hepatitis B surface antigen and 'primes' the body's immune system to produce its own antibodies. The new hepatitis B vaccines have been developed using recombinant DNA technology ('genetic engineering'); they are safe and highly effective.

Among the high-risk groups who might benefit from the vaccine are homosexual men, drug addicts, prostitutes, people who require multiple transfusions, people with immune deficiencies or malignant disease, and health care personnel. Immunization should also be considered by non-immune persons living in areas where the prevalence of hepatitis B infection is high. Strategies for immunization against hepatitis B are under review, and hepatitis B has recently been added to the childhood immunization schedule in many countries, where universal immunization against hepatitis B has been introduced.

The currently available vaccines are expensive. Vaccination of travellers is advisable if:
1. They belong to a high-risk group
2. They will remain in an endemic area for longer than about 6 months
3. They will reside in rural areas or engage in sporting or other activities that carry an increased risk of accidents, injury, or occupational exposure to blood
4. They are likely to need medical treatment abroad — such as kidney dialysis or blood transfusion.

Combined hepatitis A and B vaccine

A recent development is the availability of a combined hepatitis A and B vaccine. This vaccine, now available in many European countries, has the advantage of conferring dual protection with one course of immunization — a convenient aid for many travellers. Its profile is similar to that of the individual hepatitis A and hepatitis B vaccines; it is safe and offers protection for up to 20 years for hepatitis A and 5 years or longer for hepatitis B.

Hepatitis B and the traveller

Travellers should take commonsense precautions to reduce the risk of hepatitis B. They should employ great caution in any intimate or sexual contact (particularly male homosexual contact) with possible hepatitis B carriers; they should where possible avoid any procedure involving penetration of the skin, for example, tattooing, ear piercing, any sort of injections, blood transfusions, and many medical, surgical, and dental procedures carried out under dubious sanitary conditions.

Hepatitis C

The hepatitis C virus, which is considered to be responsible for the majority of cases of non-A, non-B hepatitis, was identified by molecular biology techniques in 1989. Although in general the illness is mild and often without jaundice, severe hepatitis does occur and in many patients the infection is followed by a persistent carrier state. Chronic liver damage may occur in as many as 50% of patients, and there is preliminary evidence of an association between hepatitis C virus and primary liver cancer in some parts of the world.

The virus is transmitted by blood and blood products and by other routes which are as yet undefined apart from intravenous drug abuse. Surprisingly, blood transfusion accounts for a small proportion of cases in industrialized countries, although between 0.01 and 2% of volunteer blood donors are carriers of hepatitis C virus. There is a very high prevalence of infection among intravenous narcotic drug abusers. Some evidence indicates transmission by the sexual route and during childbirth, but the route of infection has not been established in as many as 50% of cases.

Vaccines against hepatitis C are being developed. Methods of prevention are at present identical to those that apply to hepatitis B.

There is also considerable evidence for the existence of other non-A, non-B, and non-C hepatitis viruses.

Hepatitis D

The delta virus is a defective infectious agent that can infect actively only in the presence of hepatitis B. The infection is common in parts of southern Europe, the Middle East, parts of tropical Africa, and in parts of South America. The virus is spread in the same way as hepatitis B and precautions against it are identical. Immunization against hepatitis B will also protect against delta hepatitis.

Hepatitis E

An epidemic illness similar to that caused by hepatitis A and commonly transmitted by contaminated water has been observed in India, Burma, eastern states of the former Soviet Union, parts of the Middle East, East Africa, North Africa and parts of West Africa, and in Mexico. The virus responsible for this type of hepatitis has now been identified and characterized as hepatitis E. There is evidence that this virus is prevalent in many non-industrialized countries and where a safe piped water supply is not available.

It should be noted that although infection does not lead to chronic liver damage, it is extremely serious during pregnancy, causing a high mortality. The severity of the illness during pregnancy dictates an urgent need for a vaccine.

Methods of prevention include strict personal hygiene, not drinking untreated water, and not eating raw or inadequately cooked shellfish and raw vegetables. Immunoglobulin is not considered to afford any protection.

Non-A, non-E hepatitis

Improved laboratory diagnosis of hepatitis A, B, and C has enabled a previously unrecognized form of hepatitis, unrelated to either type A, B, or C, to be identified. It is referred to as non-A, non-E hepatitis, and it is now known to be the most common form of hepatitis occurring after a blood transfusion and the administration of blood-clotting factors in some countries. It has been found in every country in which it has been sought, has some features in common with hepatitis B, and has been detected in patients on dialysis and among drug addicts. In several countries a significant number of cases are not associated with transfusion, and such sporadic cases have been found to account for a proportion of adult patients with viral hepatitis.

In general, the illness is mild, often without jaundice or other symptoms. However, there is evidence that the infection may be followed by the development of a persistent carrier state: chronic hepatitis may occur in as many as 40–50% of patients after infection associated with blood transfusion or treatment by renal dialysis. About 10% of patients with the sporadic form of the infection may progress to chronic liver damage.

There are no known methods of preventing non-A, non-E hepatitis (beyond the precautions applicable to hepatitis B).

Treatment of viral hepatitis

No specific treatment is available for any of the types of viral hepatitis. A number of antiviral substances are available for the management of chronic liver disease associated with hepatitis B and C. Bed rest is required, and a low-fat diet is preferred during the acute phase of the disease. Alcohol should not be consumed for 6 months after recovery.

Women using oral contraceptives (the Pill or progestogen-only Pill) can carry on with this contraceptive method during convalescence and recovery from hepatitis.

Evacuation of a patient with acute hepatitis is not usually necessary unless serious complications develop, when special facilities may be required.

The different types of hepatitis virus

The five hepatitis viruses — A, B, C, D, and E — are distinct infectious agents and infection with one virus does not confer immunity against infection with a different virus. Similarly, vaccination against hepatitis A or hepatitis B does not protect against another hepatitis virus. The only exception is immunization against hepatitis B, which will afford protection against infection with the defective interfering delta virus (hepatitis D). It should be emphasized that the hepatitis viruses are common in all countries.

Summary of advice for travellers

- Hepatitis A and hepatitis E are a risk to travellers in areas of the world where hygienic and sanitary conditions are poor. Protection with hepatitis A vaccine must be considered for non-immune travellers anywhere outside the USA, Canada, northern Europe, Australia, and New Zealand. Immunoglobulin, if available, may be used to provide more rapid immunity in people who are obliged to travel to risk areas at short notice. Strict personal hygiene and avoidance of untreated water and raw or inadequately cooked food, particularly raw vegetables, shellfish, and milk, can help prevent infection. Similar precautions apply to hepatitis E.

- Hepatitis B is a risk to certain groups of people in industrialized countries, notably health care personnel, male homosexuals, and those who change sexual partners frequently. The risk increases in developing countries, where there are generally more carriers. Caution should be observed with regard to intimate or sexual contact with inhabitants of these countries. Active immunization with hepatitis B vaccine is advisable for health care personnel, members of other risk categories working in the subtropics or tropics, and frequent or long-term travellers to endemic areas.

- Penetration of the skin by any object that may have come in contact with someone else's blood or other body fluids — as in tattooing, ear piercing, sharing of razors, acupuncture, needle sharing by drug abusers, and any medical, dental, or surgical procedure, including blood transfusion and donation under dubious hygienic conditions — should be avoided.

- Hepatitis C is transmitted in the same manner as hepatitis B, and in many parts of the world is particularly associated with intravenous narcotic drug addiction.

- No preventive immunization is available for hepatitis C, and avoidance is by measures similar to those advised for hepatitis B.

- Travellers who develop a general malaise and symptoms such as right upper abdominal pain, jaundice, and dark-coloured urine either abroad or after their return should suspect viral hepatitis, and should seek medical advice immediately.

Poisons and contaminants in food

Certain foods need to be treated with caution while abroad: in the tropics, fish and shellfish pose a particular hazard.

Dr Elizabeth Driver is a medical consultant in a law firm in London, and has worked as a toxicologist at the Medical Research Council and in the Tropical Metabolism Research Unit in Jamaica.

One of the most enjoyable aspects of visiting a foreign country is the opportunity to sample the local cuisine — and provided such food is carefully prepared and cooked, this usually carries little risk.

Unfortunately, some foreign delicacies or even staple foodstuffs contain contaminants and biological toxins in their raw or uncooked form, and although local culinary methods have usually evolved for dealing with such contaminants prior to consumption, cases of poisoning still occasionally occur. This risk of poisoning is in addition to the hazards of food-borne infection considered elsewhere in this chapter.

Travellers should therefore know which foods carry a significant danger, and either avoid them completely or exercise extreme caution. The foods themselves range from cassava, eaten as a staple throughout the tropics, to 'fugu' or puffer fish, considered a delicacy in Japan and much of the Indo-Pacific.

Types of poisoning

The variety of potential food contaminants and toxins is vast and their effects range from the trivial and inconvenient to the frankly dramatic. In general, however, poisoning can be classified into 'acute' and 'chronic' varieties. *Acute* poisoning is more or less immediate in onset and may follow consumption of a single portion of contaminated food. *Chronic* poisoning is a long-term process which generally follows the repeated consumption of small amounts of a toxic substance over an extended period — so it is unlikely to appear in travellers on a short trip.

Acute poisoning

Acute poisoning may be produced by foods of either plant or animal origin.

Plant toxins

Local customs have generally developed to allow the consumption of potentially poisonous plant material by the use of particular methods of preparation which minimize the hazard. Travellers should be wary of preparing unusual foods for themselves, but may be reasonably confident, except in times of drought or famine, that food prepared by local people will be innocuous. Poisoning is much more likely to result from eating wild berries or fungi. The two most toxic flowering plants are the castor bean (*Ricinus communis*) and the rosary pea (*Abrus precatorius*). The latter is sometimes encountered in bead necklaces, usually of African origin, and should be confined to this decorative use. If seeds with broken coats are swallowed, persistent diarrhoea, often with bloody mucus, begins after a latent period of up to three days. Death may result. Many mushrooms are toxic, but generally produce gastrointestinal symptoms, sweating, or headache, which will resolve spontaneously after a few hours of discomfort. A few mushrooms have an alcohol-sensitizing effect, whilst others induce hallucinations. Only *Amanita phalloides* and similar types are likely to be fatal.

Cassava (manioc)

This is a shrub which produces starchy tubers rather like yams or sweet potatoes and also protein-rich leaves which can be used as a green vegetable. Because it is drought and pest resistant and will grow on poor soil, it is a major staple crop in tropical countries. It originates from South America but is now the major energy supply for 20–40% of the population of sub-Saharan Africa.

Cassava roots and leaves naturally contain chemicals which break down to release cyanide. The bitter varieties, which are grown in large quantities because of their drought resistance and higher yields, contain more of these toxic chemicals and must be processed before consumption, whereas the sweet varieties can be eaten fresh.

Consequently, processing methods such as soaking in water, grating, and fermenting the mash in sacks or prolonged sun-drying of the roots have developed to remove the toxins. Consumption of the unprocessed roots can result in acute cyanide poisoning.

The acute effects of eating improperly prepared cassava are abdominal pain and vomiting, progressing to mental confusion and to a variety of neurological problems. In Tanzania the neurological disorder is called 'Konzo' which literally means 'weak legs'. Konzo is caused by abrupt, symmetrical, and permanent damage to parts of the spinal cord which can lead to difficulties in walking, talking, and vision. In other parts of Africa, blindness is recognized as being related to the consumption of manioc. Deafness and loss of sensation are also features of the so-called 'tropical ataxic neuropathy'. In parts of rural Nigeria, where the staple food is cassava, the prevalence of this syndrome can be as high as 80 per 1000.

Konzo is mainly reported in epidemic outbreaks during drought years. It occurs in rural populations for whom the diet consists almost entirely of roots and leaves from bitter cassava varieties and where the availability of any other food is limited. Studies in Tanzania and Zaire have shown that the normal processing of cassava roots was less thorough in affected villages than in the areas not affected by Konzo: the resulting high cyanide exposure was indicated by frequent reports of acute poisoning within hours after the meal.

Lathyrism
A disease very similar to Konzo and characterized by the same acute onset of permanent selective damage to parts of the spinal cord. It also occurs in epidemics during acute food shortages. Lathyrism is caused by high consumption of the drought-resistant chickling pea (*Lathyrus sativus*).

Ackee
Travellers to Jamaica or Nigeria may be introduced to the delights of the fruit of *Blighia sapida*, known as the 'ackee' in Jamaica and 'isin' in Nigeria.

In Jamaica, this strange fruit is served up with bacon or salt-fish as a kind of scrambled egg look-alike. Problems arise if the fruit is eaten unripe or has been improperly prepared, as it contains a potent toxin that rapidly lowers the blood sugar level. The victim succumbs quickly to vomiting, followed by convulsions, coma, and death in the majority of cases. This is more likely to occur in the already malnourished, but unripe fruit can be lethal to anyone. Correct preparation involves boiling the fruit and then discarding the water.

Cycads
Various species of cycad grow throughout the tropical areas of the Far East including southern Japan, southern China, the Philippines, Indonesia, the East Indies, and northern Australia. Both the seeds and stems of several species of cycad are used for food, but degenerative diseases may result from eating them.

Amyotrophic lateral sclerosis (ALS) is a progressive fatal disorder of adults resulting from degeneration of cells in the brain and spinal cord. It is particularly common among the indigenous (Chamorro) population of the islands of Guam and Rota, where a clinical variant of Parkinson-like dementia (PD) is also seen. Recently, it has been shown that this disorder is associated with the consumption of the highly toxic seeds of the false sago palm (*Cycas circinalis L*). During the Japanese occupation of Guam from 1941 to 1944, when rice was hard to obtain, cycad seed represented a major source of food for the indigenous residents of Guam. Cycad flour, used to make tortillas, atole (a drink), and soup, is prepared from the endosperm of ripe (greenbrown) seeds. This is removed from the seed integument and halved, sliced, or crushed, then soaked in fresh water to remove unidentified acutely poisonous substances. It is then dried in the sun and ground to form a flour. Cycad flour products are now favoured by middle-aged and elderly traditional Chamorros living in rural communities. In addition, the fresh seed integument is chewed to relieve thirst. Improperly washed *Cycas* seed has caused acute seizures in humans but ALS and PD are the result of more prolonged ingestion.

Patients with ALS have progressive limb weakness, spasticity, and muscle atrophy. Those with PD exhibit loss of fine movements, decreased blinking, slowed movements, tremor, rigidity, and dementia. They become incontinent, unable to swallow or speak, and develop contractures of all their joints. The condition is ultimately fatal. It rarely occurs outside the Chamorro population, but one ex-marine who stayed in Guam after the Second World War developed ALS and a second was diagnosed as having Alzheimer's disease. ALS–PD also occurs in other Western Pacific islands and in the Kii Peninsula of Japan.

Plants may also be toxic indirectly, for example honey made from the flowers of mountain laurel, rhododendron, azaleas, or oleanders may contain toxins which are harmful to man. Meat roasted on oleander sticks has also led to poisoning. (In southern India and Sri Lanka, the seeds of the yellow oleander are widely known to be poisonous, and are often used by local people attempting suicide.)

Risky roots

Unless you are an experienced botanist, give unfamiliar wild plants a miss. A 23-year-old man died recently in the Maine woods while foraging for wild ginseng. He took just three bites of the root of a plant that proved to be water hemlock. His brother almost died. Water hemlock is the most toxic indigenous plant in North America; it looks like a parsnip and tastes sweet, but toxin can even be absorbed through the skin. Symptoms begin within 15 minutes, and 30% of cases are fatal.

Animal toxins

Animal toxins fall into two categories. First, a normal constituent of the animal or one of its organs may be toxic. For example, Eskimos have always known of the toxicity of polar bear liver, which contains immensely high levels of vitamin A. Second, the animal itself may be contaminated with toxins.

The vast majority of poisonings are the result of eating fish or other forms of sea food. There are approximately 1200 marine species known to be poisonous or venomous. They are found throughout the world but pose a medical or socio-economic hazard in only a few areas. Because most of the toxins are heat-stable, cooking offers no protection.

Puffer fish
The puffer fish — known as 'fugu' in Japan — is a kind of culinary Russian roulette. It is said to be sufficiently delicious to warrant the considerable risk attached to its consumption. Japanese chefs have to be specially licensed to carry out the delicate operation of removing the ovaries, roe, liver, and skin, which contain the lethal tetrodotoxin, but every year several deaths occur from eating fugu. About 40% of those who develop significant signs and symptoms die. Death is said to be preceded by a tingling sensation of the lips. Recent studies have indicated that tetrodotoxin is more widespread than was first thought: it has also been identified in crabs.

Paralytic shellfish poisoning
Rather less dramatic in onset, but none the less unpleasant, is the poisoning caused by eating fish or more often shellfish (particularly mussels, cockles, clams, and scallops) which have ingested plankton containing saxitoxin. In some areas of the world, such as the Caribbean, dinoflagellate protozoa may be present in such large numbers that the sea looks red and the amount of saxitoxin in the organs of shellfish will be correspondingly high. Fishermen in areas which are commonly affected know not to harvest the shellfish when there is a 'red tide'. Symptoms of poisoning are slowing of the heart rate, even to the point of heart failure, and muscle paralysis. Mild poisoning may result from ingesting just 1 milligram of the toxin, which could be found in a single clam. Without treatment 4 milligrams of the toxin would be fatal.

Mollusc-associated intoxications
The ability of mussels, clams, and oysters to concentrate toxins from water and pass them on to humans makes them particularly dangerous. This can occur equally in cold climates: in 1987 over 250 Canadians were poisoned when they ate mussels which had been raised in river estuaries in Prince Edward Island in eastern Canada. Nineteen patients were hospitalized, of whom 12 required intensive care because of seizures, coma, profuse respiratory secretions, or unstable blood pressure. Three patients died. Many of the patients had prolonged neurological abnormalities including memory loss, disorientation, and confusion, which had not resolved 24 months after the incident. The mussels were found to contain domoic acid, a neuro-excitatory amino acid derived from a planktonic diatom which the mussels had concentrated. In Canada steps have been taken to prevent the reoccurrence of shellfish poisoning due to domoic acid: they are tested for the presence of the toxin before commercial distribution.

Ciguatera
The most common, world-wide, food-borne illness caused by a chemical toxin. Ciguatera is a circumtropical variety of food poisoning induced by the ingestion of a

wide variety of coral reef fishes which have accumulated ciguatoxin via the marine food web. The term ciguatera was derived from a name used in the eighteenth century in the Spanish Antilles for intoxication brought about by ingestion of the cigua or turban shell. Ciguatera was recorded in the West Indies in the fifteenth century and noted in the Pacific as early as 1606, when Spanish explorers suffered from ciguatera in the New Hebrides.

Ciguatera can occur anywhere around the world in a belt from 35° North to 35° South. It is particularly common in the tropical Pacific and the Caribbean and it is also reported in Florida. Outbreaks of ciguatera occur sporadically: the problem may suddenly appear in any one location after years of absence and is not signalled by any visible change in the sea.

Ciguatoxic fish are species that feed on algae or detritus around tropical reefs, especially the surgeon fish, parrot fish, and larger reef carnivores and omnivores that prey on these, such as reef sharks, moray eels, snappers, some inshore tunas, groupers, and barracuda. In Florida, the sale of barracuda is banned. Over 400 species of fish, as well as oysters and clams, may be affected. The toxin accumulates in the flesh, skin, and viscera of the fish, but since the toxins are much more concentrated in the viscera than in the flesh, it is advised that the consumption of brain, spinal cord, intestines, gonads, and liver of all reef fish should be avoided.

Symptoms appear between one and six hours after eating the fish and are very varied, ranging from mild gastroenteritis to death. Several different toxins are almost certainly involved and symptoms depend on the relative amounts of each of these toxins. In New Caledonia, the common name for ciguatera is 'la gratte' or 'the itch'. In Samoa, the typical course for ciguatera is gastroenteritis followed by general weakness, followed by 'pins and needles' lasting three weeks or longer. Neurological symptoms can persist for months or even years. In French Polynesia, the gastrointestinal symptoms seem to be more common in victims who have eaten herbivorous fish such as the surgeon fish 'maito', whereas cardiovascular and other disorders prevail in cases caused by toxic carnivores such as snappers and groupers. In the Gambier Islands, the parrot fish causes most of the ciguatera intoxications: symptoms begin like the typical ciguatera syndrome but are followed by a staggering walk, loss of balance, and tremor, lasting a month or more.

Ciguatera is occasionally fatal. In acute cases death may be caused by respiratory failure due to paralysis of the respiratory muscles but may also result from the severe dehydration which can accompany vomiting and diarrhoea.

Recently, it has been shown that ciguatoxin may be present in the semen of men affected with ciguatera and may be capable of producing symptoms in both males and females during sexual intercourse. Two male visitors to the Bahamas developed ciguatera after eating grouper. Five days later both men had sexual intercourse and reported painful ejaculation with severe, prolonged urethritis following sex. The wives, who had not eaten any of the fish, had no symptoms until engaging in intercourse: both then reported pain immediately following ejaculation, and vaginal burning and stinging which persisted for two or three weeks. Successful treatment of some of the symptoms has recently been reported with the antiepileptic drug galapantin.

Scombroid poisoning
Some fish of the mackerel or tuna varieties may be the cause of poisoning if they are inadequately refrigerated and preserved. Cooking does not destroy the toxin. A toxic substance, originally thought to be histamine, is formed by the action of enzymes on the muscle of the dead fish. Recent research suggests that another toxin, saurine, is also formed. This causes nausea, vomiting, diarrhoea, and epigastric pain. The face of the victim becomes flushed and burning and there may be numbness, thirst, and generalized urticaria. Fortunately all these signs and symptoms, which arise within about 2 hours of the meal, subside within 12–16 hours. No treatment is required. It is said that the flesh of affected fish tastes rather peppery. This type of poisoning may occur anywhere in the world.

Abalone poisoning
This is an unusual form of poisoning in that it causes photosensitivity, so the symptoms of burning and stinging, followed by skin ulceration, only develop on the parts of the body exposed to sunlight.

Chronic poisoning
The long-term effects of food toxins are of rather less importance to travellers than acute poisons, but travellers should none the less be aware of the dangers of certain moulds and metals.

Mycotoxins
Mycotoxins, the toxins produced by moulds, have been implicated in several diseases both in tropical and in temperate climates. Mouldy foods are more commonly consumed during times of famine. Many of their effects are chronic but acute poisoning may also occur. Acute mildewed sugar-cane poisoning has been reported in China: there were 217 outbreaks of the poisoning between 1972 and 1989, affecting 884 patients and causing 88 deaths. The poison is characterized by a sudden onset of gastrointestinal symptoms followed by toxic encephalopathy. Most of the victims were children who had eaten mildewed sugar cane harvested in late October and stored during the winter. The outbreaks of poisoning usually occur between January and March, mainly in the northern part of China.

Mould-contaminated food may be consumed directly by man or by domestic animals reared for food (pigs, for example) which are capable of accumulating toxins in their flesh. Balkan nephropathy, a strange and serious disease of the kidneys confined to areas of Yugoslavia, Romania, and Bulgaria, was first recognized 30 years ago. Only recently has it been linked to consumption of a mould that grows on maize.

Aflatoxin
This is the toxin of *Aspergillus flavus*, which grows on peanuts and other crops, including pistachios, almonds, walnuts, pecans, brazil nuts, oil seeds (cotton-seed Copra), and grains (corn, grain sorghum, and millet). In tropical regions aflatoxin can be produced in unrefrigerated prepared foods. Contamination may occur in the field, especially during

times of drought and other stress which allows insect damage and predisposes the plant to mould attack, and may also occur due to inadequate storage conditions.

The toxin is highly carcinogenic and consumption of mouldy peanuts explains the high incidence of liver cancer in some parts of Africa — particularly West Africa. This has serious economic implications for many of the countries involved. Aflatoxin metabolites are sometimes present in the milk of dairy cows that have consumed contaminated feed.

Eating mouldy cornmeal may be one of the factors involved in the high incidence of cancer of the oesophagus (gullet) found in areas of China. Excessive consumption of pickles and preserved foods containing nitrites may also be contributing factors.

Poor nutritional status, particularly combined with deficiency of vitamins A and C, probably increases susceptibility to mycotoxins. The well-nourished traveller may be at rather less risk than the indigenous population, but would still be well advised to avoid mouldy foods.

Trichothecenes

These mycotoxins are produced by a number of commonly occurring moulds and occur most often in mouldy cereal grains. There have been many reported cases of trichothecene toxicity in farm animals and a few in humans. Disruption of agriculture during the Second World War resulted in millet, wheat, and barley being over-wintered in the fields in Siberia. Consumption of these grains led to an outbreak of vomiting, skin inflammation, diarrhoea, and multiple haemorrhages in inhabitants of the area around Orenburg in Siberia. The exposure was fatal to over 10% of the individuals who consumed the mouldy grain.

Metals

Various metals can be toxic. Lead from cooking pots is found in high levels in home-brewed beers in various parts of Africa, and can lead to chronic poisoning. Mercury present in seed dressing has caused poisoning in starving peasants in Iraq, forced by hunger to eat the grain intended for planting.

High arsenic content of tube well water is currently a serious problem in Bangladesh (see p. 72).

Cancer and plants

In developed countries concern has focused on the potential of food additives to cause cancer and it is often forgotten that naturally occurring constituents of plants can be much more potent carcinogens. These hazards are not unique to the traveller but may become significant if a particularly monotonous diet is consumed. For example, basil, mushrooms, celery, and lettuce all contain high levels of chemicals which are known to cause cancer when fed to experimental animals.

Safrole is a known carcinogen present in many plants eaten in various parts of the world. Oil of sassafras, which was used in 'natural' sarsparilla root beer in the USA, is about 75% safrole. Black pepper contains small amounts of safrole and large amounts of the related compound piperine.

Hydrazines are found in many mushrooms including the most commonly grown commercial mushroom (*Agaricus bisporus*); they cause lung tumours in mice.

Fucoumarins are potent light-activated carcinogens and are present in high levels in celery, parsnips, figs, and parsley. The level in celery can increase about a hundredfold if the plant is bruised or diseased.

Pyrrolizidines are known to cause liver and lung damage and tumours in animals and man. They are found particularly in herb teas such as comfrey tea and in the bush teas brewed in parts of the Caribbean.

Fortunately, many plants also contain substances which protect against the development of cancer including vitamin E, beta carotene, ascorbic acid, and selenium. Both at home and abroad it is advisable to eat a balanced, mixed diet and to avoid excessive consumption of any single food.

Radiation

Years after the accident at Chernobyl, farmers in villages in Ukraine are still being instructed not to consume the crops or milk they produce. Replacements are supposed to be delivered weekly by the government. The combination of the national food shortage and political upheavals means that this does not happen and the locally produced foods are often consumed, some reaching regional markets that cannot all be policed properly. Another bizarre government policy is to distribute modestly contaminated foods to distant regions, whilst bringing food from these regions to the contamination zone. Travellers would be well advised to avoid foods that are obviously locally produced, such as mushrooms, fruit, and vegetables.

Summary of advice for travellers

- Food toxins and contaminants are so diverse that there are no really hard-and-fast rules for the traveller to follow. Generally, where food is known to be hazardous — such as with cassava or puffer fish — traditional local methods of preparation have evolved to minimize the risk. Most such traditions have a basis in fact and are best observed.

- Obviously decayed or mouldy foods, either plant or animal, are likely to cause toxic effects.

- Problems are more likely to arise in areas of drought and famine.

---

3 Water

Safe water

Careful choice or treatment of water — whether for drinking, washing, preparing food, or swimming in — is one of the most important health precautions a traveller can take.

Dr Hemda Garelick is a Principal Lecturer in Environmental Microbiology at Middlesex University, London where she coordinates Pollution Control Master programmes. Her current research focuses on the detection and identification of faecal micro-organisms in the environment and the ecology of micro-organisms involved in bioremediation.

Water is essential for our survival: according to our size, activity, culture, health status, climate, and choice of clothing, we require between two and five litres of water (four and ten US pints) every day.

In the developed world, the availability of safe water in more or less unlimited quantities is taken for granted. This does not apply in the developing world: in many countries, easy access to a safe water supply — and that does not necessarily even mean a piped water supply — is available to only about 70–80 per cent of the urban population and to about 40 per cent of the rural population. Figures for access to sanitary facilities are even worse, so it is hardly surprising that water-related diseases remain a major problem in the developing world, where such illnesses kill at least five million people every year. Travellers to developing countries are obviously also at risk.

Water and disease

Water-related infections can be considered in four groups, according to how they are transmitted:

- Those spread by drinking contaminated water
- Those spread through lack of hygiene and sanitary facilities (lack of water)
- Those spread through *direct* contact with contaminated water (e.g. swimming) or *indirect* contact (e.g. eating fish that carry infection from contaminated water)
- Those spread through bites of insects that need water in order to breed (see particularly malaria, p. 130).

In the first two categories, the infections of greatest importance to the traveller are those transmitted by the faecal–oral route, that is from one person's faeces to another person's mouth. These include diarrhoeal diseases, dysenteries, typhoid, poliomyelitis, hepatitis A, and worm infections (see earlier chapters). In the third category, diseases transmitted through direct or indirect contact with water include schistosomiasis (see p. 104), guinea worm (p. 599), fish tapeworms (see p. 49), and liver flukes (see p. 51).

Chemical contamination (unless gross) is likely to affect travellers far less than the local population, because the harmful effects tend to be cumulative and related to duration of exposure. In contrast, biological contamination (e.g. pathogenic micro-organisms) has a more acute effect on travellers than on local people, who may have acquired partial or full immunity to locally prevalent infections.

There have recently been serious problems with chemical contamination in Bangladesh, where water from tube wells — now widely used throughout the country to reduce the hazards of microbial contamination — has a high natural arsenic content; over half the country's population is potentially at risk and many local people have become severely affected with chronic arsenic poisoning. Excessive fluoride in groundwater can be a hazard in large areas of India and the African Rift Valley.

Water and the traveller

Contamination of water supplies is usually due to poor sanitation close to water sources, sewage disposal into the sources themselves, leakage of sewage into distribution systems, or contamination with industrial or farm waste. Even if a piped water supply is safe at its source, it is not always safe by the time it reaches the tap. Intermittent tap-water supplies should be regarded as particularly suspect.

Travellers on short trips to areas with water supplies of uncertain quality should avoid drinking tap water or untreated water from any other source. It is best to keep to hot drinks, bottled or canned drinks of well-known brand names — international standards of water treatment are usually followed at bottling plants. In some countries, bottled water may be counterfeited and simply replaced with tap water. Carbonated drinks are acidic, slightly safer, and less likely to have been counterfeited. Make sure that all bottles have unbroken seals when you buy them and that they are opened in your presence.

Boiling is always a good way of treating water. Some hotels supply boiled water on request and this can be used for drinking or for brushing teeth. Portable boiling elements that can boil small quantities of water are useful when the right voltage of electricity is available. Refuse politely any cold drink from an unknown source.

Ice is only as safe as the water from which it is made and should not be put in drinks unless it is known to be safe. Drinks can be cooled by placing them on ice rather than by adding ice to them.

Alcohol may be a medical disinfectant, but should not be relied upon to sterilize water. Ethanol is most effective at a concentration of 50–70 per cent; below 20 per cent its bactericidal action is negligible. Spirits labelled 95 per cent proof contain only about 47 per cent alcohol. Beware of methylated alcohol, which is very poisonous and should never be added to drinking water.

If no other safe water supply can be obtained, tap water that is too hot to touch can be left to cool and is generally safe to drink.

Travellers planning a trip to remote areas, or intending to live in countries where drinking water is not readily available, should know about the various possible methods for making water safe.

Water treatment

The choice of processes used in a public water treatment plant depends on the physical, chemical, and microbiological characteristics of the water, but the main steps generally necessary are:

1. The removal of suspended solids by precipitation, sedimentation, or filtration
2. Disinfection — usually by chlorination or iodination — to inactivate and kill the possible pathogens (disease-causing infective agents).

Treating small quantities of water is based on similar principles but is rather easier, and a wider range of processes is possible.

Begin by choosing the purest possible source. This is likely to be tap water, well water, spring water, or collected rainwater, all of which are preferable to surface water e.g. rivers, streams, or pond water, which tend to be polluted. Rainwater can be collected from roofs, which should be clean and made of tiles or sheeting, not of lead or thatch.

Boiling

Boiling is the most effective way of sterilizing water. It kills all infective agents including amoebic cysts, which are resistant to chlorine.

This treatment is not affected by the turbidity or the chemical characteristics of the water. The only limitation of boiling is that it is not always practical and is generally suitable only for small quantities. The water should be boiled vigorously for five minutes (this is sufficient even at high altitude).

Boiling tends to make water taste flat, because it reduces the amount of dissolved gases. To improve the taste, drinking water should be allowed to cool for a few hours in a covered, partially filled, clean container, preferably in the same container in which it has been boiled.

Filtration

Filtration is a process that should be used when boiling is not practicable. It is either an initial step or can produce safe water in a single step when the right equipment is used.

Removal of suspended solids

In order to make disinfection (with chlorine or iodine) as effective as possible, suspended solids and organic matter must be removed. Organic matter interferes with the process of chemical disinfection, and pathogens adsorbed to suspended solid are less susceptible to disinfection.

Filtration through a closely woven cloth is adequate, and filtration bags such as the Millbank bag are available commercially. These can take from five to twenty-five litres (about one to five gallons). However, it is important to remember that although the water may look clear it has not yet been made safe, and requires further treatment.

Removal of pathogens

Ceramic filter 'candles' of a very fine pore size (which can be as fine as 0.5 microns — the finer the better) are available commercially, and some units can be attached to piped water supplies. They remove most pathogens found in water (bacteria, amoebic cysts, and some viruses). Some of the filters are impregnated with silver, which acts as a limited bactericide.

Manufacturers' instructions on the operation and maintenance of filters should be followed. Filters should be examined regularly for cracks and leaks. They should be cleaned by scrubbing, and boiled (unless impregnated with silver) when clogged and at weekly intervals.

Disposable paper cartridge filters are also available. They should be kept wet when in use, or the paper filter may shrink or crack.

Most activated carbon filters are not recommended for making water safe. They are normally used to improve the taste of clean water. They remove organic matter, dissolved chlorine, and pathogens by a mechanism of adsorption, not by mechanical straining. When overloaded they can shed the adsorbed material, and unless impregnated with silver, bacteria may even grow on the filter. The efficiency of the filter over a period of time will depend on the organic load of the water: travellers may find it difficult to determine when the filter is exhausted. Some ceramic filter candles have the option of adding activated carbon to improve the taste. It is important to ensure that any such combined filter does not rely on the carbon for removal of pathogens. Only in cases of high chemical contamination will addition of activated carbon to the filter be advantageous to health.

Filtered water should always be boiled or disinfected before being given to babies and small children.

There are a great many convenient-looking purification devices on the market based on filtration, and they are often recommended to travellers. And some of these are discussed in the next chapter ('Water purification units'). The manufacturers frequently make extravagant claims about the effectiveness and safety of their products without producing any objective and convincing evidence to support their claims — such as precise details of how and by whom microbiological tests were performed. Without this evidence, such gadgets must always be regarded with suspicion, however attractive they may seem. The safest purification methods remain boiling and chemical disinfection.

Chemical disinfection

Chemical disinfection is recommended when boiling or fine-pore filtration is not possible, or when extra safety is required. Cysts from protozoa tend to be more difficult to remove by chemical means, although diarrhoeas caused by these organisms represent only about 5 per cent of cases.

The two most widely used chemicals are the halogens, iodine and chlorine. There is some debate concerning which is the best to use, but chlorine is the most widely used water disinfectant in the UK, whereas iodine tends to be more popular in the US.

The ability of the halogens to sterilize water will depend upon a number of factors: how long the water is left in contact with the disinfectant before drinking, the temperature of the water, and the concentration of the disinfecting solution used. These factors can be 'traded-off' against one another: for instance, a weaker solution could be used if left in contact for longer at higher temperatures. In general, unless manufacturers state otherwise, treated water should be left for 20–30 minutes before drinking, or even longer if the water is very cold (a few hours if possible). In addition, some organisms are harder to remove, particularly amoebic cysts and *Giardia*, so that longer contact times and/or higher concentrations may be required.

The halogens also react with any other organic matter that may be present in the water, and this reduces the amount of halogen available to kill pathogens. Pathogens adsorbed to suspended solids may also be protected from disinfection. Water should thus be filtered for the removal of suspended solids before disinfection (see above). Chlorine in particular is less active if the water is alkaline, which is one possible reason for preferring iodine.

Chlorine

Chlorine kills living organisms by inactivating biologically active compounds. It is an effective disinfectant against bacteria and some viruses at reasonably low concentrations and with short contact times, although it is less effective against amoebic cysts: the amount of chlorine needed for inactivation of amoebic cysts is 10 times that needed for inactivation of bacteria.

Liquid chlorine laundry bleach can be used, but the exact constituents and concentration of the solutions should be determined. Liquid chlorine laundry bleach usually contains 4–6 per cent available chlorine, and one to two drops of such a solution (or alternatively four to eight drops of a 1 per cent solution) should be added to each litre of water. Water treated in this way should be left for 20–30 minutes before drinking.

The most popular chlorine-based product in the UK is Puritabs — tablets to sterilize 1 or 25 litres (Puritab Maxi). Halazone tablets are available for the same purpose in the US.

Chlorine in a concentrated form (e.g. bleach solution) can be highly toxic, should be handled with care, never mixed with other chemicals (particularly acidic ones), and kept away from children.

Iodine

The concentration of free iodine most widely recommended is 8 mg/litre, which should allow sterilization of water containing *Giardia* within about 20 minutes, providing the water is clear and above 5°C. However, take note of the particular instructions stated by manufacturers regarding the use of their products, as they all tend to result in slightly different concentrations of iodine and thus may require different contact times at various water temperatures.

Iodine-based disinfection tablets are available commercially as Potable Aqua tablets; they do take some time to dissolve properly and will loose potency once the bottle is opened. Tincture of iodine is more economical and usually contains 2 per cent iodine; five drops of the solution should be added to one litre of water, increasing to twelve drops if *Giardia* is suspected. One other product available is manufactured by Polar Pure and comprises a plastic cup containing crystals of pure iodine. It is used to generate saturated solutions of iodine and is probably the most economical of all methods for preparing small quantities of sterile water.

When using larger quantities of iodine the water can become almost unpalatable and some method of removing the taste is recommended. Ascorbic acid (vitamin C) removes both the taste and the red colour imparted by iodine, but also neutralizes its disinfectant properties. Manufacturers of the products will supply ascorbic acid tablets or powder for this purpose and it is important to remember to add only it after the water has been left to stand for the correct time. Also, it is advisable not to use these neutralizers in any storage container but add to a cup just before drinking.

A study of 96 Peace Corps volunteers working in West Africa found that 46 per cent of them had an enlargement of their thyroid glands. They had been using iodine-resin water purifiers — and because they lived in an arid environment, had been drinking up to nine litres a day over periods of many months. Such long-term, large-volume use is not recommended. Use in pregnancy has not been associated with harmful effects, but is probably also best avoided on theoretical grounds; anyone with a thyroid problem should consult their doctor first.

Silver

Katedyne and Micropur silver tablets and solutions are available; their main disadvantage is that they are not effective as halogen based tablets, particularly against viruses and protozoa. On the plus side, they are free of any unpleasant taste and it is claimed that they prevent recontamination of stored water. Extra care should be taken in following manufacturer instructions when using silver tablets.

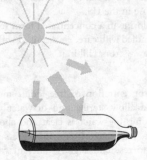

Solar disinfection works by the synergistic action of **UVA ultraviolet radiation** (wavelength 320-400 nm) and **increased water temperature**. In strong sunlight, 6 hours of exposure is sufficient. If the water temperature reaches 50°C, just one hour will suffice.

Inactivation of microorganisms by UVA-radiation and thermal treatment

Fig. 3.1 Solar disinfection

Solar disinfection

If other options are not available, a good measure of disinfection can sometimes be obtained by filling clear, plastic, soft drink bottles, preferably with their bottom sides painted black (see Fig. 3.1), with water and leaving them exposed to sunlight — a method known as SODIS. (More information about SODIS can be found at www.sodis.ch) The combination of warmth and ultraviolet radiation kills most micro-organisms. Tests have shown that 99.9 per cent of *E.Coli* bacteria in samples of contaminated water are killed when the temperature rises beyond 50°C. This is also an effective option against *Cryptosporidium* and the bacteria that cause cholera. The required exposure time ranges from six hours under bright conditions to two days under cloudy conditions. There is hope that this approach may prove very helpful in disaster relief situations in remote parts of the world.

Storage of treated water

Ideally any treated water should be consumed within 24 hours, but this may not always be practicable. Treated water should be stored in conditions that will prevent recontamination, and preferably in the same container in which it has been treated. If this is impractical, make sure that storage containers are either sterile or disinfected. They should always be covered, and should ideally have a tap at the bottom or a narrow opening, thus minimizing the risk of contamination when drawing off the treated water. Store treated water in a cool place, away from children.

Sanitation and hygiene

Sanitary facilities should be kept as far away as possible from water and food. Hands must always be washed before handling food and drink. Personal hygiene should be maintained at the highest standard possible.

Food hygiene

Food, especially fresh food obtained locally in areas where sanitary conditions are poor, should always be regarded as contaminated.

Fruit and vegetables should be washed thoroughly in clean soapy water and then rinsed with treated water. Rinsing alone is not enough — sterilizing chemicals in treated water will not kill pathogens on fruit and vegetables because contact time is not long enough.

Soaking in chlorine (e.g. using Milton tablets) or iodine — the concentration of either should be roughly three times that normally used for drinking water purification — is usually also effective, though the contact time necessary depends on how badly contaminated the food is.

Soaking in potassium permanganate, traditionally recommended for this purpose, is less reliable; permanganate has few medical uses these days.

Dipping in boiling water is a simple and effective alternative.

Avoid eating any raw vegetables or cold food prepared by others — especially in restaurants and hotels, and especially salads. (If you really must eat a salad that looks suspect, plenty of lemon juice or strong vinegar in the dressing will slightly reduce the risk.)

Seafood, fish, and meat should always be well cooked, and unpasteurized milk should be boiled or avoided.

Swimming

From the point of view of infection, swimming in the sea, away from human habitation, is usually safe. Beware of uncontrolled beaches close to sewage outfalls or highly populated areas with no proper sanitary facilities. Swimming in fresh surface water is not advised, especially in areas where schistosomiasis (bilharzia) (see p. 104) and Guinea worm (p. 596) are found.

Water purification devices

A large number of water filters and purification devices are now on the market, and claims are sometimes made for them that are difficult to assess. This chapter gives a brief personal review of some of the units currently available to travellers.

Paul Goodyer is Managing Director of Nomad Travellers Store and Medical Centre, and still travels himself. **Andreas King** was formerly Assistant Editor of *Water & Waste Treatment Journal,* and acts as an independent expeditionary adviser on water purification.

Ensuring a safe water supply to enable adequate fluid intake, especially under arduous field conditions such as tropical jungle or desert terrain, is an immensely important requirement. A supply of pure bottled water is hardly practical in such a setting, if only because of the huge amount required. The same applies to boiling, limiting factors being the difficulty of carrying sufficient fuel and the time and effort of frequent boil-ups.

A more practicable approach would be some form of treating contaminated water; chemical purification and the general principles involved have been considered in detail in the preceding chapter; this chapter gives a brief survey of specific filtration and purification products that can be used as an adjunct or an alternative, their effectiveness, and factors such as cost and weight.

Criteria to be met

Units intended to filter water should be dependable, easily maintained, and give some strong indication of when their useful life has ended. Bear in mind that nothing lasts a lifetime, and be wary of units that are claimed to be able to cope with thousands of litres. While it may be true that thousands of litres can be run through, the amount that will be treated effectively may be a different matter. Using a commonly recognized technique of 'methyl-blue' dye extraction, testing has shown that for most activated carbon units (see below), 'breakthrough' usually occurs after less than 200 litres.

Don't be misled

It is pertinent to clarify some of the terms used in manufacturers' literature that may sometimes mislead. A 'filter' removes suspended solids by mechanical straining; further purification is almost always required. However, a 'purifier' both filters and sterilizes, giving safe potable water, and obviating the need for further treatment. Product literature sometimes makes much play of a filter unit being 'bacteriostatic' — particularly in relation to activated carbon units. This merely means that bacterial growth is inhibited, NOT that bacteria are actually killed. Only a 'bactericide', defined as being lethal to bacteria, will do this.

Furthermore, virus removal test results are not always given, even though a unit may be quite effective. Such tests may require a high degree of skill, and can be expensive.

Bear in mind that no uniform, objective, agreed standards exist for such devices, and that external safeguards on quality control are generally lacking. Look, therefore, for test data from a good university department, or approval by a well-known independent organization.

Selecting a unit

The current devices on offer to travellers can generally be classified as follows.

Simple gravity filters

These are trickle filtration units, fine for pre-filtering and some removal of larger micro-organisms by adsorption. Their main advantage is aesthetic, whereby bad odours and tastes are eliminated. Heavy microbiological loading would require further chemical treatment; indeed this underscores their primary function of pre-filtration prior to adding chemical purification tablets. Be quite clear that these are filters, not purifiers.

Drinking bottle filters

These are bottles with filters attached to the top, the best-known of which is the Aqua Pure traveller (99 g, 500 ml). The bottle is filled with the water to be treated, then squeezed into a drinking cup for purification. Their appearance is slightly misleading as they look as though you should be able to drink safe water straight from the bottle. By the addition of an optional iodine sleeve to the carbon micro-filter, the Aqua Pure can be turned into a *purifier* so long as the water is left to stand for 15 minutes once it has passed through the system.

Pump-action filters

Of all the units currently available, the First Need Portable Water Purification Device (£50, 425 g; canister 7×10 cm, pump 14 cm) is the most effective against chemical contamination. The First Need comprises a pump, purifying cartridge, and a pre-filter to prevent inadvertent clogging of the purification cartridge. With 10 microns retention, the pre-filter is back-washable and cheap.

Inside the purification cartridge, three functions take place simultaneously. Ultra-filtration with 0.4 microns retention (absolute) extracts larger micro-organisms and other particles. A system of absorption materials is integrated into the matrix, scrubbing out a wide range of chemical contaminants and removing smells and tastes. Electrostatic charges remove colloidal and other ultra-small particles, binding them to the matrix without affecting the 'pass through' of water.

Although only filtering 400 litres or so before self-clogging, the First Need avoids potentially hazardous exposure to micro-organisms; these remain sealed inside the cartridge, which is then replaced when the flow rate drops to an unacceptable level. Again, it too needs to be protected from freezing and dropping, to prevent breakage of the structured matrix. If a rattle or 'thump' is heard when holding the unit up to the ear and shaking it gently, it is broken and should not be used; replacement cartridges (£20) are available.

Pumping the First Need can be quite stiff, and the little rubber stoppers on the inlet and outlet tubing can get mislaid in three seconds flat. The First Need is registered by the US Environmental Protection Agency as a 'purification device', one of very few to have this verification.

Another unit, that has been standard issue to the International Red Cross for over 50 years, is the Swiss-made Katadyn Pocket Filter (£170, 650 g, 25–155 cm), which filters raw water through a 0.2 micron microporous ceramic filter element. A built-in pump draws water up through a pipe, filtering it at a rate of 3/4 litre per minute. All pathogenic bacteria, protozoa, cysts, and helminths are extracted, including those that cause amoebic and bacillary dysentery, giardia, typhoid, cholera, and schistosomiasis. The pocket filter is much larger than the name implies, its little brother the Mini Filter is recommended for back packing.

While the Katadyn will treat heavily silted and algae-laden water, it may clog quickly. However, the ceramic 'candle' can be lightly brushed up to 300 times to restore full flow. This is best done using an old soft toothbrush, since the brush supplied is too abrasive.

A silver lining inside the ceramic candle prevents bacterial growth, so, in particular, one should not try to desalinate sea or brackish water with it. Salt would react with the silver lining and destroy its effectiveness. In freezing temperatures, the unit should be kept well insulated to prevent residual water turning to ice and cracking the candle. Likewise it should not be dropped. Furthermore, it must be stressed that brushing off the ceramic candle should be done upwind, and with care, to prevent potential exposure to disease organisms by aerosol effect.

Though viruses are far smaller than the 0.2 micron pore size of the Katadyn's ceramic candle, some viruses will be arrested during filtration by being contained in host cells, or by adsorption on to the filter medium itself. However, further chemical treatment against viral contamination is advisable.

The Katadyn should give years of continuous use, with replacement candles available (rather expensive, at £90). A larger stirrup-pump version for base-camp needs, the Katadyn Piston Filter Pump (£390) comes in a canvas carrying bag, and has a flow rate of up to 3 litres per minute.

Purifiers

Gravity purifiers

Two gravity purification units that have been independently and thoroughly tested by the London School of Hygiene and Tropical Medicine are the Travel Well Personal Water Purifier (£30, 750 g, 19 × 15 × 10 cm) and its military version, the Model PWP (£35, 500 g, 14 × 15 × 10 cm). Their effectiveness in clearing bacteriological and viral loads at extreme pH and dissolved solids levels is proven, the tests having been carried out on raw sewage. Both have a 500 litre capacity.

The Model PWP(Ranger) is adapted to fit the British Army '85 pattern' water bottle, treats 3/4 litre per unit fill in eight minutes, and comes in very strong black ABS (therefore 'unbreakable') plastic. It uses two filtration and two disinfection stages, the water bottle itself acting as the secondary disinfection chamber. A coarse foam filter extracting larger debris leads into the silver-impregnated activated carbon pre-filter, which removes finer particles and organic contamination. Colour, taste, and smell are thereby improved.

Inside the primary disinfecting chamber, a resin-iodine complex acts as a 'contact' microbicide, killing all bacteria, with very substantial reductions in virus levels. Controlled amounts of free iodine are also released, inactivating parasitic cysts and eliminating any remaining polio viruses during a two-minute 'holding period' in the water bottle. Purified water with a residual iodine level of 4 p.p.m. is held in sterile condition in the water bottle. Chemical contamination is also substantially reduced.

The Travel Well differs from the Model PWP by incorporating its own secondary disinfection chamber, and by using a final-stage activated carbon post-filter to remove the residual iodine, giving safe palatable water. The drawback of this purifier is its larger size and weight compared with the Model PWP, and the rather paltry amount of water treated per unit fill, only 180 millilitres in four minutes. Moreover, the plastic beaker included cracks easily when dropped. Be careful not to allow in too much suspended matter, which would inhibit the flow rate.

For tourists and for travellers, the Zero B (£17, 85 g, 8–15 cm) is a crystal iodine filter, which is claimed to remove 100 per cent of all waterborne bacteria and viruses. This claim should be treated with scepticism and it should be understood that this is under ideal conditions such as treating intermittent tap-water supplies; the Zero B is not designed for treating heavily contaminated or murky water under field conditions.

Easily assembled, the filter body sits on top of the beaker provided, one 250 millilitre beaker being delivered in around 30 seconds. It has a stated capacity of 500 litres equivalent to filling the beaker 2000 times. 0.5–0.8 p.p.m. of free iodine remains in the filtered water as a residual microbicide. The unit is fragile and cracks easily. On the other hand, the Zero B is light and cheap, and is a useful little standby unit.

Pump-action purifiers

Military specifications usually ensure that a unit is robust enough for operational requirements, and one such device is the Model MWP Pocket Pump or Trekker Travel Well (£20, 180 g, 4.5 × 13.5 cm). Certainly quite a compact unit, in ABS plastic, it has been developed from the model PWP referred to above, and will eliminate bacteria, viruses, and cysts from contaminated sources.

The MWP has a flow rate of 200 millilitres per minute, with a stated capacity of 250 litres, its effectiveness at this litreage having been independently verified by the London School of Hygiene and Tropical Medicine. During the three-stage operation, the source water is initially filtered to remove suspended debris as well as chemical contamination. This is followed by a resin-iodine complex which acts as a contact microbicide. A low-level residual of iodine is also released into the water for secondary disinfection during a three-minute holding period in the receiving bottle. Replacement cartridges are available (£38).

Excessive long-term use of iodine-based products is not recommended (p. 76).

Emergency units

Another emergency water filter is the Survival Straw (£6, 20 g), useful for reaching water trapped in awkward places such as rock crevices. With a slightly flexible body, if bent too much it kinks easily. Water is sucked up into the mouth, clarified and sterilized for immediate consumption.

Based on a particle filter, iodine and activated carbon, the carbon filter blocks before the iodine is exhausted, thereby avoiding the risk of drinking contaminated water. Yellow iodine discoloration on it does not detract from its performance. The Survival Straw has a capacity of 20–40 litres, towards the end of which sucking up water can be quite strenuous.

Finally the model Pockel Travel Well (£9, 60 g, 2 × 13.5 cm) is a pump-action filtration and sterilization unit, again based on the Model PWP, with size and weight kept to a minimum for inclusion in emergency ration packs. An initial filtration stage is followed by contact disinfection using a resin-iodine complex, also releasing a low level of iodine into the water for a two-minute secondary disinfection holding period in the receiving water bottle.

The Pocket Travel Well comes in ABS plastic, has a flow rate of 100 millilitres per minute, and a stated capacity of 60 litres, at which point it should be discarded. Tests carried out at the London School of Hygiene and Tropical Medicine have corroborated its effectiveness.

Choose carefully

Remember that none of the filter units reviewed here is designed for desalination.

Above all, be sure to exercise healthy scepticism when assessing manufacturers' claims.

Suppliers

1. Chlorination or iodination tablets
  Boots Co. Ltd, Nottingham NG2 3AA, UK (Chlorination tablets)
  Wisconsin Pharmacal Co. (Potable Aqua iodination tablets), 6769 North
    Industrial Road, Milwaukee, Wisconsin 53223, USA

2. Filtration bags (Millbank)
  Nomad Medical 3–4 Turnpike Lane, London N8 OPX, UK
    Tel: 020 8889 7014

3. **Filtration units, pumps, and purification units**
   First Need: Burton McCall Ltd, 163 Parker Drive, Leicester LE4 0JP, UK.
   Tel: 0116 234 4611
   Aqua Pure Traveller **www.thirstpoint.com** Abbey Business Park, Monks Walk,
   Farnham, Surrey GU9 8HT, UK. Tel: 01252 722 022
   Katadyn Filters: Katadyn (UK Warehouse), Viking Optical, Blyth Road,
   Halesworth, Suffolk IP19 8EN, UK. Tel: 01986 875315
   Model Ranger, Trekker, Pocket, Travel Well's Pre-Mac Int. Morewood Close,
   Sevenoaks Kent TN13 2HU, UK. Tel: 01732 460333
   Survival Straw: Sowester Simpson-Lawrence Stinstord Road, Nuffield
   Industrial Estate Poole, Dorset BH17 0SW, UK. Tel: 01202 667700
   Zero B: UK Products Group, The Old Forge, Woburn Road, Ampthill,
   Bedfordshire MK45 2HX, UK. Tel: 01525 406446

4. **Paper cartridge filters**
   Victoria Industrial Contract Ltd, 443–445 Holloway Road, London
   N7 6LW, UK.

5. **Boiling elements**
   Pifco Mini-boiler: Pifco Ltd, Princess Street, Failsworth, Manchester
   M35 OHS, UK.

6. **Retail stockists**
   Cotswold, Broadway Lane, South Cerney, Cirencester, Glos GL7 5UQ, UK.
   Tel. 01285 643434 **www.cotswoldoutdoor.com**
   Field & Trek plc, Langdale House, Sable way, Laindon, Essex SS156SR, UK.
   Tel. 01277 233122 **www.fieldandtrek.com**
   Nomad Travellers Centre, 3–4 Wellington Terrace, London N8 OPX, UK.
   Tel. 081 889 7014 web-site **www.nomadtravel.co.uk**
   Safariquip, The Stones Castleton Hope Valley Derbyshire S33 8WX, UK.
   Tel. 01433 620320 **www.safariquip.co.uk**

For further advice:
   Departments of Medical Microbiology and Tropical Hygiene,
   London School of Hygiene and Tropical Medicine, Keppel Street, London,
   WC1E 7HT, UK.

Recreational water and beaches

Travellers need safe water not just for drinking, but for bathing and enjoyment: possible disease hazards are considered below, though drowning and water-related accidents pose a far greater risk to health.

Dr Robin Philipp is a consultant occupational and public health physician, medical adviser to two UK water companies, and Director of the Centre for Health in Employment and the Environment (CHEE), Department of Occupational Medicine, Bristol Royal Infirmary, England. He collaborates closely with the WHO for the AESOHP programme (A European Sense of Healthy Place and Purpose).
Pamela Thorne is a research psychologist at CHEE. She works with the AESOHP programme on projects for recreational water and bathing beach quality and their impacts on public health, human needs for adequate hydration, and the importance for psychological well-being of aesthetic factors in rural, urban and workplace environments.

Beaches and the coastal environment have a natural attraction for travellers, but over the last two decades rapid and often uncontrolled development of coastal areas to accommodate mass tourism has led to a deterioration in the quality of water used for recreational purposes and in the cleanliness of beaches. Much of the pollution is attributed to increasing amounts of municipal sewage and waste and to litter left by beach visitors or thrown overboard from boats. This, and the expansion of traditional bathing and swimming activities to include scuba diving, underwater fishing, wind surfing, jet skiing, and water skiing, have increased the risks inherent in a recreational water environment.

In response, organizations such as the World Health Organization, the World Tourism Organization, and the United Nations Environment Programme encourage standards which enable travellers to make an informed choice when selecting a beach that is both **clean** and **safe**. In many places though, travellers must use their own criteria.

Water pollution

All coastal waters and some freshwaters are to some degree utilized as waste water recipients, and may be polluted by local discharges of municipal sewage or industrial effluent. Rivers may carry these wastes to the coast and may also be polluted by agricultural fertilizers and pesticides.

The risk of bacterial infections from bathing in sea water is generally low and most likely only in areas immediately around waste outlets, in estuaries, or in enclosed bays where the water is not quickly diluted. Health problems resulting from bathing are more likely to be caused by viruses, which can survive for much longer than other pathogens.

Although the risk of contracting serious illness is low, the following have been associated with bathing in contaminated waters:

- Gastroenteritis
- Hepatitis A
- Eye, ear, nose, and throat infections
- Pneumonia
- Skin infections

- Salmonellosis and poliomyelitis
- Shigellosis
- Meningitis
- Acute neurotoxicity

Freshwater swimming in some areas may carry the additional risk of schistosomiasis (p. 104) or leptospirosis (p. 371).

Pollution, particularly with high levels of phosphates, can lead to algal blooms which are intermittently toxic and may cause a range of symptoms. These are described in detail on p. 88.

The risks from dangerous and/or venomous sea creatures are described in the section on bites and stings (pp. 232–41).

Human hygiene and environmental safety

Diseases resulting from beach use may also stem from sources such as food, drinking water, toilet facilities, air and water temperature, and close contact with other people. Injury may be caused by hazardous or poorly maintained beaches and watersports equipment, or low standards of beach cleanliness. Beach surveys, for example, have reported an increasing amount of medical waste, and syringes and needles left by drug users. The latter have been found at secluded beaches, in hidden areas of sand dunes, and behind rocks near cliffs, as well as known drug-user sites such as the backs of toilet blocks or beach huts, under piers, and near sea walls. (Risks from contaminated needles are discussed on pp. 588–9.)

How to judge if a beach is clean and safe

Evidence of water quality

In most countries national legislation provides for a recreational water quality monitoring programme which meets at least the minimal standards laid down by international convention. The basic microbiological parameters are bacterial indicator organisms (primarily *E. coli* in freshwater and enterococci in marine water) and pathogens. Fungal examination of sand may also be included in some areas. In principle, where the water is found to be below standard after successive samplings, local authorities will take steps to warn users or ban bathing until the source of pollution can be controlled. Recreational water quality criteria and standards in use are however, diverse: *visual evidence of pollution* should also be checked.

Beach award schemes: criteria for cleanliness

If a beach has received an award it has passed a stringent annual assessment, and the standards which have been met should be clearly displayed with the award. The Foundation for Environmental Education in Europe, for example, has a 'Blue Flag' award scheme which denotes the following:

- Compliance with the microbiological parameters of the EEC Bathing Water Directive
- No industrial or sewage discharges affect the beach area
- No gross pollution by visible sewage-related or other visible waste

- No visible hydrocarbon pollution
- No algal or other vegetation materials accumulating or decaying on the beach area
- Freedom from litter on land and sea
- High-quality beach area management in respect of cleanliness and sanitation, covering such things as *beach cleansing* and the *provision and maintenance of toilet facilities* and *litter bins*
- Safe access to the beach
- Beach guards on duty during the bathing season and/or alternative adequate safety provisions including life-saving equipment
- First aid available and clearly signposted
- All buildings and equipment on the beach must be well maintained

Other awards, such as the 'Golden Starfish', set standards for more isolated beaches which are not actively managed and developed and include the following criteria:

- The beach must comply with nationally accepted microbiological parameters
- Beach and surrounding area must be free of litter, broken glass, oil, rotting seaweed, etc
- If toilets are on site they must be clean and in good order
- Access to the beach, and any buildings and structures on the beach, must be safe and well maintained

Notices should be displayed on or near the beach, warning that there are no safety provisions for bathers and of any dangers (steep shelving, strong currents, etc.)

It is important to note that a beach which is *not* displaying an award is *not* necessarily *un*clean or *un*safe. It is however, then more important to make a personal assessment of it.

Warning flags

Many countries world-wide have adopted flag systems on swimming beaches to advise and guide the public on sea conditions. These follow the traffic light colour code:

Green	=	Calm
Yellow	=	Caution
Red	=	Danger

A red danger flag may permanently mark an area where swimming is habitually dangerous or may replace a green or yellow flag when weather conditions deteriorate.

Zoning

Flags, buoys, and/or booms may be used to define zones for different water-based activities, for example, to segregate swimmers from water-skiing or to demarcate an area for swimming which is supervised by lifeguards.

Within a supervised system the following three zoning flags may be in operation:

1. Red over yellow rectangular flags indicate 'patrolled bathing area' — i.e. lifeguard-patrolled zone of the beach. One flag indicates a lifeguard is present; two flags denote the lifeguard-patrolled area.
2. Black and white quartered flag indicates 'surfing only area' — for the use of craft over 1.6 m in length used for the purpose of riding surf.
3. Blue and white burgee (international A flag) indicates 'divers down' — displayed from offshore diving platforms during scuba diving excursions.

These flags operate only during a prescribed and well-publicized period each day, and will also relate to seasonal activity.

If no evidence is provided
Local conditions such as tides and currents and associated prevailing winds, rocks, coral reefs, and wrecks/nets/weirs may present hazards which are not immediately obvious. Estuaries can be particularly dangerous. If information or warnings are not routinely provided, local advice should always be sought before bathing.

Unless there is clear evidence of adequate water quality, it is best to avoid:

- Any water with visible signs of sewage-related or other waste, jellyfish, dead animals, or rotting fish
- Beaches close to an obvious sewage or waste outlet or a river estuary
- Enclosed bays and inlets where the water is less quickly diluted and exchanged and where sewage outfall pipes can be seen
- Beaches and inland waters with obvious signs of algae or mucilage.

On populated beaches in developed areas avoid:

- Those contaminated with litter or where bins are inadequate or unemptied
- Those with poorly maintained or non-existent toilet facilities.

Beach and water safety risks

Drowning and swimming accidents
It has been estimated that throughout the world, 150 000 people drown each year. A major cause of drowning accidents is often ignorance, disregard, or misjudgement of danger. Currents and tides, vegetation, and the activities of other water users (for example, water-skiers) are all potentially hazardous.

Alcohol is a major factor in drowning accidents — 50 per cent are alcohol-associated. Consumption of alcohol can lead to rapid and massive heat loss if a person should fall into water, or to sudden exhaustion in swimmers. Even small amounts of alcohol can cause hypoglycaemia on a long-distance swim unless taken at the same time as a sufficient amount of food.

Water temperature Even strong swimmers may succumb in cold water and life jackets should be worn in small craft when the water is cold. Exercise in the water increases the loss of body heat. Therefore, remaining close to a sunken craft rather than striking out for shore may increase the chances of survival. Prolonged immersion in water warmer than 34–35°C is hazardous.

Diving in unfamiliar water of uncertain depth and clarity is not advisable. This applies particularly in freshwater rivers, lakes, and estuaries.

Injuries from broken glass, metal objects, or needles are best avoided by wearing footwear on the beach and avoiding secluded nooks and crannies. Footwear is needed when swimming at coral reefs.

Additional risks

A beach environment may also increase the risks of sunburn (see p. 350) and contaminated seafood (see p. 20). Hazards linked to watersports are considered further on p. 370.

Algal blooms

Pollution of sea water, lakes, and rivers with fertilizers, sewage, and organic material has caused sudden increases in the growth of microscopic plants or algae — algal blooms. The phenomenon is on the increase, with recent dramatic blooms along the Adriatic and elsewhere. The algae can be toxic or merely a slimy nuisance, interfering with swimming, windsurfing and other watersports. This chapter explains the background to the problem.

Dr Robin Philipp is a consultant occupational and public health physician, medical adviser to two UK water companies, and Director of the Centre for Health in Employment and the Environment (CHEE), Department of Occupational Medicine, Bristol Royal Infirmary, England. He collaborates closely with the WHO for the AESOHP programme (A European Sense of Healthy Place and Purpose).

Blue-green algae (BGA) are microscopic plants found in fresh and brackish waters. They have some characteristics of bacteria and are therefore described as photosynthetic bacteria, also called cyanobacteria. They are particularly common in lowland, nutrient-laden waters in the warm, sunny summer months. Mountain reservoirs generally have low numbers, except where contributory water sources drain forested areas on which phosphate or nitrogenous fertilizers have been used.

Some free-floating forms contain gas bubbles that regulate buoyancy in response to the light intensity. Normally this keeps them away from the surface, but in windy conditions that mix the water, the cells may become too buoyant and rise rapidly to the surface if the wind subsides abruptly. They accumulate downwind and at the water's edge to form scums that look like blue-green paint or jelly. In high density within the water, they can also form a visible blue-green bloom; they may also be coloured purple or red. They are an increasing problem due to nutrient enrichment of natural waters, agricultural fertilizer run-off, domestic and industrial effluents, and possibly global warming. Scums and blooms can also encourage other bacterial growth and colonization by insects.

Toxins

Toxins produced by some BGA have caused deaths in agricultural livestock, pets, wild animals, and fish. Toxicity can fluctuate daily in that BGA can be toxic one day and not the next. Blooms can also appear one day, disappear suddenly, and reappear at any time. The toxins are of three main types–those that affect the nervous system, those that damage the liver, and those that irritate the skin.

Clinical effects relating to wildlife and man

Deaths have occurred in animals venturing into thick concentrations of algae to bathe and drink the water, or licking scum and deposits off their fur when coming ashore.

Inhalation of aerosols containing desiccated algal material can also occur. No deaths have been reported in humans although harmful effects of BGA on human health have been widely reported, most commonly in developed countries with hot climates such as Australia and parts of the USA, but also from the UK, Canada, China, Scandinavia, the Baltic States, the former USSR, South Africa, Zimbabwe, India, New Zealand, Israel, Venezuela, and Argentina.

In humans, ingestion of toxic algae or body immersion in scum-containing water has been associated with dizziness, headaches, muscle cramps, runny nose, sore eyes, hay fever, asthma, pneumonia, nausea, vomiting, gastroenteritis, and liver damage; skin contact has been associated with burning, itching, and inflammation of the skin, eyes, and lips, hand and sore throat also dizziness. Outbreaks of gastroenteritis affecting travellers to countries such as Nepal have also been attributed to BGA-like organisms (p. 26).

The main exposure situations and associated risks

Drinking water
BGA can give a 'musty', 'geranium', or 'vegetable' taste and odour to drinking water. Dense blooms of blue-green algae in drinking water reservoirs have occasionally resulted in inflammation of the liver and gastroenteritis in people who have been drinking affected water.

Eating contaminated fish or meat
Some BGA toxins can accumulate in fresh-water shellfish such as the swan mussel (*Anadonta cygnea*). BGA toxins can also accumulate in some fish organs, particularly the liver. In the 1920s and 1930s, for example, outbreaks of a condition called Haff disease were common around the Baltic Coast and were linked with eating fish, in particular, fish liver from fresh waters affected by algal blooms: the livers were regarded as a delicacy if tasting of musty blue-green-algal-type flavour compounds. Haff disease was occasionally fatal and was characterized by muscular pain, vomiting, respiratory distress, and the passage of brownish-black urine. Elsewhere, there do not seem to have been any such outbreaks, even when fresh-water algal blooms have been prominent. There is no evidence at present that algal toxins can affect the flesh of fish. Fish are therefore considered safe to eat provided they are properly gutted and cleaned. The flesh of animals which have been drinking water that is affected by an algal bloom is also safe to eat.

Contact with sea-water algae and eating shellfish
Sea-water algal blooms are caused by increased nutrient loads and low oxygen levels in the water. They cause 'red algal tides' and mucilage formation. Mucilage is an amorphous, messy, viscous substance suspended in the water. It can be deposited on beaches.

The commonest toxic algae to be found in marine waters are called dinoflagellates (they are single-celled, motile algae). Their toxins are mainly a problem when they become concentrated by fish and shellfish that are subsequently eaten by humans. Toxic marine dinoflagellates can cause several illnesses.

Paralytic shellfish poisoning (PSP)
This occurs in several parts of the world. It begins with numbness and tingling around the mouth and in the hands and fingers within 5–30 minutes of eating affected shellfish, followed by numbness and weakness of the arms and legs. Usually the illness is mild and self-limiting, but in severe cases when large amounts of toxin have been eaten, paralysis of the diaphragm leads to respiratory failure, which may be fatal. There is no evidence that PSP can be caused by skin exposure, drinking sea water, or from inhaling sea-water droplets.

Diarrhoeic shellfish poisoning
Algae associated with diarrhoeic shellfish poisoning (DSP) are *Dinophysis* and *Prorocentrum* (okadaic acid). The symptoms and signs of DSP are mainly diarrhoea, nausea, vomiting, abdominal pain, and chills coming on within 30 minutes to 12 hours of eating shellfish.

Neurotoxic shellfish poisoning (NSP)
This resembles PSP but is non-fatal and paralysis does not occur. So far, blooms causing it have been reported only in the Gulf of Mexico. Sea spray containing the same algae (*Ptychodiscus brevis*) or their toxins cause an irritant aerosol that leads to inflammation of the eyes and nose, with cough and tingling lips; in windy conditions, the effects can be observed up to a few kilometres inland.

Amnesic shellfish poisoning
This is a rare illness first recognized in 1987 when a mysterious outbreak in Canada was traced to a bloom of the diatom *Nitzschia pungens*. (Diatoms are unicellular plankton with a silicified cell wall, and are widely distributed.) The illness was associated with a shellfish toxin (domoic acid) which had become concentrated in mussels. Severe headache, vomiting, abdominal cramps, and diarrhoea were followed by confusion, memory loss, disorientation, and coma. *Nitzschia pungens* is widely distributed in the coastal waters of the Atlantic, Pacific, and Indian Oceans.

Ciguatera and puffer-fish poisoning (see also p. 66)
This resembles PSP, and the term 'pelagic paralysis' has been proposed to cover all three because their neurotoxins are believed to act in the same way. Ciguatera is mainly a hazard in Pacific and Caribbean waters: the dinoflagellates involved are benthic (found at the bottom of an ocean) and therefore probably not related to blooms. It is, however, the most common form of fish poisoning and the most frequently reported food-borne disease of a chemical nature in south-east Florida and Hawaii. Puffer-fish poisoning is still a public health hazard in Japan. Both types of poisoning may occur in Europe from imported fish.

Marine cyanophyte dermatitis
This is a severe contact dermatitis known as swimmers' itch or seaweed dermatitis. It may occur after swimming or handling fishing nets in seas containing blooms of the filamentous marine cyanophyte *Lynbya majuscula*. Two of the toxic agents are known to

be potent tumour-producing compounds. Outbreaks have been reported from countries such as Japan and Hawaii. A toxic dermatitis known as Dogger Bank itch or weed rash also occurs in European trawler fishermen from the handling of trawl nets. It is caused by moss animals called sea chervils found in the North Sea, and not by algae.

Skin irritation in bathers can also be caused by jelly-fish fragments or by small crustacea in the bloom which become trapped inside bathing suits. The bloom may also dry on the skin after bathing and irritate or sensitize it if it is not washed off. Hay fever or asthma may also be provoked by bloom material drying on the shore, becoming airborne, and affecting sunbathers and others exposed to on-shore winds.

Hints for personal health

The risk of harmful effects from different patterns of exposure to BGA is not fully understood. Unfortunately, the potential toxicity of a bloom or scum cannot be determined by its appearance, odour, texture, or any other simple feature. If treated with reasonable care, there is little hazard to human health: although algal scums and blooms are not always harmful, it is sensible to regard them as such. The following points will help minimize possible risks associated with drinking water and recreational exposures.

Drinking water

Standard water treatment does not remove algal toxins from water. The toxins are heat stable and unlikely to be destroyed by boiling. There is also no evidence that water purification tablets either destroy the toxins or encourage their release from algal cells. Although an extremely uncommon and temporary phenomenon, any drinking-water supply that is obviously discoloured blue-green should be avoided. Nevertheless, there is little present evidence of particular risks from public supplies.

Shellfish are best avoided if there is doubt about the purity of the waters they came from.

In rural or wilderness areas where raw water is consumed, take the following precautions to reduce the risk of exposure.

- Where possible, take drinking water from flowing rather than still water.
- In still water, scums and decaying cells accumulate downwind on the surface, and are more likely to be associated with the release of toxins. Water should therefore be taken away from any visible scum, out from the water's edge, from below the surface, and on the windward side of a lake or reservoir.
- Brownish, peaty upland waters are less likely to be contaminated with BGA than lowland nutrient-enriched waters.
- If drinking water has been taken in the presence of a scum or algal bloom, the water should be filtered to remove particles of algal material.
- Affected water is generally safe for irrigation, but if in doubt, avoid eating leafy vegetables, or at least wash them carefully in clean, treated water.

Fresh-water recreational activities

Studies have not yet identified any particular illnesses that could be linked to BGA exposure through recreation. As a precaution though, the following guidance is recommended.

- If the water is clear there is little danger of ill-effects as a result of recreational contact.
- Toxins are more concentrated where there are visible algal scums. These areas should always be avoided. Direct contact with a visible scum, or swallowing appreciable amounts, are associated with the highest chances of a health risk.
- On a lee shore and windy day, algae and scum can be found at some distance from the water's edge — keep away from these areas.
- If sailing, windsurfing, or undertaking any other activity likely to involve accidental water immersion in the presence of scums or algal blooms, wear clothing that is close-fitting at the wrists and neck, and also boots and sailing suits that fit into the boot tops.
- Spend as little time as possible in shallow water launching and recovering boats; launching and recovery should be undertaken in areas away from thick aggregations of algae or scum.
- After coming ashore, hose, shower, or wash yourself down to remove any scum or algae.
- All clothing and bathing costumes should be washed and thoroughly dried after any contact with scums or blooms. Do not store wet clothes.
- During sailing or boating activities when scums or blooms are present, keep capsize drills to a minimum, ensure rescue boats are on hand to take crews out of the water as soon as possible, and wash boats and wet gear down immediately on coming ashore. Races should be staged away from affected areas.
- When fishing, keep away from algal scums and clean your hands after handling fish or fishing tackle.
- If any health effects are experienced subsequently, whatever the nature of the exposure, seek prompt medical attention.

Sea-water bathing
- As far as exposure to algae is concerned, sea water is generally safe to bathe in provided there is no red algal tide or mucilage, and the water is not otherwise obviously polluted.
- Avoid floating clumps of seaweed or aggregations along the shoreline.
- On the beach, do not sit downwind of any bloom material drying on the shore which could form an aerosol and be inhaled.
- If available, use beach showers after bathing, and rinse bathing costumes thoroughly in fresh water to remove salt, crustaceans, algae, or jellyfish fragments that can cause skin irritation.

4 Diseases of 'contact'

Tuberculosis

Tuberculosis (TB) is the infectious disease that causes the most deaths in the world today — it is 'the disease that never really went away'. Despite the worsening global situation and the limited options for prevention, however, it is a disease that is usually straightforward to detect and to treat.

Dr Peter Davies is Consultant Chest Physician and Director of the Tuberculosis Research Unit at the Cardiothoracic Centre, University Hospital, Liverpool. He is the editor of a major textbook on tuberculosis, an advisor to the WHO, and secretary of the UK charity, TB Alert.

A new era in the history of TB began in the mid-1980s when it was realized that the disease had not only ceased to decline in many developed countries, notably the USA, but was actually increasing. A reappraisal showed that the disease was out of control across many of the poorest regions of the world, especially Central Africa and South Asia. In 1993, the WHO took the unique step of declaring TB to be a world emergency.

Despite this intervention cases of TB are set to increase globally for the foreseeable future. One third of the world's population — no fewer than two billion people — are infected with the tubercle bacillus. Deaths from TB are expected to increase from the current level of three million a year to *five million by the year 2050*.

The global rise of TB
The main factors responsible for the massive upsurge in the spread of TB can be identified.

Population explosion
The highest incidence of TB across the globe is in central Africa, where death rates exceed 200 per 100 000 a year, and in southern Asia, particularly India, where death rates are between 100 and 200 per 100 000 a year. These are exactly the areas of the

globe where the population increase is known to be most rapid. For example, the population of India is expected to increase by 75 per cent in the next 30 years and the population of some central African countries such as Malawi, by 150 per cent.

The menace of HIV/AIDS

It is known that co-infection with HIV increases the risk of TB infection developing into disease by approximately 100-fold. The lifetime risk of about 10 per cent of infection developing into disease in a person infected with TB alone becomes an annual risk of 10 per cent in the dually infected person.

In parts of Africa, the lifetime risk of dying from AIDS is now 50 per cent. TB is the commonest cause of death in these individuals. The epidemic has overwhelmed the health services in all sub-Saharan African countries. TB causes more maternal deaths than all other causes put together: half of dually infected women die within 18 months of pregnancy.

The increase of the world's poor

The association between poverty and TB is well established. Even within the developed world the highest rates of disease are seen in the poorest sections of the community. As the world population increases in some of the poorest areas of the world so the number of people living in poverty has increased. In the last 15 years the number of people living on less than a dollar a day (the definition of absolute poverty) has increased from three-quarters to one and a third billion. More than three-quarters of these are women. The proportion of the world's wealth owned by the richest 20 per cent has increased from 65 per cent to over 85 per cent in the same time period.

Multidrug-resistant TB

Multidrug-resistant TB (MDRTB) — that is, the presence of bacteria resistant to at least isoniazid and rifampicin (the two most effective drugs in the treatment of TB) — is increasing world-wide. This makes infection extremely difficult to treat. Drug treatment may need to be prolonged from the usual 6 months to as much as 2 years. Using second line (reserve drugs) is difficult and expensive, and adverse effects are common. Some parts of the world (notably Latvia) have rates of drug resistance of almost 50 per cent. In some Russian prisons the majority of cases are drug resistant. Inmates on treatment for drug-susceptible strains have been infected with a drug-resistant strain from a fellow inmate.

Immigration: the developed world's problem

Immigration is the main factor contributing to the increase within the developed world. In England, 60 per cent of cases are in ethnic minority groups (mostly from the Indian subcontinent) which comprise only 5 per cent of the population. It should, however, be remembered that 200 years ago, TB was a disease that killed one in four people in western Europe. It was effectively exported to what we now call the developing world through trade and empire building.

The course of TB

TB is spread through the air, in the same way as the common cold. It is usually caught by inhaling air-borne bacilli, *Mycobacterium tuberculosis*, coughed into the air by an individual with infectious disease. TB tends to be less infectious than the cold virus, and contact usually has to be prolonged for a serious risk to be present. This is why TB tends to be transmitted mainly within a family or to other household members.

The primary infection of TB occurs in the lungs and usually goes unnoticed. A short period of malaise and some non-specific respiratory tract symptoms may develop. A tuberculin skin test, if performed at this time, will change from negative to positive (see below).

The great majority (probably 90 per cent) of people infected will never go on to develop the disease; it may take anywhere between a few months and a few years for '*post-primary*' disease to develop in those that do — the potential incubation period can be a lifetime. The long incubation explains why the highest incidence in the white UK population is amongst the over-60s: these people incurred infection in early adult life when TB was highly prevalent.

In the absence of pasteurization, TB can also be spread by infected milk, which can cause glandular or gastrointestinal disease.

Symptoms

TB may cause disease in any part of the body but the lung is the most usual site: the bacterium slowly destroys lung tissue. If detected early enough, such as by contact screening, there may be no symptoms.

Contact screening

Contacts of an infectious patient should be screened. This requires a skin (tuberculin) test (see below) and, if positive, a chest X–ray. The commonest early symptom is a cough. This may start as a dry, irritating cough, just like any chest infection. The cough of TB will continue for weeks or months getting progressively worse. Profuse amounts of phlegm may be brought up from the chest with each cough. If a blood vessel is damaged, blood may be coughed up. The cough of severe TB may be uncontrollable, with spasms of wracking, continuous coughing.

Weight loss is also common, the patient initially losing weight slowly but often realizing after some months that he or she is many kilograms lighter. Malaise is a usual feature, like a low-grade, flu that gradually worsens over weeks and months. A raised temperature often occurs at night, causing the patient to sweat profusely, sometimes so badly that it may be necessary to change all the bedclothes.

Sometimes the patient will complain of pains in the chest, made worse by coughing. In severe cases, where much of the lung has been destroyed, breathlessness occurs.

Confirming the diagnosis

Tuberculosis of the lung usually causes characteristic changes on a chest X-ray that will suggest (but not confirm) the presence of disease. The diagnosis must be confirmed by obtaining phlegm for bacteriological analysis. Only if the tuberculosis bacterium is found in the phlegm (sputum) or some other sample from a patient can the presence of the disease be proved. Because the bacterium is difficult to grow in culture, this process can take weeks, though molecular technology is now being developed to provide more rapid confirmation of disease.

The tuberculin skin test

In the tuberculin skin test a small quantity of protein from the tuberculosis bacillus (PPD) is injected into the skin. A reaction (swelling) will occur in someone previously infected by the tuberculosis bacterium.

There are two types of tuberculin test in use in the UK. For the Mantoux skin test a known quantity of PPD is injected using a needle and syringe. The test is read 48–72 hours later by measuring the area of swelling at the injection site. For the HEAF test the PPD solution is smeared on the skin and injected into the skin by a six-pronged multipuncture device. The test is read 3–10 days later.

A weakly positive test may be caused by mycobacteria other than TB, including the BCG vaccination. A strongly positive test usually indicates infection (but not necessarily disease) caused by *M. tuberculosis*.

Treatment

Once TB is suspected treatment should be started. This involves at least three and preferably four specific antibiotics — isoniazid, rifampicin, pyrazinamide, and ethambutol. For convenience they may be given combined in a single tablet. Treatment must continue for at least six months though the number of antibiotics can be reduced once laboratory tests have confirmed the bacterium's sensitivity to the antibiotics being used.

The family and other contacts

Individuals who are in close and frequent contact with a patient, such as family members, are at risk of disease, and need to be screened by carrying out a chest X-ray and, if positive, performing a skin test.

Preventing TB

BCG

BCG was developed at the beginning of the twentieth century by repeatedly subculturing *M. bovis* (the bacteria responsible for TB in cattle) to result in an attenuated (weakened, less virulent) strain. The vaccine provides some protection against TB by boosting the specific immunity that protects the body from *M. tuberculosis*.

Efficacy of BCG

Trials of the vaccine have been undertaken since it was first developed in the 1920s. The results have been variable. About a third of the total trials have shown no protective effect. The remainder have shown protection of up to 80 per cent* at best,

---

*Protective efficacy is a measure of the proportion of people who would have got the disease had they not had the vaccination: 80% protection means that four out of five individuals are protected. Efficacy for most vaccines exceeds 95%. BCG is therefore a relatively weak protective vaccine.

lasting a maximum of 15 years. No trials on second or subsequent vaccinations have shown any protective effect. The reasons for variability are not fully understood.

BCG in the UK
Studies carried out by the British Medical Research Council in the 1950s showed that BCG, when given to teenage school children, gave about 75 per cent protection for 15 years. Since 1953 it has been national policy to vaccinate all children aged 12–13. Thus in theory the entire population receives protection from early teenage years through to about the age of 30.

In addition to the national policy for all teenagers, BCG is given at birth to those at high risk of disease — those with a family history of TB and those from minority ethnic groups.

BCG policy in other countries
Most countries give BCG at birth to provide protection in the early years when infection can often lead to devastating widespread disease such as *miliary tuberculosis* (of the lung) or *tuberculous meningitis* (of the brain). This is particularly important in high-prevalence countries where the chance of being infected in very early life is high. Some countries such as the USA have chosen not to use it because most trials there have not shown any protective effect.

The effect of BCG on the tuberculin test
BCG converts the tuberculin skin test from negative to positive as does infection with *M. tuberculosis* (see above).

In the UK we believe it is possible to tell the difference between skin test positivity caused by BCG and by TB. BCG is not used in the USA, partly because American public health authorities do not believe it is possible to make this distinction.

BCG protection against drug-resistant TB
BCG is probably more effective in preventing disease than in providing preventive therapy to those infected (see below), a procedure for which there is no evidence of any efficacy at all. For health care workers who may be exposed to drug-resistant TB, even the low protective efficacy of BCG would make vaccination worthwhile.

BCG in low-prevalence countries
As rates of TB decline, the argument for continuing routine BCG vaccination to the whole population becomes weaker. A number of countries with very low rates of disease have stopped BCG vaccination but, due to the increase of cases that has resulted, at least one, the Czech Republic, has restarted a routine BCG programme.

The possible adverse effects of BCG
Abscesses at the site of BCG injection are frequently reported. It is often assumed that this is due to bad technique — the injection should be given intracutaneously but an accidental intramuscular injection may result. Lymph node swelling and abscess

formation may rarely occur. If the injection is given at the correct site, over the lower part of the deltoid muscle in the upper arm, the swelling will develop in the lymph nodes under the arm (in the *axilla*).

Very rarely indeed, BCG may cause disseminated infection in immunocompromised infants. This is usually fatal. For this reason, BCG should not be given to symptomatic HIV-positive individuals.

New vaccines
There is not much hope that an alternative, better vaccine can be developed within the next 20 years.

Preventive therapy
This involves giving a reduced course of antibiotics (in the UK, usually two antibiotics for three months) to people with latent TB infection (known as LTBI) — people with a positive skin test plus the established *absence* of disease.

In the USA, policy on TB prevention depends on regular tuberculin testing for those at risk of infection such as health workers, plus preventive therapy for those whose skin tests become positive. BCG is not given, as it is believed to interfere with the interpretation of the tuberculin test.

In countries like the UK where BCG is used, preventive therapy is sometimes given in addition, for example to close contacts at high risk of infection, such as children with tuberculin tests that are strongly positive.

Avoiding infection
In practice there is probably little one can do to be sure of avoiding TB, since most infections occur from unsuspected cases. Once patients start treatment they are rapidly rendered non-infectious. The exception to this is patients who have drug-resistant disease. Medical staff working with these patients should take specific precautions, including wearing special face masks.

Avoid milk unless you know it has been properly treated (though the risk of brucellosis and other infections is probably greater).

TB and the traveller
Travellers from developed countries to parts of the world where TB is endemic incur a measurable risk of being infected with and developing the disease.

BCG
Most UK citizens aged over 13 will have had BCG. There is no need for such individuals to be tested for 'tuberculin status' (i.e. a tuberculin skin test to establish whether tuberculin sensitivity is present). About 10 per cent of those who have had BCG remain tuberculin negative and there is no correlation between protective efficacy of the BCG and the presence of tuberculin positivity. Even 15 years or longer after receiving BCG, there is no need for further vaccination: second or subsequent vaccinations have never been shown to provide protection.

Children under the age of 13 who have not had BCG should be advised to have a vaccination if they are travelling for a prolonged period to an area with high endemic

TB. This would include the whole of Africa, South and Southeast Asia, parts of eastern Europe, and Central and South America. Children who have had BCG at birth do not require further testing or vaccination. (BCG is not necessary for short holidays staying in good hotels.)

BCG takes at least six weeks to give protection, plus a week beforehand for tuberculin testing. Protection therefore needs to be arranged well in advance.

Adults who have not had BCG, travelling to a high-incidence area, may wish to be tested for tuberculin sensitivity and, if negative, have BCG. However there is little evidence that vaccination in adults provides protection.

BCG should not be administered to anyone over the age of 3 months without prior tuberculin skin testing: giving BCG to a tuberculin-positive individual may result in abscess formation.

Therapy for latent tuberculosis infection (LTBI)

There are no UK guidelines for LTBI in travellers. Although not specific on the question of TB prevention in travellers, US policy suggests that tuberculin testing should be undertaken before departure and after returning to an endemic area. If there is evidence of skin test conversion, which could be attributed to infection incurred while travelling to an endemic area, preventive therapy may be advised. However, anti-tuberculosis antibiotics can cause adverse effects, particularly on the liver. This risk increases with age; thus, the risk benefit of LTBI decreases with age.

Though a course of therapy for LTBI may eliminate the current infection it will not prevent subsequent infection: approximately 10 per cent of TB occurs in previously treated individuals. Previous infection or disease does not necessarily provide protection for the future.

HIV positivity

Individuals who know themselves to be HIV positive should avoid risk of contact with TB. If this is unavoidable, primary preventive medication may be taken while in the high-risk area to prevent initial infection, but evidence for effectiveness of this precaution is scarce.

Summary of advice for travellers

For travellers going to an area of high TB endemicity:

- Children who have not had previous BCG should be tuberculin tested and given BCG if the skin test is negative.

- Adults who have not previously received BCG may wish to be tuberculin tested and given BCG, but there is little evidence for efficacy in this situation.

- Anyone with a previous record of BCG and/or evidence of a BCG scar need not have further testing or BCG vaccination.

- In special situations, such as those going to work amongst people likely to have TB, individual advice should be sought.

Further information

Davies, P.D.O., Girling, D., and Grange, J.G. (1996). Tuberculosis. In *The Oxford Textbook of Medicine* (3rd edn) (ed. D.J. Weatherall, J.G.G. Ledingham, and D.A. Warrell), pp. 630–7. Oxford University Press.

Davies, P.D.O. (ed.) (1998) *Clinical tuberculosis* (2nd edn). Chapman and Hall, London.

www.priory.com/cmol/TBpapers.htm

www.tbalert.org

Tetanus

All travellers need to be immunized against tetanus because the risks are widespread and correct treatment following injury may be difficult to obtain overseas.

Dr C. Louise Thwaites is a research registrar at the University of Oxford Wellcome Trust Clinical Research Unit in Vietnam, carrying out research into the treatment of tetanus.

Tetanus is a disease of muscle stiffness and spasms. It derives its name from the Greek word 'tetanos', meaning to contract. It occurs throughout the world and without treatment is frequently fatal. It is preventable through immunization and as a consequence is now rarely seen in the Western world. However, in countries where immunization programmes are inadequate, tetanus remains a major public health problem, responsible for the deaths of over half a million newborn babies every year as well as significant numbers of children and young adults.

In the UK, there are typically around 10 cases each year, with two or three deaths. A small number of cases have occurred following travel.

The organism that causes tetanus is found throughout the world and so travellers are not at special risk of acquiring the disease simply by virtue of being abroad. However, travellers are often more vulnerable to injury, and in many parts of the world may find appropriate treatment unavailable. All travellers should therefore ensure they are correctly immunized before leaving home.

How do you get tetanus?

Tetanus is caused by the bacterium *Clostridium tetani. Clostridium tetani* lies dormant as a spore in the soil. These spores are extremely tough and are resistant to heat, light, drying, and chemicals. They have been found in human and animal faeces, on unsterile surgical instruments, toothpicks, acupuncture needles, and needles for intravenous drug abuse.

Spores enter the body through soil contamination of wounds and minor cuts or via unclean surgical instruments and needles. In newborn babies, soil contamination of the umbilical stump is often the source of infection. Once inside the wound, if conditions are favourable, the spores germinate and the bacteria grow and multiply. *Clostridium tetani* prefers conditions where there are low oxygen concentrations, so deep wounds with a poor blood supply and/or lots of residual dead tissue are especially favourable environments for bacterial growth.

What are the symptoms of tetanus?

Clostridium tetani causes disease by producing a powerful toxin. This toxin spreads through the body in the blood, and is taken up into nerves, where it exerts its effects. A few days or weeks after the initial infection, symptoms begin to occur. The commonest early symptoms are due to stiffness of the jaw muscles causing 'lock-jaw' (inability to open the mouth) and difficulty in swallowing. Neck and back stiffness usually follow shortly afterwards. As the disease progresses, more and more muscles are affected. In very mild forms of tetanus, or in patients who are partially immunized, this may be all that the patient experiences. However, the majority of patients will go on to experience spasms. These spasms may involve all or just some muscles and vary from a brief twitch to a prolonged spasm. They are excruciatingly painful. Spasm of the facial muscles gives rise to the characteristic facial appearance of tetanus — an apparent smile — although, of course, the patient is certainly not smiling. If the spasms involve the muscles of the chest, they may interfere with breathing. In areas where artificial ventilation is not available, asphyxia is the commonest cause of death.

In severe cases of tetanus, the nerves that regulate the heart and blood pressure may be involved, resulting in dangerously high or low blood pressure, or very rapid or alternatively very slow heart rate.

Treatment

Once the tetanus toxin is bound within the nerves there is nothing to be done except to support the patient until its effects wear off. This often requires the full range of intensive care expertise.

Prevention

Tetanus is easily preventable by immunization and careful cleaning of wounds. All people, whether travellers or not, are at risk of contracting the disease and should make sure their vaccinations are up-to-date.

Adequate protection is derived from a primary course of immunization and subsequent boosters. In the UK the primary course consists of three doses of tetanus toxoid at 2, 3, and 4 months of age, usually given in combination with the diphtheria toxoid and pertussis (whooping cough) vaccine. Two boosters of diphtheria and tetanus toxoids are given at 3–5 years of age and at 13–18 years of age. In the USA, the schedule is similar, but with an extra dose at 12–18 months of age, and further tetanus boosters every 10 years. However, in the UK, the standard advice is that five doses (a primary course plus two boosters) are sufficient and that further boosters are needed only if a tetanus-prone wound occurs.

In some areas of the world, however, obtaining vaccine may be difficult, or the vaccine itself may be of poor quality. *Travellers should therefore be advised to have a booster before setting out if they have not had one within the last 10 years* (see also p. 560).

The next step in preventing tetanus is to avoid sustaining tetanus-prone wounds. These include puncture wounds, burns, animal and human bites, wounds contaminated with soil or faeces, fractures with broken over-lying skin, and any wound where treatment is delayed. So it is advisable not to go barefoot and to avoid ear piercing, tattoos, or acupuncture.

If injury does occur, the wound should be thoroughly cleaned with clean water and a mild detergent. Any splinters, foreign material, or dead tissue should be removed. This may require proper medical attention. Particular care should be paid to the tetanus-prone wounds mentioned above.

Revaccination should be considered when any wound is sustained. If the person has received a full course or a booster of tetanus toxoid within the previous 10 years, no further dose is required. If the last dose was more than 10 years ago then a booster should be given. If there is any doubt about any previous immunization or whether a full course was completed, a full primary course should be given. In this case anti-toxin (human tetanus immunoglobulin, or HTIG, 250 units) should also be given for tetanus-prone wounds. Even if the person has had a recent booster within 10 years, anti-toxin may still be given if it is thought that the risk of tetanus is very high.

In parts of the world where HTIG is not available, the older horse serum preparation, SAT, (1500 units) may be substituted. Unfortunately, this preparation causes more allergic reactions.

Summary of advice for travellers

- Tetanus is a potentially fatal disease that can be acquired throughout the world. It can be prevented by immunization and careful wound care.

- All travellers should check that they have received a primary immunization course against tetanus and that they have had a booster injection within the last 10 years. If a wound is sustained and there is any doubt about the vaccination history a booster should be given.

- Any wounds should be thoroughly cleaned. Travellers should seek medical advice about large or contaminated wounds as they may require specific medical treatment.

Further information

Further information about tetanus immunization can be found on p. 560, and can be obtained from the following web-sites plus others listed in Appendix 8.

www.cdc.gov/travel
www.phls.co.uk
www.doh.gov.uk/traveladvice

Diphtheria

Diphtheria is a significant risk for anyone travelling outside western Europe, North America and Australasia. Immunization provides complete protection, but needs to be updated during adult life.

Dr Delia B. Bethell is a paediatrician at the John Radcliffe Hospital in Oxford. She spent four years carrying out research at the Wellcome Trust Clinical Research Unit in Ho Chi Minh City, Vietnam, looking after many cases of diphtheria, the majority in children.

Diphtheria is a serious bacterial infection of the respiratory tract or skin, with potentially life-threatening complications. It is completely preventable by immunization.

In the UK there are now between one and three cases reported each year. Diphtheria is much more prevalent in poorer regions of the world, particularly Eastern Europe, the Indian subcontinent, Southeast Asia, and South America, where it remains endemic. The 1990s saw a major epidemic in countries of the former Soviet Union; this is now being brought under control by means of a voluntary mass vaccination campaign.

Diphtheria is spread by respiratory droplets or secretions and by contact with skin lesions. Carriers of the disease may harbour the organism for prolonged periods of time. In non-immune individuals the bacteria multiply in the upper respiratory tract, most commonly the throat and nostrils, causing intense inflammation and formation of the typical greyish 'pseudomembrane'. At this stage the patient has a high fever, sore throat, and feels very unwell. In severe cases complete obstruction of the airways can occur. The multiplying bacteria release a toxin, which travels through the bloodstream to affect many organs in the body, most notably the heart, kidneys, and nerves. Death from toxin damage can occur several weeks after the patient appears to have made an uneventful recovery.

The diphtheria bacilli may also colonize pre-existing skin injuries and wounds to cause cutaneous diphtheria. Seven of the eight cases of imported diphtheria in the UK between 1993 and 1998 were cutaneous. Common sites are the lower legs, feet, and hands. These infections are usually mild but chronic. They are the major reservoir of diphtheria in tropical countries.

Diagnosis of diphtheria depends on recognizing clinical signs together with culture of the organism from infected sites. Treatment consists of antibiotics (such as penicillin or erythromycin) to eradicate the organism and prevent further toxin production, and anti-toxin. There is good evidence to suggest that the efficacy of anti-toxin is reduced if administration is delayed more than 48 hours after the onset of symptoms. In a person who is unwell, treatment therefore needs to be started before a diagnosis of diphtheria has been confirmed.

Diphtheria and the traveller

Diphtheria is a significant risk to the international traveller. Because of wide disease prevalence all individuals travelling outside Western Europe, North America, and Australasia should be immunized. Serological studies from several countries, including the UK, have shown that up to 50 per cent of adults aged over 20 years are susceptible to diphtheria, with a significant trend of decreasing immunity with increasing age. Older women are least likely to be immune.

All non-immune individuals should receive a primary course of three injections at 1–2-monthly intervals. In children under 8 years this should be standard DTP (diphtheria-tetanus-pertussis) or DT (diphtheria-tetanus). In children over 8 years and adults Td (tetanus-lower dose diphtheria) is used because of a tendency in these age groups towards more severe adverse effects. Newer purer vaccines and lower pre-existing immunity mean that rates of adverse reactions are likely to be much lower than previously documented. Individuals strongly immune to tetanus will experience fewer local reactions if diphtheria toxoid alone is used. There are insufficient data on the duration of protection provided by three doses of Td as opposed to DTP.

Following primary immunization, immunity that is not reinforced by constant natural exposure wanes relatively quickly. There is good evidence that single booster doses of toxoid stimulate a strong immune response in the majority of individuals who have received a primary course of three injections. It is generally accepted that booster doses of Td in adults should be given at a maximum of 10-year intervals (see also p. 560). One study showed that seroconversion rates following a single booster dose of Td in adults aged 20 to 60 years were 45 per cent if no history of immunization was given; 80 per cent if prior immunization was unknown; and 86 per cent if they were definitely previously immunized. Based on available data, at least 70 per cent of adults who receive a booster dose of diphtheria toxoid respond with a protective level of diphtheria antibodies.

Schistosomiasis (bilharzia)

Schistosomiasis is spread by contact with fresh water. Whilst it usually causes only mild or moderate symptoms, it can be an unpleasant disease. Travellers are at risk in many tropical areas.

Dr S. Bertel (a.k.a. 'Bertie') Squire is Senior Lecturer in Clinical Tropical Medicine and Consultant Physician in the Division of Tropical Medicine at the Liverpool School of Tropical Medicine. He was Head of the Department of Medicine, Kamuzu Central Hospital, Malawi, from 1992 until 1995 and maintains close links with the Malawi Ministry of Health and the Wellcome Trust Laboratories at Malawi's College of Medicine in Blantyre.

Schistosomiasis, or bilharzia as it is also called, is present in many tropical countries. It is a grave problem in countries where it is common, because although not a 'killer' disease in the usual sense, it gnaws insidiously at the general health of entire populations. The geographical distribution of the disease is shown in Map 4.1.

At least 200 million people around the world are infected. Although some control successes have been achieved in Asia, the Americas, North Africa, and the Middle East, in other areas numbers of infections are rising rapidly. Ironically, the dams, irrigation schemes, and agricultural projects so necessary for the fight against world poverty and hunger themselves create conditions in which the disease thrives. Schistosomiasis is a special problem in young children: it hinders development and reduces life expectancy. It remains a problem in China despite a nationwide attempt at eradication.

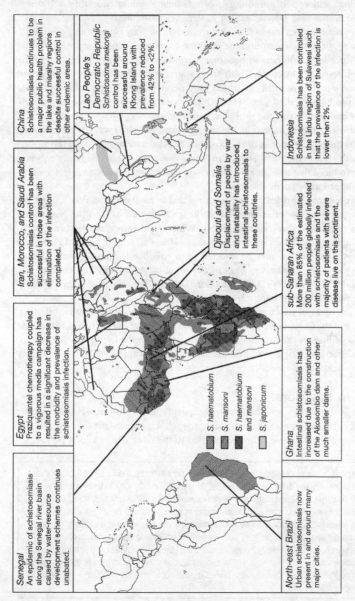

Senegal
An epidemic of schistosomiasis along the Senegal river basin caused by water-resource development schemes continues unabated.

Egypt
Praziquantel chemotherapy coupled to a vigorous media campaign has resulted in a significant decrease in the morbidity and prevalence of schistosomiasis infection.

Iran, Morocco, and Saudi Arabia
Schistosomiasis control has been successful in those areas with elimination of the infection completed.

China
Schistosomiasis continues to be a major public health problem in the lake and marshy regions despite successful control in other endemic areas.

Lao People's Democratic Republic
Schistosoma mekongi control has been successful around Khong Island with prevalence reduced from 42% to <2%.

Djibouti and Somalia
Displacement of people by war and instability has introduced intestinal schistosomiasis to these countries.

Indonesia
Schistosomiasis has been controlled in the Lindu region of Sulawesi such that the prevalence of the infection is lower then 2%.

sub-Saharan Africa
More than 85% of the estimated 200 million people globally infected with schistosomiasis and the majority of patients with severe disease live on this continent.

Ghana
Intestinal schistosomiasis has increased due to the construction of the Akosombo dam and other much smaller dams.

North-east Brazil
Urban schistosomiasis now present in and around many major cities.

■ *S. haematobium*
▨ *S. mansoni*
▤ *S. haematobium and mansoni*
▧ *S. japonicum*

Map 4.1 Global distribution of schistosomiasis

How infection is spread

Schistosomiasis is an infection with one of three kinds of worm: *Schistosoma haematobium* (urinary schistosomiasis), *Schistosoma mansoni* (intestinal schistosomiasis), and *Schistosoma japonicum* (Far Eastern schistosomiasis).

The fully grown worms live in the veins around the urinary bladder and genitals (*S. haematobium*), or the veins around the intestine (*S. mansoni* and *S. japonicum*). The worms produce large numbers of eggs that leave the body through the lining of the bladder or intestines. On contact with fresh water, larvae hatch from the eggs and infect certain varieties of snail, in which they develop further and multiply. More larvae are produced (called *cercariae*), which swim freely in fresh water, actively seeking out and penetrating the skin of a human host.

After burrowing through the skin, the young worms find their way (by an unknown route via the lungs) to the veins of the bowel or bladder once again. The adult worms lay eggs for the rest of their lives, which may be as long as 15 years. So many eggs and larvae are produced that a single infected person passing eggs daily can infect a whole river if the appropriate snails abound.

Water is necessary for drinking and washing, and in rural communities around the world, daily exposure to infection is inevitable from an early age. In the Nile valley, East Africa (especially the coastal regions), West Africa (especially the savannah), along the Euphrates and the Tigris rivers in the Middle East, and in parts of Brazil, the majority of the population may be infected from childhood. Almost all children of school age pass large numbers of eggs in the urine or stool daily, and children are mainly responsible for the spread of infection. Later in life some immunity builds up so that the worst effects of infection may be avoided.

Most of the harmful effects of the disease are due to the eggs; these cause bleeding, ulceration, and the formation of small tumours as they lodge in the tissues around the bladder and genitals or the intestine, or become trapped in the liver and other tissues. Long-term effects include severe liver damage (the eggs cause liver fibrosis), kidney failure, and cancer of the bladder.

Disease in travellers

Expatriates and travellers with no previous exposure to schistosomiasis may become seriously ill in the early stages of an infection, though it is unusual for them to suffer in the same way as local people, who are exposed to the disease over a long period.

Swimmers' itch is an intensified variety of cercarial dermatitis caused by schistosome larvae which die in the skin and do not develop further. This condition can occur in temperate as well as in tropical countries — recent outbreaks have occurred in the USA caused by non-human schistosome species. There have also been reports of cases occurring in salt water, affecting swimmers in Long Island Sound. Some hours after exposure to the water an itching sensation develops on the exposed skin surfaces, followed by a rash composed of small, red, intensely irritant papules which fade after 24 hours. Provided the infecting cercariae are not from a species of schistosome which infects humans (i.e. in a schistosomiasis-free country), no further symptoms occur and no harm results. Anti-histamine tablets (p. 585) or ointment are all that is necessary for treatment (see also p. 90).

A few hours after contact with infected water, there is sometimes tingling of the skin and a slight rash where the larvae enter the body (cercarial dermatitis or 'swimmers' itch). These symptoms subside, but weeks later, once the worms begin producing eggs, a high fever may develop. This may be severe, and may be confused with typhoid or malaria. An increased number of white blood cells (especially of a type called *eosinophils*) appear in the blood, which may give a clue to the true diagnosis — although not many doctors outside the tropics are aware of this. Travellers should always tell their doctor if they think there is a possibility that they may have been exposed to infection.

This acute schistosomiasis, sometimes called 'Katayama fever', does not always occur, and symptoms may be completely absent or no more than a general feeling of lassitude and ill health.

Once the infection becomes established, abdominal pain and blood in the urine or faeces are commonly reported. Genital symptoms caused by S. *haematobium* are rarer but have received increasing attention recently. Some female travellers have presented with small tumours on the vulva or cervix and some infected males report changes in semen consistency or blood in the ejaculate. Occasionally, severe disease, such as kidney obstruction due to obstruction of the ureters or epilepsy due to the lodgement of eggs in the brain, develops several years after the initial infection.

Safe and effective treatment

A safe drug is now available which is effective against all species of schistosomes. Praziquantel tablets are given, usually as a single dose, and side-effects are rare. The limitation of this drug is that it will not heal established scarring (for example in the liver or bladder) when heavy infection has been established for several years. Early recognition and treatment of infection are therefore very important.

Travellers at risk

Travellers to all countries shown on Map 4.1 may be in danger of infection. Especially at risk are those who swim in streams, rivers, or lakes, or who take part in watersports such as water-skiing, wind-surfing, and scuba-diving in freshwater areas; watersports are particularly dangerous because they may involve exposure to surface water over a large area. Activities such as snipe- and duck-shooting and cross-country walking safaris, where streams have to be crossed, are also hazardous.

Some areas are especially risky: the Nile valley, Lake Victoria, the Tigris and Euphrates river systems, and artificial lakes such as Lake Kariba in Zimbabwe and Lake Volta in Ghana (which are both notorious). Even small collections of water far from human habitation can give rise to serious infections since both wild and domestic animals can harbour some schistosome species.

Lake Malawi, which for many years was advertised as schistosomiasis-free, is now acknowledged to be a significant source of infection with both S. *mansoni* and S. *haematobium*, despite the fact that many tour operators and diving centres claim that it is safe. It is true that diving from boats in deep water carries less risk than swimming or snorkelling in shallow coastal water near vegetation with high snail populations. However, *no freshwater exposure in an endemic area is entirely free* of the risk of schistosome infection.

Lakes and waterfalls: look, don't swim

Lake Malawi is one of the fastest-growing tourist destinations in Africa. Scuba-diving, snorkelling, and wind-surfing — in a serene and exotic setting — are among the main attractions. The risk to visitors is made worse by the fact that the people who run these activities almost always insist that the water is safe — a false reassurance that has quickly found its way into guide books and magazines around the world. Cape Maclear, one of the most popular points on the lake, and one that is often claimed to be especially safe, is now known to carry a risk that is nearly three times higher than the risk in other parts of the lake. Between half and three-quarters of people who spend a single day swimming or diving at Cape Maclear can expect to end up testing positive for schistosomiasis. According to one recent study, at least 5000 foreign visitors to Lake Malawi go home with schistosomiasis every year, usually without realizing that they have even been at risk.

One well-documented case involved a 30-year-old Peace Corps volunteer who developed headaches, convulsions, and blindness in one eye; a brain tumour seemed the most likely cause. Only after neurosurgery did tests confirm that he was suffering from schistosomiasis. Three months earlier he had snorkelled for two days at Cape Maclear. In another case, a 26-year-old Peace Corps volunteer developed gradual paraplegia, and a spinal tumour was suspected. At surgery she too was found to be suffering from schistosomiasis; and she, too, had been snorkelling at Cape Maclear.

Elsewhere in Africa, other examples of cases include a research biologist who began passing blood in her urine, six months after a trip to Mali. She had bathed just once during the trip, at a remote waterfall, miles from anywhere. It took a month for her to recognize the symptoms — even though schistosomiasis happened to be the very subject of her own research. And an entire group of 43 Spanish tourists to Mali also came down with schistosomiasis. During the trip, their tour guide had assured them that there was absolutely no risk.

Personal protection

No vaccine is available and none is foreseen in the near future.

Never assume freshwater to be free from bilharzia in any endemic area. Infection can occur on contact with infected water from streams, rivers, and lakes. Even deep water, far offshore, cannot be regarded as safe, and it is dangerous to swim from boats in infected lakes. Salt water and brackish water are, however, safe from schistosomiasis.

Since the larvae die quickly on removal from water and cannot survive drying, quick drying of exposed skin and clothing does offer some protection, provided contact time in the water has been less than five minutes. Water that has been chlorinated or stored in a snail-free environment for 48 hours is safe, since any cercariae present will have died off.

Swimming pools that are snail-free are safe, but care must be taken that any water entering the pool has been treated. Neglected swimming pools can rapidly become colonized with snails. Dams are especially dangerous and invariably become infected within 10 years of construction.

If contact with water cannot be avoided, always observe the following precautions:
- Do not cross streams at points where there is much human contact, such as village river crossings; always cross upstream of a village.
- Wear waterproof footwear when possible.

- Always take particular care to avoid contact with water and remember the risks of animal-contaminated water. Resist the temptation to strip off and swim after a long hot hike. If you cannot resist this temptation, choose a stretch of clear water with a sandy bottom, as little vegetation as possible, and plenty of wave action.

Check-up on return home

It is advisable to have a check-up on return home (see Appendix 7) whether or not suggestive symptoms are present.

In the absence of symptoms

If, after possible or unavoidable exposure in fresh water (such as during canoeing or rafting), there are no symptoms of the kind described above, a check-up about three months after the last possible fresh water exposure is worthwhile. In these cases the simplest and most sensitive screening test is a blood test (ELISA) detecting antibodies. Such antibodies are present in patients who have been infected, but they are not reliably detectable until 3 months have elapsed from the last possible time of infection. Also, the test does not reliably revert to negative following adequate treatment.

A positive antibody test, therefore, does not necessarily indicate a currently active infection. This can be established only through demonstration of viable eggs in the urine or faeces (or, sometimes, semen). Modern egg-concentration methods should specifically be used if there is doubt about the current activity of an infection (for example, in travellers with previous infections). Not all infected travellers, however, will harbour sufficient numbers of worms to produce enough eggs for these to be detected in stool or urine samples.

A white blood cell count is advisable to look for the presence of eosinophilia, which may be a further indicator of infection.

If any of these tests indicate an infection in a person who does not have symptoms, a single course of praziquantel is advised to eradicate the infection and reduce the risks of tissue damage developing in future years.

There is some debate about whether tests to confirm infection are really necessary — why not just have treatment if you think you have been exposed? Unfortunately praziquantel is not always easily available. For example, in the UK it is not licensed and can be provided only on a named-patient basis, in which case evidence of infection is usually required. The alternative practice of swallowing some praziquantel tablets which have been obtained in the country where there has been some risk of exposure is advocated by some. The problems with this approach are:

- The drug quality and effectiveness may not be reliable.
- Praziquantel will clear only mature worms. If it is taken while worms are still maturing (i.e. within 40 days of the last possible exposure), some worms may survive to reach maturity.

If there are symptoms

Acute schistosomiasis ('Katayama fever') can be diagnosed only when other likely causes of fever (e.g. malaria or typhoid) have been excluded. There is no specifically reliable test for detecting schistosomes at this stage of infection. As most acute schistosomiasis is self-resolving and very unlikely to lead to death there will be very few occasions when presumptive self-treatment with praziquantel is necessary. It will be more important to treat for malaria and typhoid, and praziquantel can usually wait until skilled medical advice is at hand.

If there are suggestive symptoms of established infection (such as blood in the urine or stool, or a change in semen consistency), then a combination of available blood, urine, stool (and semen) tests should be carried out in order to establish if schistosomiasis is the cause. If schistosomiasis is confirmed, then follow-up after treatment, to document resolution of symptoms and clearance of eggs from samples, is advised. Once again, established schistosomiasis very rarely poses an immediate threat to life and definitive treatment can wait for authoritative diagnosis.

Research and future prospects for those in endemic regions
Although understanding of the pathology and immunology of schistosomiasis has advanced considerably through research, prospects for a vaccine in the short to medium term are bleak. In the meantime, controlling morbidity with targeted or mass drug treatment (especially in school-age children) is a feasible and effective strategy. Health education and provision of safe water are invaluable and carry benefits beyond those specific to schistosomiasis.

Further information
A range of relevant publications, maps, and information on countries affected is available through the WHO web-site **www.who.int/ctd/schisto/index.html** and its links.

Meningococcal meningitis

Meningococcal meningitis is uncommon in travellers, but can cause sudden and severe illness. Vaccination is a worthwhile precaution for people heading for parts of the world where outbreaks occur, and it is important to be able to recognize the early symptoms of infection so that prompt treatment can be arranged.

Brian M. Greenwood is the Manson Professor of Clinical Tropical Medicine at the London School of Tropical Medicine & Hygiene. He worked for 10 years in Nigeria, and then from 1980 to 1995 was director of the Medical Research Council Laboratories in the Gambia. His main research interests are malaria and infections caused by capsulated bacteria such as the meningococcus.

Meningococcal meningitis is caused by infection with the bacterium *Neisseria meningitidis*, commonly called the meningococcus. The infection is spread from person to person in respiratory droplets produced on coughing or sneezing. In the majority of people who are infected, bacteria are restricted to the nasopharynx (throat), where they cause few or no symptoms. However, such 'carriers' can pass on the infection to others. Patients with meningococcal disease are not particularly infectious, especially once they have started antibiotic treatment. Thus they do not need to be kept in strict isolation and it is safe to visit them without taking special precautions.

In a few unfortunate people, colonization of the nasopharynx is followed by invasion of the bloodstream, giving rise to meningococcal septicaemia. From the blood, bacteria invade many other tissues but especially the membranes surrounding the brain (the meninges), where they cause inflammation and the disease known as meningitis. Why some people develop severe disease whilst others experience only an asymptomatic infection is not known — genetic factors may be important.

Where it occurs

Meningococcal meningitis occurs throughout the world. In Europe and North America, a low background level of infection is augmented from time to time by small outbreaks in which several cases occur in the same community over a short period. Such outbreaks, which often receive substantial publicity, are most frequent in the winter. They rarely involve more that 20 people and large epidemics of meningococcal disease are uncommon in industrialized countries.

The situation in developing countries is different — major epidemics, often involving many thousands of people, occur frequently. Epidemics of meningococcal disease have been reported from many developing countries, but they are especially common in an area of Africa called the 'African meningitis belt', which extends from the Sudan in the east to the eastern part of the Gambia to the west, and from the Sahara in the north to the forested areas of West Africa in the south (see Map 4.2). In this area, epidemics of meningococcal meningitis occur every few years and may be very large. For example, in 1996 around 80 000 cases were reported in Nigeria alone.

African epidemics nearly always start at the beginning of the dry season (around January or February) when it is hot, dry, and dusty and subside during the rainy season (May to October), sometimes to break out again during the following dry season. Why meningococcal disease behaves in Africa in this peculiar way is not fully understood.

In the past there have also been outbreaks in Kenya, Tanzania, India, Nepal, and Brazil, but these have now declined, and several countries (including the USA) have recently stopped recommending vaccination for travellers visiting these countries.

Outbreaks have also occurred among pilgrims taking part in the annual Hajj to Saudi Arabia (who come from all parts of the Islamic world); the Saudi authorities require proof of vaccination from all people making the pilgrimage (see p. 562).

Clinical features

Meningococcal infection is greatly feared because it can strike with such rapidity. Patients who develop the septicaemic form of the disease, characterized by shock, collapse, and unconsciousness, may die within 24 hours of the first appearance of symptoms, while survivors may be left with a permanent disability. Fortunately, such cases are not common.

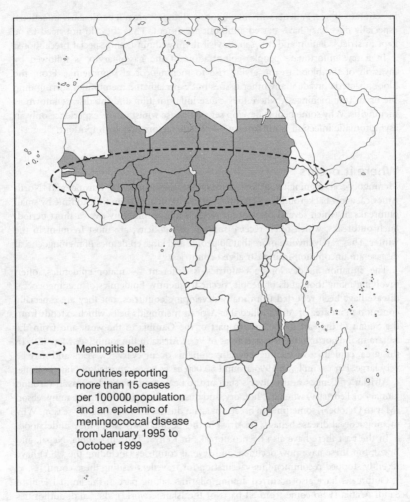

Map 4.2 The African meningitis belt

The first symptoms for most patients are those of meningitis — severe headache, a stiff neck, fever, and pain on looking at bright light (photophobia). A rash that does not 'blanch' with pressure may be an early sign of the infection but this is not always present (pressing the skin with the side of a glass can be a helpful test).

Meningitis should be suspected in anyone with severe headache and photophobia, and medical assistance should be sought urgently. If a doctor suspects meningitis, he may carry out a lumbar puncture — a needle is inserted through the back into the space around the spinal cord, and some cerebrospinal fluid is removed for laboratory examination.

Treatment

Prompt medical assistance can be life saving. If medical help is not available, and a diagnosis of meningococcal meningitis is a serious possibility (for example, in the case of severe headache and photophobia in a traveller visiting an area where an outbreak is in progress), then antibiotics should be taken without waiting for a medical consultation.

Fortunately, the meningococcus is susceptible to many antibiotics, and ampicillin, a cephalosporin, or chloramphenicol could be used, given in the recommended dose (see Table 4.1), until medical assistance can be obtained. Penicillin is probably still the most effective treatment for meningococcal meningitis but this must be given by intravenous or intramuscular injection. In Africa, an oily injection of chloramphenicol (Tifomycine) is often used to treat meningococcal meningitis; it is effective when given as a single injection. Patients with meningitis become dehydrated, so they should be encouraged to drink; they can take painkillers for their headache.

Prevention

The risk of acquiring meningococcal meningitis during a short visit to the African meningitis belt, even if an epidemic is in progress, is small. The risk is a little higher in long-term visitors, especially volunteers living with the local population. However, because meningococcal disease can be fatal and because meningococcal vaccines are safe, vaccination is recommended even when the risk of infection is only small. Thus, it is advisable for all visitors to the African meningitis belt during the dry season, and for visitors to other areas where an epidemic is occurring, to receive meningococcal

Table 4.1   Some treatment options for suspected meningococcal infection (adult doses)

Benzyl penicillin	2.4 g every 4–6 hours, by slow intravenous injection or by infusion. If available, an initial dose of 1.2 g can be given by intramuscular injection immediately the diagnosis is suspected
Cefotaxime	8 g daily in 4 divided doses, by intramuscular or intravenous injection
Chloramphenicol	750 mg every 6 hours, by mouth or intravenous injection. (Or Tifomycine as a single dose)
Ampicillin	If there is no other option, ampicillin capsules could be taken by mouth, at a starting dose of 2 g every 4 hours. (Ampicillin capsules may not be absorbed rapidly enough)

vaccine unless the visit is going to be short and/or restricted to a well-developed urban area. Visitors to the Holy Places in Saudi Arabia must be vaccinated — the ACYW vaccine is currently appropriate for travel to Saudi Arabia, and some parts of Africa, whilst elsewhere, the A+C vaccine will usually suffice.

Travellers who have had their spleen surgically removed (e.g. after trauma to the abdomen) should be immunized even if only passing through the meningitis belt, as their chances of developing meningitis are increased. (They are also at increased risk of malaria — a fact that is not widely realized.)

A single dose of a group A + C (or ACYW) polysaccharide vaccine should be given. This gives protection for at least three years in adults, but is less effective in young children. However, children over the age of one year should still be immunized if they are going to stay in a rural area in the meningitis belt (see also p. 562).

A new group C vaccine that is more effective in young children has been developed, and has been used in the UK with considerable success. Children who have received this vaccine should still have the A + C (or ACYW) polysaccharide vaccine, if appropriate (the commonest cause of meningitis in Africa is group A). Vaccines against the group B meningococcus (which causes the highest proportion of cases in the UK and elsewhere in Europe) are in development, but it is likely to be several years before such a vaccine becomes available.

Protection against meningitis should be considered for travellers to Africa's meningitis belt; and travellers who have had their spleens removed are at special risk of infection.

Legionnaires' disease

Although reports of outbreaks of legionnaires' disease occasionally receive publicity, the risks to travellers are in fact very small.

Professor Christopher Bartlett has been involved in research on legionnaires' disease and related infections since 1977, and has investigated many outbreaks. He was a member of the World Health Organization Working Group on Legionnaires' Disease.

Legionnaires' disease is named after a dramatic outbreak of respiratory illness among delegates attending an American Legion convention in Philadelphia in 1976. Despite exhaustive investigation the cause remained a mystery for nearly six months, until eventually a small bacterium now called *Legionella pneumophila* was shown to be responsible. Subsequent studies showed that the disease was not in fact new, and cases dating back to 1947 have now been identified in retrospect.

The bacterium had escaped recognition because it did not grow on the conventional nutrients used to culture micro-organisms in diagnostic laboratories at that time. *Legionella pneumophila* is found naturally in lakes, rivers, and streams. Surveys have shown that it commonly colonizes hot and cold water systems and cooling waters used for air-conditioning and industrial purposes. Other species of *Legionella* have been discovered in the same types of water environment, but have been shown to cause pneumonia much less frequently than *Legionella pneumophila*.

What is legionnaires' disease?

The principal feature of legionnaires' disease is pneumonia, with fever and cough and often shortness of breath and chest pain as the main symptoms. Diarrhoea or vomiting may also occur in the first few days, and confusion often develops at this stage; a small proportion of victims also develop difficulties with speech and balance.

Legionnaires' disease occurs both sporadically and in outbreaks, and it is the latter that have received the most attention in the media. Although legionnaires' disease is often described as a 'killer' disease, in reality the proportion of fatalities is similar to that seen in many other types of pneumonia.

The infection does not appear to be spread from person to person but is acquired from environmental sources. The investigation of outbreaks has shown that hot water systems in public buildings are an important source of infection and, less commonly, the fine water mist generated by cooling towers has also been implicated. Inadequately treated whirlpools, hot tubs and spas have also been shown to serve as occasional sources of legionella infections. There has been one outbreak from a misting device in a store. The infection is acquired by the inhalation of fine water droplets carrying *Legionella pneumophila*. Drinking water containing the germ is unlikely to cause the infection. Most people are probably in contact with low concentrations of the bacterium quite frequently at home, at work, and elsewhere, but only rarely does this exposure lead to infection.

The diagnosis of legionnaires' disease is not straightforward, because although it is not too difficult to establish that an individual has pneumonia, identification of *Legionella pneumophila* as the cause (rather than any of the other organisms which might be responsible) presents technical problems. Special nutrient media for growing *Legionella pneumophila* from clinical specimens are not used routinely in all diagnostic laboratories. Furthermore, the organism may be present only in very low concentrations in the patient's sputum, and consequently may be difficult to isolate.

The diagnosis can be confirmed by a blood test to detect the specific antibody produced by the patient to combat the infection. With this method, however, it is not possible to make the diagnosis at an early stage of the illness, because at least a week may elapse before measurable levels of antibody appear in the bloodstream. A test has been developed which detects components of the bacterium excreted in urine and this method can confirm the infection a little earlier than the blood test.

Several antibiotics, principally erythromycin and rifampicin, have been shown to be effective in treating the infection. Many doctors now include one such antibiotic in the early treatment of any undiagnosed primary pneumonia to take account of the possibility of legionnaires' disease.

Legionnaires' disease and the traveller

Only about 3 per cent of all primary pneumonias are due to *Legionella pneumophila* and the majority of these are *not* associated with travel overseas.

There have certainly been cases or indeed outbreaks in travellers to many resorts around the world and occasionally on cruise liners. Investigations into outbreaks related to travel have revealed that the hotels' or the ship's water systems have been the source of infection in most cases. Fortunately, growth of *Legionella pneumophila* can be controlled by continuous chlorination of the water or by raising the circulating hot water temperatures to above 50°C. Hotels, other public buildings, and cruise liners should have in place routine maintenance and operation procedures which help to ensure that any growth of the germ is minimized in their water services, including cooling systems and spa baths.

Summary of advice for travellers

Immunization is not available, but most people are probably not susceptible to *Legionella pneumophila*. The infection is readily treatable if the diagnosis is considered by the attending doctor, so if you should develop a chest infection it would be worth mentioning any recent travel to your doctor.

Worm infections from soil contact

Skin contact with soil contaminated by infective worm larvae can lead to localized skin problems or important gut infections.

Dr Richard Knight was a staff member at the London and Liverpool Schools of Tropical Medicine for 18 years. He has worked as physician, epidemiologist, and parasitologist in tropical countries for 17 years. He is now Associate Specialist in General Medicine, with a special interest in gastrointestinal disease, at the Royal Sussex County Hospital in Brighton, Sussex.

Several parasitic worm species have free-living stages in the soil; these are derived from the faeces of infected mammals. New hosts become infected through skin contact, usually the feet or lower limbs, with the soil. Larvae migrate through the skin and enter the circulation to be carried to the lungs, where they ascend the airways to be swallowed and take up residence in the small intestine. The two important human infections acquired in this way are hookworm and strongyloidiasis. Non-human parasites can also infect man; usually these infections are confined to the skin, producing the condition **larva migrans.**

Hookworm

An estimated 1270 million persons are infected with hookworm. There are two species: *Necator americanus* found in the hot humid tropics and *Ancylostoma duodenale* in both warm temperate and tropical areas. The adult worms measure 1 cm in length and live attached to the lining of the small intestine by their powerful jaws; they feed on blood and can live for several years.

Tourists may acquire these infections on visits to rural villages, urban slums, farming estates, and beaches — in fact, anywhere there is soil contamination by human faeces. Adequate footware will prevent most infections but in very wet situations this will not be effective. Skin lesions may resemble larva migrans (see below) but will be transient. During lung migration there may be coughing and wheezing; when worms reach the gut there is upper abdominal pain, sometimes severe enough to mimic peptic ulcer. Later, pains diminish, and if enough worms are present the patient becomes anaemic due to loss of iron resulting from the blood-sucking activity of the worms. Diagnosis is made by finding eggs in stool specimens. Treatment is with mebendazole or pyrantel.

Strongyloidiasis

This is rarer than hookworm but may have serious later consequences for the traveller. Infection is acquired in the same manner as hookworm; adult *Strongyloides stercoralis* measure only 4 mm and live within the epithelium of the upper small intestine; they do not suck blood or cause anaemia. Diagnosis is by finding larvae, not eggs, in stool specimens; most larvae develop in the soil through one generation of minute, free-living adult worms that produce infective larvae. However, freshly passed larvae can also directly penetrate the skin either around the anus or by contact with faecally contaminated soil; the former route leads to self infection which can thus be perpetuated for many years. Some Burma railway prisoners of war infected in 1945 have remained infected for 30 to 40 years.

Symptoms include episodic wheezing, upper abdominal pains, and a rapidly moving form of larval skin migration known as **larva currens** that occurs around the buttocks, lower trunk, and thighs; an abnormal white blood cell count (eosinophilia) is common. Many infections are apparently symptomless. More severe infections cause abdominal bloating, malabsorption, diarrhoea, and even bowel obstruction.

A unique feature of this parasite is internal self infection, when larvae in the faecal stream invade the gut before they reach the anus. This occurs in persons with compromised immune systems and those given steroid and other immunosuppressive treatment, including that given after organ transplants. In this context, numerous larvae in many body tissues can cause very heavy, even fatal, infection. Diagnosis is again by stool microscopy, but blood eosinophilia is absent.

This is a potentially serious infection because of its long duration and reactivation potential. The recommended drug is thiabendazole, but this has unpleasant side effects and can be toxic . A three or five day course of albendazole is a safer alternative but ivermectin, a drug used for river blindness, is being increasingly used.

Larva migrans

Itchy, red, wavy lines appear on the skin and may move several millimetres each day. Blistering and secondary bacterial sepsis are common. Untreated it may persist for many weeks. Common sites are the soles and other parts of the feet, legs, buttocks, or even the trunk or arms — anywhere in fact that comes into contact with infected soil or sand. Beaches above a high water mark, which have been fouled by dogs, and areas under stilt houses are the greatest risk to travellers. Cases occur from tropical and southern Africa, Sri Lanka, Malaysia, Thailand, Atlantic and Gulf coasts of North

America, the Caribbean, and Latin America. At least one dog hookworm, *Ancylostoma caninum,* can reach the human gut and cause eosinophilic enteritis — a serious condition presenting with abdominal pain and vomiting severe enough to warrant exploratory surgery. The Queensland coast is a recognized location for this problem, but it can occur elsewhere.

Treatment is by thiabendazole ointment, made up by a pharmacist to contain 0.5 g of the drug in 10 g of petroleum jelly. Alternatively, migrating larvae can be killed with ethyl chloride spray. Severe infections warrant albendazole tablets by mouth.

Summary of advice to travellers

- Proper footware and care on beaches polluted with human or dog faeces will minimize risks.
- Returning travellers found to be anaemic must always have their stools examined for hookworm.
- Strongyloidiasis must be excluded in former travellers who develop immune defects or receive drugs affecting the immune system.

Leprosy

Leprosy once affected every continent, and still conjures up images of mutilation and social exclusion, but it is a treatable disease and considerable progress has been made towards its elimination. It poses a negligible risk to travellers, and in particular, there is absolutely nothing to fear from people disabled by previous limb damage and scarring.

Dr Diana N.J. Lockwood is a Consultant Leprologist at the Hospital for Tropical Diseases, London; and Senior Lecturer at the London School of Hygiene and Tropical Medicine. She provides a national referral service for leprosy. She has research collaborations with leprosy centres in India, Nepal, and Ethiopia, working on understanding nerve damage in leprosy and improving treatments.

Key facts about leprosy
- It does not develop after a short visit to the tropics.
- It is not spread by touching, kissing, or sex.
- It is curable with antibiotics.
- It may cause permanent nerve damage in sufferers.

The mythology surrounding leprosy has made it a feared disease in many countries. However, it is unusual to contract the disease; it can be cured with antibiotics; and it does not eat away at one's fingers and toes.

What causes leprosy and where does it occur?
Leprosy is caused by the bacterium *Mycobacterium leprae,* an organism very similar to the tuberculosis germ. Untreated leprosy patients cough and sneeze the germ into the

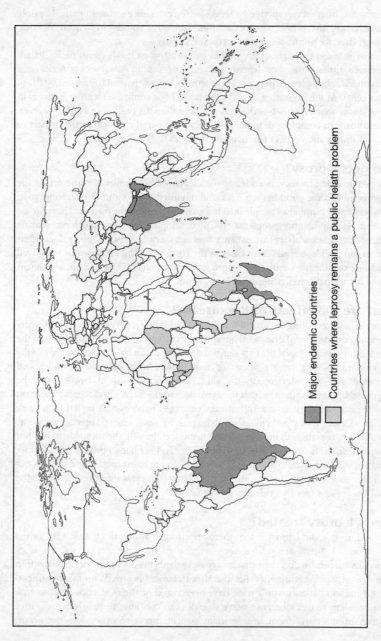

Map 4.3 Global leprosy situation (2002). (Source: WHO Weekly Epidemiological Record, 4 Jan 2002)

Major endemic countries

Countries where leprosy remains a public health problem

environment, where it can survive for weeks before entering another human. The only animals that are susceptible to leprosy are nine-banded armadillos in Central America. However, they are not important in spreading leprosy.

Leprosy is found throughout the tropics and subtropics; it was common in Britain in mediaeval times. Now, most leprosy patients are found in Asia, parts of Africa, and South America. India has 70 per cent of the world's leprosy patients, followed by Brazil (11 per cent). At the beginning of 2000, the number of confirmed leprosy patients in the world was about 750 000 — down from more than 5.3 million in 1985. However, the push towards complete elimination is being hampered by poverty, the impact of HIV, and unrest and conflict (particularly in Africa).

Who gets leprosy?

Most people living in regions endemic with leprosy have probably come across the leprosy germ at some point in their lives, and mounted a good immune response to it; only a very small number of people infected go on to develop the disease. There are no tests that reliably identify people at risk of developing leprosy. Touching, sharing meals, or having sex with leprosy patients does not spread leprosy. Leprosy does occur in Caucasian people, but all recent cases in the UK have occurred in people who lived in endemic regions for a long time (more than eight years). Thus it is not a problem that the occasional traveller needs to worry about.

What are the effects of the disease?

Leprosy has a very long incubation period — anywhere between 2 and 15 years (depending on the type of disease). The leprosy germ lives in the skin and nerves of the arms, legs, and face. One of the first signs of disease are skin patches which are usually pale and numb with no sensation for light touch, heat, or cold. Nodules and infiltration also may develop in the skin. The skin lesions in leprosy may be disfiguring, but it is the damage that the germ does to the nerves that causes long-term problems and disability. As a result of nerve damage, patients may be left with weak muscles, so that they cannot close their eyes, pick up small objects, or walk properly. They also lose sensation in their eyes, hands, and feet, leaving them unable to feel hot or damaging objects. So, a woman cooking will not feel her hand burning and a farmer ploughing will be unaware of a piece of bamboo lodging in his foot. These injuries can rapidly become infected. It is repeated episodes of trauma and infection that cause the loss of fingers and toes that one sees in beggars with leprosy.

How is leprosy treated?

The good news about leprosy is that there are effective antibiotics that kill the germs very rapidly. Patients are treated with either two or three antibiotics, for 6 or 24 months (depending on their disease type). Patients become non-infectious within three days of starting antibiotics. Relapse after treatment is rare. With this treatment, over 8.4 million patients world-wide have been cured of their infection. However, a major problem remains because nerve damage can continue to progress even after effective antibiotic treatment, and in many patients nerve recovery does not occur.

Although they have been cured of their infection, these patients remain at risk of damaging their hands and developing foot ulcers for the rest of their lives.

The stigmatization associated with leprosy also continues, and many patients will conceal their disease even from their close family. In many countries women will be excluded from the family home and even denied contact with their children.

No vaccine specific for leprosy exists, although several trials have shown that BCG vaccine protects against leprosy as well as protecting against tuberculosis.

Leprosy is no longer the feared disease that it was, but it will take decades yet to remove old prejudices. Even though there are now effective antibiotics for leprosy infection, the long incubation period means that new cases will continue to appear for many years to come.

Leprosy is a curable disease with a very low infectivity, and the chances of catching it are negligible. Beggars and other people with overt signs of the disease are not contagious and pose no threat to the traveller.

Anthrax

Although anthrax is most uncommon in travellers, certain handicrafts may be contaminated and should be avoided. Recent use of anthrax as a biological weapon has triggered renewal of interest in, and research into the disease.

Dr Arnold F. Kaufmann is an Expert Consultant, Centers for Disease Control and Prevention, Atlanta, Georgia, USA, and specializes in public health control of anthrax and other infections acquired from animals.

Anthrax is a lethal bacterial disease of livestock that is occasionally transmitted to humans. A disease of considerable historic significance, anthrax occurs or has occurred in virtually every country of the world. It is currently a relatively minor public health problem, even in developing countries, due to the wide use of animal anthrax vaccines. Lapses in local control programmes, however, can have serious consequences, such as the epidemic in the 1990s of almost 10 000 human cases in Zimbabwe. The most frequent victims of this disease are persons closely associated with raising livestock or working in industries processing animal bones, hair, and hides.

How it is spread

Anthrax is caused by *Bacillus anthracis,* a bacterium normally present in various types of soil. The anthrax bacillus has a cyclic pattern of replication, growing rapidly when environmental conditions are optimal and then forming spores to survive adverse periods. These spores are resistant to disinfectants and can remain viable for many years. Animals become infected by grazing on soils where the anthrax bacillus is in its active growth phase.

Human anthrax results not from contact with the soil but from handling the tissues of or products from infected animals.

When an animal dies of anthrax, the important control measure is either to bury or to burn the carcass. Poverty or failure to recognize the cause of death, however, frequently leads animal owners in developing countries to salvage anything of value. The meat may be eaten, and by-products such as bones, skin, and hair sold or used. Anthrax spore contamination of these by-products, which may be made into handicrafts or exported for industrial processing, can become a hazard to people far away.

Forms of anthrax

Human anthrax has three forms — cutaneous (skin), gastrointestinal, and inhalation — and these directly reflect the route of the infection.

Cutaneous anthrax, the most common, results when the anthrax bacillus is introduced beneath the skin (e.g. by a puncture, abrasion, or through a pre-existing break in the skin) while handling contaminated materials. A red, raised area develops at the site of the infection — rather like an insect bite — and characteristically progresses to a large blister, finally becoming an ulcer covered with a dark scab. This form of the disease is diagnosed easily and can be treated effectively with common antibiotics such as penicillin and tetracycline.

Gastrointestinal anthrax results from eating raw or undercooked meat from infected animals, and causes severe abdominal symptoms.

Inhalational anthrax is almost exclusively an occupational respiratory disease, associated with industrial processing of goat hair from western Asia. These last two forms of the disease are difficult to diagnose and are often fatal; however, both are so rare as to be a negligible risk.

Anthrax and terrorism

The anthrax bacillus has recently been used as a weapon by terrorists in the United States. The terrorists placed the bacillus in a powder form into envelopes that were

---

Summary of advice for travellers

- Although cutaneous anthrax may cause severe illness, the disease is only weakly contagious and presents little risk to the average traveller. Only one travel-associated case has occurred in a US citizen in the past 40 years. This patient acquired her infection from a goat-skin handicraft purchased in Haiti.

- Subsequent studies revealed that Haitian handicrafts incorporating dried or poorly tanned goat skins were commonly contaminated with anthrax spores. As a result, rugs, drums, and other handicrafts containing goat skin with attached hair (the spores are found in the hair) are not permitted to be brought into the USA. Another case, not in a traveller, was traced to a coarse goat-hair yarn produced in Pakistan.

- Travellers should not buy any item made of coarse goat hair or goat skin with attached hair in any poor country.

- General commonsense precautions of eating only well-cooked meat and avoiding unnecessary handling of dead animals also apply. Otherwise, no special precautions or immunizations are necessary.

then mailed. Victims were exposed at various points in the mail delivery system and developed either cutaneous or inhalational anthrax. Many persons who were exposed but otherwise healthy, were prescribed a 60 day course of antibiotics to prevent clinical disease. This alarming development does not present a specific threat to travellers and should not result in the need to change travel plans. Specific public health advice will be issued if the situation changes, and can be found at **www.bt.cdc.gov.**

Viral haemorrhagic fevers

Lassa fever and other viral haemorrhagic fevers periodically hit the headlines. Except in special circumstances, however, the risk to travellers is extremely small.

Dr Susan Fisher–Hoch is a virologist and medical epidemiologist at the University of Texas, School of Public Health.

Viral haemorrhagic fevers (VHFs) are 'zoonoses' — infections of animals that only occasionally affect humans. They are caused by viruses of rodents, ticks, or mosquitoes, and some of the most important infections are summarized in Table 4.2. They occur mostly in rural areas, so that infection is usually confined to the more adventurous travellers or those involved in medical care or agricultural, mining, or other projects. Infections in visitors to endemic areas are very rare: most fevers in short-term visitors to endemic areas will be due to common diseases, such as typhoid or malaria, most of

Table 4.2   Viral haemorrhagic fevers

Disease	Virus family	Geographic distribution	Host/vector	Estimated incubation period (days)	Estimates of untreated mortality
Lassa fever	Arenavirus	West Africa	Rodent	7–22	17%
Junin	Arenavirus	Argentina	Rodent	7–14	17%
Machupo	Arenavirus	Bolivia	Rodent	7–14	15%
Guanarito, Sabia	Arenavirus	Venezuela/Brazil	Rodent	7–14	60%
CCHF	Bunyavirus	Africa/Asia	Tick/small mammal	2–9	15–30%
Ebola	Filovirus	Equatorial Africa	?? bats/monkeys	3–10	60–90%
Marburg	Filovirus	Central Africa	?? bats/monkeys	2–21	20–30%
Rift Valley fever	Bunyavirus	Africa/Middle East	Mosquito/ mammals	3–6	?0–50%
Dengue fever	Flavivirus	Africa/Asia/ Central and S. America	Mosquito/human	5–8	0
Yellow fever	Flavivirus	Africa/S. America	Mosquito/ primates	3–7	10–50%
HFRS	Hantavirus	Probably world-wide	Rodent	10–35	2–50%

CCHF = Crimean-Congo haemorrhagic fever

HFRS = Haemorrhagic fever with renal syndrome

which, are eminently treatable and must therefore always be excluded.

Haemorrhagic fevers are diseases of poverty, and most sufferers are local people who have poor housing conditions and little or no access to medical care. Four VHFs — Lassa fever, Ebola, Marburg, and Crimean-Congo haemorrhagic fever (CCHF) — are capable of spreading from person to person, especially in hospitals with poor hygiene conditions or where needles or other equipment is reused. Indeed, it was the high mortality in early hospital outbreaks that led to their fearsome reputation as 'killer' diseases. More recently, several cases of hantavirus pulmonary syndrome have been transmitted case-to-case, but only in South America.

We now know that there are many mild or asymptomatic cases of these fevers and that infection can mostly be avoided by simple, basic hygiene precautions. Effective treatment is now available for some VHFs. Visitors to endemic areas who are likely to put themselves at risk by, for example, living in primitive rural conditions or working in medical facilities, should always inform themselves before travel about viruses they might encounter. Hopefully, they will then be able to avoid infection, and if this should not be possible, will at least know what immediate steps to take if they do fall ill. Physicians treating such travellers need to pay particular attention to exposure history, and be well informed about the endemicity of viruses and the treatment and management procedures they need to follow.

Lassa fever

Geographical occurrence

Lassa fever is found in West Africa, from southern Senegal to the Cameroon, principally in Guinea, Sierra Leone, Liberia, Côte d'Ivoire, Ghana, and Nigeria. Lassa fever is by far the most important VHF transmissible from human to human since very large numbers of cases occur each year in West Africa — probably more than 100 000 infections and 3000–5000 deaths. In 2000, at least four fatal cases of Lassa fever were imported into Europe, three of whom were non-residents of the endemic area, either travelling or working in health- or security-related projects in Sierra Leone.

How infection is spread

Humans are infected from the urine of a local rodent, *Mastomys natalensis* — the multimammate rat — which is larger than a mouse but smaller than the common rat. It infests village homes throughout Africa, though only in West Africa does it appear to carry Lassa virus. The disease is most common in villages in secondary bush areas, though it is also found in savannah areas. Along the coast and in the dry hinterland, Lassa fever is uncommon. The rat is peridomestic and nocturnal, and feeds on unprotected food and refuse in the house, on which it may deposit the virus. Infection can be prevented by enclosing all food in rat-proof containers, and ridding the house of rats.

The illness

The disease has an incubation period of one to two weeks, and the illness lasts about two weeks. During the first week, fever, headache, and other general symptoms develop slowly, and make the illness very difficult to distinguish from a number of common diseases. A severe sore throat is a common symptom, and this, combined with a fever and protein in the urine, is a strong indication of Lassa fever in a person in the endemic area. Many people then recover, and may not know they have been infected; others develop further symptoms, such as vomiting, diarrhoea, and in severe cases, bleeding and circulatory collapse.

The disease can be treated successfully with intravenous ribavirin, if it is started as soon as possible after the onset of symptoms. Any person who knows that they may have been exposed to Lassa fever, either from contact with rodents or patients, who then develops a fever should make sure they receive expert medical treatment as quickly as possible. Ribavirin tablets may also be used to prevent illness in individuals with a known history of exposure to the virus (the dose is 500 mg every six hours for seven days).

The risk to women during the last three months of pregnancy is very high. The baby is usually lost, and the mother may also die, especially if she is being looked after in a hospital where standards of supportive care are poor. Children, on the other hand, appear to have milder infections. Recovery in survivors is usually complete except for the risk of deafness, which is measurable in about 25 per cent of cases. Most deafness resolves but permanent loss of hearing may ensue in one or both ears.

Person-to-person spread is from contact with blood and body fluids. Lassa fever is not spread by the respiratory route, so entering a patient's room carries no risk. It can be spread, however, by sexual contact while the patient is sick or just recovering. Avoiding intimate contact with blood or other fluids from people with fevers is the most important method of avoiding infection in hospitals and clinics. There is no risk of infection from recovered persons.

Despite this knowledge, there continue to be devastating outbreaks and deaths in hospitals in endemic areas, as the result of failure to employ careful disinfection techniques and take measures to prevent blood-to-blood contact, or where surgical facilities are poor. In contrast, more than 1500 Lassa fever patients have been cared for in one rural hospital in Sierra Leone without any cross-infection, simply by disinfecting with chlorine solutions and using gloves that are disinfected and washed before reuse. In the 1990s, deteriorating political conditions in Liberia and Sierra Leone led to increased numbers of cases.

International spread

The rural areas where the disease is endemic are within reach of international airports, and the incubation period is long enough to allow ample time for displacement of infected persons before illness appears; cases have been imported into Europe and North America.

Since 1970 there have been two documented importations of Lassa fever to the USA, one of whom died; more than 10 cases imported to the UK; and one each to Canada, Australia, the Netherlands, Israel, and Japan, none of whom died. Unfortunately, a patient who died of Lassa fever in the USA in 1989 visited four emergency rooms before he saw anyone who was aware that he had recently returned from Nigeria or who knew that Lassa fever was endemic there, and that it could be treated.

It is therefore essential for travellers who fall sick to make sure their physicians have all details of travel and possible exposure to viruses, and that Lassa fever should be considered as a possible diagnosis. Simple infectious disease precautions for the care of patients in regular isolation rooms are recommended, using gloves, gowns, masks, and strict disinfection*. Patient isolators ('bubbles') are no longer considered necessary or desirable.

Prospects for a vaccine
Though an experimental vaccine has been developed and successfully tested in animals, there are currently no plans for development of human vaccines, mainly because of the high cost involved.

South American haemorrhagic fevers
At least three, possibly four, haemorrhagic fevers are recognized in South America: Junin in Argentina, Machupo in Bolivia, Guanarito in Venezuela, and Sabia in Brazil. Recently there have been reports of two possible cases of haemorrhagic fever due to a related arenavirus in North America. These diseases are caused by rodent arenaviruses (which are related to and closely resemble Lassa virus). Outbreaks are focal, and mostly involve farmers and local people in clearly defined areas coming into contact with field rodents. Most cases are therefore male agricultural workers. Little or no person-to-person spread has been reported, and no cases have been recorded in travellers.

Treatment with immune plasma and ribavirin is recommended for Junin virus infection. A vaccine for human use has been shown to be effective in Argentina.

Marburg and Ebola viruses
Marburg and Ebola viruses are related to each other. Primary human cases are extremely rare, and the reservoir in nature is not known, though in some instances monkeys may be involved in transmission. Bats have been suggested as the source, but this is not proven.

Marburg disease was first recognized in 1967, when there were 32 cases and 7 deaths in laboratory personnel working with African green monkeys recently imported to Germany from Uganda — hence the popular name 'Green monkey disease'. In 1976, simultaneous outbreaks of a lethal haemorrhagic fever, Ebola, occurred among humans in Zaire and Sudan, and another in 1979 in Sudan. These outbreaks were associated with needle sharing and poor hygiene in remote clinics and hospitals. In the 1990s, a large outbreak in the Republic of Congo (in the town of Kikwit) and two outbreaks in Gabon demonstrated the ongoing hazard of this virus. Isolated cases have also been reported in the Ivory Coast. Small outbreaks and single cases of Marburg disease continued to occur in East, Central, and southern Africa. Two were visitors to a single cave in Kenya, and one was a hitchhiker in Zimbabwe. More recently, ongoing

---

* Further details of procedures and advice on care and treatment can be found in the CDC publication: *Morbidity and Mortality Weekly Report*, 1988, Volume 37, Supplement 3 (**www.cdc.gov/mmwr/ preview/mmwrhtml/00037085.htm**)

cases of Marburg diseases have been reported in miners working illegally in gold mines in rebel-held territories in the eastern Republic of Congo. A large outbreak of Ebola haemorrhagic fever in Uganda at the end of 2000 resulted in more than 300 cases and over 150 deaths. Transmission in these recent and current outbreaks has been in hospitals and in villages. As with Lassa fever, unstable political conditions and rebel activities are heavily implicated in the spread of disease.

In 1989, monkeys infected with a virus related to Ebola were imported into the USA; many of them became sick and died. The source of this virus has also not been found, but it is clear that this Asian strain does not cause disease in humans.

The illness

Both Ebola and Marburg disease have an incubation period of less than one week, and have a very sudden, violent onset with rapid deterioration, bleeding, and shock. Like Lassa fever, patients may have a severe sore throat. No imported cases have ever been seen outside Africa. Unfortunately, there is currently no specific treatment. Recovery, in survivors, is complete.

Crimean–Congo haemorrhagic fever (CCHF)

CCHF is widely distributed throughout Africa, parts of southern and Eastern Europe, the Middle East, and Asia. Human cases are not common, but are associated with close contact with animal blood or infected humans, or with tick bites. Thus animal herders in dry areas, farmers, slaughterhouse workers, butchers, and people sleeping or working on tick-infested ground may be infected. Hospital outbreaks have been associated with high mortality, but were again invariably associated with unhygienic practices, including mouth-to-mouth resuscitation, or ill-advised surgery on a febrile patient. Good nursing techniques and care with blood and needles is sufficient to prevent transmission. Cases continue to be reported, particularly from areas of Pakistan bordering Afghanistan, where it is clear that outbreaks are not uncommon. See also p. 163.

The illness

CCHF has a very short incubation period, as little as three days, and a very sudden onset with violent headache, fever, and body pains. Patients may then bleed, and a small number may die.

CCHF may be successfully treated with ribavirin. Vaccines have been made in China and in Bulgaria, but these are not generally available, and there are no data on efficacy or safety of these mouse-brain vaccines.

Prevention is best assured by avoiding ticks and intimate contact with blood from animals or infected people. Oral ribavirin may be used to prevent illness in people who have been exposed.

Hantaviruses

These viruses are very common in parts of Asia, particularly China, where thousands of infections each year were recorded in the late 1980s, with major economic impact. In

China, the disease is seasonal, occurring mostly in the early summer and autumn. It is caused by a family of viruses of small field rodents, voles, and rats, which excrete the virus in the urine. There are rural and urban forms depending on the host rodent. Mortality in the rural disease may be as high as 15 per cent, but death is rare in the urban and European hantavirus diseases. The viruses are present throughout the former Soviet Union and most of Europe, so these are not diseases of exotic or tropical places. This is the same disease as Korean haemorrhagic fever, which affected 3000 United Nations troops in Korea during the war in the 1950s, and is closely related to an old disease in Scandinavia called nephropathia epidemica. A virus causing severe disease has been described in the Balkans.

During the 1990s we became aware of a hantavirus disease with even higher mortality (50 per cent) in North and South America, causing hantavirus pulmonary syndrome (see below). The viruses causing this syndrome are found in rodents in rural areas, and infections are therefore most common in people travelling, living, or working in rural areas.

The illness

The clinical picture is slightly different from the other VHFs, in that the incubation period may be two or three weeks and the onset is slow. Some patients may experience brief kidney failure and a very few, bleed and may die. Most make a complete recovery. Treatment with ribavirin may be effective, but must be started early in disease.

Hantavirus pulmonary syndrome is somewhat different again, in that patients usually present very acutely ill with severe pulmonary oedema, resembling adult respiratory distress syndrome. Renal involvement is less common. There have been reported cases of human-to-human spread in South America, involving at least one HIV-infected person.

Prevention

Avoidance of contact with rodent urine, directly or in dust, is the most important preventive measure. Again, these are diseases of poverty, though paradoxically, increased rural prosperity in China in the 1980s allowed expansion of rodent populations, resulting in increasing human epidemics. More recently, however, improvements in housing conditions in China appear to be associated with diminished incidence. Person-to-person spread has not been reported except with the South American virus. Vaccines are under development in China and in the USA, and have been applied in China, but satisfactory efficacy and safety data are not available.

Yellow fever, dengue, and Rift Valley fever

The viruses that cause these haemorrhagic fevers are spread by mosquitoes. Dengue is discussed in greater detail on p. 156, and yellow fever is discussed further on p. 160. Yellow fever is the oldest and one of the most severe of the haemorrhagic fevers, but there is a safe and effective vaccine. Vaccines for dengue are showing promise in clinical trials, but are not generally available at the moment. In most adults the disease is self-limiting and seldom serious.

Rift Valley fever is confined mainly to animals, though there have been two large human outbreaks in Egypt and Mauritania; in 2000 there was a large outbreak in southern Saudi Arabia. The disease is usually mild, but occasional severe cases do occur. There is an animal vaccine, but no special recommendations for protection of humans, beyond protection from mosquito bites.

Conclusion

VHFs are not viruses of humans. In fact, they are far less insidious and less lethal than HIV infection, which they resemble in their capacity for blood transmission, especially in hospitals. Like HIV, with some basic knowledge it is normally possible to avoid infection. Unlike HIV, recovery is complete within a month or two of infection, and fully effective treatment may be available. Human infection is accidental and, with care, can be avoided.

Medical staff planning to care for or be in contact with patients in areas endemic for VHFs may be at special risk. They should seek additional, thorough briefing about the fevers they may encounter in the area they are planning to visit, and ensure they understand the symptoms of the disease and appropriate protective measures and therapy. Veterinary personnel should also obtain relevant detailed information on areas they may visit.

5 Diseases spread by insects

Malaria

Malaria is the tropical disease most likely to cause severe illness or death in the modern traveller. Malaria causes an enormous amount of illness and death throughout the tropical regions of Africa, Asia, Latin America, and Oceania, where, as a single infective cause of death, it lags behind only measles, tuberculosis and HIV. The risk to travellers can be virtually eliminated by reducing exposure to infective mosquito bites and by using appropriate anti-malarial drugs.

Professor David A. Warrell is Professor of Tropical Medicine and Infectious Diseases and Founding Director of the Centre for Tropical Medicine (Emeritus), University of Oxford; Honorary Clinical Director of the Alistair Reid Venom Research Unit at the Liverpool School of Tropical Medicine; and a consultant to the WHO, the Royal Geographical Society, the British Army, and the Medical Research Council.

- If you want to know about **treatment of malaria**, turn to p. 139
- If you need advice on **malaria prevention**, turn to 'Prevention of malaria in traveller,' p. 144
- If you want to understand why malaria is such an important global problem, and such a serious hazard for travellers, read on!

The global problem

Malaria occurs throughout the tropics except in the Pacific Islands east of Vanuatu (see Map 5.1). It is the most important human parasitic disease in the world, resulting in 300–500 million clinical cases each year and causing more than two million deaths. More than 40 per cent of the world's population, in over 100 countries — more than 2400 million people — are at risk.

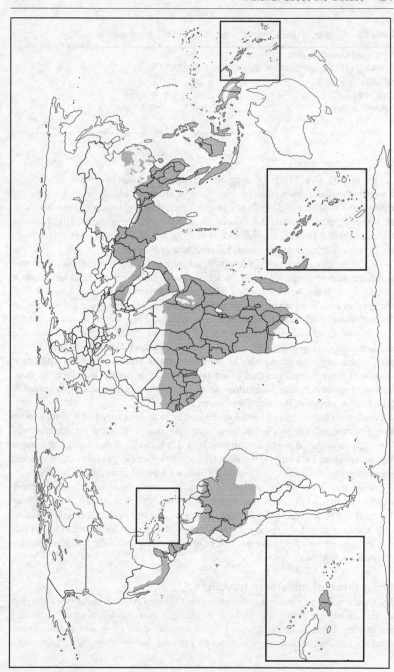

Map 5.1 Global distribution of malaria (reproduced courtesy of the WHO).

Table 5.1 Countries in which malaria remains fully sensitive to chloroquine

Mexico and Central America, northwest of the Panama Canal
The island of Hispaniola (Haiti and the Dominican Republic)
Paraguay
Egypt, Iraq, Syria
Turkey (*P. vivax* only)
Azerbaijan and Tajikistan

The WHO's world-wide programme of malaria eradication began in 1957: it eliminated malaria from Europe and some Caribbean islands and dramatically reduced the numbers of cases in the Indian subcontinent. However, there has since been a resurgence of malaria throughout most of Asia, and the spread of drug-resistant malaria (Table 5.1) from original foci in Colombia and Thailand is an increasingly important contributor to the global toll of illness and death.

The frequency and severity of infection in different age groups varies greatly from one malarial region to another. Frequent infective mosquito bites throughout life produce sustained immunity, so that infected adults may ultimately feel completely well even though they have malaria parasites in their bloodstream. However, young children may develop severe, fatal malaria before this immunity has been acquired, which explains why, in parts of sub-Saharan Africa, malaria accounts for 25–50 per cent of all deaths in children under 5 years old; a million children may die of this infection each year. In other parts of the tropics, infection may be too infrequent to create and sustain immunity: climatic or other changes can then precipitate epidemics of malaria in vulnerable, non-immune populations, with devastating effects. Such epidemics have recently occurred in Sri Lanka, Madagascar, Rajasthan, and north eastern Kenya.

People who have acquired hard-won immunity to malaria may lose it if they move away from the endemic area for anything more than a couple of years. This explains why West African or Indian migrants who have settled in Britain may develop severe malaria when they return for a visit — there are typically 500 such cases every year. In women, pregnancy, especially a first pregnancy, can cause a lapse of immunity to malaria.

For the traveller from non-malarious countries outside the tropics, however, there can be no question of immunity to malaria, even after a few attacks of the disease. Vulnerability to severe, life-threatening malaria is increased in travellers who have had their spleen removed as a result of an accident or as treatment for some blood diseases and in those whose spleens are not functioning normally following radiotherapy (for example, in Hodgkin's disease).

Importance of malaria in travellers

For the 30 million or more travellers who visit malaria endemic countries each year from non-tropical countries, malaria is the infection most likely to cause life-threatening illness or death. In the UK, about 2500 cases of imported malaria are officially reported each year, more than 60 per cent due to *Plasmodium falciparum*.

Malaria life cycle and transmission

The malaria parasite is called *Plasmodium* — four different species commonly infect humans: *Plasmodium falciparum, P. vivax, P. ovale, and P. malariae.* (Rarely, humans can also become infected with ape and monkey malarias.)

Infection occurs when a female *Anopheles* mosquito bites a human to take a blood meal. She injects sporozoites into the bloodstream. These travel rapidly to the liver and, in the liver cells or hepatocytes, the parasites divide and mature; after one to three weeks (depending on the species), merozoites are released into the bloodstream and invade red blood corpuscules (erythrocytes). In the case of *P. vivax* and *P. ovale*, some of the sporozoites remain dormant in the liver cells as hypnozoites. These are not vulnerable to the drugs usually used for prevention, and are capable of coming back to life and causing relapsing attacks of malaria, months or even years later. *Plasmodium falciparum and P. malariae* have no resting phase in the liver, but in the case of *P. malariae* merozoites may persist in the bloodstream for long periods to give rise to recrudescent attacks of malaria.

The merozoites released from the liver invade circulating erythrocytes, in which they develop from early 'ring-shaped' forms to fatter (trophozoites) containing black pigment (digested haemoglobin) and finally multinucleated schizonts, which rupture the enclosing erythrocyte. A new generation of merozoites is released which can infect more erythrocytes but cannot reinvade the liver.

At the moment of schizont rupture (schizogony or merogony), a malarial pyrogen or toxin is released that sets in train a series of reactions responsible for the violent fevers, chills, and shivering attacks which characterize a classic attack of malaria. Towards the end of the infection, some intra-erythrocytic parasites develop into the sexual forms, male and female gametocytes, which are taken up by mosquitoes during a blood meal. Inside the mosquito's gut, a sexual cycle of fusion is completed, resulting in the sporozoites which will infect a new human host when the mosquito feeds again.

(Official reports usually *underestimate* the scale of a problem.) Over the last 10 years, the number of fatal cases of imported malaria has ranged from 4 to 16 per year, increasing over the past three years (Fig. 5.1). Each year, a similar number of cases of malaria are imported into France, more than 1000 into the USA, and about 700 each into Germany and Australia. Malaria has also been identified among infectious causes of death in American and Australian travellers overseas.

The malaria parasite has a complicated life cycle, which is described in the box above and summarized in Fig. 5.2. During the cycle, each 'stage' of the parasite has entirely different behaviour and susceptibility to drugs. For travellers at risk of malaria, some key practical implications of the life cycle are:

1. The shortest period between an infective mosquito bite and the onset of symptoms of malaria is seven days for *P. falciparum* and longer for other species. This means that *a fever developing less than seven days after arrival in a malarious region cannot be caused by malaria acquired there.*

2. The time from an infective mosquito bite to the emergence of parasites from the liver into the bloodstream can be up to about four weeks; most prophylactic anti-malarial drugs act only on blood-stage parasites, so *these drugs must be*

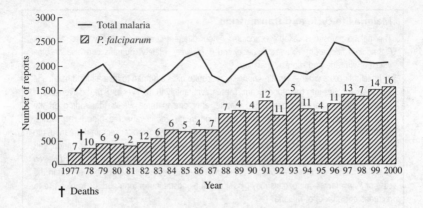

Fig. 5.1 Number of malaria cases reported to the Public Health Laboratory Service Malaria Reference Laboratory 1977–2000; and fatality rates from *P. falciparum* infections. Data reproduced by kind permission.

continued for at least four weeks after the last possible exposure to malaria if they are to be effective (Malarone is an exception — see below)

3. To eradicate hypnozoites of *P. vivax* and *P. ovale* from the liver and so prevent malaria relapses, a different drug (primaquine or tafenoquine) must be taken. (This is important mainly for people who have had prolonged, high-risk exposure or who are known to have suffered from these types of malaria.)

Malaria mosquitoes

The females of many different species of *Anopheles* mosquitoes can transmit malaria. They are distinguished from other mosquitoes by the way the body is angled up from the surface of the skin when they are taking their blood meal (Fig. 5.3). *Anopheles* mosquitoes lay their eggs on fresh or brackish water, where their larvae develop. Malaria-transmitting mosquitoes bite in the evening and night, indoors or outdoors, and these are therefore the most important times for protection against bites (see below).

Although malaria has been eliminated from Europe, several species of *Anopheles* mosquitoes capable of transmitting the infection exist in European countries, including Britain.

Malaria transmission

The vast majority of cases of malaria result from bites by infected mosquitoes in the malaria endemic areas of the world. However, infected mosquitoes can be transported, for example by aircraft, to temperate countries where they may survive long enough to bite and infect local people. This explains the occasional cases of 'airport malaria' affecting people who work in or live around busy international airports such as Schipol, Amsterdam, or Gatwick. If the climate is right and appropriate species of

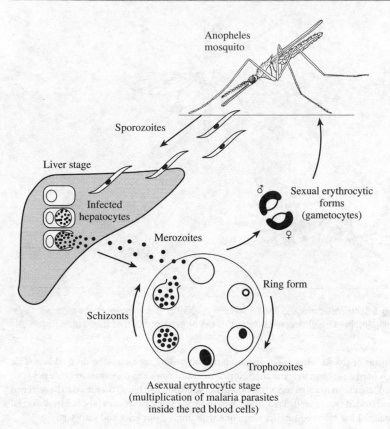

Fig. 5.2 Malaria life-cycle.

Anopheles mosquitoes are available, small outbreaks of locally transmitted malaria may result, and this has happened in New York and California (this is called autochthonous' malaria). Aircraft travelling from one non-malarious country to another may stop for a while, *en route*, in a malaria endemic area. The aircraft may stop on the tarmac with its doors open for long enough, to allow a local infected mosquito to enter the cabin and infect a passenger. This has been called 'runway malaria'. (Aircraft spraying or 'disinsection' is supposed to prevent this.) The phenomenon of 'suitcase malaria', following accidental transportation of mosquitoes in luggage, has also been reported.

Non-mosquito transmission

Blood forms of malaria can be transmitted directly, without mosquito bites, in transfusions of blood and blood products and transplants of bone marrow and other

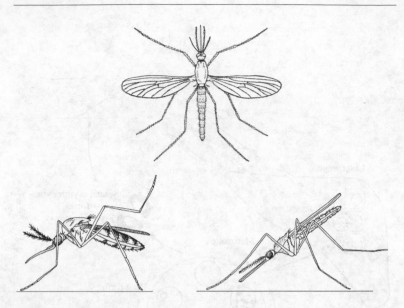

Fig. 5.3 Anopheles mosquito (female) (4–6mm long) – top. Resting positions of mosquitoes: Culex (left); Anopheles (right). Anopheles mosquitoes can be recognized by their characteristic posture.

organs or tissues. Malaria has also been transmitted by needle among drug addicts. This has been a problem in some large North American cities and continues in countries such as Vietnam. In malarial regions, blood donors and donated blood may need to be screened and treated (see p. 589). Transmission of malaria among patients in hospital (nosocomial malaria) has followed careless technique with intravenous lines and catheters.

Malaria — the disease

Except in those who have acquired immunity, infection with any of the four species of human malaria will cause fever, aches and pains, and other generalized symptoms, sometimes in particular patterns. Falciparum malaria, caused by *P. falciparum,* used to be known as 'malignant tertian malaria' — malignant because it was potentially fatal; tertian because spikes of fever might occur every third day (the asexual erythrocytic cycle takes about 48 hours). Vivax and ovale malarias, caused by *P. vivax* were called 'benign tertian malaria' — benign because they rarely kill anyone; tertian for the same reason as in falciparum malaria. *Plasmodium malariae* infection has been known as 'quartan malaria' because the spikes of fever might occur every fourth day (the asexual erythrocytic cycle takes about 72 hours).

All four species of malaria cause similar symptoms initially. However, *P. falciparum* multiplies much more rapidly than the other species and the infected erythrocytes can block small blood vessels in the brain (leading to '*cerebral* malaria'), placenta, and other vital organs, so reducing their blood supply. As a result, *P. falciparum* can cause a very severe disease, rapidly involving a number of vital organs.

The attack of malaria

Most travellers with falciparum malaria become ill within one month of leaving the malarious area. In a few, the illness may be delayed for a year or longer. Other kinds of malaria can take even longer — 10 per cent of infections with vivax malaria do not appear until more than a year after the person has returned home.

Most attacks of malaria start suddenly. The patient feels unwell and feverish with headache (often severe), aches and pains (including backache and pain in the muscles), mild nausea, and loss of appetite. Symptoms often mimic those of 'flu' but without the running nose and sore throat of true influenza. Severe teeth-rattling, bed-shaking chills, followed over the space of a few hours by high fever, profuse sweating, and exhaustion are classic features of the malarial paroxysm. Other symptoms include a dry cough, dizziness, or faintness (especially on attempting to stand up), nausea, vomiting, stomach ache, and diarrhoea. Most travellers will feel too ill, weak, and exhausted to get out of bed while the attack is on.

Signs of the infection, other than a high temperature (sometimes exceeding 40°C, 104°F) include paleness of the skin, nailbeds, tongue, and eyes, resulting from the destruction of infected erythrocytes (anaemia); jaundice (yellowness of the whites of the eyes), resulting from the breakdown of excessive amounts of blood pigment (haemoglobin) released from the destroyed erythrocytes; and an enlarged, tender spleen (felt under the left side of the rib cage).

Severe disease

In the case of falciparum malaria, severe complications can start within 24 hours of the first symptom, though usually a few days later. Cerebral malaria may begin dramatically with a generalized seizure or convulsion (like an epileptic fit), after which the victim remains deeply unconscious. In other cases it can come on more gradually and the patient sinks slowly into coma. Even with effective treatment, the patient may not wake up for several days. Other severe complications of falciparum malaria are: profound anaemia, bleeding, deep jaundice (partly the result of liver damage), low blood sugar (as in a diabetic who has taken too much insulin), and low blood pressure with shock, kidney failure, fluid leaking into the lungs (pulmonary oedema), and a complicating additional infection with bacteria (septicaemia).

Blackwater fever (famously depicted in the movie 'Out of Africa') is a rare complication of falciparum malaria, in which blood pigment (haemoglobin), released after massive destruction of erythrocytes, is passed in the urine which becomes 'coca-cola' coloured or black.

Survival and long-term complications

Even with the best modern medical care, about *1 out of 10 people who develop severe forms of falciparum malaria will die.* Most of the survivors will recover completely, even if they have been unconscious with cerebral malaria for several days; but as many as

1 in 20 of the African children who survive an attack of cerebral malaria will be left with permanent brain damage.

Rare complications of an attack of falciparum malaria are transient psychiatric disturbances ('malarial psychosis'), often attributable to medication, and a transient disturbance of balance associated with jerky movements of the eyes (post-malarial cerebellar ataxia). In rare cases, especially in Africa and New Guinea, there can be long-term immunological damage to the kidney or massive enlargement of the spleen. Repeated attacks of falciparum malaria in combination with Epstein–Barr virus (the virus that causes mononucleosis, or glandular fever) can trigger a malignant tumour (Burkitt's lymphoma).

How to recognize a malaria attack

There is no symptom or sign that is absolutely specific, so malaria must be considered, ruled out, or assumed and treated in any traveller who develops an acute feverish illness after visiting a malarious country, especially if the illness develops within three months of return. Many different infections can start with headache, shivering, chills and fevers — especially pneumonia, viral hepatitis, and ascending infections of the bile ducts in the liver (cholangitis) and urinary tract (pyelonephritis). If malaria is not considered as a possible cause of a feverish illness in a traveller, the symptoms may be mistakenly attributed to another infection and valuable time may be lost in confirming the diagnosis and starting life-saving treatment.

Confirming the diagnosis of malaria

Confirming the diagnosis requires medical and technical skills that may not always be available. The most reliable method is microscopic examination of a film or smear of blood made on a glass slide, dried, fixed with strong methyl alcohol, and treated with a special stain (such as Giemsa or Wright's stains). If there are many parasites in the blood (heavy parasitaemia) they can be found quickly and easily even in a standard thin film. In the case of scanty parasitaemias, which are usual with *P. vivax, P. ovale,* or *P. malariae* infections, a much thicker film is examined. An experienced, skilled microscopist can detect as few as 5 parasites per ml (0.0001 per cent parasitaemia) in a

---

Dangerous misdiagnoses

- Fever and jaundice might suggest viral hepatitis.
- Fever with severe headache and a stiff neck might suggest meningitis.
- Fever and headache followed by loss of consciousness might suggest viral encephalitis.
- Fever, stomach ache, and bowel disturbances might suggest typhoid.
- Fever with bleeding might suggest a viral haemorrhagic fever (e.g. yellow fever, Lassa fever, Ebola/Marburg disease).
- Fever, stomach pains, and profuse diarrhoea might suggest travellers' diarrhoea or even cholera or dysentery.

None of the tests or treatments for these conditions will detect or cure a bout of malaria. Many deaths in travellers have resulted from a mistaken diagnosis.

Beware! Some common medical pitfalls

- Do not rule out the possibility of malaria just because the traveller was taking anti-malarial drugs — no drug is 100% effective.

- Do not be put off the diagnosis of malaria by misleading symptoms such as stomach pains and diarrhoea, or if the thermometer temperature is normal on one occasion.

- Beware of unusual types of exposure such as 'runway malaria', 'transfusion malaria', and 'needlestick malaria'.

- Do not be put off the diagnosis of malaria because the traveller was born or brought up in a malarious country and is therefore assumed to be immune.

- If one person develops malaria after a family/group holiday, check on the other members in case they have early symptoms of infection.

- Always regard malaria in a non-immune traveller as a *medical emergency*; the interval between the first symptom and death may be less than 24 hours.

- If the symptoms or signs are consistent with severe malaria, start treatment immediately, even if laboratory confirmation is not possible or tests are negative.

---

thick film and 200 per ml (0.004 per cent parasitaemia) in a thin film.

New dipstick methods are now available which are almost as sensitive as microscopy and are specific for *P. falciparum,* but require less skill to use. One of the first, the ParaSight F dipstick antigen-capture assay, involves a monoclonal antibody to detect *P. falciparum* histidine-rich Protein-2 (PfHRP-2) antigen. If these tests are initially negative, they should be repeated every 4–6 hours as the numbers of parasites in the blood may fluctuate.

A routine full blood count may show a reduced haemoglobin concentration or haematocrit, a reduced platelet count (thrombocytopenia), and a normal, low, or increased white blood cell count. The serum bilirubin concentration and levels of serum enzymes (such as lactic dehydrogenase and alanine and aspartate amino-transferases) may be moderately raised. The erythrocyte sedimentation rate (ESR) and C reactive protein (CRP) may be grossly elevated.

If you develop malaria while abroad, you should bring home the results of any tests and, if possible, a blood film confirming the diagnosis; these might be helpful if you develop further symptoms.

Treatment of malaria

Treatment with anti-malarial drugs should be started as soon as possible. Those who are not vomiting and are able to swallow and retain tablets can be given anti-malarial drugs by mouth (Table 5.2). Otherwise, treatment must be given by injection, by intravenous drip, or in some cases, by rectal suppositories. Chloroquine is the drug of choice for the 'benign' malarias caused by *P. vivax, P. ovale,* and *P. malariae* and also for malaria definitely acquired in countries where the parasites are still fully sensitive to chloroquine (see Table 5.1).

Table 5.2   Treatment: Anti-malarial drugs for treating adults or children who can swallow tablets

Treatment for chloroquine-resistant *P. falciparum* or mixed infection or species of unknown origin

1. Quinine

Adults:	600 mg of quinine salt (usually quinine sulphate) 3 times each day for 7 days (Note a)
Children:	Approx. 10 mg of quinine salt per kg body weight 3 times each day for 7 days

or

2. Mefloquine (Lariam)

Adults:	1.5 g of mefloquine base given as 2 doses 6–8 hours apart (usually 6 tablets in total)
Children:	25 mg of mefloquine base per kg body weight given as 2 doses, 6–8 hours apart

or

3. Fansidar (sulfadoxine 500 mg per tablet + pyrimethamine 25 mg per tablet)

Adults:	3 tablets as a single dose
Children:	<1 year, $\frac{1}{4}$ tablet; <5 years, $\frac{1}{2}$ tablet; < 9 years, 1 tablet; <15 years, 2 tablets

or

4. Malarone (proguanil 100 mg per tablet + atovaquone 250 mg per tablet)

Adults:	4 tablets once daily for 3 days
Children:	10–20 kg, $\frac{1}{4}$ adult dose; 20–30 kg, $\frac{1}{2}$ adult dose; 30–40 kg, $\frac{3}{4}$ adult dose

Treatment for chloroquine-sensitive *P. falciparum*, or *P. vivax*, *P. ovale* or *P. malariae* (see Table 5.1)

1. Chloroquine

Adults:	600 mg of chloroquine base (equivalent to 4 x 200 mg tablets of chloroquine sulphate 'Nivaquine') on the first and second days; 300 mg of chloroquine base on the third day
Children:	Approx. 10 mg of chloroquine base per kg body weight on the first and second days; 5 mg per kg on the third day

In proven *P. vivax* or *P. ovale* infection, to eradicate liver hypnozoites and prevent malaria relapses:

2. Primaquine

Adults:	15 mg of primaquine base each day for 14 days (Note b)
Children:	0.25 mg per kg of primaquine base each day for 14 days.

Notes:

a. In Southeast Asia or elsewhere, if quinine resistance is known or suspected, add three Fansidar tablets at the end of the course of quinine or take tetracycline, 250 mg, 4 times each day, or doxycycline, 200 mg daily for 7 days, at the same time as taking quinine. **Caution: tetracycline and doxycycline should not be used in pregnant women or in children less than 8 years old who can instead be given clindamycin 10 mg per kg twice daily for 3–7 days.**

b. Larger doses of primaquine may be needed to eradicate *P. vivax* acquired in Southeast Asia or the western Pacific. Primaquine can be dangerous in patients with inherited glucose-6-phosphate-dehydrogenase deficiency (suspected in people of southern Mediterranean, African, or south Asian origin).

Chloroquine-resistant *P. vivax* malaria has been reported from New Guinea and adjacent islands, but using a higher dose of chloroquine can cure these infections.

If malaria is being treated 'blind' or if, despite a positive blood smear, the species is uncertain or a mixed infection is possible, chloroquine is still the drug of choice for the countries listed in Table 5.1. Elsewhere, the infection should be treated as for falciparum malaria, with quinine, mefloquine, Fansidar (pyrimethamine + sulfadoxine) or Malarone (atovaquone + proguanil).

In severe malaria (with the patient unable to swallow tablets and suffering jaundice, unconsciousness, bleeding, and any of the other features already described), the treatment of choice is quinine (given by slow intravenous drip infusion or intramuscular injection) or artemisinin (qinghaosu) products such as artesunate (by intravenous 'push' injection or intramuscular injection or suppository) and artemether (by intramuscular injection) (Table 5.3). Suppository formulations have proved effective in severe falciparum malaria and their ease of administration is an enormous advantage in situations where no doctor or nurse is available to give an injection. The rest of the world is learning what the French have known for many years — that suppositories are easy to use and effective!

Treatment: the most widely used anti-malarial drugs

Chloroquine
The use of this safe, synthetic anti-malarial drug is limited by the development of resistant strains of *P. falciparum*, to the point where the commercial importation of chloroquine has now been banned in countries such as Tanzania. Injections or infusions of chloroquine are potentially dangerous unless the recommended dosage regimens are strictly followed.

Quinine
This drug has been used with success for several hundred years but resistance is now beginning to appear in Southeast Asia so that combination with a tetracycline or Fansidar is now necessary for complete cure. Even when taken in the correct dosage, quinine can cause ringing in the ears, deafness, dizziness, nausea, trembling, and blurred vision. Especially when given in high doses by intravenous infusion, quinine can cause a fall in the blood sugar. In severe malaria, quinine is diluted and given as a slow intravenous drip infusion, each dose over several hours. It can also be given by intramuscular injection but this is uncomfortable and, unless full sterile precautions are observed, there is a risk of infection at the injection site.

Mefloquine (Lariam)
This is a useful treatment for uncomplicated chloroquine-resistant malaria. The single curative dose is divided into halves given 6–8 hours apart. Its side-effects are discussed below.

Table 5.3 Treatment: anti-malarial drugs for treating adults or children with severe malaria and for those who cannot swallow tablets

1. **Quinine** Adults and children should be given quinine dihydrochloride diluted in isotonic fluid (e.g. normal saline) administered by slow intravenous (drip) infusion. The standard dose is 10 mg of quinine dihydrochloride per kg body weight over 4 hours, repeated at intervals of 8 hours (from the start of the first infusion) until the patient is well enough to swallow quinine tablets and complete a full 7 days of treatment. The initial dose should be doubled (loading dose) i.e. 20 mg of quinine dihydrochloride per kg body weight if no injected quinine has been given during the previous 24 hours.

In Southeast Asia and other areas where quinine resistance is known or suspected, give a 1-week course of tetracycline, 250 mg, 4 times a day or doxycycline, 200 mg daily for 7 days, starting at the end of the course of quinine **OR** a single dose of Fansidar (Table 5.2).

Caution: tetracycline and doxycycline must not be given to pregnant women or children under the age of 8 years who can instead be given clindamycin 10 mg per kg twice daily for 3–7 days.

or (where licensed and available)

2. **Artesunate** by intravenous 'push' injection 2.4 mg per kg (loading dose) on the first day followed by 1.2 mg per kg daily for a minimum of 3 days until the patient can take oral treatment or another effective anti-malarial drug.

or

3. **Artemether** by intramuscular injection into the front of the thighs 3.2 mg per kg (loading dose) on the first day, followed by 1.6 mg per kg daily for a minimum of 3 days until the patient can take oral treatment or another effective anti-malarial drug.

If it is not possible to give drugs by the intravenous route

1. **Quinine** by intramuscular injection into the front of the thighs
   (dosage the same as for intravenous infusion)

or

2. **Artesunate** by intramuscular injection

or

3. **Artemether** by intramuscular injection

If it is not possible to give drugs by injection

1. **Artemisinin** by intra-rectal suppositories 40 mg per kg (loading dose) followed by 20 mg per kg at 4, 24, 48 and 72 hours, followed by an oral anti-malarial drug

or

2. **Artesunate** by intra-rectal suppositories 200 mg at 0, 4, 8, 12, 24, 36, 48 and 60 hours, followed by an oral anti-malarial drug

Malarone (proguanil hydrochloride plus atovaquone)
In an adult dose of 4 tablets once daily for 3 days, Malarone has proved highly effective against uncomplicated multi-drug-resistant falciparum malaria in Thailand and elsewhere. It is relatively free from side effects.

Artemisinin (qinghaosu) products
Various compounds have been extracted by the Chinese from the medicinal herb, sweet wormwood *(Artemisia annua)*. These drugs clear malaria parasites from the bloodstream very quickly and have proved safe in human patients. They are not yet licensed for use in Britain or North America (apart from Riamet — see below) but have proved as effective as quinine in treating severe falciparum malaria with the advantages that they are easier to administer (for example by suppository) and have fewer side effects.

Artemether + lumefantrine (Riamet, Co–artemether)
This recently marketed combination has proved effective where malaria is highly resistant. The adult dose is 4 tablets twice a day for 3 days.

Sulphonamide + pyrimethamine (Fansidar)
Single-dose treatment has proved to be safe and effective, but resistance is now emerging and an experimental combination drug chlorproguanil + dapsone (Lapdap) is preferred as a replacement for chloroquine in Africa.

> **Caution:** Fansidar should not be used in patients known to be hypersensitive to sulphonamides and its long-term use as a prophylactic drug was stopped because of numerous fatal skin reactions.

Primaquine and tafenoquine
These drugs are used to eliminate hypnozoites of *P. vivax* and *P. ovale* from the liver to prevent malaria relapses. Resistant strains of *P. vivax* have been found in Southeast Asia and Oceania.

> **Caution:** Primaquine and tafenoquine may cause severe breakdown of erythrocytes (intravascular haemolysis) in patients who have an inherited deficiency of erythrocyte enzymes (e.g. glucose-6-phosphate dehydrogenase deficiency). People of Mediterranean, African, or Asian origin should have a blood test before using these drugs.

Dangers of malaria in pregnancy
Pregnant women seem to be especially vulnerable to severe falciparum malaria, even if they have acquired immunity by growing up in a malaria endemic region. Falciparum malaria in pregnancy can cause severe anaemia, miscarriage, a low-birthweight baby, and sometimes the death of both mother and baby.

Pregnant travellers should be strongly discouraged from entering a malarious area, especially during the last three months of the pregnancy. If it is unavoidable, chemoprophylaxis with a safe drug combination such as proguanil and chloroquine

Table 5.4 Prevention of malaria in travellers

1. **Awareness of risk**: risk of infection in the area to be visited; high-risk activities (camping, night operations); special susceptibility (young children, pregnant women, splenectomized/immunosuppressed people)
2. **Anti-mosquito measures**: kill, exclude, repel, and avoid mosquitoes
3. **Anti-malarial medication (chemoprophylaxis)**: balance risk of malaria infection against side-effects of anti-malarial drugs
4. **Emergency stand-by treatment (for travellers to remote areas)**: treatment course with or without dipstick blood test
5. **Illness after travel**: see a doctor immediately and mention malaria

should be considered (together with careful anti–mosquito precautions), and any feverish illnesses should be investigated and treated very promptly.

Prevention of malaria in travellers

Steps that the traveller can take to prevent malaria are summarized in Table 5.4.

Awareness and assessment of risk

Risky places

Even within a single country regarded as malarious, the risk of infection may vary greatly depending on environmental factors such as temperature, rainfall, altitude, and vegetation, as well as the effectiveness of local mosquito control measures. In Africa, some large cities are free from malaria transmission because of their comparatively high altitude and cool climate (e.g. Addis Ababa and Nairobi), and in some areas, malaria transmission occurs only during a brief rainy season.

If possible, reliable local advice should be obtained about the status of malaria transmission, not only at the primary site of the visit but also along the route between there and the point of entry to the country. A visitor to Peru may be safe from malaria climbing in the High Andes, but may be infected during the overnight coach trip back to Lima. The risk of being bitten by an infected mosquito in a malarious country can vary from less than once per year to more than once per night. The chances of catching malaria during a two-week visit, without any attempt at protection, have been estimated at 0.2 per cent in Kenya and 1 per cent in West Africa.

Risky activities

What travellers do while they are in the malarious area will affect the risk of infection. Those visiting rural areas and involved in night-time military exercises or zoological studies have an especially high risk, while people back-packing, camping, and on safari run a greater risk than conventional tourists.

Vulnerable people

Pregnant women, infants, and young children, and people who have had their spleen removed or whose immune system has been supressed in any other way, are especially vulnerable to malaria and should avoid entering a malarious area.

Anti-mosquito measures

Sleeping in an insect-proofed bedroom or under a mosquito net can reduce the risk of being bitten. The protection afforded by a mosquito net against mosquitoes and other biting arthropods (e.g. sandflies, lice, fleas, bed bugs, mites, ticks) is greatly enhanced by soaking the net in a pyrethroid insecticide such as permethrin (0.2 g/sq m of material, every six months). At dusk, bedrooms should be sprayed with a knock-down insecticide to kill any mosquitoes that may have entered the room during the day. Electrical heating plates (e.g. 'No Bite' and 'Buzz Off') will vaporize synthetic pyrethroids such as bioallethrin from tablets. A methylated spirit burner can be used where there is no electricity. Burning cones or coils of mosquito repellent ('incense') may also be effective.

After dusk, high-necked, light-coloured, long-sleeved shirts and long trousers are preferable to vests, shorts, or bikinis. Exposed areas of skin should be rubbed or sprayed with repellants containing N-N-diethyl-m-toluamide (DEET). Soaps and suntan oils containing insecticide are also available, and clothes and head and wrist bands can be soaked in DEET- or permethrin-based solutions (see p. 208).

Anti-malarial medication (chemoprophylaxis)

The days of simple, safe, inexpensive, and effective chemoprophylaxis against malaria seem to have passed. In most parts of the world, except those listed in Table 5.1, *P. falciparum* is resistant to chloroquine and pyrimethamine. One important cause of ineffectiveness of chemoprophylaxis is the failure of travellers to take their anti-malarial tablets regularly and, in particular, their failure to continue taking them for four weeks after leaving the malarious area. ('Not being bitten' should never be a reason for stopping tablets early — see p. 204). During bouts of vomiting and travellers' diarrhoea, the drugs may not be properly absorbed. A high risk of contracting falciparum malaria may justify the use of a prophylactic drug that has some risk of side-effects. The recent heated debate (see below) over the use of mefloquine (Lariam) illustrates the importance of risk–benefit analysis.

The recommended doses of drugs for chemoprophylaxis are given in Table 5.5

Proguanil plus chloroquine

The safe and well-tried combination of proguanil (Paludrine) and chloroquine is, at most, only about two-thirds as effective as mefloquine in Africa, and should be avoided in parts of that continent with drug-resistant malaria, unless there is no alternative. It is a second-choice option for the Chittagong Hill Tracts of Bangladesh and for the Amazon Basin. However, it is still a suitable option for other malarious areas of South America; for Afghanistan, Iran, Oman, and Saudi Arabia; for southern Africa; for the Indian subcontinent; and for most of Indonesia. An alternative in these countries is Maloprim (see below).

The dosage is two chloroquine tablets weekly, plus two proguanil tablets daily, starting one week prior to travel and continuing for four weeks afterwards.

> **Caution:** chloroquine may cause itching in dark-skinned races and can exacerbate epilepsy and photosensitive psoriasis. Although no prescription is necessary to obtain these drugs in the UK, specialist advice is strongly recommended before using this combination of drugs in any part of the world with drug-resistant malaria.

Table 5.5 Prevention: doses of drugs recommended for malaria prophylaxis

Adults

Chloroquine	300 mg of chloroquine base once each week (equivalent to 2 x 200 mg tablets of chloroquine sulphate (Nivaquine)). Starting one week prior to exposure, and continuing for four weeks afterwards. **(See caution, p. 145)**
Proguanil (Paludrine)	2 x 100 mg tablets each day. Starting one week prior to exposure and continuing for four weeks afterwards.
Doxycycline	1 x 100 mg tablet per day. Starting one day prior to exposure, and continuing for four weeks afterwards. **(See caution, p. 148)**
Mefloquine (Lariam)	1 x 250 mg tablet (228 mg in the USA) once a week. Starting at least two weeks prior to exposure, and continuing for four weeks afterwards. **(See caution, p. 147)**
Maloprim (pyrimethamine-dapsone)	1 tablet (ONLY) each week. Starting one week prior to exposure and continuing for four weeks afterwards. **(See caution, p. 148)**
Malarone	1 tablet daily, starting 1–2 days prior to exposure, and continuing for only 7 days afterwards.

Children

Chloroquine plus	5 mg of chloroquine base per kg body weight, once a week
Proguanil	3 mg per kg body weight, once a day. Starting one week prior to exposure and continuing for four weeks afterwards.

or at age

0–5 weeks:	$\frac{1}{8}$ of adult dose
6–52 weeks:	$\frac{1}{4}$ of adult dose
1–5 years:	$\frac{1}{2}$ of adult dose
6–11 years:	$\frac{3}{4}$ of adult dose
Over 12 years:	adult dose

(See caution, p. 145)

Mefloquine	(Children over 2 years only) 5 mg per kg body weight, once a week. Starting at least two weeks prior to exposure, and continuing for four weeks afterwards.

or at age

3–5 years:	$\frac{1}{4}$ of adult dose
6–8 years:	$\frac{1}{2}$ of adult dose
9–11 years:	$\frac{3}{4}$ of adult dose
Over 12 years:	adult dose

Table 5.5 Doses of drugs recommended for malaria prophylaxis (continued)

Maloprim	(Children over 5 years only)
	6–11 years: $\frac{1}{2}$ of adult dose
	Older children: adult dose.
	Starting one week prior to exposure and continuing for four weeks afterwards.
	(See caution, p. 148)
Malarone	10–20 kg: $\frac{1}{4}$ adult tablet daily, starting 1–2 days prior to exposure, and continuing for 7 days afterwards
	20–30 kg: $\frac{1}{2}$ adult tablet daily, starting 1–2 days prior to exposure, and continuing for 7 days afterwards
	30–40 kg: $\frac{3}{4}$ adult tablet daily, starting 1–2 days prior to exposure, and continuing for 7 days afterwards
	(Paediatric Malarone tablets are available in some countries, equivalent to $\frac{1}{4}$ adult tablet. If necessary, Malarone may be crushed and mixed with condensed milk or chocolate spread to make it more palatable for children.)

After continuous prophylactic use for five or six years, sufficient chloroquine may accumulate in the eye to damage the retina.

Savarine is proguanil plus chloroquine in a single, combined daily tablet. It is not licensed in the UK but is available in many parts of the world (notably France and French-speaking Africa). Taking chloroquine daily maintains a higher and more even level of the drug in the blood and may therefore be more effective, though the total dose of chloroquine with this option is higher than that with the traditional UK regimen.

Mefloquine (Lariam)

Mefloquine is approximately 90 per cent effective against *P. falciparum* infection in Africa, but unpleasant neuropsychiatric side effects are experienced by between 0.1 and 1 per cent of those who take the drug prophylactically. Side effects are more common in women than men. They include anxiety, insomnia, nightmares, depression, delusions, convulsions (fits), and dizziness. See also p. 447. More than 75 per cent of these reactions come on by the time the third weekly dose has been taken. Travellers taking mefloquine for the first time should start three weeks before they are due to travel so that there is time to change to another drug if serious side effects develop. It is necessary to start taking the drug at least two weeks prior to departure in order to build up a sufficiently protective blood level, and to continue taking one tablet weekly until four weeks afterwards.

Caution: mefloquine should not be taken by people who have suffered from epilepsy or psychiatric disease in the past and those taking certain kinds of heart tablets.

Risks of mefloquine toxicity are outweighed by the high risk of falciparum malaria in Africa (sub-Sahara, south to Angola, Zambia, and Mozambique), Bangladesh (Chittagong Hill Tracts), malarious areas of Southeast Asia, and the Amazon Basin of Brazil, Colombia, and adjacent countries.

Many people have been so anxious to avoid any risk of side effects from this drug that they have put themselves at serious risk of malaria by taking no drug at all, or by opting for less effective drug regimens. This is borne out by the rise in numbers of malaria cases in travellers that took place between 1995 and 1997, at the height of public anxiety over this issue (see Fig. 5.1). Doxycycline and Malarone are effective alternatives, and if these are not appropriate, a trial run of mefloquine before going abroad may be worth considering.

Doxycycline

Doxycycline is a tetracycline antibiotic that has been used as an anti-malarial for many years, though it has only recently been licensed for this purpose in the UK. In Africa, its effectiveness is considered to be similar to that of mefloquine — in the region of 90–95 per cent. Its main side effects are a tendency to cause vaginal thrush in women and the possibility of a photosensitive rash — an exaggerated sunburn-like reaction that can follow exposure to bright light. (The rash occurs in roughly 3 per cent of users.)

In the border areas between Thailand, Cambodia, and Burma, mefloquine resistance is frequent and doxycycline is recommended. In New Guinea, the Solomon Islands, and Vanuatu, doxycycline is recommended, with mefloquine or Maloprim plus chloroquine as second choice.

The dosage is one tablet or capsule daily (100 mg), starting one day prior to travel and continuing for four weeks afterwards.

> **Caution**: doxycycline and other tetracyclines must not be taken by pregnant women or children under 8 years old.

Maloprim

This combination of pyrimethamine and dapsone has proved safe and effective in southern Africa and as an alternative to chloroquine plus proguanil, for example in sufferers from epilepsy, although increasing drug resistance means that this option is now less reliable.

> **Caution:** Maloprim causes blood changes and bluish-grey fingernail beds in some people whose erythrocytes lack an enzyme, NADH methaemoglobin reductases.

The adult dose of one tablet per week must never be increased.

New prophylactic anti-malarial drugs

Malarone

Atovaquone with proguanil (Malarone) is a new combination drug that may be used both for treatment and for prophylaxis of multi-resistant falciparum malaria. Unlike the drugs mentioned above, Malarone affects both the pre-erythrocytic and erythrocytic stages of *P. falciparum,* and so it is not necessary to go on taking the tablets for more than a short period after leaving the malarious area. The current recommendation is to start taking the drug one day prior to exposure to malaria, and to continue for seven days after leaving.

Malarone is an expensive drug, but is highly effective against falciparum malaria, and side effects appear to be few. The dosage is one tablet daily.

Tafenoquine
The new Walter Reid 8-amino-quinolone (WR 238,605) acts like primaquine, to eradicate hypnozoites of *P.* vivax and *P. ovale* from the liver. It is also active against blood forms of malaria parasites. This drug is at a development stage, but seems an attractive and convenient option. Taking three tablets prior to travel is all that would be necessary for a two-week trip.

For women travellers actively trying to conceive
The best advice would be to take chloroquine and proguanil (or Savarine), plus maximum anti–mosquito precautions. These are the best–tried and safest drugs in pregnancy, but it is better to avoid all drugs during the first trimester!

Emergency stand-by treatment
Travellers to remote areas where medical help is likely to be more than 24 hours away should take a treatment course of quinine; mefloquine or Malarone (unless the drugs are being used for chemoprophylaxis); or Fansidar, to use in case they develop symptoms suggestive of malaria.

As dipstick tests for malaria are introduced more widely, it may be possible for travellers to test their blood before starting emergency treatment. (The self-test kits currently available tend to have a limited shelf life and to need refrigeration, and so are not well suited to the requirements of the travellers who are most likely to need them.)

Illness after travel
All the above measures may fail to prevent malaria. In cases of feverish illness within a few months of return from a malarious area, it is vital to see a doctor immediately and to mention the possible exposure to malaria.

Expatriates and long-term visitors
Long-term expatriates in malarious countries are 'a law unto themselves' as for as far as malaria prevention and treatment are concerned. They often eschew chemopro-phylaxis and other anti-malarial precautions and not only hold wrong beliefs about malaria but promulgate them to short-term travellers. Immunity is not easily acquired

and expatriates who have spent decades living in malarious areas may continue to contract malaria and even die of it!

Long-term prophylaxis with chloroquine and proguanil is limited by the risk of retinal damage (p. 148) — periodic ophthalmological assessments are needed. Very long-term use of other anti-malarials has not been well documented; for example, with mefloquine in elderly expatriates there is an increasing risk of drug interactions (such as with beta-blockers used to control high blood pressure).

The best advice is to reduce the risk of infection through strict anti-mosquito measures, combined with judicious use of chemoprophylaxis during seasons of high transmission (usually during and after the raining season). Fevers should be treated seriously. An attempt should be made always to confirm the diagnosis of malaria by microscopy or rapid antigen ('dipstick') tests.

Many expatriates wrongly attribute all fevers to malaria and then dismiss the use of anti-malarial drugs because they fail to cure them. Confirmed attacks should be treated promptly and appropriately. Artemisinin drugs are increasingly available, often 'across the counter' in tropical countries. They should be used only in combination (e.g. as 'Riamet'or 'Co-artem') and in full dosage.

Short-term visitors should be wary of health advice from 'wise' locals. They are better guided by pre-travel advice from qualified advisers.

Ethnic minorities

Members of ethnic minorities in Western countries who return to visit their malarious countries of origin are at special risk of contracting malaria and other diseases, and are less likely to seek or receive sound travel medical advice. Many wrongly assume that they are immune to malaria, having grown up in the country. However, immunity can be lost in as little as 2–3 years away from the malarious area, or may never have been acquired at all if, for example, they lived in the Indian subcontinent in the days of near elimination of malaria. More recently many parts of the subcontinent have become highly malarious. This group of patients poses a real challenge to travel medicine practitioners.

Further reading

Bradley, D.J. and Bannister, B. (ed.) (2001). *Guidelines for malaria prevention in travellers from the United Kingdom.* Communicable Disease & Public Health, 4 (2): 84–101 (downloadable from **www.malaria–reference.co.uk**).

Warrell, D.A. and Gilles, H.M. (ed.) (2001). *Bruce Chwatt's Essential malariology* 4th edn. Edward Arnold.

Warrell, D.A., Molyneux, M.E. and Beales P.F. (1990). Severe and complicated malaria. World Health Organisation, Division of Control of Tropical Diseases. *Transactions of the Royal Society for Tropical Medicine and Hygiene,* **84 (Suppl. 2)**, 1–65.

World Health Organization (2000). Severe falciparum malaria. *Transactions of the Royal Society for Tropical Medicine and Hygiene,* **94** (Suppl. 1), 51/1–51/90.

Arboviruses: dengue, Japanese encephalitis, yellow fever and others

Arboviruses are a group of infections confined mainly to the tropics. Vaccination can be given against some of the viruses; otherwise prevention depends mainly on avoiding insect bites.

Dr Tom Solomon worked for several years on arbovirus infections in Vietnam. He continues to study arboviral diseases as a Lecturer in Neurology and Honorary Lecturer in Medical Microbiology and Tropical Medicine at the University of Liverpool; he currently holds a Wellcome Trust Fellowship at the WHO Collaborating Center for Tropical Diseases at the University of Texas, USA.

Introduction

Most medical students will tell you that the classification of viruses is something of a nightmare. They can be categorized according to shape, size, capsule, and whether they contain RNA or DNA. The official approach — the phylogenetic system — classifies viruses according to their genetic relatedness: closely related viruses are grouped into a 'genus', and closely related 'genera' into a family. However, because this tells you nothing about the illnesses they cause, or the means of transmission, alternative ways of classifying viruses are often used.

Viruses that are transmitted from one animal host to the next by insects (arthropods) are known as 'arboviruses' (arthropod-borne viruses). They have evolved from a variety of backgrounds, belong to different families, and cause a wide spectrum of diseases. Some arboviruses were named after the disease they cause, for example, yellow fever or o'nyong nyong ('joint weakening' in a Ugandan dialect). Some were named after their insect vector, for example, phleboviruses named after the phlebotomus sandfly. For many, the name includes a geographical location, either where the disease first occurred or where the virus was first isolated. However, such geographical associations are often now irrelevant: there is currently very little Japanese encephalitis in Japan.

Although there are more than 500 arboviruses contained in four viral families (the Flaviviridae, Togaviridae, Bunyaviridae, and Orbiviridae), the number of viruses of medical importance is around 25 (Table 5.6). Many of them are rapidly evolving to fill new ecological niches. They have a disarming ability to spread to new geographical locations, and cause massive outbreaks with devastating results. Collectively, the arboviruses constitute some of the most important emerging and re-emerging pathogens, and some of the greatest challenges to biomedical research. The Medscape program for monitoring emerging diseases (Pro-MED, found at **www.promedmail.org**) is a notice-board with regular bulletins giving details of the latest outbreaks.

Here, some general principles will be considered before some of the most important arboviruses are looked at in more detail.

Life as an arbovirus

Viruses comprise small pieces of genetic material (nucleic acid) whose sole purpose in life is to self-replicate. Because they don't have all the enzymes they need to do this,

Table 5.6 Medically important arboviruses*

Flavivirus, Flaviviridae	
Dengue virus Yellow fever virus	} *mosquito-borne, FAR / VHF*

Japanese encephalitis virus
    West Nile virus
    St Louis encephalitis virus
    Murray Valley encephalitis virus
	} *mosquito-borne, CNS*

Omsk haemorrhagic fever virus Kyasanur forest disease virus	} *tick-borne, FAR / VHF*

Tick-borne encephalitis virus
    Louping ill virus
    Powassan virus
	} *tick-borne, CNS*

Alphavirus, Togaviridae	

Venezuelan equine encephalitis virus
    Eastern equine encephalitis virus
    Western equine encephalitis virus
	} *mosquito-borne, CNS*

Chikungunya virus
    O'nyong nyong virus
    Ross River Virus
    Sindbis virus
	} *mosquito-borne, FAR*

Nairovirus, Bunyaviridae	
Crimean-Congo haemorrhagic fever virus	*tick-borne, VHF*
Phlebovirus, Bunyaviridae	
Rift Valley fever virus	*mosquito-borne, VHF / CNS*
Sandfly fever virus	*sandfly-borne, FAR*
Tosacana virus	*sandfly-borne, CNS*
Bunyavirus, Bunyaviridae	
La Crosse virus	*mosquito-borne, CNS*
California encephalitis virus	*mosquito-borne, CNS*
Oropouche	*mosquito-borne, FAR*
Coltivirus, Rheoviridae	
Colorado tick fever virus	*tick-borne, FAR / CNS*

*Viruses are listed by genus and family.
Key: FAR = fever arthralgia rash syndrome, VHF = viral haemorrhagic fever, CNS = central nervous system infection.

they have to muscle into 'host' cells and borrow bits of their machinery. The host develops an immune response to fight off this unwanted invasion, and the rest follows as a consequence of this eternal struggle. To avoid the host immune response viruses have two choices: hiding within the host or jumping to a new host. 'Hiding' viruses include HIV (which enters and damages immune cells) and hepatitis viruses (which sit deep in the liver). 'Jumping' viruses need a safe means of travelling from one host to the next. Respiratory viruses achieve this by jumping inside a droplet of mucus or spit; enteric viruses use the faeco-oral route; and arboviruses hitch a ride in the belly of insects that feed on the blood of host animals.

Vectors and hosts

Each arbovirus evolved to use whichever animal host and insect vector were present in that particular area. In warm, tropical climates mosquitoes are the most important vectors, whereas in cooler, northern climates many arboviruses have evolved to use ticks. After infection, an animal develops life-long immunity to that arbovirus, so a constant supply of new, unexposed, non-immune hosts is needed. Although humans are the natural hosts for a few arboviruses (dengue, chikungunya, o'nyong nyong), for the vast majority the natural hosts are birds or small mammals (often rodents) that have a high reproduction rate, providing a ready supply of non-immune hosts. For these 'enzootic' arboviruses, humans become infected only accidentally because they live or travel in close proximity to the animal–insect–animal cycle. Sometimes an 'amplifying host', such as a farm animal, is infected first, and by increasing the total circulating viral load this leads to human infection.

In general, infection does not cause severe disease in the natural host. You are not a very successful arbovirus if you have killed your host before you have had chance to move on to a new one!

Human disease

Human infection with arboviruses can result in one of four clinical syndromes.

1. Mild febrile illness

The commonest outcome is asymptomatic infection, or a mild non-specific febrile illness indistinguishable from any 'flu-like illness. This is especially true for children in areas endemic for the particular virus. Following infection the child will develop immunity to that virus and will never be troubled by it again.

2. The 'fever–arthralgia–rash' triad

There is a sudden onset of high fever, chills, headache, nausea, vomiting, and a combination of joint pains (arthralgia), muscle pains (myalgia), backache, pain behind the eyes (retro-orbital pain), and sensitivity to light (photophobia). These symptoms are often accompanied by conjunctivitis, lymph node swelling (lymphadenopathy), and a variety of rashes (exanthemas) or mouth eruptions (enanthemas). Depending on the virus, rashes may be transient blanching, erythematous, itchy maculopapular, petechial, vesicular, morbilliform (like measles), or scarlatiniform (like scarlatina).

There may also be papular or vesicular changes in the mouth, especially on the palate. The fever is often biphasic, and there may be a leukopenia (reduction in the number of white blood cells), but the fever–arthralgia–rash syndrome is usually self-limiting.

3. Viral haemorrhagic fever

Following an initial 'fever–arthralgia–rash' syndrome some arboviruses cause bleeding manifestations (sometimes after an interval of a few days). Petechiae (tiny spots of blood in the skin) may coalesce to form larger areas of purpura. There may be bruising, prolonged bleeding at injection sites, gum and nose bleeding, and in more severe disease, gastrointestinal bleeding. A variety of factors may contribute to the bleeding tendency including derangement in clotting factors (secondary to liver damage), a reduced number of platelets that function abnormally, and damage to the blood vessels. Shock (low blood pressure) may develop leading to acidosis, further clotting, biochemical derangement, and a high mortality if untreated.

The virus may attack the liver causing hepatitis (liver inflammation) and hepatomegaly (liver enlargement); deep jaundice is a sign of severe liver damage. In some infections (notably dengue haemorrhagic fever) leakage of fluid from the vessels can cause a drop in blood pressure without frank bleeding. As well as flaviviruses, phleboviruses, and nairoviruses there are many non-arboviral causes of haemorrhagic fevers (see p. 123)

4. Central nervous system infection

Following a non-specific febrile prodrome some arboviruses invade the central nervous system. Infection and inflammation of the meningeal membranes that cover the brain and spinal cord is called 'meningitis'. It is characterized by headache and vomiting, photophobia, neck stiffness, and pain on extension of the knee when the hip is flexed (Kernig's signs). Examination of the cerebrospinal fluid reveals an increased number of white blood cells (usually lymphocytes).

In encephalitis, the virus invades and destroys the brain substance with accompanying inflammation. The clinical features range from mild confusion or behavioural changes (which may be mistaken for hysteria), to focal neurological signs, convulsions, and deep coma. There are usually, though not always, increased lymphocytes in the spinal fluid. Where facilities are available, computed tomography (CT) or magnetic resonance imaging (MRI) scans may aid diagnosis by revealing characteristic areas of focal damage within the brain.

In myelitis, viruses attack the spinal cord to give weakness in one or more limbs, which are usually flaccid and areflexic.

The term 'meningoencephalomyelitis' is used to reflect the fact that many viruses attack all three components of the central nervous system. The differential diagnosis for arboviral encephalitis includes members of the *Alphavirus, Flavivirus, Bunyavirus,* and *Phlebovirus* genera as well as many other causes.

Most arboviruses are known by just one or two of these four syndromes, but it is becoming apparent that some arboviruses have a disarming ability to cause different clinical presentations in different settings.

Diagnosis

Broadly speaking, viral infections are diagnosed by either demonstrating that the virus is present or that it was present and the host now has an immune response against it. Culturing virus from clinical samples (the traditional 'gold standard') requires a sophisticated laboratory, highly trained personnel, and the maintenance of cell lines (or a supply of small mammals) in which to isolate the virus — not very practical in most rural tropical settings.

Newer methods for detecting minute amounts of viral nucleic acid using the polymerase chain reaction have been developed for many arboviruses. Although frequently used in specialized research laboratories, most have yet to prove their worth in a routine diagnostic service. The older serological techniques for demonstrating anti-viral antibodies, such as the haemaglutination inhibition test, are technically fiddly, and since they require both acute and convalescent sera, are not useful for making an early diagnosis or for diagnosing patients that die soon after admission.

The development of new IgM- and IgG-capture ELISAs to allow early detection of anti-viral antibody in single serum or cerebrospinal fluid samples has been a major advance. These tests have become the accepted standard for diagnosis of many arboviral infections. Some have recently been adapted into simple bedside kits requiring no specialized laboratory equipment, making them even more appropriate for rapid diagnosis in the field.

Treatment and prevention

For a few arbovirus infections (Crimean–Congo haemorrhagic fever, Rift Valley fever) specific antiviral treatment is available, but for the majority there is none. In these cases current management consists of treating the complications of the disease such as high fever and aches, low blood pressure, blood loss, convulsions, or raised intracranial pressure.

Vaccines are available against some arboviral infections (yellow fever, Japanese encephalitis, tick-borne encephalitis) and are being developed against others. However, the simplest preventive measure is to avoid bites from the insects that carry the viruses. This means wearing long sleeves and trousers (especially during the time of day when that particular insect bites), using an insect spray containing at least 30 per cent DEET, and sleeping under bed-nets. Although this might be practical for the short-term visitor, it is rarely possible for residents.

In the following sections, arboviruses are classified according to their most important clinical presentation, though to some extent these divisions are artificial because of the considerable overlap.

Haemorrhagic arboviruses

Dengue

Dengue (genus *Flavivirus*, family Flaviviridae) is now numerically the most important arbovirus world-wide, with an estimated 100 million cases per year and 2.5 billion people at risk. The virus has spread dramatically since the end of the Second World War, in what has been described as a global pandemic. Virtually every country between the tropics of Capricorn and Cancer is affected (Map 5.2), and it is the arbovirus that travellers are most likely to encounter, though thankfully usually in its mildest form.

Dengue is unusual among arboviruses in that humans are the natural host. There are four slightly different types of dengue virus (distinguished serologically). The expansion of dengue has been linked to a world-wide resurgence of the main mosquito vector *Aedes aegypti* (Fig. 5.4), overcrowding of human populations, and increasing human travel. Intercontinental transport of used car tyres containing eggs of *Aedes albopictus*, has also been implicated in dengue resurgence.

Dengue tends to occur in cities — particularly poor, overcrowded areas on the edge of cities — rather than in the countryside, where the human population may be widely dispersed. The mosquito breeds in clean water, for example, in water storage jars and in rainwater accidentally collected in tyres and other rubbish.

In endemic areas, most of the population is infected by dengue viruses during early childhood, when most infections are asymptomatic or cause a non-specific 'flu-like illness. When the virus spreads to new areas, adults and children are both affected, since neither group has pre-existing immunity. Infection with dengue viruses can cause one of two diseases: dengue fever and dengue haemorrhagic fever.

Dengue fever

Named 'breakbone fever' by William Rush, 200 years ago, this is a classic 'fever–arthralgia–rash' syndrome. In young children it is often an undifferentiated febrile illness. In older children and adults there is an abrupt onset of high fever, muscle and joint aches (which may be severe), often with retro-orbital pain, photophobia, and lymphadenopathy. There may be a transient mottling rash, or sometimes petechiae (spotty bleeding into the skin). Occasionally there is frank bleeding in dengue fever, but in most cases the disease is self-limiting and hospital admission is not necessary.

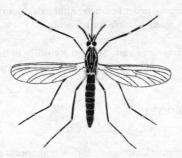

Fig. 5.4 Female *Aedes aegypti* mosquito (4–6 mm long)

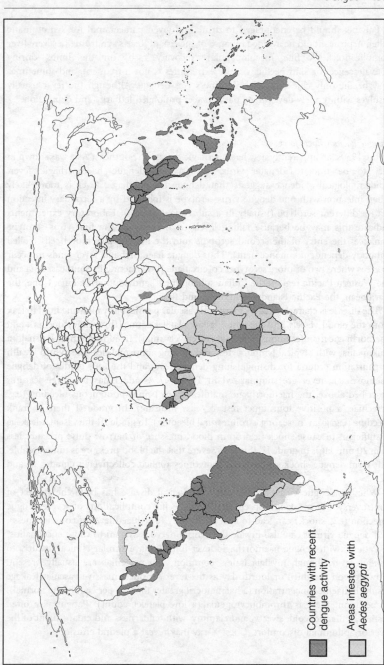

Map 5.2 World distribution of dengue viruses and their mosquito vector *Aedes aegypti* (2000).

Countries with recent
dengue activity

Areas infested with
Aedes aegypti

Patients should be encouraged to drink and given paracetamol for symptomatic relief. Aspirin should be avoided because of the risk of Reye's syndrome (a severe liver complication). A fine maculopapular 'recovery rash' on the limbs during convalescence, or skin peeling on the extremities is not infrequent, and sometimes may be the only clue that a febrile illness was dengue. Although the fever usually resolves within a few days, many patients feel prolonged lethargy and depression.

Dengue haemorrhagic fever

In the 1950s, an apparently new haemorrhagic disease in Southeast Asia was shown in fact to be due to dengue virus, and named dengue haemorrhagic fever. Epidemiological evidence suggests that dengue haemorrhagic fever is more likely when infection with one dengue virus serotype is followed by a secondary infection with a different serotype (usually in a subsequent season). Laboratory experiments indicate this may be because falling levels of antibody to the first virus serotype enhances the entry of the second serotype into the macrophage blood cells (called antibody-dependent enhancement). Thus dengue haemorrhagic fever tends to occur in areas where two or more serotypes co-circulate. It is endemic in Southeast Asia and the Western Pacific region, the Indian subcontinent, and southern China, Cuba, the Caribbean, the Pacific Islands, Venezuela, and Brazil.

The disease is characterized by increased vascular permeability allowing fluid to leak from the blood vessels into the tissue, a low platelet count (thrombocytopenia), and haemorrhagic manifestations (which are often very mild). In addition there is usually a leukopenia, with atypical lymphocytes, and clotting abnormalities The World Health Organization criteria for distinguishing dengue fever and the four grades of dengue haemorrhagic fever are summarized in Table 5.7. Grade I has the three features described above, the haemorrhagic manifestations being spontaneous bleeding (e.g. petechiae, a positive tourniquet test, or easy bruising). In grade II there is frank bleeding (e.g. gum, nose, or gastrointestinal bleeding). In grade III the vascular leakage is sufficient to cause shock (a drop in blood pressure or narrow pulse pressure less than 20 mm Hg). In grade IV this is so severe that the blood pressure is unrecordable. The term dengue shock syndrome is sometimes applied collectively to grades III and IV.

Whether dengue viruses can cause neurological disease has been the subject of controversy, but most now accept that non-specific complications of severe dengue infection (e.g. shock) can lead to encephalopathy (a reduced level of consciousness), and dengue viruses can also invade the central nervous system to cause encephalitis.

Patients with dengue haemorrhagic fever initially have similar clinical features to dengue fever, though myalgia is less common, and petechiae are usually present. However, on the third or fourth day as the fever subsides, massive vascular leakage results in haemoconcentration (a haematocrit greater than 20 per cent of the normal). In addition, there is thrombocytopenia (a low platelet count). Patients are often restless, lethargic, cold, sweaty, and clammy, with tenderness and enlargement of the liver or abdominal discomfort. Chest X-ray may reveal a pleural effusion.

Table 5.7 WHO criteria for distinguishing dengue fever (DF) and dengue haemorrhagic fever (DHF) grades I–IV

		Plasma leakage*	Platelets (μL)	Circulatory collapse	Haemorrhagic manifestations
	DF	No	Variable	Absent	Variable
	DHF I	Present	<100 000	Absent	Positive tourniquet test (or easy bruising)
	DHF II	Present	<100 000	Absent	Spontaneous bleeding^ with or without positive tourniquet test
DSS {	DHF III	Present	<100 000	PP<20 mm Hg#	Spontaneous bleeding and/or positive tourniquet test
DSS {	DHF IV	Present	<100 000	Pulse and BP undetectable	Spontaneous bleeding and/or positive tourniquet test

^ skin petechiae, mucosal or gastrointestinal bleeding

*identified by haematocrit 20% above normal, or clinical signs of plasma leakage

pulse pressure less than 20 mm Hg, or hypotension for age

DSS = Dengue shock syndrome

Patients with grades I and II dengue haemorrhagic fever are encouraged to drink and need to be monitored closely for a deterioration with repeated haematocrit measurements as well as observation of vital signs. For treatment of grades III and IV (dengue shock syndrome), the WHO recommends initial intravenous crystalloid (e.g. Ringer's lactate solution) at 10–20 ml/kg/h, followed by a colloid solution (e.g. dextran 40) at 10–20 ml/kg/h if shock persists. Only rarely are blood products needed. If possible, oxygen should be given. The rate of infusion needs to be carefully tailored according to the vital signs, haematocrit, and urine output. Even cautious treatment may precipitate peripheral and facial oedema, ascites, pleural effusions, and pulmonary oedema; diuretics and ventilatory support are sometimes needed.

Although there are no anti-viral drugs against dengue, in expert hands the mortality of dengue haemorrhagic fever has dropped from around 10 per cent untreated to less than 1 per cent.

Diagnosis of dengue infection is possible by virus isolation or PCR detection in the first few days of the illness. After this, viral titres are low, but anti-dengue antibodies can be measured in serum by ELISAs. A range of diagnostic kits is now commercially available (Table 5.8).

Prevention

There is currently no commercially available vaccine against dengue, though this remains the subject of active research. Vaccines have proved hard to produce because of concern that antibodies raised against one virus serotype might enhance infection with a different serotype. Vaccines equally effective against all four serotypes are being developed and several are in trial; it is likely that one will be available in the future.

Preventive measures against dengue include steps to limit the breeding of *Aedes* mosquitoes around the house (e.g. removing stagnant pools of water collected in tyres and other rubbish), and steps to avoid being bitten. But given that *Aedes* mosquitoes bite during daylight hours, this is almost impossible for those living in endemic areas. Some comfort may come from the fact that although most of the European staff I have known working in tropical units in Asia have been infected with dengue at some time, none has come to serious harm.

Yellow fever

In the early 1900s, American efforts to link the Atlantic and Pacific Oceans with the Panama Canal were being severely hampered as hundreds of labourers succumbed to yellow fever. A local physician, Dr Carlos Finlay suggested that the disease was transmitted by mosquito bites (a revolutionary idea at the time), and a team of US Army physicians, headed by Dr Walter Reed, was sent to investigate. To prove the point, one of the team, Dr Jesse Lazaer, allowed a mosquito that had just fed on a yellow fever patient to bite him: he subsequently developed the disease and died. The vigorous mosquito-control efforts that followed enabled the Panama Canal to be completed; and subsequent virological studies established that yellow fever was caused by a virus. It was the first arbovirus identified, and gave its name to the flaviviruses (in latin, flavus = yellow).

Table 5.8 Commercially available diagnostic kits for arbovirus infections

	Format	Kit	Comment
Dengue	96 well ELISA, requiring ELISA reader	PanBio Dengue Duo IgG and IgM Capture ELISA (DEC-400)[1]	IgM and IgG ELISA distinguishes primary and secondary infection
		Focus Technologies Dengue Fever IgM and IgG ELISA[2]	
	Visible colour change, requiring no specialized equipment	Venture Technologies Dengue Blot-IgM and IgG Capture Dot Enzyme immunoassays (MAC DOT)[3]	Distinguishes primary and secondary infection; suitable for small numbers of samples
		PanBio Dengue Rapid (DEN-25)[1]	Distinguishes primary and secondary infection; suitable for single samples
		denKEY™ and denTYPE™ Antigen Enzyme Immunoassays[4]	For detection of dengue virus antigen during early febrile phase of illness
Yellow Fever	96 well ELISA, requiring ELISA reader	PanBio Yellow Fever IgM ELISA[1]	
Japanese encephalitis	96 well ELISA, requiring ELISA reader	PanBio JE IgM Capture ELISA (JEM-200)[1]	Distinguishes JEV from dengue
	Visible colour change, requiring no equipment	Venture Technologies JEV Blot-IgM Capture Dot Enzyme immunoassay (MAC DOT)[3]	Distinguishes JEV from dengue

[1]Microgen Bioproducts Limited, 1 Admiralty Way, Camberley, Surrey, GU153DT, England, Tel 01276-600081, Fax 01276-600151, email pberry@microgenbioproducts.com **www.microgenbioproducts.com**

[2]The Binding Site, PO Box 4073, Birmingham B29 6AT, UK Tel 0121 414 2000, Fax 0121 472 6017 email info@bindingsite.co.uk **www.bindingsite.co.uk**

[3]Genelabs Diagnostics S.A, Halle de Fret/Aeroport, P.O. Box 1015, 1211 Geneva 5, Switzerland. Tel 41-22 788-1908. Fax 41-22 788 1986. email salesgva@genelabs.ch **www.genelabs.com.sg**

[4]Globio Corporation, 100 Cummings Center, STE 424A, Beverly, MA, USA. Tel 1-978 921 6488, Fax 1-978 232 9084, email info@globio.com **www.globio.com**

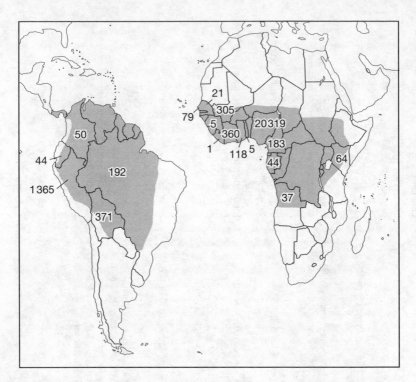

Map 5.3 Distribution of officially reported yellow fever cases by country (1986–95).

Yellow fever occurs in jungle and urban cycles in West Africa and South America (Map 5.3). In South American 'jungle yellow fever', *Haemagogus* mosquitoes transmit the virus between monkeys. Humans become infected by entering this cycle, and carry the disease to populated areas. Here, *Aedes* mosquitoes are responsible for transmission between humans to give 'urban yellow fever'. In West Africa, *Aedes* mosquitoes are responsible for both jungle and urban transmission.

Clinically, yellow fever is characterized by the abrupt onset of high fever, headache, back and muscle aches, nausea, and vomiting. The majority of infections are mild, but in more severe disease there is liver failure causing the mild jaundice by which the disease is known. Bleeding into the stomach produces characteristic black vomit and darkened stool (melaena). There may also be bleeding from the eyes, nose, bladder, and rectum, and renal failure, and, occasionally, nervous system involvement. Faget's sign (failure of the heart rate to rise with a rising temperature), is indicative of damage to the heart muscle. Laboratory tests confirm elevated liver enzymes, leukopenia, thrombocytopenia, and clotting abnormalities. The diagnosis is confirmed by virus isolation in the first few days, or ELISA after that. Councilman bodies, found in the liver at autopsy, were thought to be pathognomic (i.e. unique to yellow fever), but they also occur in Crimean–Congo haemorrhagic fever and Rift Valley fever.

The vaccine against yellow fever was one of the first live attenuated vaccines, and is essential for visitors to all endemic areas — even if no cases have recently been reported. A single 0.5 ml dose of 17D yellow fever vaccine confers immunity for 10 years or more (see also p. 539). Be sure to obtain an International Certificate of Vaccination, because travel to and from certain countries may be restricted without it. In addition, travellers should take standard measures to limit mosquito bites (see p. 208)

Crimean–Congo haemorrhagic fever (CCHF)

Crimean–Congo haemorrhagic fever (genus *Nairovirus*, family Bunyaviridae) is unusual among arboviruses in that direct human to human transmission can occur without the need of an insect vector. The name reflects the fact that 'Congo virus', isolated from a febrile child in the Belgian Congo (now Zaire) in 1956, proved to be identical to the filterable agent identified in 1944 as the cause of 'Crimean haemorrhagic fever'.

The virus is transmitted naturally between mammals by *Ixodes* ticks, and is widely distributed through Africa, Asia, the former USSR, eastern Europe, and the Middle East. Humans become infected when bitten by an infected tick, but secondary cases can occur in health care workers and others in direct contact with blood from infected patients. Hence, such patients should be barrier–nursed. Similarly, abattoir workers may become infected from the carcasses of infected animals.

The clinical features are similar to other haemorrhagic viruses (see also pp. 123–9), but patients sometimes undergo surgery for profuse upper gastrointestinal bleeding before the diagnosis is suspected. In milder forms the disease is usually self-limiting, but the mortality can be high (up to 50 per cent) in epidemics. However, prompt treatment with the anti-viral drug ribavirin, administered intravenously or even orally, can be life saving.

Rift Valley fever

As its name implies, Rift Valley fever (genus *Phlebovirus*, family Bunyaviridae) is endemic in the Rift Valley and much of eastern Africa. Although genetically close to the viruses transmitted by sandflies (and hence a member of the phlebovirus genus), the virus is principally mosquito-borne. *Aedes* and *Culex* mosquitoes are the most important vectors. Epidemics are associated with the explosive increases in mosquito populations that follow heavy rainfalls and new irrigation projects.

Rift Valley fever virus causes disease in sheep, cattle (causing abortions), and other farm animals, as well as humans. There were 200 000 human cases during an epidemic in Egypt in the late 1970s. Most human cases have a febrile illness, which is clinically indistinguishable from other arboviral fevers, but 5–10 per cent have haemorrhagic manifestations, meningoencephalitis, or ocular complications (reduced visual acuity due to exudates). This triad of symptoms during an epidemic of a febrile illness may provide a clue that Rift Valley fever is the cause, especially if it is associated with concurrent disease in animals. Intravenous ribavirin is effective treatment for severe disease.

Omsk haemorrhagic fever

Omsk haemorrhagic fever is a flavivirus of rodents (particularly musk rats) in the Omsk area of Siberia, transmitted to humans by *Dermacentor ticks*. The disease can also be contracted by direct contact with infected carcasses. Most infections are asymptomatic, but there may be a papulovesicular eruption on the soft palate, and mucosal and gastrointestinal bleeding. Kyasanur forest disease is caused by a closely related tick-borne flavivirus found in forest rodents in western India. Most cases consist of a febrile illness, but haemorrhagic disease, and even meningoencephalitis can occur.

Central nervous system arboviruses

Japanese encephalitis

Can there be anything more devastating than watching a previously well child deteriorate from a mild 'flu-like illness to severe coma and death within the space of a few days? Although considered by many in the West to be a rare and exotic infection, Japanese encephalitis is probably the most important viral encephalitis world-wide. Around 50 000 cases and 15 000 deaths are reported every year, but the true numbers may be much higher.

Japanese encephalitis virus (genus *Flavivirus*, family Flaviviridae) is transmitted between birds, chickens, pigs, and other animals by *Culex* mosquitoes. The most important, *Culex tritaeniorhynchus*, breeds in rice paddy fields. The geographical area affected by the virus has expanded in the last 50 years and now includes all of Southeast Asia, most of the Indian subcontinent, and much of China and the Pacific Rim (Map 5.4). In addition, there have recently been epidemics in the Kathmandu Valley of Nepal and, in 1998, Japanese encephalitis was reported for the first time in northern Australia. The reasons for this expansion are incompletely understood, but probably include increased irrigation facilitating mosquito breeding and changing farming habits (e.g. more animal husbandry). The situation would probably be far worse were it not for the use of Japanese encephalitis vaccine in some countries (see below).

In northern temperate regions (China, Nepal, and northern parts of India, Thailand, and Vietnam) Japanese encephalitis occurs in summer epidemics. In southern tropical climates (Indonesia, Malaysia, and southern India, Thailand, and Vietnam) the virus is endemic, with sporadic cases occurring throughout the year. These two patterns probably relate to mosquito numbers, rainfall, and temperature, though different viral strains are also a possible explanation.

In many parts of rural Asia, Japanese encephalitis virus is so abundant that it is almost impossible to avoid. Serological studies (looking for antibody to the virus in the blood) show that by early adulthood almost all people living in rural Asia have already been infected. Thankfully, the majority of infections do not cause disease. Only about 1 in 30 to 1 in 300 infected people develop symptoms. These may range from a mild

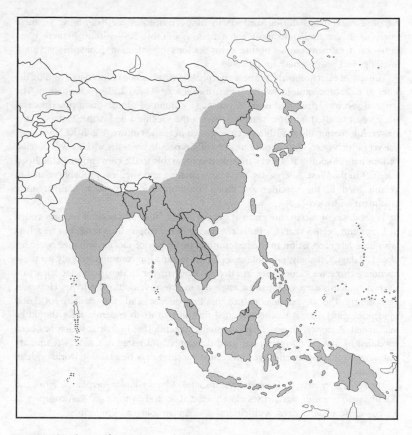

Map 5.4 Distribution of Japanese encephalitis in Asia 1970–98).

'flu-like illness to a severe meningoencephalitis leading to death. Patients typically present with a few days of fever, headache, nausea, and vomiting, followed by a reduced level of consciousness (often heralded by convulsions). In addition, a new variant of the disease has recently been described in which the predominant lesion is in the spinal cord (myelitis) causing an acute flaccid paralysis which looks very similar to polio. Whether viral or host factors determine which symptoms develop following infection remains to be determined.

In endemic areas, most new cases of Japanese encephalitis occur in children, because the majority of adults have already been infected. However, adults who have not previously been exposed to the virus (including travellers) are equally susceptible. This was amply demonstrated by the many Western troops who succumbed to

Japanese encephalitis during conflicts in Asia. Techniques for diagnosing Japanese encephalitis are similar to those for dengue (see Table 5.8). Although there is no anti-viral treatment, some of the complications of infection (convulsions, brain swelling, and pneumonia) are treatable.

The risk of infection with Japanese encephalitis virus can be reduced by avoiding the bites of *Culex* mosquitoes (which bite from dusk to dawn) and by vaccination. The original vaccines, produced over 30 years ago, contained mouse-brain proteins, and occasionally caused immune reactions, giving the vaccine a bad name. However, the newer, internationally available vaccines grown in tissue culture (e.g. BIKEN vaccine) are very much safer. Only about one per million people given the vaccine will develop serious neurological side-effects, making it comparable to the conventional childhood vaccines in the West. Allergic-type reactions (itching and swelling, probably related to gelatin used in the vaccine) are more common, and very occasionally require treatment with steroids.

Three doses of vaccine are given at days 1, 7, and 30, with a booster recommended at 1 year and every 3 years for those remaining in the tropics long term. For travellers who have left vaccination to the last minute, two doses of vaccine will give cover for about 30 days. Officially, Japanese encephalitis vaccine is recommended only for those spending three weeks or more in affected areas, or for those on shorter trips to a known epidemic area, or for those engaging in extensive outdoor activity. However, considering the devastating nature of the disease and the paucity of good epidemiological data, it has been argued that all visitors to endemic areas should be vaccinated. A newer, cheaper, live-attenuated vaccine (i.e. live virus which has been modified to make it harmless) has been developed and tested in China. Preliminary data suggest it is highly effective and related vaccines may be available world-wide in the future.

West Nile fever virus, St Louis encephalitis virus, Murray Valley encephalitis virus, and *Kunjin virus* are four flaviviruses closely related to and in the same serocomplex as Japanese encephalitis virus, with clinical and epidemiological similarities.

West Nile fever virus

This virus (genus *Flavivirus*, family Flaviviridae) was first isolated from the blood of a febrile Ugandan in 1937. It was subsequently shown to have a very wide area of distribution that included most of Africa, southern Europe, the Middle East, and even parts of the Far East. In its natural cycle, the virus is transmitted primarily between pigeons and crows by *Culex* mosquitoes.

Classically, West Nile fever virus causes a non-specific febrile illness, and until recently nervous system manifestations were considered a rarity. However, in recent years the epidemiology has changed, with the virus spreading to new areas and causing different disease patterns. In 1996 an epidemic of West Nile encephalitis affected several hundred people in Romania, and in 1999 the virus caused an epidemic in New York. Although there were only around 60 cases, this outbreak of West Nile encephalitis caused considerable alarm because the virus had not previously reached the Americas, or indeed anywhere in the western hemisphere. How it arrived there is the subject of much speculation, but via birds migrating from Israel now seems most likely. Since then the virus has spread across much of America and continues to cause sporadic disease.

St Louis encephalitis

St Louis encephalitis (genus *Flavivirus*, family Flaviviridae) is the most important arboviral encephalitis in the USA. The arbovirus branch of America's Center for Disease Control was founded following outbreaks of the disease in the 1930s in St Louis, Missouri. The virus occurs naturally in many birds and is transmitted by *Culex* mosquitoes. Up to 3000 cases have been reported during epidemics in some years. However, the continuing surveillance for St Louis encephalitis virus and intensive mosquito spraying in affected areas reduce the chances of such epidemics in the future. In recent years there have been approximately 130 cases annually, mostly in Florida and Texas.

Murray Valley encephalitis virus

This flavivirus causes sporadic cases of encephalitis every year in Australia, and occasionally causes small outbreaks (up to 20 cases). The disease is transmitted between wild birds by *Culex* mosquitoes, but the means of over-wintering is uncertain. The virus has also been found in New Guinea.

Tick-borne encephalitis (TBE)

In cooler climates flaviviruses evolved to use the more abundant tick vector as their means of transmission. Tick-borne encephalitis virus circulates in small wild animals, mostly rodents, and is transmitted by *Ixodes* ticks. Humans may also become infected by drinking goat's milk. It has a wide area of distribution across Europe and the former Soviet Union, and its seasonal incidence is reflected in one of the many pseudonyms, 'Russian spring–summer encephalitis' (Map 5.5).

Genetic sequencing has allowed Western tick-borne encephalitis virus, which is endemic in Germany, Austria, and much of Europe, to be distinguished from Far-Eastern tick-borne encephalitis virus which is found across the former Soviet Union. The number of cases is rising; 40 per cent of victims have no recollection of having been bitten by a tick. Austria is currently attempting to vaccinate its entire population against the disease.

After one to two weeks' incubation the virus causes a sudden onset of fever, headache, nausea, and photophobia. In mild cases this resolves after a week, but in more severe cases there is a second phase of illness with meningoencephalitis or myelitis. The latter tends to cause flaccid paralysis of the upper limb and shoulder girdle. Respiratory muscle and bulbar (brainstem) involvement lead to respiratory failure and death. Far-Eastern tick-borne encephalitis has a higher case fatality rate; the Western form is often associated with neurological damage. Overall, there is a 10 per cent risk of death or disability.

An inactivated vaccine given as two doses, 4–6 weeks apart, is recommended for those likely to be exposed in the endemic forested areas of Europe and the former Soviet Union (this includes walkers, campers, and hikers) and a TBE immunoglobulin injection can provide rapid immunity for people travelling at short notice.

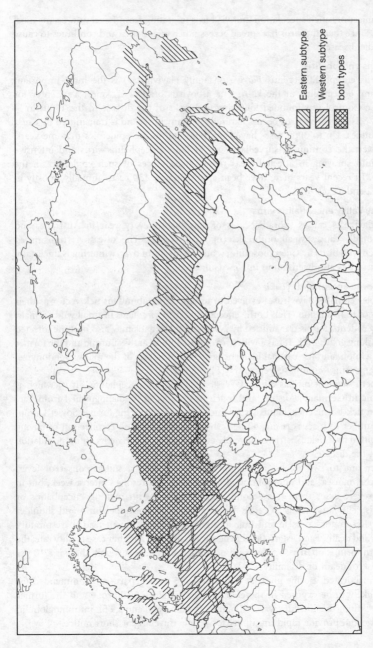

Map 5.5 Distribution of Western and Eastern subtypes of tick-borne encephalitis

Eastern subtype
Western subtype
both types

Louping ill

This virus is a closely related tick-borne virus, notable for being the only flavivirus found naturally in the British Isles (as well as Scandinavia). It occurs among small mammals (hares, wood-mice and shrews), but is also transmitted to highland sheep which develop encephalitis. The disease is named after the leaping (or louping) demonstrated by the encephalitic sheep. Very occasionally the virus infects humans, causing meningoencephalitis, which can be severe. Powassan virus is a distantly related tick-borne flavivirus found principally among small mammals in Canada that has occasionally caused meningoencephalitis in humans.

Equine encephalitis viruses

These mosquito-borne alphaviruses (genus *Alphavirus*, family Rubellaviridae) cause epidemics of encephalitis in horses and humans in the Americas. Venezuelan equine encephalitis virus is normally transmitted in an enzootic cycle involving small mammals and *Aedes* and *Culex* mosquitoes. Following high rainfalls, the number of circulating mosquitoes increases and horses become infected. They act as amplifying hosts, and human infection follows. Massive outbreaks of human and equine disease occur every few years in Venezuela and neighbouring central and southern American countries. In 1995, there were up to 100 000 human cases, most of which had a mild, non-specific febrile illness; but 300 of these were fatal. Recent work has shown subtle genetic differences between enzootic and epidemic strains of the virus.

Eastern equine encephalitis virus is found along the eastern coast of North America, Central America, and northern countries of South America. It is transmitted between wild birds by *Culiseta* and *Aedes* mosquitoes. Although it currently only causes only a handful of cases each year, large epidemics have occurred. Western equine encephalitis virus is transmitted between wild birds by *Culex* and *Culiseta* mosquitoes. It has a wide area of distribution across much of the USA, but only rarely gives human disease.

Bunyaviruses

These viruses (genus *Bunyavirus*, family Bunyaviridae) are widely distributed mosquito-borne, tick-borne, and biting fly-borne viruses, named after Bunyamwera, the village in Uganda where the first one was isolated. Most cause non-specific febrile illnesses, but the mosquito-borne American bunyaviruses of the California serogroup also cause encephalitis. The most important, La Crosse virus, is transmitted between chipmunks and squirrels principally by *Aedes* mosquitoes. It causes up to 200 cases of encephalitis in the USA annually, but the case fatality rate is low. Other members of the same serogroup include California encephalitis virus and viruses with such unlikely names as Jamestown Canyon and Snowshoe hare. Toscana virus (genus *Phlebovirus*, family Bunyaviridae) is transmitted by sandflies, and is an important cause of viral meningitis and encephalitis in children in Italy.

Colorado tick fever virus

This virus (genus *Coltivirus*, family Rheoviridae) is transmitted among small mammals (chipmunks and ground squirrels) by *Dermacentor* ticks in the Rocky Mountain states of the USA. Because of its geographical distribution, vector, and symptoms it is often confused with the rickettsial disease, Rocky Mountain spotted fever. Infection presents with a non-specific fever, myalgia, and maculopapular rash, and up to 10 per cent of children may develop neurological features (from mild meningitis to severe encephalitis). A haemorrhagic disease is also occasionally reported.

Fever–arthralgia–rash arboviruses

Many of the viruses described above as 'haemorrhagic' can also cause a febrile syndrome, with arthralgia and rash. However, for other arboviruses the triad of fever, arthralgia, and rash is the only significant clinical presentation. The 'old world' alphaviruses (genus *Alphavirus*, family Togaviridae) are the most important ones amongst these. Chikungunya virus ('that which bends up' in a Tanzanian dialect) is very widely distributed across Africa, India, and Southeast Asia, and is transmitted by *Aedes* and *Anopheles* mosquitoes. Humans and non-human primates are the only hosts. The virus causes massive epidemics of an illness very similar to dengue fever, some of which can last for years. O'nyong nyong virus is a closely related alphavirus that causes severe arthritis, often with conjunctivitis; epidemics are far less frequent. *Anopheles* mosquitoes are the vectors and humans are the only natural host.

Ross River fever virus (genus *Alphavirus*, family Togaviridae) is numerically the most important arbovirus in Australia, and is responsible for 'epidemic polyarthritis'. There are approximately 5000 cases per year in adults, but when the virus spread to the Pacific in 1979 there was a massive epidemic of 50 000 cases. Ross River fever is characterized by arthralgia (joint pain) and myalgia (muscle pain), with fever and rash apparent in only 50 per cent of cases. Occasionally, the disease progresses to give chronic arthritis (joint inflammation). *Aedes* and *Culex* mosquitoes are the main vectors, and the natural hosts are thought to include kangaroos and wallabies.

Other fever–arthralgia–rash arboviruses include Sindbis (an alphavirus found in South Africa) and Oropouche (a bunyavirus from Brazil). Sandfly fever viruses (genus *Phlebovirus*, family Bunyaviridae) are transmitted by sandflies across Africa, Asia, and Europe. They cause a non-specific febrile illness with myalgia, retro-orbital pain, and marked conjunctival infection; 'dog disease' was an early description because of the resemblance to the eyes of a bloodhound.

Summary of advice for travellers

- Minimize the risk of mosquito, tick, and sandfly bites by wearing appropriate clothing and using DEET insect repellent and impregnated bed-nets.

- Where vaccines are available (yellow fever, Japanese encephalitis, tick-borne encephalitis), the benefits of vaccination usually outweigh the possible risks.

- Anti-viral treatment is available for a few arboviruses (Rift Valley fever and Crimean–Congo haemorrhagic fever), but for most the treatment is symptomatic.

- Dengue is the arbovirus infection you are most likely to encounter, but it is usually no worse than a very nasty bout of 'flu.

Filarial infections

This is a group of worm infections transmitted by biting insects. Filarial worms live in the tissues and can survive several years.

Dr Richard Knight was a staff member at the London and Liverpool Schools of Tropical Medicine for 18 years. He has worked as a physician, epidemiologist, and parasitologist in tropical countries for 17 years. He is now Associate Specialist in General Medicine, with a special interest in gastrointestinal disease, at the Royal Sussex County Hospital in Brighton, Sussex.

Adult filarial worms are long, thread-like, whitish in colour, and up to 30 cm in length. Those infecting man live in the lymphatic system or in the deeper layers of skin, and are found only in tropical latitudes.

The female releases numerous embryos called microfilariae that either circulate in the bloodstream or persist in the skin. The transmission cycle begins when biting insects ingest blood from intact capillaries or from blood pools from damaged capillaries. Larval worms develop in the insect, a process speeded up at higher temperatures. At a later bite, the insect releases infective larvae into a new host, where they mature over a period of about a year. Those species with blood microfilariae usually show a pattern of periodicity of their numbers in the circulation that coincides with the day- or night-biting cycle of the vector insect.

Nearly all human disease occurs in heavily infected local residents living in high transmission areas over long periods of time. However, travellers and short-term residents may also develop symptoms, sometimes long after exposure. Special diagnostic methods are needed and self-treatment is not recommended.

Lymphatic filariasis

Two parasites are involved: *Wuchereria bancrofti,* which infects 115 million persons and occurs throughout the tropics, and *Brugia malayi,* which infects 13 million and occurs on the Indian subcontinent and Southeast Asia (Map 5.6). Adult worms live in the lymphatic vessels and nodes, particularly those of the legs and male genitalia. Microfilariae are in the bloodstream, usually at night.

Transmission is by several species of mosquito including *Anopheles gambiae* in Africa (where it also transmits malaria) and *Culex fatigans,* which breeds in pit latrines and is common around many habitations in most of the tropics, even in urban areas. In the Pacific area, microfilariae are not periodic and the vectors are *Aedes,* with a 24-hour biting cycle.

In the early stages of infection, sometimes after only three months, there is recurrent painful swelling of lymph nodes and lymph vessels, especially in the groin and spermatic cord, with fever, malaise, and sometimes transient limb swelling. After many such episodes, usually over a period of many years, there may be permanent swelling of a limb with skin changes that earn the condition its name *elephantiasis.* Fluid can also collect around the testis — producing hydrocele. Diagnosis is by blood films but, in the early stages, antibody tests are used. Treatment is with diethylcarbamazine.

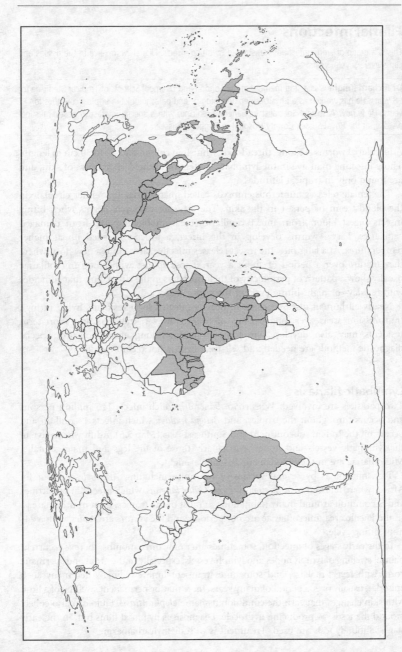

Map 5.6 Distribution of lymphatic filariasis. The disease is endemic in over 80 countries in Africa, Asia, South and Central America and the Pacific Islands. More than 40% of all infected people live in India and one-third live in Africa.

Some patients, who usually have few lymphatic features and no microfilariae in the blood, develop a lung problem called **tropical pulmonary eosinophilia** with cough, breathlessness, and wheezing. Diagnosis is made by an antibody test and very high blood eosinophilia (an abnormal white blood cell count); response to treatment is good.

River blindness (Onchocerciasis)

About 18 million persons are infected with *Onchocerca volvulus*, most live in tropical Africa, Central and South America, and Yemen. In Africa it occurs both in dry savannah and thickly forested areas.

Adult worms live in the deeper skin and connective tissue; most are within smooth, non-tender nodules, up to 4 cm in diameter, which can be felt or even seen and occur especially over bony prominences such as the hips, knees, and skull. Several pairs of worms live in each nodule. Microfilariae live in the upper dermis, where they are taken, up by small biting *Simulium* blackflies (see Fig. 5.5), which breed in swift-flowing, well-oxygenated streams and rivers. *Simulium* bites during the daytime or at dusk; bites are painful and often numerous; most will occur within 1 km of a breeding site.

Heavily infected people develop a disfiguring skin condition called onchodermatitis; initially there is skin thickening, then atrophy and depigmentation. Microfilariae in the eye cause damage to the cornea and also a choroidoretinitis at the back of the eye. Blindness is a common sequel in endemic populations. Diagnosis is by finding microfilariae in skin shavings. Treatment is with ivermectin, but this must be continued at six-monthly intervals until the worms produce no more microfilariae; nodules containing adult worms can be removed surgically.

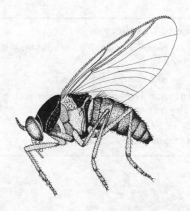

Fig 5.5 *Simulium* fly (1.5–4 mm long)

Travellers may develop itchy rashes on the trunk or limbs a year or more after exposure and some will experience eye irritation and minute snowflake opacities in the cornea. With proper treatment, lightly infected persons suffer no permanent eye damage. Control of this infection is by regular insecticidal treatment of river breeding sites together with annual rounds of treatment with ivermectin which kills microfilariae. Since adult worms can live up to 15 years, vector control without mass chemotherapy must continue for this long.

African eye worm (Loiasis)

This occurs in the tropical rainforest areas of West and Central Africa. Adult *Loa loa* worms live under the skin and in connective tissues. The microfilariae occur in the bloodstream during the daytime to coincide with the biting of the vector *Chrysops* which resembles a very large, brown horsefly and inflicts a painful bite. This fly breeds in the mud of forest pools and is attracted to wood smoke.

Adult or maturing worms can migrate across the white of the eye beneath the conjunctiva producing severe itching, lacrimation, and transient swelling of the eyelids; no permanent eye damage results but the appearance of a wriggling worm certainly causes alarm. More commonly the worms cause **Calabar swellings**. These are painful red lumps, often several centimetres in diameter and lasting for several days, which are most common on the forearms and wrists but can occur anywhere. Diagnosis is made by finding microfilariae in daytime blood films. Treatment is with diethylcarbamazine, but supervision is necessary as severe allergic complications can occur.

People staying in high–risk areas for Loiasis can take 300 mg of diethylcarbamazine weekly as a prophylactic measure; this drug has no known preventive action against other human filarial infections.

Summary of advice to travellers

- In endemic areas, risks can be minimized by the use of insect repellents and bed-nets (see p. 212).
- Symptoms can appear long after leaving endemic areas.
- A blood eosinophilia and unusual skin manifestations or tender lymphatic tissues should raise suspicion of filariasis. Early male genital lesions may be wrongly attributed to a sexually transmitted infection.
- Diagnosis and treatment require specialist attention.

Lyme disease

Lyme disease is transmitted by tick bites, and although the risk in the USA has been widely publicized, the disease in fact occurs throughout the northern hemisphere.

Dr David M. Wright is former Director of the Lyme Disease Laboratory at Charing Cross Hospital and Consultant Microbiologist and Reader in Medical Microbiology at the Department of Medical Microbiology, Imperial College of Science, Technology, and Medicine, London.

The characteristic feature of Lyme disease is an expanding skin rash (erythema migrans), which is often accompanied by headache, muscle pains, joint aches, and low-grade fever. There are sometimes more serious complications involving the nervous system, heart, or joints.

Most cases occur in the summer or early autumn. The disease is acquired through the bites of hard ticks. Female ticks bite to obtain blood from man (or other mammals) so as to undergo their next phase in development. A few ticks survive the winter and then bite in the following spring. The causative bacteria, *Borrelia burgdorferi,* reside in the tick's salivary glands, and are transmitted to the victim when the tick bites. To ensure transmission of *Borrelia,* the tick should remain continuously attached to the host for at least 24 hours. In Europe, and in Sweden in particular, there may be a skin recurrence many years after the initial rash. Unlike the early skin changes, this late manifestation, termed acrodermatitis chronica atrophicans, tends to result in occlusion of the blood vessels and nerve damage in the locality of the bite.

Distribution

There have been more than 150 000 confirmed cases in the USA since 1980, coming from almost every state; some estimates put the true number of cases very much higher — perhaps at two million (Map 5.7). Though often thought of as a North American problem, Lyme disease is found throughout the northern hemisphere; cases — though not laboratory-confirmed reports of being able to grow the causative microbe — have even been reported from coastal areas of Australia.

The species of tick able to transmit the disease differs slightly with geography; *Ixodes pacificus* being found on the western US seaboard, while *Ixodes scapularis* (formerly *dammini*) is found in the Atlantic coastal areas of America. The main vector in Europe is *Ixodes ricinus* and in Asia, *Ixodes persulcatus.* Other ticks implicated are *Ixodes hexagonus* (the hedgehog tick), the sheep tick, and *Amblyomma americanum* (the Lone Star tick). Small mammals (such as field mice, voles, and badgers) or birds tend to be the repository of the infecting organism. Ticks which usually feed on these species bite man or his pets only accidentally. Wild deer, whilst carrying large numbers of ticks, tend not to suffer from the disease but, being 'nomadic' animals, tend to disperse the ticks, and hence the disease, more widely than other animals. Although mosquitoes and other insects can spread the disease by biting, their role tends to be minimal as disease transmission depends on their mouth parts being transiently infected (like a contaminated needle), unlike ticks where *Borrelia* survive inside the ticks' bodies.

The illness

Mercifully, subclinical infections are the rule. Symptoms can begin between 3 and 32 days after the tick bite (typically after 14 days), but only about 15 per cent of patients remember having been bitten. This is partly because the tick may be too small to be noticed or because with each tick bite, anti-inflammatory and anaesthetic substances are injected into the victim, so that there is little or no reaction. The ticks are often first observed following their blood meal, when they enlarge, sometimes to the size of a small thumbnail.

The first sign to appear is a red area on the skin surrounding the tick bite. Over the next few days the rash may expand in a circular fashion, the centre of the ring returning to normal skin colour. The rash is usually painless and non-irritating. If left untreated, the rash may resolve in a few weeks or continue to expand for up to a year, with the ring approaching a metre in diameter. Multiple tick bites can cause multiple red circles on the skin — a finding more common in the USA.

In less than a fifth of patients, the rash may be accompanied by mild 'flu-like symptoms, muscle paralysis, particularly on one side of the face (a Bell's palsy), and nerve pain in specific areas supplied by the nerves either in the head or body. Rarely, the patient complains of an insidiously developing stiff neck — a sign of chronic meningitis. This may be associated with a degree of unsteadiness brought about by the involvement of the nerves from the brain passing to the cerebellum. In children and the over 60s, attacks of delirium have been recorded. In a smaller number of patients, inflammation of the tendons and joints occurs, particularly of the lower limb, although no joint or tendon is immune. Occasionally, arthritis may persist. In less than 1 in 30 of those patients with a rash, irregularity of the heart beat may be detected. This may require urgent antibiotic treatment as well as the insertion of a temporary pacemaker.

There are many patients who do not have, or fail to notice, any rash and may present with just one complication of Lyme disease. Blood tests like ELISA and immunoblot tests may confirm the diagnosis. These tests may not become positive for six weeks from the time that the initial skin signs appear, while supervening antibiotic treatment may prevent these blood tests from ever becoming positive. In endemic areas of Lyme disease, a positive blood test may occur in many patients who either do not remember exposure to anything that could be Lyme disease, or who have had the disease many years previously, or who have had a subclinical exposure.

On the Baltic Island of Wisby, some 80 per cent of the population have a positive blood test for Lyme disease, whereas less than 3 per cent give a history of having had the infection. This makes the diagnosis of Lyme disease somewhat questionable without the hallmark of the initial specific rash. Unfortunately, there are an increasing number of residents in Lyme endemic areas with non-diagnostic general symptoms of Lyme disease like fatigue, fibromyalgia, loss of concentration, and a feeling of 'pins and needles' — all of whom have a positive blood test for Lyme disease but in whom the relationship to the clinical manifestation remains doubtful. In fact, labelling them as suffering from Lyme disease may lead to more appropriate psychiatric or physical treatments being withheld. In early cases of Lyme disease, when the standard blood test may be negative, the polymerase chain reaction on tissue taken from the specific rash or body fluids, other than blood, may sometimes prove helpful in establishing the diagnosis.

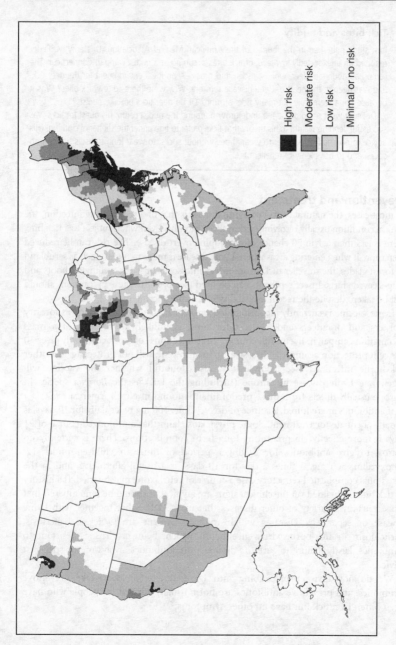

Map 5.7 US National Lyme disease risk map with four categories of risk.

High risk

Moderate risk

Low risk

Minimal or no risk

Tick bites and nudity

In a study published in the Journal of the American Medical Association, Dr Henry M. Feder reported an unexpectedly low level of tick bites occurring at a nudist camp in Connecticut. The camp had abundant deer, woods, rocks, and grass — an ideal environment for the deer tick, and was deep in the heart of Lyme disease territory. Why were there so few tick bites? Was it because there were truly not many ticks around? Or do deer ticks not like nudists?

Dr Feder went on to probe the undergrowth around the nudist camp: his quest for ticks was successful, lending weight to his theory that ticks prefer to bite under the shelter of clothing. (His advice to non-nudists is never to wear shoes without socks, to wear long trousers tucked into socks, and to use plenty of repellent.)

Prevention and treatment

In most cases, the natural course of Lyme disease is that of a self-limiting infection, the clinical condition usually resolving within three months. Even when subject to a tick bite, there is less than a 1 in 50 chance of developing overt disease. The risk can be reduced even more if when entering areas where Lyme disease is more frequent, such as scrubland or forest glades, the traveller tucks trouser legs into socks or wears wellington boots and long-sleeved shirts. Insect repellents can be used (see p. 208). These precautions should still be taken, despite the recent availability of a Lyme vaccine in the USA.

Lyme vaccine is currently recommended only for high-risk groups such as forestry workers and orienteers and, at least for now, is unlikely to be used in a mass vaccination campaign. Even a full course (three injections) of the vaccine only gives 70 per cent protection against the disease and, in any event, will not protect against other tick-borne infections (see below). It is also doubtful whether the vaccine will ameliorate Lyme disease in Europe (including the UK) as the *Borrelia* species in Europe usually differs from those predominantly found in North America.

If antibiotics are required, a course of doxycycline, 100 mg twice daily for 10 days, is usually adequate for treatment. Some physicians claim that a prolonged course of 21 days is more effective in preventing long-term complications. There is certainly no reason to give antibiotics for a longer period of time. In children under 12, amoxycillin, 500 mg, 3 times a day for 10 days, is a useful alternative, and in the occasional complicated refractory case a course of ceftriaxone may be tried. If a history of tick bite is obtained yet the clinical signs are atypical, it should be remembered that ticks transmit a variety of other diseases that may occur either together with Lyme disease or separately. Diseases which may be present are Q fever, babesiosis, ehrlichiosis, or tick-borne virus encephalitis which, being a virus, is resistant to antibiotics. Lastly, failure to cure the disease with antibiotics always merits specialist advice.

We do not advise people going into Lyme disease areas to take preventive antibiotics, and preventive antibiotics are not normally advised for people who have been bitten by a tick but have no other symptoms.

Further reading

Rahn, D.W. and Evans, J. (ed.) (1998). *Lyme disease*, pp. 1–254. American College of Physicians, Philadelphia.

Leishmaniasis

Leishmaniasis occurs in Mediterranean countries, the Middle East, India, Nepal, East Africa, and Central and South America. The internal (visceral) form is fatal if untreated; the skin (cutaneous) form is a persistent nuisance; the rare mucocutaneous form is serious and disfiguring. Avoiding sandfly bites, the main protective measure, is difficult. Fortunately, all forms of leishmaniasis are uncommon in travellers.

Dr Robert N. Davidson is a Consultant in Infectious Diseases and Tropical Medicine at Northwick Park Hospital, Harrow. He has done much research on treatment of leishmaniasis, and works with Médecins Sans Frontières. He has written many journal papers and contributed to several medical textbooks on the subject of leishmaniasis. He is happy to answer queries about leishmaniasis (r.n.davidson@ic.ac.uk).

Deforestation, irrigation, war, and famine have all led to an increase in leishmaniasis, which occurs widely (Maps 5.8–5.10). Each year, there are about 10 million cases of cutaneous leishmaniasis, and 400 000 cases of the internal form, visceral leishmaniasis (also called kala-azar). Mucocutaneous leishmaniasis, in which the nose and lips become swollen and gradually destroyed, is rare. Because it is uncommon in travellers, whenever it does occur the diagnosis is often missed or delayed until a specialist is consulted.

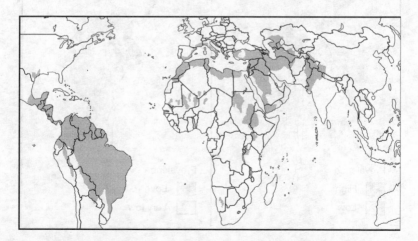

Map 5.8 Prevalence of cutaneous leishmaniasis (European, African, and Asian forms)

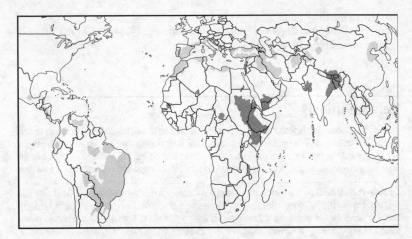

Map 5.9 Prevalence of visceral leishmaniasis (kala-azar)

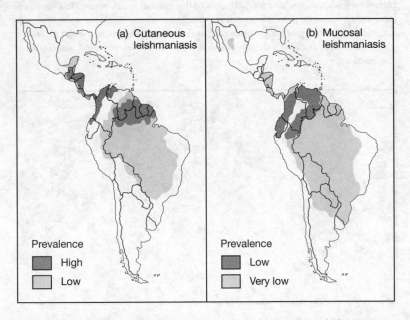

Map 5.10 Prevalence of American cutaneous leishmaniasis and mucocutaneous leishmaniasis.

What is leishmaniasis?

Leishmania are single-celled organisms, about the same size as the malaria parasite, which infect macrophage cells (part of the immune system) in the skin, spleen, liver, bone marrow, and lymph glands. They are carried in the salivary glands of certain types of sandfly (Fig. 5.6), which have themselves become infected when feeding on an infected animal or human. Sandflies do not live on the beach, as one might suppose from their name, but, according to their species, live in bush, forests, the cracks in stone or mud walls, animal burrows, or termite mounds. Sandflies are small (~2 mm) and beige-coloured, so that they are scarcely noticed. They fly silently, and their bites may itch but are not painful. They usually bite at night, sometimes indoors but more often outdoors.

Wild or domestic animals such as rodents, dogs, foxes, and jackals can be carriers of certain species of *Leishmania*, with which man is 'accidentally' infected. Other *Leishmania* species affect mainly humans, and are transmitted from man to man in towns or rural areas

Cutaneous leishmaniasis (European, African, and Asian forms)

Cutaneous leishmaniasis consists of one or several persistent nodules or ulcers, most commonly on the face or limbs. They occur at the site of the sandfly bites and start about 2–8 weeks after being bitten. The transmission season is during and after the rains — in Europe and the Middle East it is the summer, and in Africa, the months of June to October. Ulcers are relatively painless and not particularly 'pussy', unless secondarily infected with bacteria. Without treatment, lesions usually eventually heal in about 3–12 months, leaving a scar. Throughout the Middle East and Afghanistan, many people have obvious scars of cutaneous leishmaniasis on their faces.

An urban species (*Leishmania tropica*) is common in cities such as Kabul, Aleppo, Baghdad, Damascus, and Tehran. The best protection against this is to sleep in an air-conditioned room or use an impregnated mosquito net. A rural, semi-desert species

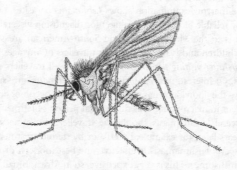

Fig. 5.6 *Phlebotomus* sandfly (2–5 mm long)

(*Leishmania major*) is common in Israel, Jordan, Libya, Tunisia, Algeria, Morocco, Iran, Iraq, and some parts of Saudi Arabia. When camping in the desert, keep your tent away from gerbil burrows (these are the animal carriers of cutaneous leishmaniasis) and always use an impregnated bed-net and insect repellents on your skin. Uncommonly, cutaneous leishmaniasis is acquired in regions bordering the Mediterranean, including the islands.

The diagnosis is made by recognizing the characteristic lesions, and confirmed by a smear from the cut edge of an ulcer; success depends upon the skill of the microscopist. Treatment is not necessary in every case: if the ulcers are small and few, they may heal naturally. Some forms of cutaneous leishmaniasis require injections of an antimonial drug, either into the edge of the sore or intravenously.

Visceral leishmaniasis (kala-azar)

Visceral leishmaniasis is widespread throughout large areas of India, especially Bihar state, and also in Bangladesh and Nepal. There have been massive epidemics in India and Sudan, and it remains common in parts of Sudan, Ethiopia, Kenya, Eritrea, and Somalia. In all these areas, the spread is man to man by sandflies, and the parasite is called *Leishmania donovani*.

In Brazil, and all the countries bordering the Mediterranean, dogs are commonly infected with *Leishmania infantum* (confusingly called *Leishmania chagasi* in the Americas). *Leishmania infantum* can cause visceral leishmaniasis in man, but requires a bite from an infected sandfly — close contact with pets does not spread *Leishmania*. The numbers of canine cases outnumber human cases by thousands to one.

In visceral leishmaniasis, the *Leishmania* parasites spread internally, invading cells in the spleen, bone marrow, liver, and lymph glands. The symptoms start weeks to months after being bitten and are of prolonged fever, weight loss, abdominal discomfort, weakness, and anaemia. The spleen, liver, and, sometimes, lymph glands, all become enlarged. *When it occurs in travellers, visceral leishmaniasis is usually suspected as being lymphoma or leukaemia, which it mimics.*

Fortunately, bone-marrow examination shows *Leishmania* parasites, not malignancy. There is also a fairly reliable blood test (serology) for diagnosing visceral leishmaniasis. Visceral leishmaniasis in the Mediterranean and South American areas chiefly affects infants and young children and is not common in travellers of any age. *The illness may begin up to two years after visiting the endemic area* — unwell travellers should remind their doctors of this. Of interest, many infections with *Leishmania* are 'silent': although bitten by a sandfly, the individual has no symptoms and becomes immune; a few parasites remain latent in macrophage cells during that person's lifetime. These parasites can then cause visceral leishmaniasis should the traveller's immune system become suppressed many years later, for example, by HIV or by steroid treatment.

Treatment of visceral leishmaniasis is effective: the best modern drug is liposomal amphotericin B (AmBisome). This is very expensive, so in Africa, Brazil, and India, the older pentavalent antimony drugs, sodium stibogluconate (Pentostam) and meglumine antimoniate (Glucantime), are used.

Occasionally, visceral leishmaniasis has been spread by needles shared between HIV-infected drug users; very rarely by blood transfusion or transplantation; and even more rarely from mother to unborn child.

American cutaneous leishmaniasis and mucocutaneous leishmaniasis

Travellers to Belize, and other parts of rural Central and South America, may contract cutaneous leishmaniasis from the bite of a sandfly. Archaeologists, tourists, and soldiers are at risk, especially if spending evenings in the forest. The parasites responsible are *Leishmania mexicana* and *Leishmania braziliensis*. The nodules or ulcers of both species of *Leishmania* resemble cutaneous leishmaniasis lesions from the Middle East. Lesions will usually heal spontaneously over several months. Cutaneous leishmaniasis caused by *Leishmania braziliensis* can occasionally progress to, or recur as, the disfiguring mucocutaneous leishmaniasis. In this disease the nose and lips become swollen and over the course of months or years the lesions ulcerate and spread along the cartilage of the nose, progressively destroying the tissues. For this reason only, cutaneous leishmaniasis from the Americas needs specialist attention and very careful treatment. Fortunately, mucocutaneous leishmaniasis is rare.

Summary of advice for travellers

- Awareness of leishmaniasis is very low outside the regions where the disease is a problem — and this is despite the fact that the disease is named after a Scot. However, the disease is unpleasant, and efforts to prevent it are worthwhile.

- The key precaution is to try to avoid sandfly bites by using an impregnated mosquito net. Sandflies bite in darkness, and although small enough to pass through the mesh of a mosquito net, they will not do so if the net is impregnated with permethrin, deltamethrin, or lambda cyhalothrin. If in a highly *Leishmania*-endemic area, permethrin can also be impregnated into clothing.

- If camping in the Middle East, in semi-desert country, look out for the communal burrows of gerbil colonies, and camp as far away from them as you can. In areas where there is a high prevalence of leishmaniasis, and if sleeping indoors, you should also use your net — sandflies are well-adapted to living in and around poorly constructed dwellings. Repellents containing DEET (see p. 208) should be applied to exposed skin in the evening, and re-applied as instructed.

Sleeping sickness

Sleeping sickness is a potentially serious infection spread by biting flies in Africa. Infection in travellers is unusual but visitors to game parks or those visiting rural areas may be at risk and should protect themselves from the bite of the tsetse fly.

Dr David Smith† was Senior Lecturer in Clinical Tropical Medicine and Head of the Division of Tropical Medicine of the Liverpool School of Tropical Medicine. He died in May 2000 and is greatly missed by his colleagues both in Liverpool and around the world. His wisdom and breadth of experience in the discipline was much admired and he was particularly involved with investigating bypanosomiasis in Uganda in the early 1990s.

Sleeping sickness (or human African trypanosomiasis) occurs in some 36 countries in sub-Saharan Africa (Map 5.11). It is transmitted by tsetse flies (Fig. 5.7). In recent years large epidemics have recurred in Central Africa, largely as the result of instability

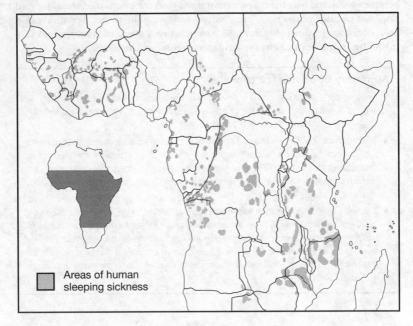

Areas of human
sleeping sickness

Map 5.11 Human trypanosomiasis distribution. Although confined to historical foci, human trypanosomiasis continues to affect many of the 37 tsetse-infested countries in sub-Saharan Africa. In recent years, a resurgence of the disease to epidemic proportions has been experienced in several countries, notably, Sudan, Angola and the Democratic Republic of Congo. The acute form of the disease, caused by *Trypanosoma rhodesiense*, is generally confined to eastern and southern Africa, with the chronic form, *T.gambiense*, being found in western and central regions (source: WHO).

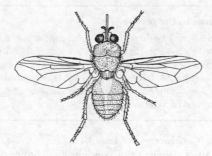

Figure 5.7 Tsetse fly (female) (6–15 mm long)

and unrest. Estimates by the WHO suggest that between 300 000 and 500 000 people have the disease — especially in parts of Sudan and Congo–Zaire. In East and southern Africa, travellers to game parks are potentially at risk from this infection, which is both difficult to diagnose and complicated to treat. A number of recent cases have been recorded in European travellers. Trypanosomiasis is also an economically important infection of cattle in much of Africa.

The disease

What causes it?
Sleeping sickness is caused by a motile, single-celled organism. Infection is acquired from the bite of a tsetse fly. There may be redness and swelling at the site of the bite, followed by illness with fever, and eventually the organisms enter the central nervous system where they cause fatal encephalitis. The disease gets its name from the characteristic sleep disorder where individuals fall asleep at inappropriate times.

How is it spread?
Sleeping sickness is spread by tsetse flies infected with trypanosomes. The flies are sturdy, about the size of a housefly, and the bite is painful. Characteristically, they rest with the wings folded across their back. Tsetse flies require shade and humidity and tend to occur in association with game animals in East Africa and along rivers and lake shores in Central and West Africa. They are attracted to moving vehicles, the scent of animals, and contrasting colours.

What are the features of the disease?
There are two forms of the disease: one type occurs in rural areas of West and Central Africa, and the other in East and southern Africa. The infection is fatal if not treated.

Unwanted facial hair to the rescue

Eflornithine, a powerful treatment for sleeping sickness, but one that was in dwilndling supply because it was commercially non-viable, has been given a new lease of life. It's been discovered that the drug has a remarkable effect on reducing unwanted facial hair in women — sold as a facial cream called Vaniqa in the USA. This enabled production of an intravenous form of the drug to resume, to combat sleeping sickness. The manufacturers have donated 60 000 doses to Médecins Sans Frontières and the WHO.

West and Central Africa (Gambian trypanosomiasis)
In Central and West Africa sleeping sickness is initially a chronic disease, with mild early symptoms, but leading to extensive brain disease after months or years. It may be difficult to diagnose. People are infected in rural areas, close to water, and all age groups and both sexes are affected. Over the past decade there has been a dramatic increase in this infection especially in rural areas of Central African countries including Congo–Zaire, southern Sudan, northern Uganda, and Angola, partly as a result of civil disturbance. There are believed to be several hundred thousand people currently infected. Longer-term visitors to rural areas and aid workers are more at risk than tourists or short-term visitors.

East and southern Africa (Rhodesian trypanosomiasis)
The infection in East and southern Africa is much more acute and presents as a severe febrile illness, often with a lesion at the site of the tsetse bite (a chancre), severe fever, and early onset of central nervous system abnormalities. This form of trypanosomiasis occurs in game animals and tourists are at special risk visiting game parks and game lodges. Recent epidemics of this form of the infection have occurred in Busoga, in south-eastern Uganda.

The diagnosis
Sleeping sickness should be considered in travellers who have recently visited game parks in East or southern Africa (including Kenya, Tanzania, Zambia, and Zimbabwe) and who have a severe fever. A characteristic inflamed lesion at the site of the tsetse bite (the chancre) may be present. They will give a history of tsetse bites whilst viewing game and may have a skin rash.

Sleeping sickness should also be considered in travellers from rural parts of Central or West Africa, who may present with a more chronic febrile illness or symptoms suggestive of an infection of the central nervous system, including the typical sleep disorders, behavioural changes, or neurological abnormalities. This form of infection may not present for months or even years after periods of travel. Among travellers, it is more common in those working for extended periods in endemic areas.

The parasite can be detected in the blood, though often only in small numbers. A range of concentration techniques may be required to establish the diagnosis, especially with the Gambian form. Progression of the infection to involve the brain can be confirmed by examining the cerebrospinal fluid.

Treatment

The treatment options for trypanosomiasis are limited to the drugs suramin, melarsoprol, pentamidine, and eflornithine. All need careful specialist prescription and monitoring, and have high side effects profiles.

Summary of advice for travellers

- There are no vaccines or prophylactic drugs available to prevent infection.

- In game areas, prevention therefore depends on avoiding tsetse flies bites. Tsetse bite during the daytime; they often follow moving vehicles, for example on game-runs. Keep the windows closed and kill tsetse that enter the vehicle with an insecticide spray. Insect repellents have only a short-lived effect. In Central Africa, tsetse flies live along rivers and lake shores.

- Travellers who become ill after travel to areas where sleeping sickness occurs should ensure that their doctor knows the areas visited and, if there is a possibility of tsetse bites, it is important to exclude sleeping sickness. In view of the difficulties of diagnosis, suspected cases should be referred to specialists.

Chagas disease (South American trypanosomiasis)

Chagas disease is widespread in Latin America and in parts of the southern USA (Map 5.12). Around 16 million people are thought to be infected. It is a potentially serious infection, but large-scale control campaigns have substantially reduced the risk of transmission, especially in the southern cone countries such as Chile, Argentina, Uruguay, and central and southern Brazil. Elsewhere, travellers to rural areas may be at some risk if they sleep in huts infested with the insect transmitters. Transmission can also occur through blood transfusion from infected donors; again, this is of declining importance in many countries but transmission of unscreened blood should be avoided. Eating raw or undercooked small mammals — especially opossums — should also be avoided since these are often infected with the causative parasite.

Dr C.J. Schofield has carried out research on Chagas disease and its control throughout Latin America for over 25 years. Since retiring from the World Health Organization in Geneva, he has been based at the London School of Hygiene and Tropical Medicine and co-ordinates the ECLAT research network in support of Chagas' disease control activities.

What is Chagas disease and how is it spread?

The disease takes its name from the Brazilian clinician, Carlos Chagas, who first described it in 1909. It is caused by a microscopic protozoan parasite, *Trypanosoma cruzi*, which is mainly transmitted by large blood-sucking insects sometimes known in English as cone-nosed bugs or kissing bugs, but known by a variety of local names in Latin America (e.g. 'vinchucas' in the southern cone countries, 'barbeiros' in Brazil, 'chirimachas' in Peru, 'chinchorros' in Ecuador, 'pitos' or 'chipos' in Colombia and Venezuela). Most species of kissing bug live in sylvatic habitats, associated with small

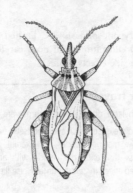

Fig. 5.8 Triatoma (average size of adult is 2.4 cm long; species range from 5 mm to 4.5 cm)

nest-building mammals or birds, but a few have adapted to live also in rural dwellings. These domestic species pose greatest risk, emerging from cracks and crevices at night to suck the blood of the sleeping occupants. The bite of these species is generally painless and often unremarked. Sylvatic species of kissing bug sometimes fly into rural houses, probably attracted by light; their bite tends to be more noticeable. All the developmental stages of the kissing bugs, including the small wingless nymphs, will feed on vertebrate blood and can transmit *T. cruzi*. See Fig 5.8.

Unusually amongst insect-borne parasites, *T. cruzi* is not transmitted by the bite of the insects, but instead passes out in the insect's faeces, which are often deposited while feeding on the host. If this is seen to occur, the dark faecal droplets should be washed off — preferably with alcohol, or with copious soap and water. This type of transmission is inefficient. It has been estimated that, on average, over 1000 contacts with infected bugs are required to produce one new human infection.

The parasite can also be transmitted to cold food or drinks by contamination with the insect faeces, and is readily transmitted by blood transfusion from infected donors (see also p. 589). Most Latin American countries now have strict screening procedures to eliminate infected blood donations, but unscreened blood is still a risk in some countries, particularly Bolivia, Peru, Ecuador, and parts of Central America and Mexico.

Symptoms
The infection proceeds through two phases. The initial acute phase lasts up to eight weeks, during which time the parasites are mainly circulating in the peripheral bloodstream. There may be no obvious symptoms, but fever, lymph node swellings, and diffuse heart pain are common. Unilateral swelling around one eye (known as Romaña's sign) is strongly diagnostic of the acute phase, but is not always apparent.

The acute phase declines as the parasites enter cells of most of the vital organs — particularly heart muscle and nervous tissue. The parasites reproduce inside the cells, eventually destroying them and so producing chronic tissue destruction. In general, however, the chronic infection will remain without obvious symptoms, but about 30 per cent of infected people may develop serious lesions — often 10–20 years after the initial infection. The most serious lesions involve the heart (e.g. arrhythmias, conduction difficulties, aneurysms). Parasite strains found in the southern cone countries can also cause important intestinal problems (e.g. megaoesophagus, megacolon).

Treatment

There are two drugs that can be used to treat the early acute phase of infection — nifurtimox (marketed by Bayer as Lampit) and benznidazole (marketed by Roche as Rochagan or Radanil). However, neither drug should be given without medical supervision because of the risk of side effects. Treatment with either drug is lengthy; 10 days' treatment may be sufficient if the infection is diagnosed immediately, but 30–60 days' treatment is more usual. Both drugs are generally well-tolerated by children up to 10 years old, but side effects in adults are frequent, generally starting after the eighth day of treatment. Common side effects include intense itching and skin-shedding, anorexia, malaise, and loss of concentration. In extreme cases anaemia and destruction of white blood cells can occur, which require suspension of treatment.

Chronic infections in young children can also be treated with benznidazole or Lampit; the cure rate is much lower, but prompt treatment does seem to reduce the likelihood of severe lesions later in life. For adults in the chronic stage of infection, only supportive treatment can be given, such as antiarrythmic drugs and/or vasodilators. Extreme cases may require surgical intervention such as a pacemaker implant.

If a new infection with *T. cruzi* is strongly suspected (for example, due to a laboratory accident) seek immediate treatment with benznidazole or nifurtimox. The sooner treatment begins, the greater the likelihood of successful cure without severe side effects.

Prevention and personal protection

In general, Chagas disease represents a very low risk to travellers, especially since the intensive control campaigns in most Latin American countries. Most at risk are those who sleep in rural dwellings infested with kissing bugs. How can you tell? Ask the local residents if bugs are present, and if in doubt, sleep elsewhere. If this is not possible, sleep in the middle of the room away from the walls and check the bed and mattress for insects. Insect repellents will discourage the bugs from feeding, and a bed-net should protect you from those falling from the roof. Most importantly, check in the morning for any dark deposits that may be insect faeces, and wash these away with alcohol or soap and water.

Blood transfusions from unknown sources should be avoided, not just for the risk of Chagas disease but also HIV(AIDS), hepatitis, and syphilis. In some rural clinics, blood for transfusion is treated first with gentian violet in order to clear any possible parasites. This gives the blood (and the recipient) a blue colour that can last for several days.

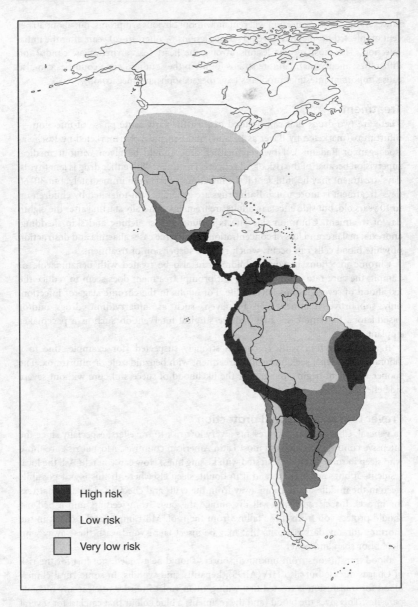

High risk

Low risk

Very low risk

Map 5.12 Approximate distribution of human Chagas disease. Broad lines mark approximate northern and southern distribution limits of Triatominae and of silvatic *T.cruzi*.

Check-up

The parasite is difficult to detect directly in the bloodstream even during the early acute phase. Instead, serological tests are carried out on a sample of blood taken by finger-prick. These tests (indirect fluorescent antibody test, indirect haemagglutination test, or ELISA) are now extremely accurate, and may be recommended to anyone having received a blood transfusion while in Latin America. Treatment with benznidazole or nifurtimox can then be given. These tests are also important if you are considering becoming a blood donor and also for pregnant women, because there is a small risk that the parasite can be passed across the placenta to the developing foetus. In such cases, the newborn baby can be treated, with a high chance of eliminating any infection.

Plague

Perhaps remarkably, the ancient scourge of plague is still with us, though the risk to travellers is extremely small.

Dr Tom Solomon has studied the history of plague and worked for several years in Vietnam, where plague is endemic. He is a Lecturer in Neurology and Honorary Lecturer in Medical Microbiology and Tropical Medicine at the University of Liverpool.

There are few diseases that strike more fear into the hearts of men than the plague, and few organisms have affected the globe with such devastating consequences. Although a disease compatible with plague was described in the eleventh century BC, the first of three pandemics (global epidemics) occurred in the sixth century AD. The second pandemic, known as the 'Black Death' wiped out between a third and a quarter of the European population during the fourteenth century. At this stage the communicable nature of the disease was appreciated, and so was the importance of overcrowding and poor sanitation — but the cause was unknown. The third pandemic began in China in the mid-nineteenth century.

By 1894 it reached Hong Kong, where the causative organism, a small gram-negative cocco-bacillus was first identified. Who deserves the credit for this has been one of the most famous and prolonged controversies in medical history. Although Kitasato, a Japanese investigator, lay claim to the discovery for many years, the taxonomic name of the bacillus *Yersinia pestis* reflects the fact that ultimately a Frenchman, Alexandre Yersin, was credited with it. It was subsequently shown that the disease spread to man from infected rats, via the bites of fleas — particularly *Xenopsilla* species. The flea's proventriculus (gullet) becomes blocked by the replicating bacterium, and it thus regurgitates the organism whilst feeding on mammals.

Epidemiology

During the third plague pandemic the disease reached South America, Africa, and Asia. Although urban plague was largely controlled by sanitary measures, plague spread to forest rodents (rats, rabbits, squirrels, chipmunks), and has persisted as a rural disease ever since. In its natural cycle, the bacterium is transmitted between these rodents, which remain relatively free from symptoms. Sporadic human cases occur when individuals (usually forest and field workers) encroach on this cycle and are incidentally bitten by infected fleas.

Under certain circumstances, however, probably related to climate and the availability of host animals, the flea population can suddenly grow. The bacterium is spread to urban rats, particularly the black rat (*Rattus rattus*) and the brown sewer rat (*Rattus norvegicus*), which act as *amplifying* hosts. In these rats infection causes severe illness, and as they die, the fleas jump to new hosts, including humans. Hence urban plague epidemics are associated with large numbers of dead rats, and 'rat fall' has been recognized as an indicator of impending plague for over a century.

During the 1980s and early 1990s there were approximately 1000–2000 plague cases globally every year. Since then the number of cases reported to the WHO has gradually increased (Fig. 5.9). In 1997, there were 5500 cases. Areas particularly affected include China, most of Southeast Asia (especially Vietnam), much of Africa (particularly Madagascar, Tanzania, Congo, Zaire, Uganda, and Botswana), South America (especially Peru), and India, where there was a large outbreak of pneumonic and bubonic plague in 1994 (Map 5.13). There were also a handful of cases in eastern Europe and North America.

Clinical features

Three main clinical syndromes are recognized: *bubonic plague, septicaemic plague,* and *pneumonic plague.* Two to seven days after the bite of an infected flea, patients develop a high fever, rigors, headache, and muscle aches. In bubonic plague, the bacterium moves through the bloodstream to the local lymph nodes (usually in the groin), where it causes a painful swelling known as a 'bubo'. Occasionally bleeding into the skin causes a patchy dark discoloration (purpura) giving rise to the name 'Black Death'.

In some patients, rather than being confined to the lymph nodes, the bacterium spreads into the rest of the bloodstream causing septicaemia. The symptoms of septicaemic plague are indistinguishable from septicaemia due to other gram-negative bacteria. Patients have fever, malaise, and headaches, and, if untreated, rapidly deteriorate into shock (low blood pressure), dying in a few days.

In other plague patients, the bacteria spread into the lungs to give pneumonic plague. A severe pneumonia develops, with shortness of breath and a cough productive of bloodstained sputum. It is this cough, and in particular droplets infected with bacteria, that are responsible for the direct spread of pneumonic plague between humans. Untreated, pneumonic plague can be rapidly fatal. Persons, seemingly fit and well, may be dead within a day — hence the children's nursery rhyme: 'Ring o' ring o' roses, a pocket full of poses, atishoo, atishoo, we all fall down.'

Diagnosis, treatment, and prevention

Plague is diagnosed by identifying the bacillus in bubo aspirate or sputum using a light microscope, and by culturing the organism. More recently, antibody detection tests (ELISAs) have been developed.

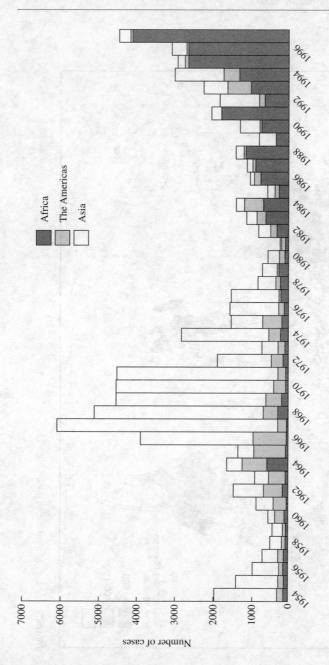

Fig. 5.9 Number of cases of plague reported to the World Health Organization (1954–97)

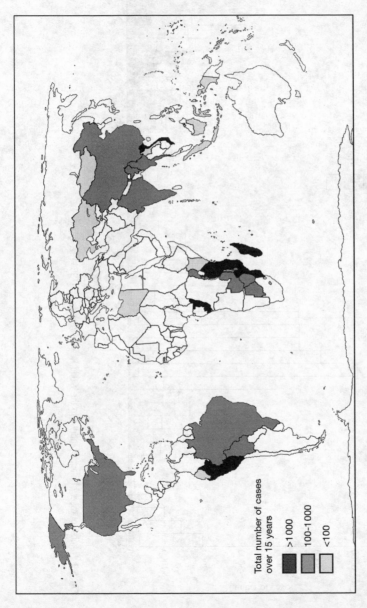

Map 5.13 Countries reporting human plague, 1983-97.

Total number of cases
over 15 years

>1000

100–1000

<100

Surprisingly, given the panic associated with plague outbreaks, the disease is easily treated with antibiotics, so long as they are started early enough. In suspected cases treatment should therefore be started as soon as diagnostic samples have been taken, without waiting for the results. Streptomycin, tetracycline, and chloramphenicol are all effective. However, antibiotic resistance has been documented, and fluoroquinolones (drugs like ciprofloxacin) may have a role in the future. Patients with pneumonic plague should be nursed in isolation, if possible, and prophylaxis (preventive treatment) with tetracycline is recommended for their close contacts.

Although there is a formalin-inactivated vaccine, this is only given to individuals at an especially high risk of exposure e.g. laboratory personnel working on the bacterium, or field-workers whose occupation brings them into regular contact with rodent fleas in affected areas. In endemic areas regular insecticide and rodenticide use around the dwelling is recommended. Flea powder should be used on dogs, cats, and other pets that might come into contact with infected rodents. During epidemics, flea and rodent control measures are used to limit the spread of the disease. It is important that the fleas are killed before the rats, so they don't simply jump onto humans.

Summary of advice for travellers

- Despite the fear associated with it, plague is a relatively rare disease that is easily treatable if caught early. Those going to endemic areas should minimize exposure to fleas from rats, use an insect repellent containing DEET, and seek medical advice early if they develop fever or other symptoms of the disease.

Typhus

Typhus can occasionally be a risk to travellers on walking holidays or to medical aid workers in refugee camps.

Dr George Cowan was Dean of Postgraduate Medicine in the University of London and is past President of the Royal Society of Tropical Medicine and Hygiene. For over 20 years he was a consultant physician in the British Army and practised hospital medicine on four continents (not all at once!).

Each of the four main types of typhus fever is spread by a different insect; all are potential hazards to travellers to the tropics. They are caused by small bacteria called *rickettsiae*. In all cases the illness consists of high fever, muscle pains, severe headache, and a rash (mainly on the trunk of the body), although the severity varies between the four types. Fortunately, all respond quickly to treatment with doxycycline (200 mg in a single dose, for adults, is usually sufficient) or other types of tetracycline (250 mg 6-hourly for a week). *No* useful vaccines are readily available.

Epidemic typhus

Epidemic typhus is a serious illness spread by the faeces of the human body or clothing louse (inhaled or rubbed into the louse bite), and especially occurs in time of war and social upheaval in prisons and refugee camps. Huge epidemics occurred in the past, notably in the aftermaths of both the Great Wars of the twentieth century, and it remains a risk in all the cooler mountainous parts of the tropics, especially in refugee camps, where it can pose a risk to expatriate health workers and NGO members. An epidemic in Burundi in 1995 at altitudes over 1500 m, caused 50 000 cases in prisons before spreading to the general population, in which it remains a problem. Other countries recently affected have been Ethiopia, Nigeria, and Peru, and the potential for epidemics exists in the troubled areas of the Balkans (e.g. Kosovo).

Control depends on rapid treatment of all cases with doxycycline and vigorous delousing of the populations at risk (e.g. all refugees in a camp) by the provision of clean clothing and the use of dusting with 1 per cent malathion or 1 per cent permethrin powder. Volunteer workers should wear clothing thus dusted, and can take preventive doxycycline, 200 mg once weekly.

Endemic typhus

Endemic typhus is spread by the bites of rat fleas and is especially associated with markets, food stores, breweries, and garbage dumps. It is usually a mild illness, but can become severe in refugee villages. A recent case in Newcastle had been acquired in India; and it has occurred also in Central America, West Africa, and Southeast Asia. In suburban Los Angeles the infection is present in fleas living on cats and opossums.

Tick typhus

Tick typhus occurs in different forms in different parts of the world. In the African veldt it is transmitted by ticks living on cattle, rhinos, and hippos, and is a risk to visitors to game parks. A small black scab develops at the site of the tick bite, and a general rash occurs. In the Mediterranean area, dog ticks are the vector and the illness can be acquired especially in the South of France, Spain, and Tunisia. A recent human case in Lille was caused by a tick from a dog recently imported from Marseille. In North America, the illness is called 'Rocky Mountain spotted fever' because of the site of its original discovery, but it now has the potential for severe illness in the Atlantic states in the summer, especially in hunters and trekkers exposed to wild animal ticks. Cases also occur in South America (notably around Sao Paulo), India, and Southeast Asia. Prevention is helped by the impregnation of travellers' clothes with permethrin.

Scrub typhus

Scrub typhus is a hazard for travellers to rural Japan, Southeast Asia, the Indian subcontinent and Indian Ocean islands, Papua New Guinea, and North Queensland, who spend time in rural areas of secondary jungle covered with spiky, waist-high *imperata* grass (known as *lalang* in Malaysia and Indonesia, *kogon* in the Philippines, *kunai* in Papua New Guinea, and *illuk* in Sri Lanka). The responsible insect, a tiny mite larva, lives on the grass and hops on to passing humans, eventually biting painlessly in the armpits, groins, and trouser belt areas. The fever comes about 10 days later, with a skin rash and a small black scab at the site of the mite bite. Prevention is helped by clothing impregnation with permethrin, the use of DEET repellents, and by wearing jungle boots and gaiters with long trousers. People who have to pass through known infected areas (e.g. soldiers) can also take prophylactic doxycycline, 200 mg (e.g. Vibramycin, 2 capsules) once weekly.

Summary of advice for travellers

- There are no commercially available vaccines against any variety of typhus.

- Anyone walking through tropical bush should inspect their skin carefully at the end of the day and remove any attached ticks (see p. 203). Repellents give useful protection against ticks and mites.

- Dogs are a potential source of a number of infections. It is wise to remove any ticks from pet dogs before they can transfer their infections to you.

Maggot infestation (myiasis)

Travellers to tropical Africa and South America may occasionally come across this unpleasant condition.

Dr John Paul is Consultant Medical Microbiologist and Director of Brighton Public Health Laboratory. Dr Paul provides an insect identification service and previously worked in Kenya.

Invasion of the body by the larvae (maggots) of *Diptera* (flies) is called myiasis. Myiasis may be accidental, such as when maggots are consumed in contaminated food, or spurious, as when rapidly hatching larvae are seen on faeces. A few species of fly specialize in infesting living tissues (specific or primary myiasis). These include species whose larvae actively penetrate the skin to cause dermal myiasis and species which invade wounds or orifices.

Dermal myiasis is quite a common complaint of travellers to the American and African tropics. Dermal myiasis in the Americas is caused by the human bot fly, *Dermatobia hominis*. The fly deposits her eggs on mosquitoes. When the mosquito bites, the larva hatches and invades the skin. The larva grows subcutaneously to form a boil. As the spiny larva grows (Fig. 5.10), the lesion becomes more uncomfortable for the patient. Secondary bacterial infection may occur.

There are many local remedies for removing larvae, including the application of glue, bacon, and steaks, but these methods are unreliable. It may be possible to express (squeeze out) larvae but incomplete removal may cause granuloma formation. It is safest to extract the larva though a simple incision. Left unmolested, the larva will grow to about 2 cm in length in 10 weeks and leave the host to pupate.

Dermal myiasis in Africa is caused by the tumbu fly, *Cordylobia anthropophaga*. The female fly lays eggs in shady conditions on dry sand or on clothes left out to dry; (ironing will kill eggs on clothes). Larvae (Fig. 5.11) penetrate the skin and grow subcutaneously to form boils which ooze fluid. Boils may be single or multiple, are

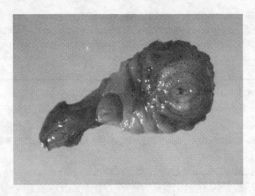

Fig. 5.10 Second instar larva of *Dermatobia hominis*

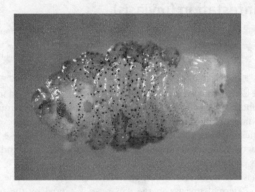

Fig. 5.11 Second instar larva of *Cordylobia anthropophaga*

uncomfortable, and may be associated with secondary bacterial infection and fever. Left untreated, larvae will grow over about 10 days to a length of approximately 1 cm and exit the host to pupate on the ground. It may be possible, after spreading petroleum jelly over the boil, carefully to squeeze out the larva. Larvae may be removed through a simple incision.

Many species of fly have been associated with wound myiasis. These are mostly species whose larvae normally feed on carrion or necrotic tissues. In wounds they restrict themselves to dead tissues and cause little or no harm and may actually be beneficial. However, there are some species which actively invade living tissues. Such species include the screw-worms (*Cochliomyia hominivorax* in the Americas and

Chrysomya bezziana in the Old World) which may invade wounds or orifices. Burrowing groups of larvae may be highly destructive and are sometimes lethal.

To avoid myiasis, wounds should be kept clean and dressed. As initially it is difficult to distinguish between different causes of wound myiasis and because benign and destructive species may frequent the same wound, any infested wound should be examined, cleaned, and if necessary debrided.

> • In the tropics, laundered clothes should always be ironed.

Fleas, lice, bugs, scabies, and other creatures

These insects and mites can cause irritation and annoyance to some travellers but are often mistakenly blamed for reactions resulting from attack by other unrelated insects. The majority do not carry infections, but in some countries there is also a disease risk. Most problems can be avoided by an awareness of the problem and simple protective measures.

Dr Ian F. Burgess is a public health entomologist and parasitologist who has specialized in personal ectoparasites of humans and animals.

Insects and related creatures that feed on humans can be divided into two groups. The first are micro-predators like mosquitoes and other biting flies that may also bite other species. The second are those that feed from us almost exclusively, or are totally dependent upon us for food and shelter, and these are mostly parasites. Whilst some of these may be encountered in any country, or even in your own home, there are others that may be met only whilst travelling, especially in more tropical climates.

In general, few of the problems are related to hygiene. The main reason that some insects cause greater problems in developing countries is that the environment provides optimum conditions that favour their survival and growth, coupled with a local economy that prevents most people from employing anything more than the most rudimentary control measures against the pests.

Fleas

The majority of flea species are highly host-specific and will never bite humans; others bite with varying degrees of avidity. The majority of flea species are only found in and around the nests of their preferred hosts so exposure is unlikely unless you sit nearby or else the fleas have jumped off a sick animal.

Fleas are mostly small (2–4 mm long), brownish, wingless insects that are flattened from side to side. They jump using their powerful hind legs (Fig. 5.12). All species have larvae, like caterpillars, that forage on the detritus in the host nest. Some species (e.g. cat fleas) emerge from their pupae when stimulated by vibration.

Tropical rat fleas, and a few other species, are able to transmit bubonic plague (see p. 191). This disease is common in rural parts of Africa and Asia and parts of

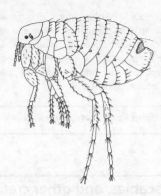

Fig. 5.12 *Pulex irritans* flea (male) (2–3 mm long)

North and South America. Most infections occur when people work or play near the infected rats' holes (ground squirrels in North America). Epidemic plague only occurs in urban areas when rural rat populations spill over to accidentally infect town rats that are susceptible to the disease.

In some heavily populated urban areas, urban rat fleas may transmit 'murine' (endemic) typhus (see p. 196). In this case the infection is usually associated either with urban squalor or else affects workers in infested warehouses.

Most fleas just cause irritating bites, but the Chigoe fleas are true parasites. These normal-looking fleas are usually found in dry sandy places in parts of West Africa and Central and South America. After attaching to the skin, the female flea burrows beneath it and then swells up with eggs to form a sac about 10 mm across. If left untreated, secondary infections, including gangrene, may result in loss of toes.

Lice

All lice are highly host-specific and will never transfer from animals to humans or *vice versa*, so a puppy crawling with lice is not a risk for anyone touching it, although the insects may crawl onto you temporarily. The three lice found on humans are of world-wide distribution and all feed on blood. They must all feed more than once each day in order to survive. All three species are spread by direct contact between people. In the case of head lice this requires physical head to head contact. In the case of crab lice (see pp. 455 and 467), which live amongst the hairs on the body, the contact is usually rather more intimate. Clothing, or body lice, live in the seams of clothing and only visit the skin of the body to feed. In the main, lice are harmless and only produce irritant reactions around the sites where they bite.

Lice are wingless insects that are flattened from top to bottom (Fig. 5.13). Those found on humans are all pale in colour with some pigmentation along their sides which

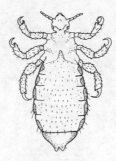

Fig. 5.13 *Pediculus humanus* the human body (or clothing) louse (2–3 mm long).

helps camouflage them. Head and clothing lice are 2–3 mm long and cigar-shaped, but crab lice are short and triangular with large claws on the rear two pairs of legs.

Clothing lice are the most important because they can spread classic (epidemic) typhus and louse-borne relapsing fever. These two diseases are currently restricted mainly to tropical upland areas (e.g. Ethiopia, Rwanda, Burundi) and also to parts of southern Sudan. Other tropical uplands such as the Himalayas and Andes may also be affected. These are all areas where for economic or cultural reasons people do not completely change their clothing regularly or else do not launder them at high enough temperatures to kill the insects. Typhus is spread by inhalation or exposure to infected louse droppings that have accumulated in folds of clothing. Consequently it is possible to contract the disease without having lice. In contrast, relapsing fever is only caught by people with lice. The infective spirochaetes that cause the disease are found in the blood of the louse and only released if the insect is crushed.

Clothing lice are mainly passed between fully clothed people sleeping huddled together for warmth. It is most unlikely that clothing lice could be contracted simply by sleeping in a bed in which someone else has previously slept. Outbreaks of louse infestation have occurred recently following social disruptions in the Balkans, where there have also been a number of cases of the less serious quintana fever, spread in a similar way to typhus.

'True' bugs

Bugs are flattened insects with a proboscis that is held beneath the front of the body. Most bugs feed on plant sap but a few suck blood, most notable of which are the bed bugs and the triatomine, or cone-nosed bugs. Neither of these groups is host-specific: they feed on a wide range of hosts.

Bed-bugs

Bed-bugs (Fig. 5.14) are oval, brown, wingless, and 4–6 mm long when fully grown. They live in crevices in furniture and walls and the architrave of doors and windows.

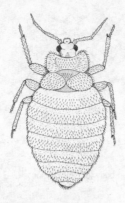

Fig. 5.14 *Cimex* bed-bug (male) (6–10 mm long).

They mainly feed at night, although in some local cinemas in tropical countries they may bite at any time. There are several species of bug in this group, some of which are associated with poultry, other birds, or bats. They are found world-wide and appear to be increasing in distribution. They are often found in moderate hotels for international travellers and it is not uncommon for one or more insects to hitch a ride in luggage. They do not carry disease but their biting can be a considerable nuisance. They can generally be deterred from biting by use of insecticide-impregnated mosquito nets and by leaving the bedroom light on at night — the bugs prefer to feed in the dark.

Triatomine bugs
These bugs are mainly found in Central and South America. They are common in rural areas and some species have adapted to urban life. The insects are relatively large (adult size 15–40 mm, depending upon the species). They have narrow heads, brown or black bodies, often ornamented with red or orange at the edges, and large wings. Some species fly readily. The bugs shelter in crevices in thatch, adobe, or broken plaster during the day and bite at night.

Some triatomines are capable of transmitting South American trypanosomiasis (Chagas' disease, see p. 184). The parasites are excreted in the insects' droppings, which are often deposited on the skin of the host after feeding, whence they can enter any scratch in the skin.

Scabies

Scabies is an allergic reaction to a parasitic mite (*Sarcoptes scabiei*) that burrows in the skin. It is passed from one person to another by moderately prolonged physical contact. The infection is long-lasting and the intensely itchy symptoms appear only after about 4–8 weeks in most people. Scabies is widespread in developing countries, where it mainly affects children. It is not highly infectious and it is unlikely that travellers will contract the infection from chance contacts with local people. Scabies mites die rapidly when removed from their host and so the infection is not contracted from bedding or towels.

Biting mites

Several species of mites that normally parasitize animals can bite humans. The most common of these are the red poultry mites and related species that affect rodents (*Dermanyssus* and *Ornithonyssus,*). *These animals crawl around the vicinity of the host nest and bite anything suitable. They do not live on the body.*

In several parts of the world, the larvae of 'harvest' or trombiculid mites can cause highly itchy lesions that may last for weeks. Older stages of the mites are free-living and do not affect us, so the biting season is usually limited to the late summer/early autumn period. In parts of Asia, these mites can carry 'scrub' typhus (see p. 192) and are sometimes known as 'jiggers'.

Ticks

Ticks of several species can be both serious biting nuisances and vectors of disease. There are two main groups of ticks.

Soft ticks

These mainly feed on birds, but some species will attack any suitable host. They often hide in crevices in buildings or in thatch and crawl out at night to feed. These animals feed rapidly and leave the host before it rises in the morning. They are important for transmission of tick-borne relapsing fever in North, South, and Central America, Africa, and Asia.

Hard ticks (Fig 5.15)

These are found away from nesting sites and are usually picked up from tall grasses or other undergrowth. Although the life cycle of all hard ticks is essentially the same, each species varies in the number and type of hosts it requires. Consequently, you may pick up tiny larvae not much bigger than 'full stops on legs', though as adults they may be 6–8 mm before engorgement. All hard ticks are slow feeders and it usually takes about a week for an adult tick to complete feeding. At the end of feeding the tick may have increased in size three- to five-fold.

Disease transmission by hard ticks usually happens near to the end of feeding when the ticks are expressing excess water from their enormous meal. Lyme disease is one of the most widely distributed tick-borne infections, being found in Europe, North America, and parts of Asia (see p. 175). More serious infections, such as Rocky Mountain spotted fever (see p. 196) and the Russian and European tick-borne encephalitides (see p. 167) are relatively more restricted in distribution. Ticks also transmit malaria-like organisms between cattle and occasionally these can be transferred to humans.

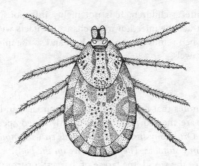

Fig 5.15 Hard tick (about 3 mm long, but up to 20 mm when engorged with blood)

Some species of tick may release a toxin that affects the central nervous system, resulting in a condition known as 'tick paralysis'. Children are affected more often than adults, and this occurs most usually when they attach to the neck or head. The problem resolves when the tick is removed.

Any tick attached to the skin should be removed as soon as possible. There are several possible ways to remove them but the most effective is to grasp the animal close to the skin with either finger tips or forceps, push slightly to disengage the teeth, twist it back and forth a quarter turn once, and then remove with a slight twisting action. If possible the animal or wound should be examined to see if any of the mouthparts have been left behind. Any fragments left in the wound should be removed in the same way as for removal of a splinter of wood. It is a good idea to flush the wound with hydrogen peroxide or an iodine-based antiseptic. Keep the tick in a sealed container, with a note of the date, for future reference and identification if any disease symptoms appear.

Bites

It is virtually impossible to examine an isolated bite and decide what type of arthropod delivered it. Anyone who claims otherwise is exaggerating their knowledge. However, it may be possible to make an educated guess about the cause of an itchy reaction from its location on the body and the circumstances in which you are staying, and this in turn may enable you to decide upon ways to avoid further problems. Generally speaking, unless you have been bitten by a particular type of insect in the past, you may not show any reaction to bites initially. *You may not develop itchy red reactions until several hours, and up to three to four days, after being bitten.* It may therefore be impossible to pinpoint what was actually doing the biting and where.

Fleas
Fleas do not bite humans except in the total absence of their normal host. Consequently, if cats live in the house they will almost certainly have fleas at some

time. Similarly, if there are rat holes near where you sit for your lunch, there will probably be some rat fleas — but you are most unlikely to be bitten by either whilst staying in a fourth-floor hotel room. Most fleas do not jump high nor crawl upwards very far, so the majority of bites are likely to be around the lower legs. The only exception to this is when bird fleas enter rooms from nests in roof voids, when they usually bite the head and shoulders as they fall onto sleeping persons.

Fleas do not usually hide in beds or other fabrics. It is, therefore, normally possible to see them hopping about if you disturb them by stamping or banging around along the junctions of walls and floor in a room.

Bed-bugs and triatomine bugs

These usually bite whilst you sleep. The most likely places to be bitten are the face, shoulders, arms, and legs, where these protrude from beneath bed clothes. These bugs all defecate whilst feeding, or soon after, to eliminate excess fluid from their bodies. This black liquid material may be found dried onto the skin, bedding, or around the entrance to the cracks where the insects shelter.

Lice

Contrary to popular opinion, the bites of lice do not itch much, particularly in the early stages of infestation. Clothing lice cause more irritation and are difficult to find but, since they congregate in the seams of clothing, most bites are likely to be in the vicinity of these clusters and the louse eggs will also be found there.

None of the human lice is able to survive away from its host for more than a few hours. Consequently it is most unlikely that any of them can be acquired other than through close physical contact with an infested person. Despite much popular anecdote that lice can be transmitted via inanimate objects such as combs, bed linen, and toilet seats, there is no scientific evidence in support of any of these conjectures.

Scabies

Scabies is characterized by an intense itch that is worse at night or after clothing has been removed. The first physical symptom is a rash that appears around the midriff and down the insides of the thighs. This is away from where any mites may be found, which is mainly on the hands and arms. If scabies is contracted in a tropical climate it is more likely that the mites may also spread to the head than would be the case in cooler conditions.

Biting mites and soft ticks

These are virtually never seen and identifying them as a source of irritation is extremely difficult and often largely circumstantial, except in the case of the trombiculids, which leave a characteristic dark scar (eschar) at the bite site. Similarly, soft ticks may come and go without leaving any demonstrable sign of their presence.

Table 5.9 Treatments for insect bites and parasitic arthropods

Problem	Treatment	Method of application
Insect bites: fleas, bed-bugs, mites; also mosquitoes, midges etc.	Topical creams or lotions: dilute ammonia (Afterbite), antihistamines, hydrocortisone 1%.	Dab or spread on affected parts as soon as symptoms are experienced. Repeat application once or twice only. If symptoms persist seek medical advice.
Head lice	Topical lotion: [malathion 0.5%, Prioderm (EU), Ovide (USA), Lice Rid, KP24 (AU)]; créme rinse [permethrin 1% (Lyclear (UK), Nix (worldwide)]; or shampoo [pryethrum 0.16%–0.4%, Rid (USA), many others worldwide except UK]	Apply lotion to dry hair, leave minimum 8 hours, then wash. Apply créme rinse to damp hair, leave 10 mins, rinse. Apply pyrethrum shampoo to dry hair, leave 10 mins, add water, lather, rinse. In all cases repeat treatment after 7 days
Crab lice	Topical cream: [permethrin 5%, Lyclear dermal cream (UK), Elimite (USA), other brand names elsewhere].	Apply to whole body below neck.
Clothing lice	Hot laundering or drying of clothes. Hot pressing of seams. Dry cleaning	Wash clothes in hot 55°C water (too hot to keep hands in) for at least 15 mins. Alternatively tumble dry on hottest setting for 15 mins or dry in full tropical sun. Rotate complete sets of clothing so no cross-contamination at 1–2 week intervals. Do not use insecticides on the person
Scabies	Topical cream: [permethrin 5% cream, Lyclear dermal cream (UK), Elimite (USA), other brand names elsewhere]; lotion [malathion 0.5% aqueous liquid Derbac-M (UK), Filvit (Sp)]; or suspension [benzyl benzoate, Ascabiol (EU)].	Apply to whole body below neck. Benzyl benzoate requires 3 applications over 3 days. Repeat other preparations after 7 days
Ticks	Physical removal (keep the tick for reference in case of disease).	Hold the tick firmly close to the skin, press, twist slightly and then remove with a twisting action. Treat the wound with a topical antiseptic e.g. iodine. If inflammation occurs or other disease symptoms follow seek medical advice

Hard ticks
These are usually discovered by their hosts only some time after feeding has commenced and often only a short time before they are due to drop off, when fully engorged. Subsequent to dropping off there is usually little to see apart from a reddish area with a small puncture in the middle. It is good practice, therefore, if visiting an area known to have ticks, to use a repellent product, to wear long trousers, and to tuck them into socks to prevent the animals climbing up the legs. Regular checks of the surface of the clothing to remove climbing ticks, and also of skin at the end of each day, can help prevent them attaching or engorging. See also p. 414.

Treatment
Recommended treatments for the various types of bites are summarized in Table 5.9

Personal protection against insect pests

Many serious diseases in the tropics and elsewhere are spread by insects. Personal protection against insects is thus an important health precaution for travellers.

Professor Christopher Curtis qualified in genetics, and has worked for several years on the application of genetics to tsetse fly and mosquito control. He is now involved in developing 'appropriate technology' for mosquito control.

Several types of insect — as well as related creatures like ticks and mites — obtain all their food by sucking blood from humans or animals i.e. 'biting'. In certain other kinds of insects, including mosquitoes, the females require a blood meal in order to produce each batch of eggs. (See Fig. 5.16 for method of distinguishing male and female mosquitoes.)

The pain and discomfort that insect bites cause is due to an allergic reaction to saliva introduced by the insect during blood-sucking. Such bites should be distinguished from the stings of bees, wasps, or ants, which have a different biological function, namely to deter intruders from approaching their nests (see p. 244). This distinction

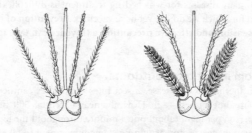

Fig. 5.16 Heads of female (left) and male (right) *Anopheles* mosquitoes. Unlike the females, male mosquitoes do not bite and can be recognized by their bushy antennae

may appear somewhat academic to the unfortunate victim. The severity of skin reaction in different people to bites and stings varies greatly, and people also differ widely in their apparent attraction to biting insects. (For treatment, see p. 206 and p. 584.)

This attraction is due to warmth at close range, but at longer range, carbon dioxide in the breath and components of body odour attract different species of insect to different degrees. The dangerous African mosquito *Anopheles gambiae* is attracted by the foot odour in some individuals which is caused by bacterial action on the sweaty skin. If this is washed off with anti-bacterial soap, the mosquitoes will simply bite any other exposed warm skin.

Diseases spread by insects

The nuisance of biting insects can be at least as great in the arctic summer as it is in the tropics. It is mainly in the tropics that insect-borne diseases are still an important health hazard, though more has been heard recently of two tick-borne diseases and one mosquito-borne disease that are a slight risk in certain parts of Europe and/or North America — Lyme disease (p. 175), tick-borne encephalitis (p. 167), and West Nile fever (p.166). The viruses, bacteria, protozoa, or worms responsible for these diseases take advantage of the biting habits of insects and ticks to enable themselves to be transported from the bloodstream of one victim to another.

Some ticks and insects hatch from their eggs already infected with viruses or somewhat larger organisms called *Rickettsiae* (see p. 195), which can cause human disease, but this is the exception rather than the rule. Most insects become infected when biting an infected individual; the infection develops inside the insect and is passed on to someone else during a subsequent feed or, with some diseases, by defecation on to the skin.

Table 5.10 gives a summary of the commoner biting insects and the diseases they may carry. The list of diseases may appear daunting, but the only ones commonly contracted by visitors to the tropics are malaria (see p. 130) and, in certain places, dengue (see p. 156), and cutaneous leishmaniasis (see p. 181). Of these, malaria presents by far the most serious risk. The other diseases need be considered only by travellers who will be living for a considerable period in a tent, or in tropical villages, urban slums, or refugee camps. In such cases it would be wise to take local advice about the particular risks and possible counter-measures.

Insects spread many diseases for which drug treatment is difficult, dangerous, or non-existent, and for which we do not yet have vaccines. **Prevention of insect bites is the single most sensible and effective precaution a traveller can take to avoid these diseases.**

Protection from insect bites outdoors

Quite apart from the hazard of disease, insect bites themselves can be more than a trivial nuisance in some places — in Howrah, near Calcutta, 500 bites by *Culex* mosquitoes per person per night (about one a minute throughout the night) are usual – and in such situations few visitors would need encouragement to take measures for personal protection.

Table 5.10 Insects, mites, and ticks that bite or burrow in the skin, and risk of disease transmission in different tropical and subtropical areas (also some parts of Europe and N. America in the case of two tick-borne and one *Culex*-borne diseases)

Pest	Rough guide to identification of adult	Time and place of biting or burrowing	Disease	Risk of disease transmission (x = slight risk; xx = moderate risk; xxx = high risk)			
				Africa	Asia	Americas	Western Pacific
Mosquitoes:							
Anopheles	Head and body in straight line and at an angle to surface (Fig. 5.3, p. 136)	Night; indoors or out; mainly rural	Malaria Filariasis	xxxx x	xx	x	xx x
Culex	Body parallel to surface, head bent down, whining flight; dull brown (Fig. 5.3, p. 136)	Evening and night; indoors or out; urban or rural	Filariasis Encephalitis West Nile fever	x	x x	x x	x
Aedes	Body shape as for *Culex*; but tropical species are black and white (Fig. 5.4, p. 156)	Day; indoors or out; urban or rural	Dengue Yellow fever Filariasis	x x	xx	x x	x xx
Mansonia	As *Culex*; but patterned wings and legs	Night; outdoors; rural	Filariasis	x	x		
Tsetse flies	Brown fly with proboscis projecting in front of head (Fig. 5.7, p. 185)	Day; outdoors; rural; tropical Africa only	Sleeping sickness	x			
Blackflies	1.5–4 mm, stout and black with humped body (Fig. 5.5, p. 173)	Day; outdoors; rural	Onchocerciasis	x		x	
Phlebotomine sandflies	Tiny hairy flies (Fig. 5.6, p. 181)	Evening; indoors or out; rural or urban	Leishmaniasis Sandfly fever Bartonellosis	x x	x x	x x x	
Biting midges	Tiny flies with spotted wings	Evening; outdoors; rural	No significant human disease — only nuisance				

Table 5.10 (Continued)

(x = slight risk; xx = moderate risk; xxx = high risk)

Pest	Rough guide to identification of adult	Time and place of biting or burrowing	Disease	Africa	Asia	Americas	Western Pacific
Gadflies, horse-flies, stable-flies	As large or larger than house-fly; fast flying	Day; outdoors; rural	Loiasis	x			
Ticks	Eight-legged creatures which attach tightly to the skin and swell up with blood to pea size (Fig. 5.15, p. 204)	Day or night; cling to long grass or hide on cave floors and attach to passers-by or sleepers	Relapsing fever Typhus Lyme disease [1] Encephalitis [2]	x x		x x	x x
Bed-bugs	1 cm; brown beetle-like; but wingless (Fig. 5.14, p. 202)	Night; in beds	No proven disease transmission-only a nuisance				
Triatomine bugs	1–4 cm; cone-like head; long legs (Fig. 5.8, p. 188)	Night; in beds	Chagas disease			x	
Fleas	2–3 mm; brown; flattened sideways; run and jump (Fig. 5.12, p. 200)	Night or day; indoors or out	Bubonic plague	x	x	x	
Lice	2–3 mm; cream or brown; claws often visible; flattened top to bottom; crawl (Fig. 5.13, p. 201)	Night or day; on body hair or clothes for their whole life cycle	Typhus Relapsing fever	x	x x	x	
Tumbu fly	9–12 mm; robust; yellow-brown; non-biting fly	Larvae attach to clothing while it is being dried on the ground and burrow into skin (Fig. 5.10 and 5.11, p. 198)	Larva creates a large boil	x			
Mites	Tiny eight-legged creatures	Climb on to skin from undergrowth or from other people and cling to or burrow in skin	Typhus Scabies	x	x x	x	x x

Notes: 1. Northeast USA and Europe   2. East and Central Europe

Repellents

A chemical repellent is the best, and perhaps *only* suitable personal protection against outdoor biting insects. As far as is known, repellents act by interfering with the sense organs with which insects locate their victims. Most of the commercially available insect repellent preparations contain diethyltoluamide (commonly known as 'DEET' or DET), ethylhexanediol, or hydroxymethyl isobutyl piperidine. These preparations come as lotions, sticks, gels, creams, or in aerosol cans or pump-action dispensers. In Australia, a mosquito repellent soap called 'Mosbar' has been developed by Simmons Pty Ltd, Box 107, Chadstone, Victoria 3148. This leaves a residue on the skin that can be washed off with water when no longer required. Recent trials in Kabul, Afghanistan, have shown a significant reduction in malaria risk among 'Mosbar' users.

DEET is harmful to some hard plastics and paint, causes a stinging sensation if it gets into the eyes, and tastes unpleasant: it should be applied with care. Conventional toxicity tests when DEET first came on to the market in the 1950s were reassuring, and DEET has been used without harm by millions of people. More recently, however, occasional reports have appeared of serious reactions in a few individuals. Anyone who suspects an adverse reaction to DEET should stop using it immediately and seek medical advice.

DEET is apparently effective against all free-flying biting insects, although the dose required may depend on the species of insect.

Clothing treatment

When applied to the skin, DEET remains effective for only a few hours. However, when impregnated into cotton (not synthetic) material it remains effective for several weeks, if the material is kept in a plastic bag or tin when not in use. The chances of an adverse skin reaction are presumably much reduced if DEET is impregnated into clothing rather than applied direct to the skin.

Clothing can be impregnated with the pyrethroid insecticide, permethrin, by the same method as treatment of bed-nets (see below). Studies in the USA showed that such treated clothing, plus DEET-treated skin, reduced mosquito biting more than either method on its own. Data are also available from the Colombian army using permethrin-treated uniforms and from Afghanistan using permethrin-treated Islamic shawls (chaddurs) and bed-sheets. These data show significant reductions in the risk of both malaria and cutaneous leishmaniasis when universal usage of these materials was backed up by military discipline or strong religious traditions.

When one is sitting on a chair, most mosquito bites occur on the ankles or feet. Cotton anklets (ankle bands), 10 cm wide and each impregnated with 4 ml DEET, have been found to give 80–85 per cent reduction in biting by several species of tropical night-biting mosquitoes. One impregnation remains effective for several weeks if the anklets are kept sealed up when not in use. One can make anklets for oneself or purchase ready-impregnated sets (see Appendix 8).

Alternative repellents

Citronella oil is distilled from a tropical grass and is used as a soap perfume. It has long been sold as an insect repellent but does not remain effective for as long as DEET.

However, p-methane-diol is an extract of lemon eucalyptus and is as long-lasting a repellent as DEET; it is sold under the brand name 'Mosiguard Natural' and, unlike DEET, does not attack plastics. Some people prefer its lemony smell to the less agreeable smell of DEET.

Mosquitoes tend to be diverted away from a person wearing a repellent (or naturally unattractive to mosquitoes) towards a nearby person not using repellent (or naturally more attractive to mosquitoes). This might suggest that the best protection would be to sleep with someone more attractive to mosquitoes than yourself!

Methods that don't work: buzzers and vitamins

'Repellents' that don't repel are dangerous, because they not only fail to give protection but they also promote a false sense of security. Buzzers which are advertised as repelling mosquitoes have been repeatedly shown to be completely useless and in the UK, vendors have been successfully prosecuted under the Trades Descriptions Act. Taking large doses of vitamin B_{12} is believed by some to make one repellent to mosquitoes, but two separate studies have failed to confirm this. Eating garlic has also been claimed to offer protection, but there is no evidence to support this.

Clothing

Long sleeves and long trousers have for many years been recommended to be worn after dark to minimize the risk of mosquito bites. Canvas mosquito boots can be purchased that make it impossible for mosquitoes to bite the ankles. Denim jeans are thick enough to be impenetrable to the probosces of blackflies, which prefer to attack the lower legs. Blue clothing is said to be very attractive to tsetse flies and should be avoided in the tsetse-infested areas of Africa.

However, the frequently-given advice to avoid dark-coloured clothing to prevent mosquito bites is not well-founded, since mosquitoes respond more to olfactory than to visual stimuli.

Protection from insect bites indoors

In addition to the repellents already described, several other useful counter-measures can be employed when the 'target area' is confined to a house or hotel room.

Tight closure of well-fitting windows keeps out most mosquitoes but would be an uncomfortable proposition in a hot climate unless the room is air-conditioned. Ceiling fans help to distract the blood-seeking flight of insects, especially weak fliers such as phlebotomine sandflies.

Screens

Windows kept open for ventilation should be screened: fibreglass netting coated with PVC (e.g. brand T685 sold by Simpkin Machin, Eckington, Sheffield S31 9BH, UK) is more durable, more easily fitted, and less expensive than wire netting. The netting should have six or seven threads per centimetre width to keep out mosquitoes and should be closed before sunset, when *Culex* and *Anopheles* mosquitoes become active.

Similar netting should be used to keep mosquitoes from laying eggs in domestic water containers, in which their larvae could flourish. In cities such as Mumbai the screening of roof water tanks, etc. has been a strictly enforced legal requirement to prevent the breeding of the urban malaria mosquito *Anopheles stephensi* and the dengue-carrying mosquito *Aedes aegypti*. The screening of vent pipes and other apertures to cesspits, septic tanks, and pit latrines helps to prevent the mosquito *Culex quinquefasciatus* from breeding in these collections of polluted water, to which it is attracted. A 1 cm thick floating layer of expanded polystyrene beads (as used in the manufacture of packing material) is highly effective in preventing mosquito breeding and lasts for years in such sites.

Sprays, coils, and vaporizing mats

Screening windows is seldom completely effective in keeping mosquitoes out of rooms, so other lines of defence may also be needed. Aerosol spray cans of insecticide are available in many tropical countries. They usually contain pyrethroids, which are synthetic near-relations of the natural product pyrethrum and are very safe, although they should not be used over uncovered food. They do not harm pets or domestic animals.

Air passengers from the tropics may notice the aircraft being sprayed after take-off. This is a reasonable precaution as almost every year there are malaria cases near European airports that are attributed to infected mosquitoes arriving from the tropics on improperly sprayed aircraft. (A summary of countries' disinsection policies can be found at **www.ostpxweb.dot.gov/policy/safety/disin.htm**)

Aerosols are good for clearing out mosquitoes that are lurking in a room before one goes to bed, but they have no residual effect on mosquitoes that enter later on during the night. The old-fashioned, but still effective, way of dealing with these insects is to light a slow-burning 'mosquito coil' which will smoke gently, giving off pyrethrum or pyrethroids for 6–8 hours. These are available cheaply in many tropical countries. However, tests have shown that some fraudulent brands contain no pyrethrum or pyrethroids. Local advice should be sought about good local brands, or some simple tests carried out for oneself.

A more modern version of the same idea is a small mains-operated heating plate that slowly vaporizes a mat containing pyrethroids. They are more effective than mosquito coils, but a reliable electricity supply and a supply of the mats may not be available in some parts of the tropics. It is also possible to heat the mats by placing them a few centimetres above an oil lamp.

The smoke emitted by coils kills mosquitoes in unventilated rooms, but in comfortably ventilated rooms the smoke may do no more than repel or stun insects so that they do not bite. Care may be needed to achieve even this — for example, on a porch or verandah one should always place the source of vapour upwind of those to be protected and perhaps at floor level, to deter mosquitoes heading for the ankles.

The pyrethroid vapour from vaporizing mats is more effective in draughty conditions and less offensive to the user than the smoke from coils. The mats are manufactured and used on a very large scale in India.

Mosquito nets

The use of a mosquito bed-net is strongly recommended wherever there is any risk of bites from *Anopheles* mosquitoes that carry malaria and bite at night, or the nuisance of *Culex* mosquitoes. It is well worth buying a good-quality net, because slippage of the weave would allow mosquitoes to enter. Tears should be repaired or blocked with cotton wool, and the net should be tucked in carefully under the mattress.

The net should be checked after getting into bed, using an electric torch to make sure that no gaps are left. Take care not to sleep with any part of the body resting against the net — mosquitoes feed through nets, and never miss an opportunity. Rectangular nets are safer in this respect than the 'tent' type. Increased security can be achieved by impregnating nets with a pyrethroid such as permethrin, which is effective for several months in killing or repelling mosquitoes which contact it. A dose of 0.2 gm/m^2 is sufficient, which can be achieved by dipping the net in a 1 per cent emulsion made by diluting in water an emulsifiable concentrate of permethrin (see Appendix 8 for suppliers). The net is wrung out and laid to dry on a plastic sheet. Because many of the mosquitoes making contact with a permethrin-treated net are killed, one person using such a net has been shown to provide some degree of protection to a companion in the same room, but not using the net. This contrasts with the situation where only one person uses a repellent (see above) or an untreated net. There is a communal benefit when almost all the inhabitants of a village are using permethrin-impregnated nets — the risk of a malaria infective bite to those in the village, but temporarily or permanently not using nets, was found to be greatly reduced in experiments in Tanzania.

Pyrethroid resistance has been detected in malaria vectors in some parts of Africa (e.g. Ivory Coast) but the evidence is still equivocal about whether this resistance is at a sufficient level to nullify the effect of net treatment on malaria.

Many hotels in the tropics provide mosquito nets. If in doubt it may be worth taking your own, and if suitable anchorage points are not available you should ask the management to provide some or to provide poles of sufficient height that can be lashed to the bed legs.

Other methods

Ornamental ponds should be stocked with small fish to eat any mosquito larvae that may start to develop there. Other water containers around houses are likely to be rubbish and should be either carted away, flattened, and buried or punctured so that they cannot hold water and become breeding sites for *Aedes* mosquitoes.

It almost goes without saying that residents should always co-operate with any community-wide insect control measures run by local authorities e.g. house spraying against malaria vectors in parts of India and South America, or elimination of *Aedes* breeding sites in Cuba and Singapore.

Traps
Very effective traps have been developed for tsetse flies based on visual and/or olfactory stimulants. They are used to prevent tsetse invading places where people come to collect water or where cattle are vulnerable. The charity Caritas is making available a tsetse trap for use in sleeping sickness endemic areas in Angola.

Various types of baited trap for mass killing of houseflies have been developed including a very cheap one based on discarded bottles*. As yet, there are no cheap traps for effective elimination of mosquitoes, although traps using a light or carbon dioxide as attractants are useful to monitor control campaigns.

Control of domestic non-biting pests
Although they do not bite, houseflies, cockroaches, ants, and termites are often worrying pests in the tropics, and some may be a serious health hazard. Flies, for example, are able to carry more than 100 different types of harmful disease-producing organisms, and may transfer them directly from excreta to food and children's faces. There is now evidence that community-wide fly control operations reduce the risk of diarrhoea and the blinding disease, trachoma. In the kitchen, exposed food, unwashed plates, crumbs, and rubbish are an open invitation to flies, cockroaches, and ants. Very attractive foods such as sugar and jam should be kept in the refrigerator and others, such as breakfast cereals, biscuits, or bread, should be kept in screw-topped containers.

Flies, ants, and cockroaches
Houseflies breed in rotting rubbish, and if refuse is not regularly collected by the local authorities it should be buried under a thick layer of soil. Screening of the vent pipes of pit-latrines and cesspits is a most effective measure against *Chrysomya* blowflies, because light attracts them into the pipes, and they are unable to escape. Mothballs on bathroom drain grilles discourage cockroaches from emerging from the drain. Ants' nests can often be located by following the trail of ants back to its source, and can then sometimes be destroyed with boiling water or, if the nest is in a small object such as a book, by placing it in an oven.

Old-fashioned sticky fly paper can help to keep a fly infestation in check but, in the event of a persistent fly problem, periodic use of insecticide aerosol spray cans may be necessary. These pyrethroid insecticides may also be effective in irritating cockroaches and driving them out of the crevices in which they hide. Otherwise, the best insecticidal approach for a cockroach infestation is to scatter a carbamate insecticide such as 'Baygon' in powder form or 'Maxforce' gel, containing hydromethylnone, near crevices, drain-inspection covers, and in the bottoms of cupboards and closets.

Termites
In the many tropical areas where there is a serious termite problem, houses should be protected by pouring a persistent insecticide such as dieldrin into a trench around the

* Details available from TALC, see Appendix 8.

foundations and impregnating timber with this insecticide (for further information see Overseas Building Notes No. 170, obtainable from Building Research Station, Garston, Watford WO2 7JR, UK). Before starting long-term occupation of a house, it is wise to enquire whether such precautions have been taken. For the short-term resident, termite infestation will be revealed by sinuous earth-covered tunnels adhering to the walls.

Termites can completely destroy books and other objects from within and before this happens, the trails should be followed to where they reach ground level and liquid 'Baygon' or a similar insecticide should be poured down any crevices. As an additional precaution, bookcases can be stood on bricks placed in basins of water covered in an oil film to reduce evaporation and prevent them becoming breeding places for *Aedes aegypti* mosquitoes.

6 Animal bites; rabies; venomous bites and stings

Snake bites and scorpion stings may be perceived as the greatest zoological hazard to travellers, but in practice, dog bites are a much more common problem: in many countries they carry the terrifying risk of rabies, and in all cases require prompt and careful treatment. Bathers and swimmers in the tropics should be aware of the various types of venomous marine animals, and anyone who is allergic to bee and wasp stings should also take special precautions.

Professor David A. Warrell has treated animal bites and stings in five continents. He is Professor of Tropical Medicine and Infectious Diseases and Founding Director of the Centre for Tropical Medicine (Emeritus), University of Oxford; Honorary Clinical Director of the Alistair Reid Venom Research Unit at the Liverpool School of Tropical Medicine; and a Consultant to the WHO, the Royal Geographical Society, and the British Army.

Encounters with animals can produce the following medical problems, all of which are uncommon but potentially fatal: mechanical injury, envenoming, poisoning, infection, infestation, and allergic reactions. Only the first two of these will be discussed in detail in this chapter.

Injuries: attacks by large animals

Many species of animals have claws, teeth, tusks, horns, or spines capable of inflicting potentially fatal mechanical injuries. With the one exception of bites by domestic dogs, these accidents are rare and are easily avoided by treating all large animals with respect and avoiding unnecessarily close contact with them.

Most wild animals, unless they are ill or starving, avoid confrontation with humans. Visitors to game parks in the tropics or to safari parks in the temperate zones should take local advice about where and when it is safe to walk. Strolls between dusk and dawn without a light invite attacks by large carnivores. It is usually safe to approach large carnivores in a hard-topped vehicle, but this may not be a safe place from which to view elephants or rhinoceroses (see also p. 440). In Tsavo East National Park, a French tourist was recently trampled to death by a lone bull elephant he had followed on foot, during a lunch stop.

Animals in zoos or safari parks should not be assumed to be tamer and therefore safer. Several keepers have been killed by tigers and elephants in British zoos or safari parks during the last few years; over a period of 15 years, tigers killed 659 people in Sunderbans Reserve Forest, in West Bengal; between 1967 and 1986, 12 people were killed by grizzly bears in Banff, Glacier, and Yellowstone National Parks; and 126 attacks by these bears in North American national parks were recorded between 1900 and 1980. A British visitor to Yosemite was badly mauled by a bear in 1993, and another was killed in 1992 in Alberta, Canada. A recent study of animal-related

---

Bear attacks

Visitors to national parks in the USA are at occasional risk of encounters with black and grizzly bears, especially if they go hiking or camping off the beaten track. The danger comes when the bear is caught by surprise, and the most likely encounters are with adult females tending their cubs or protecting a carcass. Bears are attracted by food and may demolish tents or even vehicles if they smell something edible.

Bear attacks, and the injuries they cause, have been studied in detail. Bears are a formidable foe: their claws are typically as long as human fingers, so that even what might in human terms be a friendly pat would be capable of inflicting severe damage. Their jaw muscles are enormous. They are extremely agile; in any encounter with a bear there is simply no point in running away or attempting to climb a tree — sudden movements or running away prompt the bear to chase or attack.

The best course of action is probably to keep still, and to lie curled up on the ground. If you are wearing a backpack, keep this on — it provides protection. Interlock your fingers behind the neck and tuck your elbows in, in front of your face. This position affords maximum protection for the hands, neck, and face, which is where the most serious injuries occur. People who adopt this position are much less likely to sustain serious injury. In the case of black bears, fighting back and putting on an aggressive display has proved effective on occasions.

Defensive aerosol sprays containing capsicum (red pepper extract) have been used with some success for protection against bears. They may be effective at a range of approximately 5–7 metres; if discharged upwind or in a vehicle, they can disable the user. Take appropriate precautions. If you carry a spray can, keep it handy and know how to use it.

---

injuries in Yellowstone National Park also revealed at least 56 bison-goring injuries over a 15-year period. A British spectator at an elephant display in Thailand was gored to death in 2000.

Other mammals known to have killed or severely mauled humans include lions, tigers, leopards, wild cats, wolves, hyaenas, hippopotamuses, camels, buffaloes, and wild pigs. Deaths from ostrich attacks have also been reported.

Sharks claim about 5–15 lives each year out of 70–100 reported attacks, mostly between latitudes 30°N and 30°S. In 2000 there were 24 reported shark attacks in Australia with three deaths. In 2001, a spate of shark attacks off the Florida coast attracted much publicity, with a significant impact on the local tourist industry. More than 25 attacks were reported, but there were no fatalities. Much smaller fish can also kill! In parts of the Indo-Pacific Ocean, garfish or needle-fish (Beloniformes) (which have long, spear-like snouts) have been known to leap out of the water and impale fishermen. Moray and conger eels, groupers, barracudas, and stingrays can also produce severe mechanical injuries with their teeth or spines.

Fish capable of delivering electric shocks are found in fresh-water rivers of South America (electric eel — *Electrophorus electricus*) and Africa (electric catfish — *Malopterurus electricus*) and in the sea (e.g. torpedo rays). The electric eel can discharge up to 650 volts at one ampere 400 times per second and is capable of killing an adult human. The electric catfish can discharge 90 volts at 0.1 amps and is not dangerous, but the torpedo ray produces a dangerous shock in salt water of 80 volts at high amperage. Victims should be given cardio-respiratory resuscitation as in other cases of electric shock.

It is foolhardy to wade, bathe, or swim in rivers or lakes in the tropics unless they are known to be safe — not only from bilharzia (see p. 104) but from crocodiles as well. Crocodile attacks caused 51 deaths between 1990 and 1994 in one small district in Tanzania — and 18 of them occurred during the first four months of 1994 alone. Crocodiles recently killed a Scottish tourist on a camping safari near a water hole in East Africa, and an English gap-year student who went swimming in a lake reputed to be 'safe'. Riverine populations in the Sudan, Central Africa, and Southeast Asia are at greatest risk, and the total annual mortality from the Nile crocodile in Africa exceeds 1000. River pollution reducing the fish supply is thought to be a factor in the growing attack rate. Saltwater or estuarine crocodiles have attacked people in Indonesia and Sarawak, and in northern Australia 27 deaths from 60 attacks have been reported since 1876.

The giant pythons (reticulated python of Indonesia, African rock python, and boa constrictor and anaconda of South America) are certainly capable of killing and swallowing humans, and there are a few reliable reports of fatal attacks.

Travellers are, however, far more likely to be bitten by a dog before leaving their home country than by a wild animal during their travels.

In the USA there are now more than a million dog bites each year requiring some sort of hospital attention; the number is increasing. In Liverpool and Sunderland, about 500 people per 100 000 population attend hospitals each year because of dog bites. Reports of 11 deaths from dog bites were collected in a two-year period in the USA, and there have been several in the UK during the last few years. Domestic cattle (especially bulls), rams, pigs, cats, and even ferrets have also killed people.

In Edinburgh, 1 per cent of animal bites requiring hospital treatment are caused by grey squirrels in public parks — literally biting the hands that feed them.

Types of injury

Teeth and claws produce lacerating and destructive injuries to soft tissues. Tusks, horns, and antlers can tear and produce serious penetrating injuries resulting in blindness, pneumothorax and haemothorax (leakage of air and blood into the lining of the lungs), perforation of the intestines, and bleeding from the liver and spleen. Even dog bites can cause compound fractures (where the broken bone ends protrude through the skin).

All bites, gorings, and maulings carry a heavy risk of infection with bacteria, viruses, and other micro-organisms present in the animal's mouth or contaminating its claws, horns, etc. Large mammals may trample and kneel on the human victim, producing severe crush injuries.

First-aid

A guide to the treatment of mammal bites, licks, and scratches is given in the box below. Mild superficial injuries should be cleaned thoroughly. Anyone who has suffered a serious attack should be taken to a hospital for proper assessment. The use of antibiotics, anti-tetanus, and anti-rabies treatments may need to be considered.

Treatment of mammal bites, licks, and scratches

First-aid

- Scrub with soap or detergent, preferably under a running tap, for at least five minutes.

- Remove foreign material (e.g. dirt, broken teeth).

- Rinse with plain water.

- Irrigate with a virucidal agent, such as povidone iodine (Betadine), 0.01 per cent aqueous iodine, or 40–70 per cent alcohol (gin and whisky contain 40 per cent). **Note:** hydrogen peroxide, mercurochrome, and quaternary ammonium compounds — the brightly coloured antiseptic dyes still popular in some countries — are not ideal for this purpose.

At the hospital or dispensary

A medical attendant should:

- Check that first-aid measures (above) have been carried out.

- Explore and irrigate deep wounds (if necessary, under local or general anaesthesia). Dead tissue should be cut away, but wound excision is rarely necessary.

- Avoid immediate suturing (stitches) and occlusive dressings.

- Consider tetanus risk and treat accordingly: booster dose of tetanus formol toxoid (0.5 ml by intramuscular injection) for those fully immunized in the past and boosted within the last 10 years; human tetanus immunoglobulin (250 mg by intramuscular injection) for severe or grossly contaminated wounds that have been left untreated for more than four hours in a previously unimmunized person. In the case of serious or neglected wounds, antibiotics such as penicillin or metronidazole should be given to kill tetanus bacteria.

- Consider risk of infection with other bacteria, viruses, and fungi particularly associated with mammal bites. Preventive antibiotic treatment is advisable for severely contaminated wounds e.g. a broad-spectrum antibiotic such as amoxycillin (500 mg, three times a day for five days) (see p. 228 for other options).

- If the exposure occurred in a rabies-endemic area, consider full post-exposure rabies prophylaxis (see below).

Rabies

Rabies or 'hydrophobia' is a virus infection of mammals that can be transmitted to humans in a variety of ways, but usually as the result of a bite by a domestic dog.

In 1997, the WHO estimated 60 000 deaths from dog-mediated rabies and the use of 50 million ampoules of rabies vaccine in post-exposure prophylaxis. In the UK, the last human death from indigenous rabies occurred in 1902. There were two human cases of rabies in the UK in 1988 and 2001, and one in 1996, all acquired abroad. At least 12 human cases are known to have occurred in travellers returning to the USA between 1981 and 1998; and three further American travellers died of rabies whilst abroad.

In areas where rabies exists, the infection is usually established and circulates only in a few particular mammalian species. These may include domestic mammals

In 1996, an English navy veteran was bitten by a dog. He had been working in Indonesia as a diver, and the dog belonged to a friend. He knew about the risk of rabies, but he decided not to seek treatment because he hated injections. He kept a diary of his last days, cataloguing in graphic detail the onset of his symptoms, hydrophobia, and terminal rabies. He was 32 years old.

A French couple visiting Mexico were both bitten by a dog lying injured by the roadside that they had stopped to attend. No preventive measures were taken. Forty-seven days later, back in France, the young man developed fever, diarrhoea, and strange behaviour. He died 10 days later. His companion was given a course of rabies vaccine and survived, but had probably not been infected.

(particularly dogs), cats, and/or wild mammals (for example, skunks, raccoons, foxes, and insectivorous bats in North America — in the USA, rabid bats have been reported from every state except Alaska and Hawaii, and have caused rabies in at least 18 humans); foxes in the Arctic; mongooses and vampire bats in the Caribbean; vampire bats in Central and South America; foxes, wolves, raccoon dogs, and insectivorous bats in Europe; wolves, jackals, and small carnivores such as mongooses and civets throughout most of Africa and Asia; and flying foxes (fruit bats) in Australia.

Humans may contract rabies from any rabid mammal, domestic or wild, but because of the particularly close association between humans and dogs the most common source of human rabies world-wide is the bite of a rabid domestic dog (which may itself have been infected by another dog, cat, or rabid wild mammal). In the USA, canine rabies has been largely eliminated through measures such as immunization, but there is still a risk to people who come into contact with rabies-affected wild-mammal populations — naturalists, animal trappers, and people on expeditions. Thus a bite from a skunk in the mid-western USA or from a jackal in Africa could involve a risk of rabies.

Geographical distribution

Rabies occurs in most parts of the world, in Greenland, Canada and North America, throughout Russia and the territories of the former Soviet Union, China, and New Territories of Hong Kong, as well as in the main tropical regions. See Table 6.1 for details.

The following areas are free of rabies at present: Britain and Ireland, mainland Norway, Sweden, Finland and Iceland, Cyprus, Bahrain, Singapore, peninsular Malaysia, New Guinea, Taiwan, Japan, Oceania, Antarctica, and New Zealand. Human and animal rabies is most common in the Indian subcontinent, Thailand, the Philippines, and parts of South America.

How infection occurs

Rabies infection can occur when the normal protective barrier provided by healthy, unbroken skin is breached by a bite or scratch and the wound is contaminated with the animal's saliva containing rabies virus. Rabies virus can penetrate unbroken mucous membranes such as those covering the eye and lining the mouth or nose. On a few occasions, rabies has developed after the virus had been inhaled — in the air of bat-

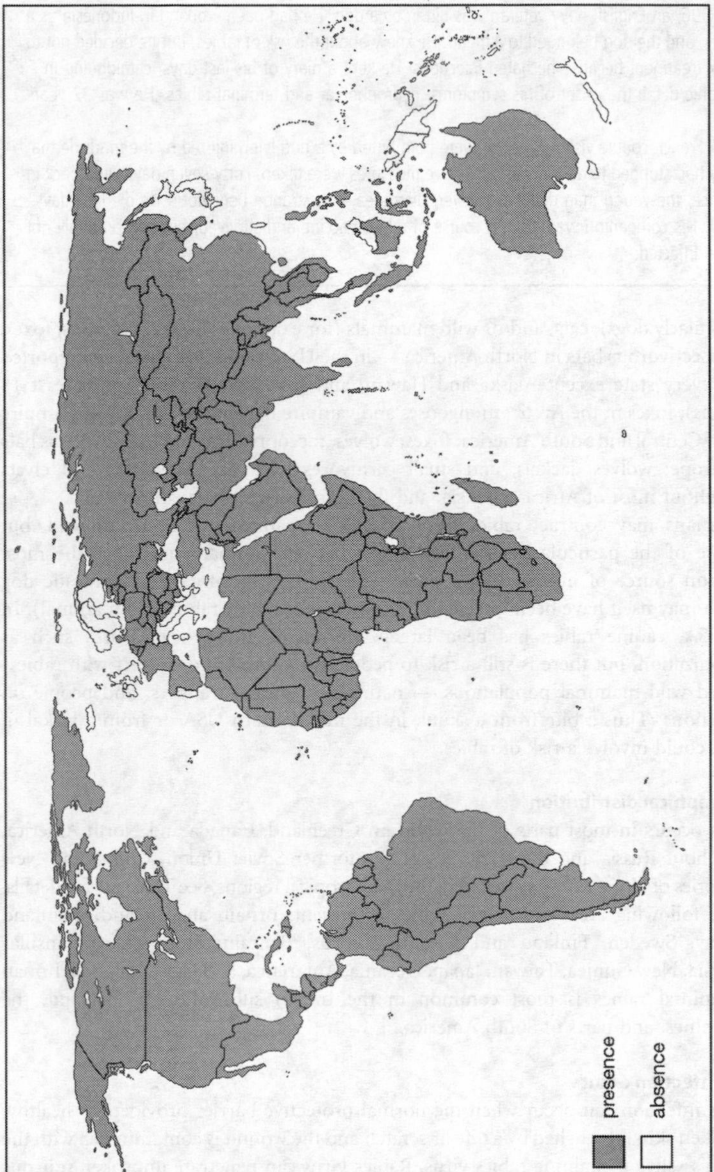

Map 6.1 Presence/ absence of rabies (1997).

presence

absence

Table 6.1 Geographical distribution of rabies.

Country	Rabies?	Remarks
Afghanistan	yes	
Albania	no	
Algeria	yes	
Andorra	no	
Angola	yes	
Antigua and Barbuda	no	Rabies has never been reported.
Argentina	yes	
Armenia	no	
Australia	yes	Australian bat Lyssa virus
Austria	yes	
Bahamas	no	
Bahrain	no	
Bangladesh	yes	
Barbados	no	Rabies free for more than 100 years.
Belarus	yes	
Belgium	yes	
Belize	yes	
Bhutan	yes	
Bolivia	yes	
Botswana	yes	
Brazil	yes	
Brunei Darussalam	no	
Bulgaria	yes	
Burkina Faso	yes	
Cameroon	yes	
Canada	yes	
Cape Verde	no	
Central African Rep.	yes	
Chad	yes	
Chile	yes	
China	yes	
Colombia	yes	
Congo	yes	
Cook Islands	no	
Costa Rica	yes	
Côte d' Ivoire	yes	
Croatia	yes	
Cuba	yes	
Cyprus	no	
Czech Republic	yes	
Denmark	yes	
Dominican Republic	yes	

Table 6.1 *(continued)*

Country	Rabies?	Remarks
Ecuador	yes	
Egypt	yes	
El Salvador	yes	
Eritrea	yes	
Estonia	yes	
Ethiopia	yes	
Fiji	no	Rabies has never been reported. Stringent quarantine restrictions are in place to prevent entry of rabies into Fiji.
Finland	no	
France	yes	No fox rabies for two years; occasional case of European bat Lyssa virus.
French Guyana	yes	
French Polynesia	no	
Gabon	yes	
Gambia	yes	
Germany	yes	
Ghana	yes	
Gibraltar	no	Gibraltar has been rabies free since 1971.
Greece	no	
Grenada	yes	
Guam	no	Rabies was eradicated in the 1970s.
Guatemala	yes	
Guinea	yes	
Guyana	yes	
Haiti	yes	
Honduras	yes	
Hong Kong	no	
Hungary	yes	Vaccine for human use is imported from Germany, from the firm Chiron-Behring (Rabivac, Rabipur).
Iceland	no	
India	yes	
Indonesia	yes	Rabies has mainly been reported in Java, Sumatra, and Kalimantan. Not in Irian Jaya.
Iran	yes	
Iraq	yes	
Ireland	no	
Isle of Man	no	
Israel	yes	

Table 6.1 *(continued)*

Country	Rabies?	Remarks
Italy	no	
Jamaica	no	
Japan	no	
Jersey, Channel Islands	no	Rabies has never been recorded.
Jordan	yes	Vaccine usage suggests many cases needing post-exposure treatment.
Kenya	yes	
Kiribati	no	
Korea Republic of	yes	
Kuwait	no	
Laos Peoples Democratic Republic	yes	
Latvia	yes	
Lebanon	yes	
Lesotho	no	
Libyan Arab Jamahiriya	no	
Lithuania	yes	Most rabies cases in animals were diagnosed in Silutes, Taurages, Siauliu, Pakruojo, Joniskio, Jubarko districts.
Luxembourg	yes	
Madagascar	yes	
Malawi	yes	
Malaysia Peninsula	yes	
Malaysia Sabah	no	
Malaysia Sarawak	no	
Maldives	no	
Mali	yes	
Malta	no	Rabies free since 1911. Quarantine of dogs and cats on import is ongoing.
Mauritius	no	Rabies has not been reported in Mauritius since 1896.
Mexico	yes	
Moldova Republic of	yes	
Mongolia	yes	
Montserrat	no	
Morocco	yes	
Mozambique	yes	
Myanmar	yes	
Namibia	yes	
Nepal	yes	

Table 6.1 *(continued)*

Country	Rabies?	Remarks
Netherlands	yes	Only bat rabies. Apart from EBL rabies in wild bats, 260 bats (*Rousettus aegypticus*) from the Blijdorp Zoo in Rotterdam were investigated for rabies after the confirmation of EBL in the colony present in an artificial cave. The artificial cave was depopulated and closed to the public as a result.
New Caledonia	no	
New Zealand	no	Rabies has never been reported.
Nicaragua	yes	
Niger	yes	
Nigeria	yes	
Norway	no	Svalbard Islands: rabies has been sporadically diagnosed, last in 1992.
Oman	yes	Foxes and wolves.
Pakistan	yes	
Palau	no	
Panama	yes	
Papua New Guinea	no	
Paraguay	yes	
Peru	yes	
Philippines	yes	Since 1996, surveillance has been improved through the regional and Provincial Rabies Coordinating Units and the National Epidemiological Surveillance System which submits surveillance reports to the Communicable Disease Control Service, Department of Health every quarter.
Poland	yes	
Portugal	no	
Qatar	no	
Reunion	no	
Romania	yes	
Russian Federation	yes	
Saint Kitts and Nevis	no	
Saint Lucia	no	
Samoa	no	
Saudi Arabia	yes	
Senegal	yes	
Seychelles	no	
Singapore	no	
Slovakia	yes	

Table 6.1   *(continued)*

Country	Rabies?	Remarks
Slovenia	yes	
South Africa	yes	
Spain	no	Occasional bat rabies.
Sri Lanka	yes	
Sudan	yes	
Suriname	yes	
Swaziland	yes	
Sweden	no	
Switzerland	no	
Syria	yes	
Tanzania	yes	
Thailand	yes	
Togo	yes	
Trinidad and Tobago	yes	
Tunisia	yes	
Turkey	yes	
Turkmenistan	yes	
Uganda	yes	
Ukraine	yes	
United Arab Emirates	no	Rabies has not been recorded since 1984, no surveillance in place.
United Kingdom	no	
United States of America	yes	
Uruguay	no	
Vanuatu	no	Rabies has never been reported
Venezuela	yes	
Vietnam	yes	
Yemen	yes	
Yugoslavia	yes	
Zambia	yes	
Zimbabwe	yes	

infested caves in Texas — and as the result of a laboratory accident. On several occasions, recipients of corneal transplants from patients dying of unsuspected rabies have later developed rabies themselves.

After the virus has entered the wound it may be killed by antiseptics used to clean the wound or by the person's own immune defence mechanisms. Unless this happens within a few days of the bite, the virus may invade the nerves which lead to the brain and spinal cord; it then multiplies and causes a severe infection of the central nervous system (called an encephalomyelitis) which is almost invariably fatal.

The incubation period — the time interval between the bite and the first symptoms of rabies — is usually two to three months, but can vary from a few days to many years.

The earliest symptom of rabies infection of the central nervous system is itching, irritation, tingling, or pain at the site of the healed bite wound. The disease advances rapidly, producing headache, fever, spreading paralysis, and episodes of confusion, aggression, hallucination, and hydrophobia (literally, fear of water). Attempts to drink water induce powerful contractions of the neck muscles and the muscles involved in swallowing and breathing in. These spasms are associated with indescribable terror. The patient dies in a few days.

Some species of animals such as mongooses, skunks, and vampire bats can recover from rabies encephalomyelitis, but in humans the infection is almost invariably fatal. During the last 20 years, a few patients with probable rabies, and only one with proven rabies, have survived after prolonged intensive care, but all but two of them were left with severe long-term effects.

The prospect of an agonizing death from this untreatable disease should encourage everyone to do everything possible to prevent rabies.

Pre-exposure vaccination

Pre-exposure vaccination against rabies should be considered in the case of travellers who run a high risk. These include cave explorers, animal collectors, zoologists, botanists, hunters, and also those whose work involves walking and cycling in urban or rural areas, as well as travellers spending a prolonged period in endemic areas. One of the safe, comparatively new cell-culture vaccines should be used, such as Aventis Pasteur human diploid cell strain vaccine (HDCSV), purified vero cell rabies vaccine (PVRV), or Chiron purified chicken embryo cell vaccine (PCEC) (see Box, p. 230).

Expense can be reduced by giving one-tenth of the normally recommended dose by intradermal rather than intramuscular or subcutaneous injection, but this regimen is not satisfactory if chloroquine is being taken (e.g. for malaria prophylaxis) at the time of immunization.

Travellers within a rabies-endemic area should avoid close contact with domestic or wild mammals. They should be particularly wary of wild animals that appear unusually tame, for this change in behaviour is a common early sign of rabies in animals.

Action following a bite

Irrespective of the risk of rabies, all mammal bites, scratches, and licks on mucous membranes or broken skin should be cleaned immediately and vigorously (see Box, p. 220). Mammal bites (including human bites) are usually contaminated by a variety of bacteria, some of which can cause serious infections.

In the case of deep penetrating or contaminated wounds, it is wise to take a prophylactic antibiotic (such as amoxycillin, 500 mg, three times a day for five days; tetracycline, 500 mg, four times a day for five days; or cefuroxime axetil (Ceftin), 250 mg, twice a day for five days — all **adult** dosages). The risk of tetanus should always be considered: all travellers should be fully protected with a course of tetanus toxoid before starting their journey. An animal bite warrants a booster dose of tetanus toxoid (tetanus formol toxoid 0.5 ml) (see also p. 560).

Post-exposure vaccination

The aim of post-exposure vaccination is to neutralize the rabies virus introduced by the bite before it can enter the nervous system. Treatment should be started as soon as possible, but although the chances of preventing rabies decrease with delay, vaccination is still worthwhile even weeks or months after the bite. The decision about vaccination should be made by a doctor, who will need the following information:

1. When, where, and in which locality the bite occurred; the circumstances — was it unprovoked?
2. The severity and site of the bite.
3. The species, appearance, behaviour, and fate of the biting animal, and whether it had been vaccinated against rabies during the previous year.

This information should allow some assessment of the risk of exposure, but if there is any doubt it is safest to give a full course of vaccine, if possible with passive immunization — rabies immune globulin (see Box, p. 230). The first dose of vaccine should be doubled or divided between several sites intradermally on the body if there has been more than 48 hours' delay in starting vaccination; if passive immunization has been given more than 24 hours before vaccine; if the patient is elderly, malnourished, or believed to be immunodeficient or immunosuppressed; and if passive immunization is not available.

The newer cell-culture anti-rabies vaccines, such as HDCSV, carry no serious risk of reactions, unlike the older vaccines, which consisted of animal nervous tissue.

Passive immunization

Passive immunization (see Box, p. 230) should never be omitted in cases of severe bites or high risk of exposure unless the patient has had pre-exposure vaccination. 'Ready-made' rabies-neutralizing antibody in the form of human rabies immunoglobulin (HRIG) or equine rabies immune globulin (ERIG) is necessary to provide immediate activity against rabies virus during the interval of about seven days between vaccination and the first appearance of antibody produced by the body itself in response to the vaccine. HRIG is free from side-effects, but ERIG is complicated by reactions such as serum sickness in up to six per cent of those treated. (**There is currently a global shortage of both, which is why pre-exposure immunization is generally a better option.**)

Travellers who are exposed to the risk of rabies (mammal bites, licks, scratches, etc) should seek immediate help at the time of the incident, and not wait for days (or even months) until they return home before considering post-exposure treatment.

Only orthodox/Western medical practitioners should be consulted about rabies, *not* herbalists, homeopaths, traditional practitioners, monks, priests, or other practitioners of 'fringe medicine'. In some countries, even Western-style practitioners may not give adequate treatment.

Rabies immunization schedules

Pre-exposure vaccination

Aventis human diploid cell strain vaccine (HDCSV)

    0.1 ml by intradermal (id) injection or 1 ml by intramuscular (im) injection on days 0, 7, and 28
    + boosters of 0.1 ml by id injection or 1 ml by im injection every 2 years

Post-exposure vaccination

(Do not forget wound cleaning! See Box, p. 220)

1. For those who have been given pre-exposure vaccination

- No passive immunization (human or equine rabies immune globulin) is needed

- HDCSV, PVRV or PCEC— one ampoule by intramuscular (*im*) injection on days 0 and 3

2. For those not given pre-exposure vaccination

- HDCSV, PVRV or PCEC — one ampoule by *im* injection on days 0, 3, 7, 14, and 28.

and

- Human RIG, dose 20 units/kg: At least half infiltrated in and around the bite wounds (dilute with sterile water/saline if bites are numerous) the rest by intramuscular injection elsewhere but distant from the site of vaccine injection.

or

- Equine RIG, dose 40 units/kg: At least half infiltrated in and around the bite wounds (dilute with sterile water/saline if bites are numerous) the rest by intramuscular injection elsewhere but distant from the site of vaccine injection, beware of (rare) anaphylactic and serum sickness reactions. Test dose not necessary.

- The following economical regimen is effective and recommended by WHO: 8-site intradermal regimen: 0.l ml HDCSV or PCEVC given at 8 sites (deltoids, suprascapular, abdominal, and thighs) on day 0; 4 sites on day 7 (limbs); and single sites on days 28 and 90. This is very economical and induces antibody rapidly

Rabies prevention following exposure in a risk area

Minor exposure

— including licks of the skin, scratches or abrasions, minor bites, or unprovoked attack by cat or dog, or attack by wild animal or by domestic cat or dog unavailable for observation

- Vaccine

- Stop treatment if animal remains healthy for five days

- Stop treatment if tests on animal proves negative

- Administer RIG on positive diagnosis of animal and complete the course of vaccine

Major exposure

— including licks on mucosa or major bites (multiple or on face, head, fingers, or neck), or unprovoked attack by cat or dog, or attack by wild animal or by domestic cat or dog unavailable for observation

- RIG and vaccine

- Stop treatment if domestic cat or dog remains healthy under observation for five days

- Stop treatment if test on animal's brain proves negative for rabies

> **Rabies in Thailand**
>
> A recent estimate puts the number of stray dogs on the streets of Bangkok at more than 110 000 (of a total of 630 000). A few per cent of dogs in Thailand are rabid. Of all attendances at the largest emergency unit in Bangkok, 5 per cent are for animal bites — some 50 animal bites per day, mostly in children. Rabies causes at least 200–300 human deaths each year, and more than 150 000 people receive courses of post-exposure vaccination.
>
> Airport surveys of departing visitors indicate that 1.3 per cent of visitors are bitten and 8.9 per cent of visitors are licked by dogs during their stay.

No one exposed to rabies should allow themselves to be fobbed off with tablets or a single injection.

In the UK, expert advice and materials for post-exposure treatment are available from the Communicable Disease Surveillance Centre (CDSC) (Tel: (020) 8200 1295), or in the USA, from local or state health departments or from the Division of Viral Diseases at the Centers for Disease Control and Prevention (Tel: (404) 329 3095 — 24-hour service). (see also Appendix 8.)

Venomous animals

Many animals possess venoms that can be injected into the unfortunate traveller by a variety of mechanisms. The normal purpose of envenoming is to discourage enemies or to immobilize and digest prey.

Some people become sensitized to venoms after one or more stings or bites. In this case, the allergic (anaphylactic) reaction to the venom may prove far more dangerous than its toxic effects, and in some parts of the world, such as Europe and North America, there are more deaths from such anaphylactic reactions to bee and wasp stings than from lethal snake, scorpion, and spider venoms.

Tropical regions have the richest venomous fauna, and travellers to these areas often regard snake bites and scorpion stings as the two greatest medical hazards of their journey. However, it is nearly always the indigenous human population, rather than the traveller, that falls victim to venomous animals.

In the USA in 1995, 1370 snake bites were reported with only one death. Snake bites kill many South American Indians who hunt barefooted in the jungle and many rice farmers in Southeast Asia who work barefooted and bare-handed in the paddy fields. Travellers are usually less exposed and better protected, and there have been only two reports of American travellers dying from venomous bites in recent years. A German tourist came close to death after being bitten by a cobra in central Bangkok, and several other Europeans have been severely envenomed in the jungles of South America and Southeast Asia.

Anyone planning to travel off the beaten track in a tropical country should find out about the venomous fauna well before leaving home. Those visiting a particularly remote and snake-infested area should be trained in first-aid techniques and consider taking the necessary equipment including their own supply of antivenom. Usually, this can be supplied only by a national centre of antivenom production in the capital; contact will have to be made with the centre well in advance. Some anti-venoms available in Western and in tropical countries are of dubious potency. Information supplied with commercial antivenom (the 'package insert') may be misleading. It is also important to find out something about the quality of local medical services or referral centres in the larger cities.

Information and advice about venomous fauna and availability of anti-venoms can be obtained from some specialist institutions and poisons centres, such as those listed at the end of this chapter.

Venomous snakes

Venomous snakes have one or more pairs of enlarged teeth, the fangs, in the upper jaw. Venom passes from the venom gland just behind the eye, through a duct to the base of the fang, and then through a channel or groove to its tip.

Dangerous species

Important venomous snakes belong to two families:

The *Elapidae*, which include cobras (Figs. 6.1b and 6.2), kraits (Fig. 6.3), mambas (Fig. 6.4), coral snakes, Australasian snakes and sea snakes (Fig. 6.1a). The South African ringhals and African and Asian spitting cobras can eject venom from the tips of their fangs towards the eyes of an aggressor as a defensive strategy.

The *Viperidae*, which is the largest family of venomous snakes and includes the sub-families *Viperinae*, the Old World or typical vipers and adders (Figs. 6.1c and 6.5); and

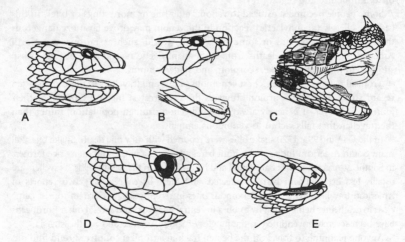

Fig. 6.1 Fangs of the five families of venomous snakes. A: sea snake (*Hydrophis cyanocinctus*, family Elapidae, subfamily Hydrophiinae), very small front fangs; B: Thai spitting cobra ('*Naja siamensis*,' family Elapidae), erect front fangs; C: Gaboon viper (*Bitis rhinoceros*, family Viperidae), long, hinged front fangs; D: boomslang (*Dispholidus typus*, family Colubridae), rear fangs; E: burrowing asp or stiletto snake (*Atractaspis aterrima*, family Atractaspididae).

Crotalinae, the New World rattlesnakes, moccasins and lance-headed vipers (Fig. 6.6), and Asian pit vipers, all of which possess a heat-sensitive pit organ situated between the eye and the nostril.

Less important groups are:

The *Colubridae,* of which some members have small fangs at the back of their mouth (Fig. 6.1d). Effective bites in humans are very uncommon but a few species, such as the African boomslang and bird, twig, tree, or vine snake, and Asian keel backs have caused some fatalities.

The *Atractaspididae,* (burrowing asps or stiletto snakes) are found in Africa and the Middle East. They strike sideways, with one long fang protruding from the corner of their mouth (Fig. 6.1e).

Dangerously venomous snakes do not occur at high altitudes (more than 5000 metres or about 16 000 ft), in the Antarctic, nor in a number of islands such as Ireland, Iceland, Crete, New Zealand, and Madagascar, and most Caribbean and Pacific islands (see Map 6.2). Sea snakes inhabit the warmer oceans within latitudes 40°N and 40°S, but not the Atlantic (see Map 6.3).

The incidence and medical significance of snake bite have been underestimated because it is a problem of the rural tropics, often little known to academic centres in the capital cities even of countries where it is particularly common. However, snakes still cause more than 50 000 deaths each year and disable half a million or more people because of complications such as limb gangrene and kidney failure. As mentioned above, the incidence of snake bite is highest among native populations who are forced to live and work, relatively unprotected, in snake-infested environments. Epidemics of

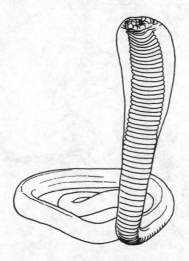

Fig. 6.2 Egyptian cobra (*Naja haje*) in typical threatening/defensive posture

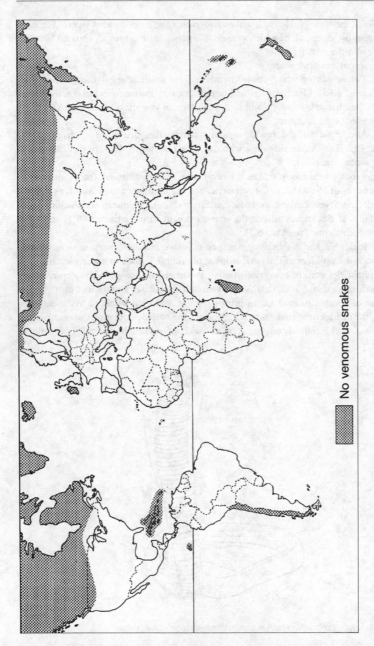

No venomous snakes

Map 6.2 Areas where there are no venomous snakes

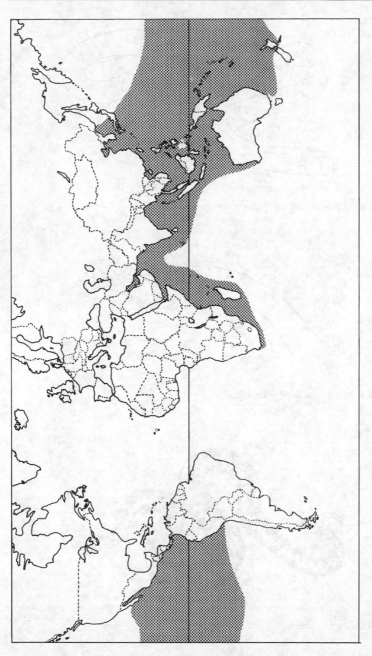

Map 6.3 Distribution of venomous sea snakes

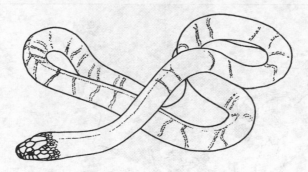

Fig. 6.3 Common (Indian) krait (*Bungarus caeruleus*)

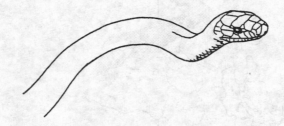

Fig. 6.4 Black mamba (*Dendroaspis polylepis*)

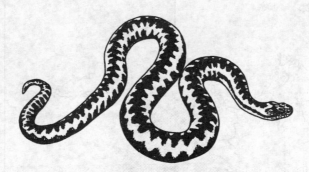

Fig. 6.5 European adder (*Vipera berus*)

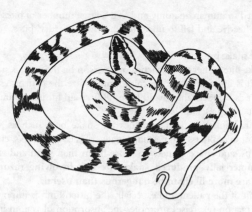

Fig. 6.6 Jararaca (*Bothrops jararaca*).

snake bite have resulted from flooding and invasion of snake-infested regions by a large human work force.

Effects of snake venom
Snake venoms contain 20 or more different toxins. The main clinical effects of snake venoms are summarized below:

- *Local pain, swelling, bruising, blistering, and necrosis (gangrene) in the bitten limb* with enlargement of local lymph glands (e.g. in the armpit or groin) are seen particularly with *Viperidae* and some cobras. Fluid and blood leak into the tissues of the bitten limb. Swelling starts soon after the bite and may spread to involve the whole limb and adjoining area of the trunk.

- *Bleeding and blood-clotting disorders* occur mainly in patients bitten by *Viperidae*, *Colubridae*, and Australasian elapids. The commonest sites of bleeding are the gums, nose, stomach, bowels, and genito-urinary tract.

- Shock *(fall in blood pressure)* may occur in patients bitten by *Viperidae*.

- *Paralysis ('neurotoxicity')* is first noticeable as drooping of the eyelids (ptosis), but later spreads to other muscles, particularly those responsible for swallowing and breathing. The *Elapidae*, and a few of the *Viperidae* have neurotoxic venoms. Venoms of sea snakes, Australasian elapids, and of several species of the *Viperidae* damage muscles causing painful, tender, stiff muscles and paralysis and leakage of muscle pigment (myoglobin) into the blood and urine which turns black.

- *Kidney failure* resulting from clotting of blood in the small blood vessels, prolonged shock, or a direct action of the venom is a major feature of bites by Russell's viper and some of the New World pit vipers and sea snakes.

Despite this formidable repertoire of toxic effects, 20–80 per cent of people bitten by venomous snakes suffer negligible or no envenoming. It may be that the snake's strike is not well adapted to human anatomy and that a large number of bites are therefore mechanically ineffective and fail to inject much venom — 'dry' bites.

Management of snake bite

First-aid for snake bite, either by the victim or a person on the spot, is summarized in the box below. It is important to keep calm, immobilize the patient, especially their bitten limb as far as is practicable, avoid harmful first-aid measures, and get them to hospital or a dispensary as soon as possible.

Most of the traditional first-aid remedies for snake bite, such as suction, local incisions, application of potassium permanganate crystals, cold packs, electric shocks, tourniquets, herbs, and snake stones, do more harm than good and should not be used. **Most commercially–produced snake-bite kits involving razor blades and suction devices are more likely to be dangerous than useful.**

Immobilization of the patient and especially the bitten limb is important, because any muscle contraction (exercise) promotes the absorption of venom into veins and lymphatics and its spread throughout the body.

Snake bite: first-aid

1. Reassure the patient.
2. Immobilize the bitten limb with a splint or sling.
3. Move the patient to hospital or a dispensary as quickly as possible.
4. Avoid harmful measures such as incisions, suction, potassium permanganate crystals, electric shocks, and tourniquets (except as below).
5. If the patient has definitely been bitten by an elapid snake (e.g. cobra, mamba, krait, coral snake, Australian elapid, sea snake but *not* an African spitting Cobra) use pressure immobilization (see below).
6. Use paracetamol, codeine, or dihydrocodeine not aspirin to treat pain.
7. If you have your own supply of antivenom, take it with you to the hospital or dispensary.
8. Do not attempt to pursue or kill the snake, but if it has been killed take it along with you to the hospital or dispensary; do not handle it with your bare hands, even if it appears dead.

Reassurance

This is a most important part of treatment. Most snake-bite victims are terrified, but only a minority of bites, even by dangerously venomous species, produce serious envenoming.

The speed of the lethal effects of snake venoms has been greatly exaggerated. To kill a man, lethal doses of venom usually take hours in the case of neurotoxic species such as cobras, mambas, and sea snakes, or days in the case of vipers and rattlesnakes — not seconds or minutes as is commonly believed. This interval between bite and death is usually sufficiently long to allow effective treatment.

Pain

If pain is a problem, safe pain-killing drugs for snake-bite victims are paracetamol — the dose is one or two 500 mg tablets for adults — or codeine (30–60 mg) — or dihydrocodeine (30 mg). Aspirin should *never be used* in snake-bite victims as it may cause stomach bleeding.

Medical treatment
At the hospital or dispensary, medically trained staff should examine the patient (and dead snake if available) and decide about further treatment. The only specific remedy for snake bite is antivenom (also known as antivenin, antivenene, or antisnake-bite serum) which is made in horses or sheep by immunizing them with increasing doses of snake venom. Although most modern antivenoms are refined and purified, injection of 'foreign' protein (i.e. from another species of animal) always carries the risk of potentially serious anaphylactic reactions. To be optimally effective, antivenom must be given by a slow intravenous injection or infusion.

Not all people bitten by snakes require antivenom. Since the decision about antivenom treatment, the administration of antivenom by the intravenous route, and the treatment of antivenom reactions all require clinical skill, lay people should not undertake the medical treatment of snake bite except under most unusual conditions (for example, a serious bite in a member of an expedition in a very remote area).

As a *life-saving measure*, antivenom may be given by intramuscular injection (the dose divided between several sites in the front of the thighs), followed by massage to promote absorption of the antivenom into the bloodstream. *However, this is certainly not recommended as a general rule.*

Patients who need antivenom are those in whom there is evidence that venom has been absorbed and is circulating throughout the body to produce severe general effects ('systemic envenoming'). The important signs are low blood pressure, failure of the blood to clot, bleeding from the nose or gums or vomiting or passing blood, generalized pain and stiffness in the muscles, and paralysis.

The earliest sign of neurotoxic poisoning is an inability to raise the upper eyelids when the bitten person tries to look up (ptosis). Slight bleeding from the site of the bite and mild local swelling and bruising are not normally regarded as justification for antivenom treatment. However, rapidly extending swelling and swelling involving more than half the bitten limb (for example, above the knee and above the elbow in bites of the foot and hand respectively) indicate that enough venom has been injected to warrant antivenom, especially if the snake is known to have a venom that causes necrosis (gangrene).

Administration of antivenom by a medically qualified person
For intravenous injection, freeze-dried antivenom is dissolved in sterile water for injection (usually 10 ml per ampoule) and liquid antivenom is given neat. The injection should be given slowly, at a rate of not more than 2 ml per minute. A method that is easier to control, but requires more equipment, is to dilute antivenom with 'normal'/isotonic saline or 5 per cent dextrose solution, making up the volume to 200 ml. This is administered through an intravenous giving-set and is infused over about 60 minutes, starting slowly (30 drops per minute), then speeding up after about

10 minutes if there is no reaction. The dose of antivenom varies with the manufacturer and the severity of envenoming. **THE SAME DOSE SHOULD BE GIVEN TO CHILDREN AS TO ADULTS.**

Antivenom should never be given, even by medically qualified staff, unless adrenaline (epinephrine) (0.5 ml of a 1 mg/ml or 1 in 1000 solution by intramuscular injection) is available to treat anaphylactic reactions.

The commonest symptoms of an antivenom reaction are itching, the appearance of a raised, reddened nettle rash (urticaria), and a throbbing headache. More serious symptoms include coughing, vomiting, wheezing, and fall in blood pressure leading to unconsciousness. At the first sign of a reaction, andrenaline should be given.

An antihistamine drug should also be given, preferably chlorpheniramine maleate (Piriton, Chlor-Trimeton), 10 mg by intravenous injection. Allergic patients (those suffering from asthma, hay fever, and eczema) are more likely to develop severe antivenom reactions than other people. Skin tests are not reliable in predicting whether or not someone will develop a reaction.

Although I would strongly discourage lay people from giving antivenom themselves, it may be worth some expeditions taking a small supply (5–10 ampoules) of antivenom to be given by a local physician or dispensary if the need arises. The supply of antivenom to rural hospitals and health centres in the tropics is often very unreliable.

There is an alarming global shortage of antivenom, a problem that has become much more serious since production in many countries has passed from government to the private sector (since there is little profit to be made). Perhaps the best solution for the future would be internationally-sponsored production of 'polyvalent' antivenoms, effective against all of the major snake species in a particular region.

Infection
There is a small but definite risk of tetanus and secondary bacterial infection following snake bite. Patients should be given a booster dose of tetanus toxoid and a course of penicillin or metronidazole, especially if the wound has been interfered with.

The special danger of early paralysis after bites by some elapid snakes
Bites by cobras, king cobras, kraits, Australasian elapid snakes, and sea snakes have, on rare occasions, led to the rapid development of life-threatening paralysis of the breathing muscles. This paralysis might be delayed by slowing down the absorption of venom from the site of the bite. The most effective and acceptable way of doing this is by '**pressure immobilization**'. An elasticated, stretchy, crepe bandage, approximately 10 cm wide and at least 4.5 metres long, is bound firmly around the entire bitten limb, starting around the fingers or toes and moving up towards the armpit or groin, binding in a rigid splint. The bandage is applied as tightly as for a sprained ankle, but not so tightly that the hand or foot becomes cold, pale, and pulseless, or that a finger cannot be slipped easily between its layers. The bandage should be left in place until the patient has reached hospital and antivenom treatment has been started.

Compression immobilization may increase the local effects of necrotic venoms such as those of *Viperidae*.

Prevention of snake bite

Fortunately, travellers can virtually exclude the risk of being bitten by a snake if they heed the following advice.

Snakes and snake-charmers should be avoided as far as possible. If you happen to see a snake, do not disturb, corner, or attack it, and never attempt to handle a snake even if it is said to be a harmless species or appears to be dead. *Even a severed head can bite!*

If you should happen to find yourself confronted with a snake at close quarters, try to keep absolutely still until it has slithered away: snakes strike only at moving objects.

Never walk in undergrowth or deep sand without boots, socks, and long trousers; and at night always carry a torch. Unlit paths are particularly dangerous after rainstorms or floods. Never collect firewood or move logs and boulders with your bare hands, and never push your hands or sticks into burrows, holes, or crevices. Avoid climbing trees and rocks that are covered with thick foliage and never swim in overgrown rivers or lakes (there are a good many other reasons for not swimming in lakes and rivers in the tropics.).

If you are forced to sleep in the open or under canvas, use a hammock or try to raise your bed at least one foot off the ground or else use a sewn-in ground-sheet or mosquito net that can be zipped up or well tucked in. Snakes never attack man without provocation but will strike if grabbed, trodden on, or even if someone rolls onto them in their sleep. Snakes are sometimes attracted into houses in pursuit of their prey (chickens, rats, mice, toads, and lizards). Sea snakes bite only when they are picked out of fishing nets or trodden on by waders.

It has not proved possible, nor would it be desirable, to exterminate venomous snakes. The Burmese rice farmer may regard the Russell's viper as his enemy, but in fact the snake protects his livelihood, the rice crop, by controlling the rats and mice attracted to the harvest.

Venomous fish

Fish sting with venomous spines that may form part of the dorsal and pectoral fins and gill covers or may be separate appendages situated in front of the dorsal fins or on the tail. Tropical coral reefs, especially of the Indo-Pacific region, harbour the greatest number and diversity of venomous fish. Stings by weeverfish can also occur in temperate waters such as along the coasts of the UK and Europe (e.g. Adriatic and Cornish coasts).

Dangerous species

Members of several families of fish have caused human deaths: sharks and dogfish, stingrays and mantas, catfish, weeverfish, scorpionfish, and stargazers.

Stingrays cause many stings around the coasts of North America and in the rivers in South America. Waders and bathers may tread on these fish as they lie in the mud or sand. The tail, armed with a formidable spine up to 30 cm long in some species, is lashed against the intrusive limb, causing severe mechanical trauma and releasing venom into the wound, which is usually on the ankle.

Weeverfish (Trachinidae) occur in temperate waters of the North Sea, south coast of England, Mediterranean, and north coast of Africa.

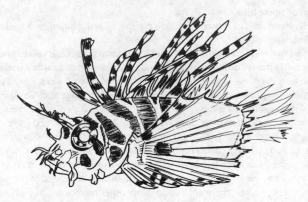

Fig. 6.7 Lionfish (*Brachirus species*, family *Scorpaenidae*) *from Papua New Guinea*

Scorpionfish (Scorpaenidae) include the very dangerous stonefish (which lies motionless and well camouflaged on the bottom, resembling a roughly textured lump of rock) and the attractive zebra or lionfish (Fig. 6.7). They occur throughout the Indian and Pacific oceans.

Effects of fish venom
Fish stings can produce excruciating pain radiating from the wound, some local swelling, vomiting, diarrhoea, sweating, fall in blood pressure, and irregularities of the heartbeat.

Treatment
To relieve the intense pain, the stung limb, finger, or toe, should be immersed in water that is hot enough to be uncomfortable but not scalding (just under 45°C). Alternatively, a local anaesthetic such as procaine (Novocain) or lignocaine can be injected. The most effective way of anaesthetizing a stung finger or toe is to apply a 'ring block' of local anaesthetic — a simple procedure that any doctor should be able to perform. The stinging spine and membranes should be removed to prevent secondary infection of the wound. If the patient loses consciousness, stops breathing, and no arterial pulse can be felt, mouth-to-mouth respiration and external cardiac massage should be used.

> If hot water is not available to treat a fish sting, make a hot compress by heating a wet towel on the engine block of a car or boat motor that has recently been used, and then apply its clean side to the wound. Alternatively, a heat lamp effect can be achieved by using a boat spotlight: hold the affected area close to the spotlight. Be careful, however, not to allow the skin to touch either the spotlight or the engine block directly, because this can produce a burn. A glowing cigarette end may be advanced close to the sting.
>
> Dr Stanley Schwartz, Fort Myers, Florida

Antivenoms for *Scorpaenidae* and *Trachinidae* are manufactured in Australia and Yugoslavia. Waders and bathers can avoid stepping on stinging fish by adopting a shuffling gait in sand or mud, and prodding in front of them with a stick. Footwear is protective, although not against stingray spines. Divers should be aware of the dangers of stinging fish, especially in the neighbourhood of coral reefs.

Food poisoning and marine animals (ciguatera, tetrodotoxic, and scombroid fish poisoning)
See pp. 65–68 (poisons and contaminants in food).

Venomous jellyfish and related animals
Jellyfish, sea wasps, Portuguese men-o'-war, polyps, hydroids, sea anemones, sea nettles, and corals all belong to a group of animals called Cnidarians (formerly *Coelenterates*). The tentacles of these often brightly coloured and beautiful animals are armed with millions of stinging capsules (called nematocysts) which discharge when touched by a swimmer. In many cases the worst that can occur is an itchy rash, but some jellyfish can cause very painful stings with severe envenoming. The most dangerous species is the box jellyfish (*Chironex fleckeri*) of the north coast of Australia and Indo-Pacific region. Severe stings produce violent shivering, vomiting, and diarrhoea with fall in blood pressure, paralysis of breathing muscles, and fits.

Treatment
Fragments of tentacles must be removed from the skin as soon as possible without causing a further discharge of stinging capsules. Commercial vinegar or dilute acetic acid effectively inactivates the capsules of box jellyfish. A wet compress of baking powder (sodium bicarbonate) is the best first aid for the Atlantic sea nettle, *Chrysaora quinquecirra*.

What to do if you are stung by a box jellyfish
The best instant remedy is to splash vinegar onto your skin — lots of it, and fast. Vinegar inactivates tentacle fragments still in contact with your skin, preventing further stinging (it doesn't help much with damage that has already occurred).

In Asia and the Pacific, this treatment can save lives — the sting of the Australian box jellyfish causes cardiac arrest — so medical teams have been testing out alternatives to vinegar that are easier to find on an Australian beach. They have studied wine, beer, fruit juices, and tea. Wine worked best — but only when it was about four days old and had turned mostly to vinegar anyway. Next best treatment: Coca-Cola, which reduced further stinging by 30 per cent and also reduced pain by 25–70 per cent.

In several cases of box jellyfish stings in Australia, resuscitation (CPR) on the beach has proved effective. The most severe effects of the toxins may be extremely transient. An antivenom for box jellyfish is manufactured in Australia.

Prevention

Cnidarian stings could be prevented if swimmers stayed out of the sea during seasons when large numbers of jellyfish are washed ashore. Warning notices on beaches should not be ignored!

Coral cuts are the commonest injuries in snorkellers and scuba divers. They are part venomous and part mechanical. Calcareous fragments may remain embedded in the painful wounds and secondary infection with unusual marine bacteria is common. Cuts should be thoroughly cleaned, explored for coral fragments, debrided of dead tissue, and dressed with antiseptic. Systemic antibiotics may be needed.

Other venomous marine animals

The venomous spines and grapples of echinoderms (starfish and sea urchins) can produce dangerous envenoming, and their spines can be a painful nuisance. All spines and grapples should be removed methodically from the wound after softening the skin with 2 per cent salicylic acid ointment.

A few molluscs (cone shells, and octopuses) are also venomous. Cone shells and the Australian blue-ringed octopus (Fig. 6.8) can produce fatal envenoming. No specific treatment is available.

Bees, wasps, and hornets

Stings by bees, wasps, hornets, yellow jackets, and their relatives are very common events throughout the world. Transient pain, local swelling, and redness are usually

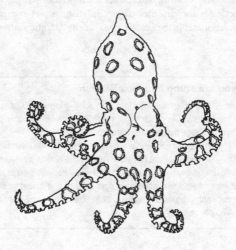

Fig. 6.8 Venomous spotted octopus (*Haplochlaena lunulatus*) from Papua New Guinea (similar to the Australian blue-tinged octopus *H. maculosa*)

the only effects. People are occasionally attacked by swarms of bees. A rock-climber in Nigeria fell to his death when attacked by bees, and in Thailand one child died of kidney failure and another of swelling and blockage of the windpipe after being stung hundreds of times. In Zimbabwe, however, a man survived after being stung 2243 times by an angry swarm.

Allergy
About 1 in 200 people become hypersensitive (allergic) to bee or wasp venom, so that a single sting may produce a severe and even rapidly fatal effect. In the USA, many more deaths occur from severe allergic reactions (anaphylactic reactions) to insect stings than from snake bites. Anyone who is allergic to bee or wasp venom may notice itching of the scalp, flushing, dizziness, collapse and loss of consciousness, wheezing, swelling of the lips, tongue, and throat, vomiting, colic, diarrhoea, and hives ('nettle rash') over the whole body. The diagnosis of venom hypersensitivity can be confirmed by special skin tests or blood tests (measurement of venom-specific IgE by RAST).

Treatment
Embedded bee stings should be removed immediately. Aspirin is an effective painkiller. Insect-sting anaphylaxis should be treated with adrenaline 1 mg/ml (0.1 per cent) solution in a dose of 0.5–1 ml given by intramuscular injection. People who know they are allergic to stings should carry an identifying tag such as provided by Medic-Alert Foundation International (In the UK: 1 Bridge Wharf, 156 Caledonian Road, London N1 9UU; tel: (020) 7833 3034; fax: (020) 7278 0647; **www.medicalert.co.uk**; In the USA: P.O. Box 1009, Turlock, CA 95381; tel: (209) 668 3333, **www.medicalert.org**) in case they are found unconscious. They should always carry equipment for self-injection of epinephrine (adrenaline) (e.g. 'Epi-Pen', 'Ana-Kit', 'Min-i-Jet'). Desensitization using purified specific venoms is safe and effective.

Venomous spiders
Almost all spiders have venom glands associated with a pair of small fangs near the mouth, but only about a hundred species have caused severe envenoming in humans.

Dangerous species
The most important species from the medical point of view are the following:

Latrodectus tredecemguttatus, which occurs in Mediterranean countries and was known historically as tarantula

Latrodectus mactans, the black widow spider of North America and related species in South America (*L. curasaviensis*) and South Africa (*L. geometricus*)

Latrodectus hasselti, the Australian red-back spider

Loxosceles reclusa, the brown recluse spider of North America (*L. laeta, L. gaucho*) and related species in South America

Phoneutria, (Fig 6.9) the banana spider of South America

Atrax robustus, the Sydney funnel web spider of Australia

Spider venoms cause two groups of symptoms — neurotoxic, with painful muscle spasms and stimulation of the autonomic nervous system to produce local sweating and goose flesh *(Latrodectus, Phoneutria,* and *Atrax)*, or local necrosis (gangrene) and haemolysis *(Loxosceles)*.

Treatment
Local infiltration of lignocaine (1–2 per cent) is effective for painful bites (e.g. *Phoneutria*)

Neurotoxic symptoms may develop very rapidly in some cases, so 'pressure immobilization' (see p. 236) should be applied to delay spread of venom until the patient reaches hospital.

Spider antivenoms are manufactured in a number of countries. Calcium gluconate (10 ml of 10 per cent solution given by slow intravenous injection) is said to relieve painful muscle spasms dramatically in cases of *Latrodectus* bite.

Venomous ticks
In north-western North America, eastern USA, and eastern Australia, children and sometimes adults have become paralysed following attachment of hard or soft ticks. The tick may not have been spotted because it is hidden in a hairy area or even inside the ear. The victim may vomit and eventually die from paralysis of the breathing muscles unless the tick is found and removed. The tick should be detached without being squeezed: either paint it with ether, chloroform, paraffin, gasoline, or turpentine or prise it out between partially separated tips of a pair of small curved forceps. In Australia, an antivenom is available against the venom of the common dog tick.

Venomous scorpions
Dangerously venomous scorpions are found in South Africa, North Africa, the Middle East, India, North, Central, and South America (Fig. 6.10), and the Caribbean. In

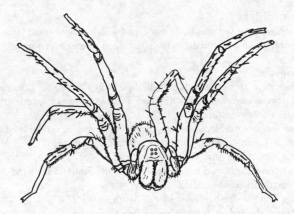

Fig. 6.9 Banana spider (*Phoneutria keiserlingi*) from Brazil, in defensive posture

Mexico, scorpions kill ten times more people than do snakes. Mortality is particularly high in young children. Scorpion venoms produce symptoms such as sweating, vomiting, and diarrhoea (due to the stimulation of the autonomic nervous system). Damage to the heart muscle may cause a fall in blood pressure, irregular heartbeat, and development of heart failure.

Treatment
Local pain is very severe in all scorpion stings, even those that are not particularly dangerous. This is best treated with local anaesthetic given by a ring block in the case of stings on fingers or toes (see p. 242). Emetine is effective but may cause necrosis. If this does not control the pain, a powerful analgesic such as pethidine (50–100 mg by intramuscular injection for an adult) or even morphine may be needed. Antivenoms are made in the USA, South America, the Middle East, North Africa, and South Africa.

Millipedes and centipedes
Millipedes can secrete an irritant liquid that may produce blistering of the skin or more severe effects if it gets into the eyes. Centipedes can produce painful venomous stings but are rarely, if ever, dangerous.

Ants, beetles, and caterpillars
Ants, beetles, some hairy caterpillars, and a variety of other insects and their larvae can produce irritation of the skin and conjunctiva on contact, with pain, inflammation, and blistering. Serious effects caused by fibrinolytic caterpillar venoms are common in some parts of Venezuela and Brazil. Haemolymph of blister beetles (family *Meloidae*) contains the vesicant substance, cantharidin, which is emitted in defence or if the insects are crushed. Beetles may be trapped inadvertently in body crevices and skin

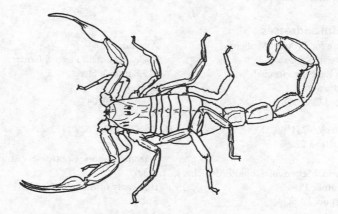

Fig. 6.10 Scorpion (*Tityus serrulatus*) from Brazil

creases such as under the arm or in front of the elbow. Painful blisters are produced. The most famous species is *Lytta vesicatoria*, misleadingly known as 'Spanish fly'.

Leeches

Leeches can be a severe nuisance to travellers, particularly in damp rainforest regions of Southeast Asia.

Land leeches wait in low vegetation near game tracks or paths until a large, warm-blooded animal approaches. With incredible speed and efficiency they sense their victim and attach themselves. In humans, they usually suck blood from the lower legs or ankles, easily penetrating long trousers, socks, and lace-up boots. An anticoagulant is secreted so that even after the leech has been removed or has fallen off, engorged with blood, there is persistent bleeding.

Aquatic leeches attack swimmers and crawl into the mouth, nostrils, eyes, and other body orifices such as the vagina or urethra.

Treatment

Leeches are best removed by application of salt, alcohol, vinegar, or a lighted match or cigarette. If they are pulled off forcibly their mouth-parts sometimes remain in the wound, which may then become infected.

Prevention

Infestation with leeches can be prevented to some extent by smothering boots, socks, and trouser-legs with dibutylphthalate or *n,n*-diethylmetatoluamide (DEET, see p. 214). Coarse tobacco rolled into the top of the socks and kept soaked is also effective. Aquatic leeches are best avoided by refraining from swimming or bathing in forest streams and pools.

Useful addresses

Centre for Tropical Medicine
University of Oxford,
John Radcliffe Hospital,
Headington,
Oxford OX3 9DU,
UK
Tel: 01865 741166/220968/221332
Fax: 01865 220984

Liverpool School of Tropical Medicine
Pembroke Place,
Liverpool L3 5QA,
UK
Tel: 0151 708 9393
Fax: 0151 7088733

Poisondex
Rocky Mountain Poisons Center
645 Bannock Street,
Denver,
Colorado 80204,
USA
Tel: 001 (303) 629 1123

Arizona Poison Control & Antivenin Index
University of Arizona,
Tucson,
AZ 85721,
USA
Tel: 001 (602) 626 6016

Principal antivenom manufacturers

Instituto Clodomiro Picado
Universidad de Costa Rica,
Ciudad Universitaria,
Rodrigo Facio,
San Jose,
Costa Rica
(Central America)

Instituto Butantan
Caixa Postal 65,
05504 Sao Paulo,
Brazil
(South America)

Aventis–Pasteur
1541 Av. Marcel Merieux,
69280 Marcy I'Etoile,
Lyon,
France
(Europe, Middle East, Africa)

Institute of Immunology
Rockerfellerova 2,
Zagreb,
Croatia

South African Institute for Medical Research
P.O. Box 1038,
Johannesburg 2000,
Republic of South Africa
(Africa)

Haffkine Biopharmaceutical Corporation Ltd
Acharya,
Donde Marg,
Parel,
Mumbai 400012,
India
(Indian subcontinent)

Thai Red Cross Society
Queen Saovabha Memorial Institute,
Rama IV Road,
Bangkok,
Thailand
(Southeast Asia)

Commonwealth Serum Laboratories
45 Poplar Road,
Parkville,
Victoria 3052,
Australia
(Australasia).

7 Air and sea travel

Air travel

Most health problems in air travellers are minor, and can usually be anticipated. All travellers should know about the possible effects of reduced cabin pressure, and should know how to minimize the risk of DVT.

Dr Richard Harding is co-author of the book *Aviation Medicine*, published by the British Medical Association, and author of *Survival in Space*, published by Routledge. His past research interests included advanced oxygen systems and the medical problems of manned spaceflight; and he is currently a consultant in biomechanics and injury causation with Biodynamic Research Corporation, San Antonio, Texas.

On 11 September 2001, four airliners were hijacked by 19 suicide terrorists intent on causing the greatest number of casualties possible. American Airlines Flight 11, carrying 92 people, was deliberately crashed into the North Tower of New York's World Trade Center. United Airlines Flight 175, with 65 people on board, was crashed into the South Tower; American Airlines Flight 77, carrying 64 people, hit the Pentagon, and United Airlines Flight 93, carrying 43, crashed in Shanksville, Pennsylvania. Aware of the hijackers' intentions, passengers on Flight 93 are believed to have wrested control of the aircraft, crashing into open land. The exact death toll on the ground from the impact of the other aircraft may never be known, but was close to three thousand.

On 4 October 2001, in the tense aftermath of these atrocities, a Russian passenger jet was shot down by a missile — during a Ukrainian military exercise, killing all 78 on board. A further crash on 12 November 2001, of American Airlines Flight 587 shortly after take-off (254 on board) was found not to be due to terrorism, but to mechanical failure.

Much is being done to learn from these events, particularly in terms of improved security procedures. Despite these tragic incidents, air travel remains remarkably safe: it is a tribute to the technological and practical skills of aircraft designers, airlines, and air-traffic controllers that of more than 1.6 billion people who travelled on scheduled passenger flights world-wide during 2000, a total of 1126 died in 37 fatal accidents (see Fig. 8.1, p. 296).

This chapter, however, is concerned with the less dramatic but no less important aspects of the health of the vast majority of people who travel by air, whether for business or pleasure. A measure of the increasing awareness of the truly huge scale of human migration by air around the world each year, and of the need for this movement to be as safe and healthy as possible, was the publication in November 2000 of the UK House of Lords Science and Technology Committee's wide-ranging inquiry into 'Air Travel and Health' (see Further Reading).

Preparation for the journey

Immunizations and medicines

Even the seasoned air traveller should double-check requirements and recommendations for immunization and malaria prevention — not just for the ultimate destination, but also for any stop-over points *en route* (see p. 130, and Appendices 1 and 8). Don't forget to carry any medical supplies you may need for the trip in hand luggage at all times, and it may also be sensible to take along a prescription or certificate, signed by your doctor, confirming the details of your medical treatment. Passengers taking regular medication (such as those with diabetes mellitus or epilepsy) should remain on 'home time' during a long journey, and readjust timings only after arrival.

Fear of flying

Flying is an exciting and exhilarating experience but many people are also anxious and, occasionally, frightened by it. This is particularly likely in inexperienced passengers, and at times when security and safety concerns are much in the news, although fears usually abate very quickly once they are air-borne.

For the habitually fearful passenger, mild sedation may be advisable for a few days before and during the flight. Such treatment can be discussed and prescribed on a pre-trip visit to your doctor, and minimizes the personal misery that can surround an impending air journey. Remember that sedatives enhance the effects of alcohol, so avoid alcohol when taking these drugs.

Once at the airport, the hustle and bustle increase tension for many people, particularly the elderly, and if at all possible a 'dummy run' to the airport some weeks before flying is one way to reduce this. So too is arrival in good time on the day of travel, and prompt transfer to the departure lounge, where the surroundings are usually much calmer.

Increasing awareness of the fear of flying, which is believed to affect millions of people in the UK alone — perhaps between 10 and 40 per cent of air travellers — has led to the establishment of support groups (especially on the Internet) and of professional (usually psychological) programmes to address the problem. The latter often involve a course of gradually increasing exposure to the aviation environment, and so are based at or near airports.

Pacemakers

The security devices through which passengers must pass in most international airports work by detecting changes in an electromagnetic field made by metal objects passing through them. The intensity of the field is set, in the UK and other Western countries, at a level that will not induce changes in the electrical components of pacemakers, but machines used in developing countries may not be so innocent. People fitted with pacemakers should mention the fact to security officials: this will enable a personal body check instead, and remove any possibility of interaction.

Fitness to fly

The presence of a pacemaker and indeed of *any* other serious medical condition should be notified to the airline at the time of booking. This useful precaution is as much for the benefit of the passenger as for the airline and, if in doubt about whether or not to notify a condition, ask your doctor to contact the airline's medical department for advice. In addition, a medical information form (termed MEDIF) is available from travel agents and airlines upon which the intending passenger and their doctor can provide advance information to the airline.

Patients may well be advised not to fly when suffering from a disease or condition that will be affected by the environmental changes produced by ascent to altitude. Ascent carries with it certain physiological problems, the most important of which is a *fall in atmospheric pressure* from 760 mm mercury (mmHg) at sea level to about 600 mm Hg at 6000 feet (a realistic 'cabin altitude' for a civil aircraft, maintained by the pressurization system regardless of the actual altitude of the aircraft).

The fall in *total* pressure may cause problems for passengers because it allows gases in body cavities to expand. But the associated fall in pressure of each constituent gas in the air, and in particular the reduced pressure of oxygen, is also highly important.

At sea level, the *partial* pressure of oxygen contained in the lungs is about 103 mm Hg, and this pressure allows healthy individuals to function normally. At 10 000 feet, however, the partial pressure of oxygen falls to only 60 mm Hg. In fact, because of the peculiar way in which oxygen is bound to blood, healthy people are virtually unaffected by this reduction, but the health of people who have any difficulty obtaining sufficient oxygen at sea level will be further compromised by the fall in partial pressure, and may develop symptoms of *hypoxia* (lack of oxygen).

Aircraft designers build in a safety margin which ensures that cabin altitude is held well below 10 000 feet and, as mentioned above, typically at 6000 feet, where the partial pressure of oxygen in the lungs is a 'safer' 74 mmHg. If the cabin was not pressurized in this way, passengers would be obliged to breathe oxygen from face masks whenever the aircraft altitude exceeded 10 000 feet. In addition, they would be unable to enjoy any freedom of movement within the cabin. Cabin pressurization systems also allow the cabin temperature and humidity to be controlled.

Medical conditions unsuited to flying

Table 7.1 lists many of the pre-existing medical conditions that may be affected by hypoxia and/or pressure changes associated with even the modest cabin climb to 6000 feet. It also lists certain other conditions that should be discussed with a doctor before a flight is contemplated *and* about which the airline's medical department would wish to know.

Such prior notification enables the airline to support needy passengers during embarkation/disembarkation procedures, and to provide wheelchairs and escorts if appropriate. Extra seats and special arrangements may be required for those wearing large plaster casts or with orthopaedic problems, or for whom a stretcher is needed. The cabin staff will also wish to know of any passengers who might need oxygen during the flight. The airlines normally make no additional charge for such supporting services, but passengers are expected to pay for any extra seats occupied.

You will see from Table 7.1 that it is advisable to restrict newborns from flying until they are 48 hours old (both because of the risk of hypoxia if the baby's lungs are not fully functional and of undiscovered medical problems in that early period). The suggestion, in a research paper published in 1998, that the hypoxia associated with air travel could be linked to sudden infant death syndrome (SIDS) has not subsequently been given credence in the medical literature.

Physiological effects of flight

Fortunately, the vast majority of passengers do not have a serious pre-existing illness and are fit to withstand the rigours of air travel. They are not, however, immune from certain other risks.

Hypoxia

Hypoxia may affect those who are heavy smokers (because carbon monoxide in cigarette smoke reduces the oxygen-carrying capacity of the blood); it may also affect drinkers (because alcohol enhances and mimics the effects of hypoxia) as well as those who are fatigued or have minor illnesses such as acute head colds. The last group should avoid or delay flying if at all possible, while heavy smokers and drinkers should avoid these vices, at least while airborne! Acute irritation of the respiratory tract, and the effects of 'secondary smoking' on non-smoking passengers, are minimized by both segregation of smokers and by efficient cabin air-conditioning. The International Civil Aviation Organization (ICAO), in its 1999 annual report, noted that smoking is now banned on all flights in Australia, New Zealand, Scandinavia, and North America; on most flights in Europe, the Middle East, and Asia; and on many in Africa; but only on a minority in South America. This world-wide effort has met with widespread approval.

The symptoms and signs of mild hypoxia are subtle and insidious, and resemble the early stages of alcoholic intoxication: personality change, euphoria, impaired judgement, mental and muscular incoordination, and memory impairment may all be features, along with blueness of the lips, ear lobes, and nailbeds. The treatment is administration of oxygen, and this should be given by the cabin staff whenever hypoxia is suspected.

Hyperventilation

A more common, but happily less sinister, problem is hyperventilation, which may best be described as inappropriate overbreathing. The symptoms and signs of this condition are similar to those of hypoxia and, indeed, hypoxia can cause hyperventilation. But the commonest cause is emotional stress, and the picture is

Table 7.1 Pre-existing medical conditions unsuited to or requiring special consideration for air travel

Condition	Severity	Reason	Advice
Conditions made worse by hypoxia (lack of oxygen)			
Respiratory disorders		Lower partial pressure of oxygen at altitude compromises already impaired oxygenation	May fly if able to walk about 150 feet and climb 10–12 stairs without symptoms
Chronic bronchitis			
Emphysema	Causing breathlessness at rest		
Bronchiectasis			
Severe anaemias of any sort			
Cardiovascular disorders			
Severe heart failure			Should not fly within 2 weeks
Severe angina			
Heart attack			Risk improves with time but wait at least 21 days
Neurological disorders			
Stroke			Should be accompanied
Hardening of the arteries in the elderly	Causing confusion at night		
Epilepsy			Drug dose may need to be increased
Conditions made worse by pressure changes			
Recent ear surgery			
Inner (stapedectomy)		Risk of severe damage	Wait at least 2 weeks, ideally 2 months
Middle			Wait until eardrum healed
Recent eye surgery		Gas expansion	Wait at least 21 days — see p. 432
Recent abdominal surgery		Gas expansion may cause disruption of the wound	Wait at least 10 days
Recent gastrointestinal bleeding		Re-bleeding may occur	Wait at least 21 days
Recent chest surgery		Trapped gas may expand and reduce lung function	Wait at least 21 days
Collapsed lung (pneumothorax)		Trapped gas may expand and reduce lung function	Wait until lung re-expanded

Table 7.1   (continued)

Condition	Severity	Reason	Advice
Recent cranial procedures		Trapped gas may expand and compress brain tissue	Wait at least 7 days
Fractured skull (with air entry)		Trapped gas may expand and compress brain tissue	Wait at least 7 days
Retinal surgery		Trapped gas may expand and cut off retinal blood supply	Seek specialist advice
Plaster casts		Trapped air in plaster may expand and compress limbs	Consider splitting plaster for long journeys
Other conditions requiring special consideration			
People with colostomies/ileostomies		Increased gas venting may occur	Carry extra bags and dressings
Psychiatric disorders		Novelty of airport and flight environments may exacerbate conditions	Trained escort needed
Diabetes mellitus		Problems with control may occur, possibly complicated by motion sickness	Remain on 'home' time during flight; consider anti-nauseant treatment
Facial surgery		At risk of asphyxia if jaws are wired and vomiting occurs	Should be accompanied by a person trained to release wires quickly
Pregnancy		Aircraft are not ideal delivery suites	No flying after 34–35 weeks of pregnancy on international routes and after 36 weeks on domestic routes
Newborn infants		At risk from hypoxia if lungs not fully expanded	Should not fly until over 48 hours old
Terminally ill		Death in-flight is distressing to other passengers and is legally most complex	May be allowed to fly on humanitarian grounds or for urgent treatment but not if likely to die on board
Infectious disease and disease characterized by offensive features such as vomiting, diarrhoea, copious sputum, or severe skin disfigurement		Cabin staff have neither the training nor the time to act as nursing attendants; they also have to handle food	

usually one of an obviously anxious passenger who becomes increasingly agitated, breathes rapidly, and then complains of light-headedness, feelings of unreality and anxiety (which reinforce the condition), pins and needles, and visual disturbances.

All of these features are the result of an excessive loss of carbon dioxide by overbreathing and, since carbon dioxide controls the acidity of the body, this loss leads to increasing alkalinity of the tissues.

The treatment is to re-breathe the expired air (traditionally from a paper bag!), which will minimize the loss of carbon dioxide. Reassurance, explanation, and firm instructions to breathe more slowly should also be given. Habitual hyperventilators may require mild sedation during the flight.

Gas expansion

Gas expansion on ascent may manifest itself in healthy individuals by a tighter than normal waistband, particularly if much alcoholic or carbonated drink is consumed or if gas-producing foods such as beans, cabbage, turnips, and curries are eaten. Moderation in drinking and gastronomic habits is therefore advisable, and comfortable, loosely fitting clothes are recommended. (Women who are susceptible to cystitis should in any case not wear tightly fitting trousers for long flights.)

Dehydration

Continuous plying with drinks is partly a legitimate attempt by the cabin staff to counteract any dehydration caused by the dry circulating cabin air and other factors associated with flying. Water or juices are the preferred means of fluid replacement because of the problems with alcohol, tea, coffee, and some carbonated drinks (see p. 259). The dryness of cabin air may also affect wearers of contact lenses and such passengers should be aware of accelerated drying of both soft and hard lenses (see pp. 433–5). Dehydration increases the risk of thrombosis (considered on p. 257).

Ears and sinuses

During ascent, gas expansion will also take place in the middle-ear cavities and the sinuses, and some gas must escape to the outside; the middle-ear cavities vent gas via the eustachian tubes, which open into the back of the throat, and the sinuses vent via tiny holes, called *ostia*, into the back of the nose. Such venting during ascent is entirely normal, and will be noticed when the ears 'pop': it should be neither unpleasant nor painful and does not require the help of chewing or other manoeuvres.

Unfortunately, the same cannot be said of the pressure changes that take place in these cavities as the aircraft descends. The volume of a gas decreases as the pressure increases, so that there is a 'contraction' of gas inside the middle-ear cavities and sinuses on descent. If the eustachian tubes and ostia are reasonably clear, air passes freely into the cavities, and the pressure inside rises to equal the pressure outside. If, however, the tubes and ostia are closed or are only partially clear — because, for example, they are inflamed and swollen as the result of a cold — air cannot enter the cavities and a *pressure differential* develops.

In the case of the middle-ear cavity, this differential is across the eardrum, which is pushed inward: slight deafness and feelings of fullness are followed by discomfort and increasingly severe pain. Similarly, if the ostia are blocked, severe pain develops in the sinuses above the eyes or in the cheeks. Such barotrauma (trauma due to pressure) may happen to anybody, but is more likely in those with a severe head cold.

Prevention of this kind of problem is one of the principal reasons for the slow rates of descent adopted by passenger aircraft. Sinus involvement is uncommon, but middle-ear barotrauma is a relatively frequent event.

Fortunately, the ability to 'clear the ears' by forcible opening of the eustachian tubes relieves the pressure differential, and correct use of manoeuvres for achieving this will prevent much airborne misery. Helpful manoeuvres include pinching the nose and, with the mouth shut, blowing out hard or swallowing; pinching the nose and drinking; moving the lower jaw from side to side; yawning, or simply opening the mouth wide. Such techniques should be repeated during descent at regular intervals when pressure on the eardrum is felt, and it is therefore advisable not to be asleep during this time.

Nasal decongestant sprays or drops may help keep both the eustachian tubes and ostia clear, but there is no voluntary means of opening the latter. Babies and small children are less affected by barotrauma because of the anatomy of the ostia and eustachian tubes, but crying or sucking will also help.

Mechanical help is also available in the form of ear plugs (called Earplanes, in sizes both for children and for adults). A special ceramic valve-like insert is said to limit excess pressure build-up on the eardrum during descent, so allowing any problems with tardy eustachian function to be balanced by a similarly but temporarily reduced external pressure.

Children

A method of relieving ear pain that I have found to work well with my own children is to gently pinch the child's nose, placing your lips around the child's mouth as if to give artificial ventilation; now blow gently! This may need to be repeated a number of times during a descent, but the relief is immediate. I am thinking of calling this the 'Dawood manoeuvre' — unless anyone else lays claim to it!

R.D.

Air sickness

Many people worry about motion sickness, but only a small number of passengers suffer symptoms.

Prevention with medication is a realistic approach, and motion sickness is discussed further in the chapter on pp. 271–7.

Immobility and travellers' thrombosis

Prolonged sitting encourages swelling of the feet and legs (*postural oedema*) (see below), which in turn is responsible for the familiar sight of people struggling to

---

Deep vein thrombosis and flying: how great is the risk?

Some passengers travelling by air undoubtedly do develop blood clots that can cause long-term damage to the leg and that may rarely travel to the lung (pulmonary embolism) causing difficulty in breathing and perhaps fatal complications. Of the millions of passengers travelling each year, relatively few are aware that they have developed blood clots in the leg and even fewer are aware that they have pulmonary embolism.

The problem is much more common than previously supposed: most passengers, once they land, get up from their seat and become mobile; the clots dissolve without the person ever being aware that they have had a clot, and without long-term consequences.

In a recent study, 12 out of 116 (one in ten) long-haul passengers developed a clot in the deep veins detectable only by scanning. None of these passengers had any symptoms, although a small number did require treatment. As part of the study, another group of 115 passengers wore class I elastic compression stockings; none of these passengers developed blood clots.

Our current state of knowledge is such that we believe that passengers who travel long distances on aeroplanes are at risk of developing clots in the deep veins detectable only by scanning. The risk will increase for older passengers and for passengers who have pre-existing illnesses such as heart disease, lung disease, cancer, or recent surgery. We would endorse a recent recommendation from the House of Lords that airlines make passengers aware of the risk and offer simple advice, pending definitive clinical studies.

If you are planning to travel, and you have medical concerns, then you should seek the advice of your GP. For the normal, fit, healthy traveller, buy a pair of elastic compression stockings and wear them for the duration of your flight. During the flight avoid excess alcohol, drink plenty of water, and move your legs frequently.

John Scurr, Consultant Vascular Surgeon, Lister Hospital, London.

---

replace footwear at the end of a flight. Postural oedema and stasis or stagnation of blood flow in the legs predispose to development of deep vein thrombosis (DVT) — painful clotting of blood in the deep veins of the calves — especially in those with a history of such problems. This may, on rare occasion, lead to pulmonary embolism (caused by movement of the clot from the leg to the lungs), which is a very serious and potentially fatal condition. The potential occurrence of DVT in aircraft passengers, whilst rare, was considered by the House of Lords, in its report, to be the most serious in-flight medical issue facing the industry.

Research by doctors from the German airline Lufthansa has shown that many symptoms experienced by long-haul passengers can be linked to airline seating conditions. Some term this the 'economy class syndrome'; others (including the House of Lords Committee) feel this is a seriously misleading term, since no passenger is immune from the risk (there are documented links with first- and business-class seating) Their Lordships preferred the terms 'flight-related DVT' or 'travellers' thrombosis'.

The Lufthansa team used a mock-up of a Boeing 747 interior; they studied 12 volunteers in economy-class seating on four simulated 12-hour flights (two daytime and two night-time), during which physiological tests were performed. The experiments were then repeated at 35 000 ft, in a real 747 on a 10-hour flight, using the same volunteers. A total of 35 000 samples were taken and analysed.

Key observations included significant movement of fluid out of the bloodstream and into the tissues of the lower body — evident as the ankle swelling with which many air travellers are all too familiar. Volunteers' weight increased significantly during the flights, some individuals gaining as much as 2 kg — an increase attributed almost entirely to the tissue fluid. There was remarkably little difference between the measurements in the air and those recorded from the 'passengers' on simulated flights, but there were significant differences between passengers who stayed in their seats and those who walked about the cabin or took exercise.

These findings suggest that the dehydration or fluid loss usually associated with flying, responsible for so many other symptoms, is in fact caused or made worse by sequestration of fluid in the tissues by gravity, during prolonged immobility in a seated position under cramped conditions.

The ideal solution would be to provide air travellers with much more space and freedom of movement, with (horizontal) sleeping facilities on long-haul flights. Few airlines do this, so here are some tips for comfort:

• Avoid crowded flights; travel the highest class you can afford.

• Choose an aisle or bulkhead seat, or find empty seats and put your feet up.

• Bring your own pillow or cushion.

• Perform isometric exercises in your seat, or use an in–seat exerciser such as the Airogym or the Push-Cush; and stand up, stretch, and walk about the cabin every hour if at all possible.

• Request prompt removal of your meal tray when you have finished eating.

• Drink plenty: most people drink less when they fly. Ideally you should drink at least 1 pint (water, fruit juice) every 3 hours. Small 'airline-sized' cans of soda are not enough. Alcohol, tea, and coffee have a diuretic (fluid-losing) effect; if you drink them you'll need to drink extra water to compensate not just for the losses they cause, but for the water you should have been drinking instead. Airline food is low on water content and low in fibre: consider bringing your own picnic, including, where regulations permit, items such as fresh fruit.

It is very clear that some travellers are at increased risk, and need to take special precautions. The House of Lords report (November 2000) and new guidelines from the UK Department of Health (November 2001), have identified some of these (see Box).

Emergencies in the air

Accidents (see also pp. 290–304)

When in your seat, it is always advisable to keep the lap strap loosely fastened: this not only prevents injury should the aircraft suddenly encounter turbulence, but also prevents any likelihood of being sucked out of the aircraft should it decompress rapidly.

Airborne emergencies are very rare, but do occur occasionally. So pay attention to safety briefings given by cabin staff before take-off, and take careful note of the description of the emergency oxygen system (some masks deliver oxygen only after they have been firmly pulled on to the face), the location of emergency exits, and to any other advice offered. You should also be aware of the danger of fires on board caused by illegal smoking in the lavatories.

Travellers at increased risk of DVT

Moderately increased risk

Women on the Pill or hormone replacement therapy
Smokers
Overweight, very tall, or very short
Over 40 years old
Varicose veins, or previous or current leg swelling from any cause
Pregnancy or recent childbirth
History of cancer or vascular disease

- Compression stockings and, perhaps (on medical advice), a low-dose aspirin tablet to help counteract any tendency to clot should be considered

Higher Risk

Previous DVT
Inherited clotting tendency
Recent major surgery or surgery involving hips or knees
Stroke and cardiovascular disease
Current malignant disease or chemotherapy
Paralysed lower limb(s)

- Compression stockings and, perhaps (on medical advice), an anti-coagulant injection (low molecular weight heparin) should be considered.

Further information: **www.doh.gov.uk/dvt** and Appendix 8.

In the unfortunate event of an in-flight emergency, passengers can do little more than follow instructions carefully, stay calm, and help one another. Should a crash landing be announced, pay particular attention to crash posture since survival will depend upon being fully conscious and mobile immediately after landing; most crash landings are survivable, but deaths have commonly occurred because of toxic fumes generated by post-crash fires. Again, in the aftermath of several 'survivable' tragedies of this nature, the regulating bodies have acted to insist upon the use of fire-blocking and less toxic materials for cabin furnishings, and upon the assessment of other aids to survival and escape (e.g. fire extinguishers, exit route lighting, smokehoods, etc). Speedy and panic-free evacuation is of the greatest importance, however. Once at the

Most accidents are survivable

In a study of 568 commercial aircraft accidents between 1983 and 2000, 96 per cent of those on board survived. In 26 serious accidents, 56 per cent survived.

foot of the escape slide, move quickly out of the way of following passengers in order to avoid the risk of a collision injury.

For extra safety on an airline flight:

* Buy tickets for children under two and place them in child-restraint seats. Do not carry an infant on your lap throughout a flight to avoid the cost of a ticket.
* Choose an aisle seat for faster evacuation in an emergency; there is no evidence that one section of the aircraft is safer than any other.
* Memorize the number of rows between your seat and the nearest emergency exit door, as well as an alternate exit (remember that your closest exit may be behind you).
* Read the emergency card in the seat pocket, and learn how to open the emergency exit doors — but don't be tempted to practise, even on the ground.
* In an emergency evacuation, leave all possessions and move quickly toward the exit, keeping your head as low as possible if the cabin fills with smoke or toxic fumes. Don't get down on your hands and knees — you might be trampled.
* Keep your seat-belt buckled during the flight: even in fine weather, the plane could hit clear-air turbulence and you could be thrown about the cabin.

Flying on private aircraft

Between 1995 and 1999, an average of 652 people died each year in accidents involving private aircraft, accounting for 85 per cent of all aviation deaths in the USA. An investigation into the causes found significant differences in accident rates among male and female pilots (female pilots were safer), and also between younger and older pilots (older pilots were safer). Poor decision-making and risk-taking, such as flying under adverse conditions or with faulty equipment, were more likely to be a problem with male pilots, while female pilots were more likely to mishandle the controls or stall during take-off or landing.

Illness during a flight

The available statistics are difficult to interpret, but the 'attack rate' for illness in passengers during a flight is of the *order* of 1 in 13 000, increasing to 1 in 350 for passengers who have a previously notified disability. This means around one medical emergency in every four or five flights.

The most common problems are associated with the central nervous system, including stress and anxiety, the gastrointestinal system, the cardiovascular system, and the respiratory system. Of these, the cardiovascular disorders are the most serious and include angina, heart attacks, and heart failure.

The chances of a doctor being on board any flight have been variously estimated at 40 per cent on domestic routes to 90 per cent on international flights. The all-important decision, after any necessary or possible first-aid has been administered, is whether or not to divert the aircraft if help can possibly be obtained sooner than at the intended destination — an expensive and inconvenient course to take. The decision is ultimately that of the aircraft captain, but he or she will naturally take advice from any available professional source. And increasingly, such advice is given via *telemedicine*: the pilot and/or an available on-board doctor can discuss the case with medical experts on the ground (even to the extent of transmitting an electrocardiogram and other medical data for analysis and subsequent treatment options).

Decompression sickness following scuba diving

An unusual form of in-flight medical emergency, normally only a risk to subaqua (scuba) divers, is decompression sickness (often known as the 'bends'), which is caused by the release of nitrogen bubbles in body tissues as pressure is reduced. Decompression sickness does not occur in healthy individuals at altitudes below 18 000 feet and is very rare below 25 000 feet. Passengers within a pressurized aircraft are not, therefore, at risk *unless* they have been subaqua diving shortly before undertaking a journey by air.

Diving allows compression of more nitrogen than normal into the body tissues, some but not all of which will evolve on return to the surface; the rest may evolve during ascent in an aircraft. Symptoms and signs include joint pains, itching, and rashes (see also p. 379).

Subaqua enthusiasts should avoid any dive requiring a decompression 'stop' in the 24 hours preceding their flight and should not dive at all during the two to three hours preceding their flight. Most divers will be or should be aware of these precautions, and what constitutes a dive requiring 'stops', but if in any doubt, a foolproof rule is to avoid diving to a depth greater than 9 m (30 feet) in the 24 hours before flight.

The risk of decompression sickness affecting passengers after a failure of cabin pressurization is also remote, since the aircraft will rapidly be flown to a safe altitude.

Aircraft medical kits

Although not of obvious importance to the healthy traveller, it is comforting to know that all airlines are now required to maintain an on-board medical kit or kits for use by trained persons (cabin staff who have undergone paramedical-type instruction or serendipitously available medically-qualified passengers). Airlines have long had some form of first-aid material available, and many have for some time provisioned their aircraft with kits for use solely by (medically qualified) doctors. But new regulations are being introduced to require kits of a minimum standard and content to be provided; and many airlines have already equipped long-haul aircraft with automatic external defibrillators (AEDs).

Jet lag

Modern air travel can cause disruption or desynchronization of many physiological and psychological rhythms. These circadian rhythms are governed or entrained in part by environmental cues — clock hour, temperature, day and night. Rapid passage across several time zones outstrips the ability of environmental factors to readjust these rhythms: desynchronization occurs and 'jet lag' develops.

Jet lag is discussed in detail in the next chapter. Simple methods to minimize its effects include sleeping on the aircraft, with or without the effect of short-acting sleeping medication (but remember the interaction with alcohol) (see also p. 270), avoiding heavy meals and excessive alcohol, avoiding important commitments for at

Air rage

There is increasing concern in the airline industry about the problem of disruptive passenger behaviour, and recent media reports suggest that incidents are becoming more frequent and more violent. Our own research confirms increasing concern among commercial airlines and a move towards formulating policies and procedures for dealing with incidents.

The earliest recorded incident of passenger disruption on a commercial flight occurred in 1947, on a flight from Havana to Miami. Two crew members who intervened were also injured, as was a flight deck crew member who was bitten by the passenger; he was able to walk away from any charges because the matter of jurisdiction on board aircraft flying international routes had not yet been established.

Between 1994 and 1995, American Airlines reported a 200 per cent increase in passenger interference with flight attendants' duties, and there were 450 similar incidents on board United Airlines flights during 1997. One of the more spectacular incidents occurred on a British Airways flight from London to Nairobi in December 2000, when a disruptive passenger gained access to the flight deck; loss of the aircraft was only narrowly avoided. A number of incidents have resulted in death of passengers or crew.

Tempers can also run high on the ground. One recent fracas in Newark left a Continental Airlines employee with a broken neck.

Results of our own survey of the **causes of 'air rage'** are shown in the chart below, based on responses from the airlines. More than a third of airline staff have no training in dealing with air rage; in 10 per cent of airlines, there was no requirement to report incidents, and in 40 per cent only a verbal report was necessary. A third of airlines had no policy on whether or not crew were permitted to leave the flight deck to deal with incidents.

'Air rage' is not just a passenger problem: airlines need to train their staff to manage difficult or violent passengers; to give clearer passenger briefings about air rage and the airline's policy on disruptive behaviour, at the start of the flight; and to do more to prevent such situations arising in the first place.

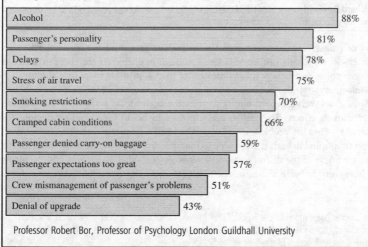

Alcohol	88%
Passenger's personality	81%
Delays	78%
Stress of air travel	75%
Smoking restrictions	70%
Cramped cabin conditions	66%
Passenger denied carry-on baggage	59%
Passenger expectations too great	57%
Crew mismanagement of passenger's problems	51%
Denial of upgrade	43%

Professor Robert Bor, Professor of Psychology London Guildhall University least 24 hours after arrival, and generally being aware of the inevitable reduction in performance for a few days. Sensible behaviour along these lines will help make your trip a successful one.

The passenger milieu

Finally, as will be clear from the above, there is today an increasing 'official' awareness of passenger health issues which surround what the International Labour Office has defined as the goal of the civil aviation industry: 'the safe passage of an aircraft through a physiologically and physically hostile environment'. More and more attention is now being paid to the safety, health, and comfort (that is, to the milieu) of those who travel by air. But much remains to be done.

Other topical areas addressed by many national and international regulating and advisory bodies include: the quality of cabin air, the risk of transmission of disease, exposure to cosmic radiation (see p. 489) and the handling of in-flight medical emergencies. The last has been considered above and is amenable to timely advancement but, while both are believed to present little risk to the general travelling population, the possible dangers of poor cabin air and of the spread of disease are universally agreed to require urgent study.

Jet lag

Jet lag is a difficult problem for large numbers of air travellers. Understanding the factors that control the human 'body clock' is the key to helping travellers develop a personal strategy for overcoming or reducing its effects.

Dr Richard Dawood runs a busy travel clinic in Central London. A large part of his work is devoted to looking after frequent fliers and business travellers.

Years of painstaking research* into the behaviour and mechanisms of the human 'body clock' are paying off: we now know enough to enable air travellers to adapt to new time zones as much as three times faster than is possible by nature alone.

While many strategies can help alleviate some symptoms of jet lag, there are only two known factors with a proven ability to reset the body clock, addressing the problem rather than its effects. The factors are exposure to bright light, and small doses of melatonin — but the problem is to know when and how to use them effectively. With correct timing and dosage, it is possible to manipulate and adjust the body clock, and to eliminate much of the discomfort, inconvenience and other symptoms and problems that have come to be an almost inseparable part of the experience of modern air travel.

---

* This chapter owes much to the work of Dr Al Lewy, Director of the Sleep and Mood Disorders Laboratory at Oregon Health Sciences University, Portland, Oregon, who has conducted extensive research into the function of the human 'body clock'.

The body clock: taking control

Almost every living creature exhibits circadian rhythms. In humans, every natural process within the body shows some variation in pattern between night and day. The most obvious patterns are sleep and wakefulness, but an internal body clock (located in a portion of the brain known as the suprachiasmatic nuclei) also controls alertness, hunger, digestion, bowel habits, urine production, body temperature, secretion of hormones, and even blood pressure.

These rhythms differ in their ability to be altered by external factors (such as light and darkness, social cues like mealtimes, and the ambient temperature and apparent time of day — known as *zeitgebers*). Rapid air travel across several time zones outstrips the ability of the body to re-synchronize these rhythms. The resulting physiological desynchronization causes symptoms such as malaise, gastrointestinal disturbance, loss of appetite, tiredness during the day, disorientation, memory impairment, and reduced mental performance, that every air traveller recognizes only too readily as 'jet lag'.

In turn, these external factors differ in their ability to influence the body clock and draw it back into line — some are much more powerful than others. Experiments confirm that the two most powerful factors are exposure to light, and melatonin.

Light

Exposure to light during the mid-portion of the day, not surprisingly, has no effect on the body clock. Experiments show that light exposure earlier in the day will shorten (i.e. bring forward or advance) the normal circadian cycle, whereas light exposure occurring later in the day has the effect of lengthening (delaying) it. By experimenting with the timing and duration of the light exposure, it is also possible to determine the times when light exposure reaches its maximum 're-setting' effect. The effect in fact turns out to be greatest during the night: during the first half of the night, light causes a delay; during the second half, light causes an advance. The same experiments show that prolonged exposure is not necessary — relatively short pulses of bright light (as short as 30 minutes) are all that are needed to achieve the same effect.

Melatonin

Melatonin is the so-called 'hormone of darkness' — a naturally occurring substance secreted in the brain by the pineal gland during the hours of night. The pineal gland was once believed to be a functionless evolutionary remnant, like the appendix; but in a primitive creature called the lamprey, the pineal is actually a third eye, and is directly responsive to light. In the human body, melatonin levels in the blood rise as darkness descends, reaching a peak around 4.00 a.m., and falling again as morning approaches.

Melatonin is known to be a major regulator of circadian rhythms, and 20 years ago, experiments demonstrated that bright light suppresses human melatonin production. Experiments with the timing of a dose of synthetic melatonin show a pattern that is an exact mirror image of the re-setting power of light. A dose of melatonin taken during the night has little effect on the body clock. By experimenting with bringing the dose forward, or delaying it, it is possible to advance or delay the circadian cycle, and to calculate the

To achieve phase advances:

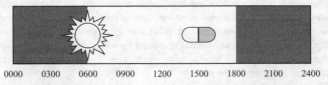

To achieve phase delays:

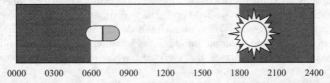

Fig. 7.2 Phase-shifting effects of light and melatonin. In order to cause a phase advance light should be scheduled in the morning and melatonin administered in the afternoon. In order to cause a phase delay, light should be scheduled in the evening and melatonin should be administered in the morning. By permission of Dr. A. Lewy

most effective timing. The effect is greatest during the day (Fig. 7.2). Experiments with dosage show that, with correct timing, only tiny doses of melatonin are needed to achieve a powerful effect.

Melatonin is not licensed or readily available in the UK, though it is sold in many countries as a 'nutritional supplement' (see Box on p. 269). Very little is known of its effects in children or pregnant woman, in whom it should therefore not be used.

Overcoming jet lag

Most long-haul travellers who travel across time zones can expect to adjust naturally to their new 'local time' at a rate of approximately one hour per day. For example, a traveller flying between Portland, Oregon, and Amsterdam (a difference of nine time zones), would probably take around nine days to adjust fully, and another nine days to adjust back to home time at the end of the trip. For most people, such a trip therefore represents an 18-day commitment to jet lag.

Two additional factors can make the situation slightly better than this, or substantially worse. The first is that, left to their own resources, our bodies have a natural tendency towards operating on a cycle that is 25 hours long, not 24 hours. (If you are a 'late-night' person rather than an 'early-morning' person, your natural cycle may be even longer.) This means that it is generally much easier to adapt to a longer day (as in westward travel) than to a shorter one (as in eastward travel). The second is that inappropriately timed light exposure following arrival can reset the body clock in the wrong direction, making jet lag considerably worse.

Travellers who use **either** correctly timed light exposure **or** correctly timed low-dose melatonin can generally adjust to their new local time at a rate of approximately two hours per day — twice as fast as by nature alone. By combining both methods, a rate of three hours per day can be accomplished.

Instructions for overcoming jet lag can be followed to different levels of complexity.

Using melatonin

The 'simple' solution:

If you are eastbound
- Before you travel east, begin by taking 0.5 mg of melatonin at 2.00 p.m. (this advances your 'phase'). Ideally, do this the day before and on the day of travel.
- Following arrival at your destination, depending on the number of time zones you have crossed, take melatonin at the local equivalent of the same time. For example, for a trip from Portland to New York (a time difference of 3 hours), you should take your dose of melatonin at 5.00 p.m. (equivalent to 2.00 p.m. in Portland). Do this each day until you have adjusted.

If you are westbound
- Before you travel west, begin by taking 0.5 mg of melatonin when you wake up (this delays your 'phase'). Do this the day before and on the day of travel.
- For westbound travel — up to a time difference of three hours — continue taking the melatonin on awakening. For a time difference any greater than this, take the dose of melatonin at bedtime (to avoid having to wake up to take it). If you wake up during the night, take a further dose of 0.5 mg. Continue until you have adjusted.

The more complex solution
As you begin to adjust to your new time zone, the optimal timing for your dose of melatonin will change. If you are sufficiently motivated, it is possible to 'fine tune' your melatonin dosage by advancing or delaying its timing by one to two hours each day, until you again reach the timing you started with.

Tip: getting the dosage right
It may be worth trying a dose of 0.5 mg of melatonin at 2.00 p.m., at a time when you are not travelling; after 2 or 3 days you should find that you begin to wake up earlier. If you don't see this effect, the brand you are using is not giving you the full 0.5 mg, and you may need to adjust the dosage accordingly.

Using light exposure

For a time difference of six hours or less:

If you are eastbound
At your destination, you need light in the morning, as soon as you wake up; 30 minutes of bright light is sufficient. Avoid light later in the day.

If you are westbound
At your destination, you need light at the end of the day. Avoid light earlier than this.

For a time difference of more than six hours:

- Get light exposure during the middle of the day, regardless of your direction of travel.
- Avoid light in the morning, if you have travelled east, or at the end of the day, if you have travelled west.
- One final tip: if your travel is eastward by 10, 11, or 12 time zones, treat this as westbound travel, because it is easier to delay your cycle than to bring it forward.

An alternative, simpler approach

If you can't cope with following complex instructions, one simple option is just to take a dose of melatonin at bedtime following arrival at your destination. This is generally suitable for journeys across more than three or four time zones, and also takes advantage of the fact that melatonin has a mildly soporific effect. This is by far the most widely followed regime for taking melatonin. A recent survey of subscribers to the American travel magazine, *Condé Nast Traveler* (melatonin is readily available in the USA) showed that approximately 30 per cent of its readers who had tried taking melatonin found this helpful.

Other ways to beat jet lag

A recent internet search revealed over 66 000 web pages on jet lag, offering advice from the tediously conventional to the utterly spurious. Remedies proposed include:
- Aromatherapy
- Homeopathy
- Diet
- Stimulation of energy meridians
- Kinesiotherapy
- Magnetic therapy/use of rare earth magnets
- Pendants with mysterious properties
- Pressure-point massage.

Other popular remedies include massage, exercise, and a good hot bath. While some of the above may go part way to helping the disorientated traveller feel better, less

Is melatonin safe?

Melatonin is not currently licensed in the UK or in the USA (though it is widely and cheaply available as a nutritional supplement in the USA and other countries). Among many reasons for this are that melatonin is easy to produce, already in the public domain, and cannot be patented. There is therefore no commercial incentive for any pharmaceutical company to take melatonin through the costly and complex process of licensure. (However, several drug companies are interested in developing melatonin 'analogues' — drugs that behave in a similar manner to melatonin — that could be exploited commercially.)

In the USA, 'nutritional supplements' and vitamins are not subject to the same degree of control as pharmaceutical products, and this is a potential source of concern over safety and purity. During the late 1980s, contamination of L-Tryptophan (also classed as a nutritional supplement) in the USA caused many cases of illness, and heightened awareness of the possible dangers of non-regulation.

The published research on the benefits of melatonin for jet lag is extremely convincing. However, a variety of exaggerated and ridiculous claims have been made relating to its role as a seeming panacea, for conditions ranging from impotence to senility; these have tended to tarnish its image.

According to estimates by the Mayo Clinic, more than 20 million Americans now regularly take melatonin supplements, spending $200–$350 million every year. If there was a genuine health hazard arising from its use, this might be expected to have become apparent by now.

The dose of melatonin advocated in this chapter for occasional short-term use in alleviation of jet lag is 0.5 mg — one tenth of the dose typically advised for melatonin's other 'effects'.

stressed and more relaxed, melatonin and light are the only two methods of speeding adaptation to a new time zone that have attained any level of scientific proof.

Jet lag is bad for your health

Shift work has many similarities with jet lag, and is easier to study objectively. Shift work is known to have a definite link with coronary heart disease, as well as more predictable problems such as reduced alertness and an increased risk of accidents (fatigue resulting from shift work was the likely cause of the Chernobyl disaster).

Studies in volunteers show that a meal taken at an inappropriate time, during the middle of the night, has a completely different effect on the metabolism compared with an identical meal taken at an appropriate time during the day.

Effects include raised blood levels of fats and sugars — which are also known to be associated with heart disease. These effects disappear following readjustment to the new time zone, suggesting that there may be significant health benefits from re-synchronizing the body clock as soon as possible, particularly for frequent flyers, as well as from avoiding heavy meals at inappropriate times.

A study of breast cancer in flight attendants from California shows a 30 per cent increased risk (they also had double the risk of skin cancer), whilst another in Finland shows an 80 per cent increase. The hormonal effects of time zone changes are an important possible factor, though in-flight radiation exposure and lifestyle factors may also be significant.

Sleeping medication

Sleeping medication **does not** speed up adaptation to a new time zone, but several studies suggest that taking medication results in better next-day performance, compared with sleep of questionable quality using no medication. Medication can be extremely useful in reducing fatigue arising from delayed or interrupted sleep during the nights after travel across time zones, and possibly in ensuring a good night's sleep during a flight that is long enough (though deep sleep in an awkward position may add to the risk of deep vein thrombosis — see pp. 257–260).

Most sleeping tablets are intended to provide eight hours' sleep, so it is unwise to take medication for flights that are much shorter than this. Sleeping medication should generally not be used during a flight unless you are able to stretch out in a horizontal position; it may otherwise contribute to immobility and restriction of the circulation.

Following eastbound travel, most people have difficulty falling asleep; a short-acting drug, such as zaleplon (Sonata), is most suitable — it works quickly and is rapidly eliminated from the body. For westbound travel, where the tendency is toward early waking, some longer-lasting medication (such as temazepam) is more appropriate. Such medication requires a prescription and should of course be discussed carefully with your doctor.

Summary of advice for travellers

- Appropriately timed exposure to bright light can help speed adjustment to a new time zone.
- Appropriately timed small doses of melatonin can also help, but remember that melatonin is unlicensed, not widely available, and little is known of its long-term use.
- Adjust your itinerary to minimize sleep loss and fatigue.
- Adjust night-time flights when possible and, if you can't, build a rest period into your schedule.
- Recognize that your performance may be reduced through jet lag, and avoid important business activities for at least the first 24 hours following arrival.
- Travel in the highest class that you can afford.
- Avoid eating inappropriately timed large meals or any other activity inappropriate to your daily routine.
- Consider using sleeping medication to reduce sleeplessness during the adjustment at your destination.
- For short trips, stay on home time.

Motion sickness

Motion sickness is one of the commonest and most familiar problems relating to travel itself, and it is helpful for sufferers to understand the underlying mechanisms and treatment.

Dr Alan Benson was a Consultant at the RAF School of Aviation Medicine, Farnborough, and has a special interest in vestibular and allied problems in conventional and space flight.
Dr Rollin Stott is a Principal Medical Officer (Research) at the Centre for Human Sciences, QinetiQ, Farnborough and has been involved in research on motion sickness for many years.

About half the adult population admit to having felt travel sick at some time in their lives. Most commonly this will have been car and coach sickness or sea sickness in stormy conditions aboard a passenger ferry. Air sickness on passenger aircraft is nowadays relatively infrequent as cruising altitudes tend to remain well above the weather, but it can still occur in turbulent weather conditions during take-off and landing. Less familiar forms of travel sickness are associated with riding on camels and elephants (though not horses), and among that highly select group, the space travellers, more than half suffer the effects of space sickness. Though hardly a form of travel, many individuals have experienced nausea and perhaps vomiting following fairground rides, and some may also have found that watching implied motion on a wide-view cinema screen, or in a flight simulator, can also provoke nausea. While for some, travel sickness is a minor but dispiriting experience, for more susceptible individuals it has the potential to ruin a holiday or discourage them from continuing with activities such as gliding or sailing.

Despite the diversity of possible causal situations and environments, the stimuli that result in symptoms have essential characteristics in common — all provoke what is termed sensory conflict, either between the eyes and the balance organ of the inner ear or between the functional components within the balance organ itself. Pedestrian man has the expectation that his movements will be against a background of a predominantly fixed visual world, plus a force of gravity which remains fixed in direction and intensity. Motion sickness tends to occur when the combined signals from the body's sensors of motion — the eyes and inner ear — fail to reflect these expectations.

While there is now a good understanding of the principles that relate the motion environment to the likelihood of motion sickness, it remains unclear what underlies the wide differences in susceptibility between individuals. However, motion sickness must be regarded as a normal response. Virtually everybody can be made motion sick given a sufficiently provocative environment, and only those rare individuals who have lost all function in the balance organs of the inner ear are totally immune.

A further feature of motion sickness is that, with repeated exposure to a stimulus that initially provokes nausea, an individual will gradually adapt and become less susceptible to its effects. This state of adaptation tends to be specific to the type of motion involved and is temporary, lasting for several days or perhaps weeks after the last experience of the provocative stimulus. There is probably also a short-term adaptation that occurs, for example, during the course of a rough sea crossing lasting only a few hours. The implication of this is that *preventive measures are best undertaken early in the voyage* and, all being well, can later be relaxed.

Signs and symptoms

The development of motion sickness follows a sequence, the time scale of which is determined by the intensity of the stimulus and the susceptibility of the individual. It is worth being aware of the early symptoms, since at this stage preventive measures may still be effective. In circumstances where the onset of motion sickness is gradual, the first indication may be an increasing lethargy often accompanied by a tendency to repeated yawning. Stomach awareness is usually the next symptom, and this progresses to nausea of increasing severity. The face becomes pale and the individual begins to sweat and to feel the need for cool air. There may also be a feeling of light-headedness, dizziness, or headache, and an increasing sense of depression and apathy may have significant consequences if, as a result, individuals fail to carry out some essential task.

With continued provocative motion, well-being can deteriorate quite rapidly — the so-called 'avalanche phenomenon'. Vomiting is then generally not long delayed, though some individuals can remain severely nauseated for long periods without vomiting. Once vomiting has occurred there is often an improvement in well-being for a time, before the cycle of increasing nausea and vomiting begins again. The increasing nausea sometimes provokes hyperventilation (overbreathing) and this can contribute to the light-headedness; it sometimes leads to numbness and tingling sensations in the hands and feet and around the mouth.

With continued exposure to provocative motion, as for example when aboard ship in a storm, most individuals experience a progressive reduction in the severity of symptoms as they adapt to the motion environment. After two to three days most have obtained their 'sea legs' and are relatively symptom-free, although a minority of the population (estimated at about 5 per cent) are 'non-adapters' and continue to have problems as long as the rough weather persists.

Adaptation to the motion of a ship may carry a penalty on return to dry land, for the sensory conflict between actual and expected motion stimuli can engender a recurrence of symptoms — the so called 'mal de débarquement' phenomenon (see also p. 284). Although readaptation to the familiar, stable environment of dry land is usually rapid and sickness is rarely severe, transient illusory sensations of motion may persist for a day or more.

Incidence

The incidence of sickness in a particular environment is influenced by several factors. These are the physical characteristics of the stimulus (frequency, intensity, duration, and direction), the natural susceptibility of the individual, the nature of the task performed, and environmental factors such as the ability to view a stable visual world.

The incidence of air sickness ranges from a fraction of 1 per cent in large civil passenger aircraft, which usually fly above the worst turbulence, to almost all in the crew of aircraft that deliberately fly into bad weather to collect meteorological data.

Likewise, the incidence of sea sickness varies widely. An extensive questionnaire study of sickness on various ferries operating around the British Isles in different sea states found overall that 7 per cent of passengers had vomited and 21 per cent had experienced less severe symptoms; the incidence of sickness on any one journey ranged from 0 per cent to 40 per cent, dependent on the sea state. In rough seas, all the occupants of a life raft or an enclosed survival craft may be sea sick.

Susceptibility appears to be a relatively stable and enduring individual characteristic; those who are sensitive to one type of motion are more likely to succumb when exposed to another. Motion sickness is rare below the age of 2 years, but susceptibility increases rapidly to reach a peak between the ages of 3 and 12 years. Over the next decade there is a progressive increase in tolerance that continues, albeit more slowly, with increasing age. This reduction in susceptibility with age has been recorded for both sea sickness and air sickness, though the elderly are not immune. About a fifth of those suffering from sea sickness on a British Channel Island ferry were aged 60 years or more.

Females are more susceptible to motion sickness than males of the same age, and a higher incidence of vomiting and malaise is reported by female passengers on ferries. The difference in susceptibility between men and women is in the ratio of about 1 to 1.7. The reason for this, which applies both to children and to adults, is not clear. It may be that females are more ready to admit to having symptoms. Hormonal factors may also play a part as susceptibility is highest during menstruation and is increased in pregnancy.

Prevention
Behavioural aspects

Avoiding provocative motion is the only certain way of preventing motion sickness, the possible, but not practicable, exception being the bilateral destruction of the vestibular apparatus of the inner ear. In the modern world, however, few are prepared to forego travel by car, plane, or boat, or to tolerate the restriction of their mobility imposed by the 'go sit under a tree' approach to prevention. Nevertheless, there are a number of things an individual can do that may prevent the development of symptoms.

The passenger aboard ship should seek out a position in the vessel where the motion is least, usually near the middle of the ship, and on a low deck if there is much roll motion. The intensity of motion can also be influenced by the way a vehicle is controlled. The driver of a car should take bends gently and avoid frequent and powerful braking and acceleration; the captain of a boat may be able, by regulating its speed and heading, to provide a more comfortable passage. Likewise, the pilot of an aircraft can attempt to avoid flying through turbulent air and making high-rate turns that may incommode his passengers.

There is evidence that head and body movements potentiate susceptibility to motion sickness. Restriction of head movement by pressing the head firmly against the seat or other available support is therefore likely to be beneficial; adopting a recumbent position can also reduce head movements. It is a common observation that those suffering from sea sickness have less malaise when made to lie down with their eyes closed.

Procedures to reduce visual/vestibular sensory conflict can also be helpful. When below deck in a boat or in the enclosed cabin of an aircraft, it is better to close the eyes than to keep them open. On the other hand, when able to see out, one should fixate on the horizon or some other stable external visual reference. Passengers in a car should, like the driver, look at the road ahead. Susceptible coach passengers should likewise choose a seat with a good forward view. For children confined to the back seat of a car the use of a booster cushion may improve their view of the road ahead, and on winding roads they could be usefully encouraged to lean into the corners as a means of getting them to anticipate the motion of the vehicle. Reading in a car is well known to precipitate motion sickness, so tasks involving visual search and scanning within the vehicle should be avoided.

The person in control of a car, boat, or plane is less likely to suffer from motion sickness than other passengers, presumably because of a greater ability to anticipate the motion and to make appropriate postural adjustments so that sensory conflict is reduced. A further benefit of being in control may derive from the mental distraction that it provides. There is experimental and anecdotal evidence that symptoms are reduced by mental activity that directs the subject's attention away from features of the provocative motion and introspection about lack of well-being.

Dietary factors

Dietary factors do not play an important part in the prevention of motion sickness. The avoidance of food before a rough sea crossing makes little difference to the likelihood of sea sickness, and many express the preference to have something in the stomach to vomit rather than suffer unproductive retching. Motion sickness sufferers tend, however, to avoid alcohol before and during a voyage, and are probably correct in assuming that alcohol would increase their susceptibility, though there is surprisingly little experimental evidence on this topic. Root ginger, a traditional oriental remedy for sickness, has been shown in sea trials to reduce the incidence of vomiting, but to have little effect on the degree of nausea.

Adaptation

In addition to the behavioural measures outlined above, a further important factor in reducing susceptibility is adaptation to the provocative motion. The phenomenon is familiar to many mariners in whom symptoms of sea sickness commonly abate during the first few days at sea. Likewise, astronauts and cosmonauts who develop space sickness on initial exposure to weightlessness are usually free of symptoms by the third or fourth day in space. Adaptation is 'nature's own cure' and in many respects is the ideal prophylaxis, although the specificity of adaptation can be responsible for the return of symptoms on transfer from one motion environment to another.

Therapeutic programmes that build up an individual's level of protective adaptation by graded exposure to progressively more intense provocative stimuli, have proved to be very successful in controlling air sickness in student pilots and other flying personnel. The procedure is time consuming (typically three to four weeks of twice daily, ground-based exercises and 10–15 hours in the air) and costly. There is a

possibility, however, that a self-administered, ground-based desensitization programme could be of benefit to the weekend sailor or the light aircraft or glider pilot,
whose frequency of exposure to provocative motion is often insufficient to promote an
adequate degree of adaptation.

Acupressure

Claims have been made that pressure applied to a point above the wrist, known to
acupuncturists as the P6 or Nei-Kuan point, is an effective prophylactic against
motion sickness. Unfortunately, these claims have not been substantiated in
controlled trials in which pressure to the P6 point was applied by elasticated bands,
sold as 'Sea bands' or 'Acubands'. Nevertheless, the placebo effect of any form of
treatment, prescribed with conviction, can be beneficial to some individuals. The same
argument can be applied to the conductive strips fitted to the rear of cars.

Preventive drugs

Oral medication

Over the years, many medicinal remedies have been proposed for the prevention of
motion sickness, but relatively few are effective and none affords complete protection
to all individuals in severe environments. Nevertheless, a number of drugs have been
shown to increase tolerance to provocative motion, and allay the development of the
motion sickness syndrome, especially if used in conjunction with behavioural
measures and not instead of them. It should be noted, however, that a number of the

Table 7.2 Anti-motion-sickness drugs

Drug	Route	Adult dose	Time to take effect	Duration of action (hr)
Hyoscine				
— hydrochloride (Joy-rides, Kwells)	Oral	0.3–0.6 mg	30 min	4
(Scopoderm)	Patch	One	6–8 hr	72
	Injection	0.2 mg	15 min	4
Cinnarizine				
— hydrochloride (Stugeron)	Oral	15–30 mg	4 hr	8
Promethazine				
— theoclate (Avomine)	Oral	25 mg	2 hr	24
— hydrochloride (Phenergan)	Oral	25 mg	2 hr	18
	Injection	50 mg	15 min	18
Dimenhydrinate (Dramamine)	Oral	50–100 mg	2 hr	8
Cyclizine				
— hydrochloride (Valoid)	Oral	50 mg	2 hr	12
Meclozine				
— hydrochloride (Sea-legs)	Oral	12.5–25mg	2hr	8

drugs that are used to treat nausea and vomiting from other causes are either not effective or are of doubtful value in motion sickness prophylaxis; these include metoclopromide, prochlorperazine, domperidone, and ondansetron. Table 7.2 lists currently used drugs, with brand name, dosage, time of onset, and duration of action.

The choice of drug to be used depends in part upon the expected duration of exposure and the susceptibility of the individual. In practice, if one drug is not effective or not well tolerated then another drug or combination of drugs should be tried. Where the objective is to provide short-term protection, oral hyoscine (scopolamine USP) (0.3–0.6 mg) is the drug of choice. This acts within about 30 minutes and provides protection for about four hours. Side effects from oral hyoscine are frequent, in particular, sedation and dry mouth. Blurring of vision, and occasionally hallucinations, can occur with repeated administration of the drug. Hyoscine is not recommended for children under the age of 14 years or the elderly, especially those with glaucoma or prostate gland problems.

Protection over a longer period is provided by drugs like cinnarizine, promethazine, dimenhydrinate, and cyclizine, which have anti-histaminic properties. As may be seen from Table 7.2, most of these drugs are not effective until about two hours after ingestion, the exception being cinnarizine which should be taken at least four hours before exposure to provocative motion. The duration of action ranges from about eight hours for dimenhydrinate to about 24 hours for promethazine. None of the drugs is without side-effects; sedation is common with promethazine and dimenhydrinate, but somewhat less so with cinnarizine and cyclizine, although the latter drug, in common with hyoscine, can give rise to hallucinations in excessive or repeated dosage. The drug ephedrine has been shown to have a small beneficial effect in motion sickness when used alone. However, its value is in its combination either with hyoscine or the anti-histamine group of drugs when its alerting properties counteract the sedative side-effects of these drugs.

Skin patches

An acceptable alternative to the repeated oral administration of drugs for extended prophylaxis, such as during a long sea voyage in rough weather, is the transdermal delivery of hyoscine by means of a skin patch (Scopoderm TTS). This delivers a loading dose of 200 micrograms of hyoscine and controlled release at 20 micrograms per hour for up to 72 hours after the patch is applied behind the ear. Therapeutic blood levels are not reached until some six hours after application of the patch, so it is necessary to anticipate the requirement for prophylaxis or to take 0.3–0.6 mg hyoscine orally at the time the patch is applied if exposure to provocative motion is more imminent.

Although the characteristic side-effects of oral hyoscine are less when the drug is administered transdermally, they are not necessarily absent. In addition to dry mouth and drowsiness there may be impairment of vision (difficulty focusing) particularly in long-sighted individuals, and this effect tends to increase with the length of time the patch is in place. Side effects may persist for several hours after removal of the patch because a fraction of the drug binds to the skin under the patch. As noted earlier, hyoscine is unsuitable for prophylaxis in young children or the elderly, and this constraint is even more relevant when the drug is administered transdermally. Hallucinations, extreme agitation, and psychotic reactions have been reported in children who have received the drug by means of a dermal patch.

Because of the central action of all effective anti-motion-sickness drugs, irrespective of the route of administration, it is inadvisable to drink alcohol, drive a car, or operate dangerous machinery when under the influence of the drug. Under no circumstances should the sole pilot of an aircraft take any of the drugs detailed above.

Treatment once vomiting has started

Once vomiting induced by motion is established, treatment by orally administered drugs is unlikely to be effective because of delayed gastric emptying or elimination on vomiting. If the individual has no duties to perform, as for example a passenger aboard ship, an intramuscular injection of 25–50 mg promethazine hydrochloride is the best treatment. However, if the degree of sedation produced by promethazine is unacceptable, effective blood levels of hyoscine can be achieved by absorption directly through the mucous membrane of the mouth, by simply allowing tablets to dissolve in the mouth. At the same time, one or two transdermal hyoscine patches can be applied if exposure to the provocative motion is likely to be prolonged. Hyoscine may also be given by intramuscular injection, but in small doses (0.2 mg), since it is about six times more effective when administered by this route than when taken orally.

Summary of advice for travellers

- If you suffer from motion sickness, always carry a suitable remedy at times when you will be vulnerable, and start using it *before* symptoms appear.
- Don't drive when taking a remedy that causes drowsiness.

Cruise ship medicine

The cruise industry has more than doubled in size over the past decade. Its growth has been accompanied by substantial improvements in the medical facilities that the major cruise lines now offer, and cruise ship medicine is now a medical specialty in its own right.

Dr Alastair Smith trained as a surgeon and as a GP, and has worked as a ship's doctor and at an airport medical practice. He was Vice-President and Medical Director of P&O and Princess Cruises for eight years, before setting up his own independent consultancy to the cruising and maritime industry.

On the 1st June 1867, 65 passengers boarded the *Quaker City* for an extraordinary voyage — a five and a half month cruise through history. They would visit ancient cities and distant lands from the comfort of a first class steamer. They would tour Europe and the Holy Land in safety and in good health.

> BROOKLYN, February 1st, 1867
> 'Grand Holy Land Pleasure Excursion'
> An experienced physician will be on board.
> The ship will at all times be a home, where the excursionists, if sick, will be surrounded by kind friends, and have all possible comfort and sympathy. Should contagious sickness exist in any of the ports named in the program, such ports will be passed, and others of interest substituted.
>
> *The Innocents Abroad*, Mark Twain

Cruises would retain their leisurely and exclusive style until the late 1960s when an unwanted ocean liner and two ferryboats were refitted and refurbished as the *Mardi Gras*, the *Sunward* and the *Princess Pat*. Their casual three and four day cruises from the United States to the Caribbean and the Mexican Riviera revolutionized the industry, which has become more and more popular every year.

In 2001 over six million travellers joined friends, family and new acquaintances on sea voyages to exotic lands.

Mega-liners and intimate luxury vessels offer the comfortable familiarity of home, but cannot entirely remove the risks of international travel. Without careful planning those with an infirmity, pre-existing disease, or disability may be particularly susceptible to harm.

For most passengers, cruising poses few health risks and these can be minimized by sensible planning and a few precautions before, during, and after the voyage.

Preparation / planning

Travel insurance and medical assistance

Most illnesses and injuries can be treated on board, but patients with serious problems must be disembarked for specialist care. An experienced medical assistance company will select, plan, and co-ordinate all of the shore-side care while their agents resolve language problems, financial difficulties, and provide accommodation, solace, and support for travelling companions.

Treatment on board normally carries a cost: all travellers, and especially those with pre-existing medical conditions or those intending to participate in high-risk activities such as scuba diving, should ensure that they purchase an insurance policy that provides timely medical assistance and covers the treatment and evacuation costs of any illness or injury.

Travel medicine check-up

Travellers are advised to contact their doctor or a specialist travel clinic for appropriate advice. The initial consultation should ideally be six to eight weeks before the scheduled date of departure.

Vaccinations, medicines, and health precautions

Most cruise lines will advise their passengers of any vaccination certificates that are *required* by the International Health Regulations, and in particular, a yellow fever vaccination certificate is *required* for some itineraries to South America and Africa. Cruise lines do not routinely provide information on *recommended* immunizations, or on prophylactic medications (such as for malaria).

Additional information is available from the sources listed in Appendix 8.

Pre-existing medical conditions

A cruise is often thought to be the perfect place to convalesce — a getaway with fresh sea air and attentive service. But a ship is more than just a getaway — it is an isolated international community. Access to quality medical care is not always easy and what starts out as a minor complication can become a costly setback.

Anyone with a pre-existing medical condition, or a known health problem that may require medical care on board (including pregnancy), should first:

- Consult their doctor or usual health care provider
- Complete all scheduled medical, surgical, or dental investigations and treatments
- Recuperate from any major illness or surgery
- Adapt fully to any recent modifications in their treatment program
- Understand that specialist medical care might not be readily available
- Advise cruise line medical department of any conditions that may require medical care onboard

Cruise line medical departments can provide prospective travellers or their health care providers with information on a variety of topics including:

- The ship's medical and nursing staff
- The ship's medical facilities
- The limitations of cruise ship medicine
- *Required* vaccination certificates
- Medical insurance and medical assistance companies
- Travel medicine resources for recommended immunizations and prophylactic medicines
- Medical evacuation and disembarkation procedures
- Cruise line's policy regarding infants and pregnancy
- Medical device resources for travellers
- Medical device safety requirements e.g. maintenance certificates / CE mark
- Medical device compatibility with shipboard systems e.g. plug type / voltage / cycles / wattage
- Medical oxygen resources for travellers
- Medical oxygen (international) cylinders and connections
- Medical gas safety in the shipboard environment
- Peritoneal dialysis and haemodialysis
- Assistance animals
- Food allergies — anaphylaxis.

Table 7.3 Examples of medical records and information to carry with you

Traveller's Identification & Personal Contact Information

	Traveller	Travelling companion	Next of kin
First Name:			
Last Name:			
Address:			
Tel No. Day:			
Tel No. Night:			
E-mail address:			
Nationality:			
Passport No.:			
Relationship to self:			

Medical Contact Information

	Name	Tel No. (Day)	Tel No. (Night)	E-Mail
Primary healthcare provider:				
Specialist — type:				

Insurance Policy

Insurance Company: Policy No:

Medical Assistance Company:

24 Hr. Contact No:

Table 7.3 (*continued*) Examples of medical records and information to carry with you

Medicines list (regular) — prescribed, OTC, herbal and homeopathic

	Generic Name	Formulation	Strength	Dosage Instructions
Example:	Propranolol	Tablet	40 mg	One tablet three times each day
Example:	Echinacea	Tablet	Unknown	One tablet twice each day

Medicines list (travel) — prescribed, OTC, herbal and homeopathic

	Generic Name	Formulation	Strength	Dosage Instructions
Example:	Atovaqone + Proguanil	Tablet	250 mg/ 100 mg	One tablet each day with meals. Start two days before and take until seven days after travel to malarial zone

Medical history & copy of medical records

- List of allergies
- Medical problem list
- Copy of recent ECG / EKG
- Copy of recent laboratory results with units of measure NB. Prothrombin times should be recorded as the International Normalized Ratio (INR)
- Copy of recent hospital discharge letters or summaries
- Vaccination certificates

Dental checkup

Travellers with any dental problems should consult their dentist. Most cruise ships do not carry dentists and shore-side dentists with appropriate facilities are not always readily available.

Medical documentation

Travellers are advised to carry a summary of their medical records and contact information. In an emergency, this information and documentation may be of great assistance to ship's medical staff (see Table 7.3).

Cruise ship medical staff and facilities

There are no international standards of care for cruise ships, but many have medical facilities that are staffed and equipped in accordance with guidance provided by the American College of Emergency Physicians (ACEP Health Care Guidelines for Cruise Ship Medical Facilities) or the International Council of Cruise Lines (ICCL).

Both ACEP and ICCL recommend that the ship's medical facilities are staffed and equipped to:
- Provide onboard medical care 24 hours a day
- Handle common medical ailments and injuries
- Provide reasonable on board emergency medical care
- Initiate appropriate diagnostic and therapeutic measures for patients who are critically ill
- Facilitate the evacuation of seriously ill or injured patients to the nearest appropriate shoreside medical facility
- Credentialing process to verify the medical staff's experience and qualifications
- Internal and external audits.

Updates to these guidelines can be reviewed at :-
ACEP: **www.acept.org/1,594,0.htm**
      www.acep.org/1,593,0.html
ICCL: **www.iccl.org/policies/medical2.htm**
      www.iccl.org/policies/medical3.htm

The aftermath of the September 11th 2001 terrorist attacks caused a downturn in the cruising industry that has undoubtedly had an impact on the levels of investment in medical resources that cruise lines are able to make. Hopefully, this situation will only be temporary.

Onboard medical care

A ship's medical centre is not a hospital, there are no operating rooms, blood banks, CT scanners, nor MRI machines. The small well-equipped clinic is usually staffed by one or two doctors and several nurses. A typical medical centre has a couple of consulting rooms, a simple laboratory, an X-ray machine, and several wards for the treatment and isolation of passengers and crew. At least one of the wards will have an intensive care bed for the initial treatment of life-threatening illnesses. The ACEP guidelines recommend that the ship's medical centres should be equipped with defibrillators, external pacemakers, ECG / EKG machines, cardiac monitors, infusion pumps, respirators, pulse oximeters, and a comprehensive range of medications including thrombolytics.

The vast majority of cruise ship passengers do not seek any medical treatment while they are onboard: one out of every 250 passengers experiences a serious illness that requires in-patient care. The onboard staff can treat heart attacks, strokes, and chest infections in the intensive care ward and when necessary they will obtain advice from specialist shore-side colleagues via fax or telephone.

Telemedicine

On some of the newer ships, shore-side specialists can review a patient's X-rays, interpret ECGs, and provide real time audio-video consultations via satellite links.

Emergency medical disembarkation or evacuation

Helicopter evacuations are dramatic but they are often impractical and rarely improve the medical outcome. If a ship is within the rescue helicopter's range, the weather and lighting are adequate, and the patient can be efficiently transferred to an appropriate hospital, the ship's doctor has to decide whether or not an immediate evacuation will benefit their patient. Does the time factor justify the risks? Is the helicopter safe? How will the patient respond as they are winched aboard? Will the noise or vibration cause any problems? Are there any doctors or nurses onboard? Do they have enough space and equipment to provide treatment during the transfer? For all but a few, the patient is much better off being managed in the ship's medical centre until they can be disembarked at the next port.

Specific diseases and health problems

Seasickness

"Sailing on the sea proves that motion disorders the body"

Hippocrates

"The best cure for seasickness is to go and sit under a tree"

Spike Milligan

La maladie de la mer is the body's natural and yet terrible reaction to the heaving, pitching and rolling motions that accompany sea travel. Seasickness is therefore predictable. Children, teenagers, and young adults suffer more than infants or the elderly. Women get sicker than men. Previous experience predicts future susceptibility. Small boats are more provocative than mega-liners and the roughest seas affect everyone.

Modern cruise ships passengers are rarely bothered by the ship's motion but anyone planning a cruise should have a 'seasickness prevention strategy' based on the itinerary, the season, and the ship's size and reputation. Fresh air and a distant horizon may be all that a seasoned seafarer needs but herbal medicines, tablets, patches, and acustimulation devices are a comfort to many. (Seasickness and its remedies are also considered on pp. 271–7.)

Scopolamine tablets and patches may cause confusion in the elderly but they are very effective for those that don't mind feeling a little sleepy.

Divers and anyone else who needs to remain alert may want to experiment with ginger root (*Zingiber officinale*) or acustimulation. High dose ginger root (1G every eight hours) and stimulation of the nei-guan (P6) acupuncture point at the wrist have both been shown to be helpful in a few small trials but their effectiveness is still debated. The Relief Band (**www.reliefband.com**) generates low level electrical pulses while the Sea-Band (**www.sea-band.com**) applies simple acupressure.

The common travel sickness pills (antihistamines — Avomine, Stugeron, Dramamine and Sea-Legs) are often misused and then disparaged as 'useless'. When taken as a last resort they have no effect. I usually recommend starting with a low dose a couple of days before leaving home but if that is not possible the first dose should be taken at least eight hours before embarkation.

A doctor may prescribe ondansetron (Zofran), a non-sedating, selective 5-HT$_3$ antagonist if the usual prophylactic medications are ineffective and the patient can afford the exorbitant price, but the benefits are questionable.

Once symptoms have begun, the ship's physician can provide rapid relief, usually with a 'shot' of intramuscular promethazine.

Medications and herbal remedies can produce unpleasant or even dangerous side-effects. Read package inserts carefully and discuss treatment options with a registered pharmacist or licensed health care provider (p. 275).

Mal de débarquement (sickness of disembarkation)

This is a rare condition in which a traveller continues to sense a rocking or swaying motion long after disembarking from ship.

Infectious diseases

A cruise ship's population is ever changing and its stores are constantly being replenished with local food and water. If the joining passengers and crew are infected or the food and water supplies are contaminated, an infection can spread rapidly throughout the entire community and cause severe disease in the frail and elderly.

During the last few years, onboard surveillance programmes have identified cases of food poisoning, Norwalk virus, *Legionella*, chickenpox, German measles, and influenza A & B. Vaccination programmes and additional hygiene strategies have been implemented to prevent future outbreaks.

In spite of these precautions, cruise ship travellers may be exposed to a variety of infectious diseases. Most of these infections can be prevented or cured by vaccinations, prophylactic medications, or timely treatment.

Food and water-related problems

The vessel sanitation programmes that have been developed over the last thirty years have been very successful in minimizing food and waterborne disease. Only three outbreaks were reported to the CDC's Vessel Sanitation Program in 1999.

Cruise ships undergo regular health and hygiene inspections and the CDC and Health Canada publish each ship's scores on their web-sites:

- CDC VSP **www.cdc.gov/nceh/vsp/vsp.htm**
- Health Canada **www.hc-sc.gc.ca/ohsa/shipinsp.htm**

HACCP (Hazard Analysis Critical Control Point) programs which were originally designed to monitor NASA astronaut's food and water from source to consumption have been effectively used onboard ships, but strict control of hygiene in shore-side hotels and restaurants is more difficult.

Eating and drinking ashore increases the risk of gastro-intestinal disease and recent cases of cholera and typhoid have been linked to shore excursions in Asia and Oceania. Advice on food and hygiene precautions given elsewhere in this book should be followed carefully.

Quarantine regulations require all cases of gastro-intestinal disease (diarrhoea and / or vomiting) and all on-board sales of anti-diarrhoeal medications to be documented. To ensure full compliance, most cruise lines do not permit the sale of anti-diarrhoeal medications (including Pepto Bismol) without a medical consultation.

Norwalk virus and related infections
Norwalk virus is highly infectious form of gastro-enteritis characterized by vomiting and prostration.

Some cruise ship outbreaks of Norwalk and Norwalk-like gastro-enteritis have been caused by ice, shrimp, and fresh cut fruit. Infected passengers and crew and environmental contamination may have contributed to the outbreaks in which no food or water source could be identified. Even if the source is unknown, secondary spread can usually be halted if the index cases are recognized and a rapid response program initiated.

If intensive cleaning reduces but does not eliminate new cases, environmental contamination, person-to-person contact, and airborne transmission can still infect each new group of passengers and crew shortly (24–36 hours) after they join the vessel. In this way, the outbreak can be extended. In these prolonged outbreaks a cruise may have to be cancelled in order to interrupt the chain of transmission.

Airborne disease / droplet spread
The HVAC (Heating, Ventilation and Air Conditioning) systems on modern cruise ships deliver 70–100 per cent fresh air and pose little health risk. Poorly maintained air ducts on older vessels may harbour moulds such as *Aspergillus* which can cause a variety of lung diseases.

Legionnaire's disease
Legionella pneumophilia can cause severe pneumonia and death especially in the frail and elderly. *Legionella* species are found in many rivers, lakes, and streams and they can find their way into a ship's potable water systems. Without inadequate chlorination or poor temperature control this fastidious bacterium needs inadequate chlorination or poor temperature control to survive and multiply. Outbreaks on the MV *Horizon*, the SS *Edinburgh Castle*, and several other vessels have shown that a ship's spas, fountains, and showers can generate the aerosols that are necessary to spread this disease.

The spas, water distribution systems, and air conditioning units on most cruise ships are now carefully maintained and monitored to minimize the risk of further outbreaks. *Legionella* (*pneumophilia sero group 1*) urinary antigen test help with rapid diagnosis.

Influenza
Influenza ('flu) causes a mild disease in healthy adults, but can cause severe illness or even death in the frail and elderly.

In the northern hemisphere, 'flu tends to occur between November and March, but in the southern hemisphere the 'flu season runs from May to October, while in the tropics (including the Caribbean) 'flu can occur all year round. Cruise passengers come increasingly from all over the world thus making it easier for the virus to be carried into the closed environment of a modern ocean liner, where it can pass freely between passengers and crew, and from one cruise voyage to the next.

In addition to the usual seasonal cases, cruise ship surveillance programmes have detected emerging strains and summer time outbreaks of both influenza A and B. These programmes have also detected several outbreaks that began on land tours.

Anyone travelling to regions where 'flu is prevalent (see WER and FluNET, Appendix 8) should be vaccinated, or should discuss the use of standby anti-viral agents with their doctor. These medications can shorten a patient's illness, reduce viral shedding, and reduce the transmission of disease to fellow travellers.

Many ship's physicians regularly perform rapid influenza A and B tests on all cases of acute respiratory illness (ARI) and treat cases of influenza with rimantidine (influenza A) or one of the neuraminidase inhibitors (influenza A or B).

During outbreaks, the viral cultures are compared with the latest (N & S hemisphere) vaccine strains so that any unprotected populations can be identified are advised to carry 'stand-by' medications.

Effective crew vaccination programs shorten outbreaks by reducing the ship's pool of susceptible individuals.

Vaccine-preventable diseases

(Though vaccine-preventable, influenza is discussed above; the WHO-recommended vaccine is not normally available during the summer months.)

Varicella (chickenpox)

Varicella is highly infectious and travellers may be exposed at home or abroad. Shipboard outbreaks usually start with infection passing from a child to a crewmember from a tropical country where childhood chickenpox is not as common as it is in temperate climates. The infection then spreads rapidly amongst all non-immune passengers and crew.

Chickenpox contracted during the first 20 weeks of pregnancy or during the neonatal period can cause congenital abnormalities, severe illness, or even death.

Contact with chickenpox may cause *Herpes zoster* (shingles) in the elderly or immuno-compromised. Those with severe immunodeficiency may develop systemic zoster — a serious generalized infection.

Acyclovir or Varicella-Zoster Immune Globulin (VZIG) may be used to treat some cases. Varicella vaccine can help protect susceptible individuals who have been exposed, but neither VZIG nor Varicella vaccine are normally available on board cruise ships.

International travellers (passengers and crew) who are not immune should consult their doctor for advice. Chickenpox vaccine (Oka strain) is available in several countries (including the USA) and is being considered for more widespread use in the UK.

Rubella (German measles)

Rubella is moderately infectious and travellers may be exposed at home or abroad. Shipboard outbreaks have occurred amongst crewmembers.

Infection during the first 20 weeks of pregnancy can cause congenital rubella syndrome — a group of birth defects including deafness, cataracts, heart defects, and mental retardation.

Female travellers (passengers and crew) of childbearing age who do not have documented immunity should consult their doctor. The live attenuated RA 27/3 vaccine is available as a single antigen or in combination with other vaccines including measles and mumps (MMR).

Vector-borne diseases
Malaria / Dengue fever
Travellers may not necessarily need anti-malarial medication even if the cruise-ship visits a malarial zone. The use of protective clothing, insect repellents, and anti-malarial medication should be based on general recommendations and the specific exposure risk.

Personal risk is determined by:
- The ship's itinerary, including arrival and departure times
- The individual's onboard activities (A/C public room vs. open deck)
- The individual's shore-side activities (sunbathing vs. city tour or safari)
- The individual's pre- and post-cruise activities

Yellow fever
A valid International Certificate of Vaccination is *required* for entry to some ports. A certificate's validity begins ten days after the date of vaccination and extends for a period of ten years. Cruise ships are not designated yellow fever vaccination centres and they are not authorized to issue valid yellow fever vaccination certificates. **Travellers lacking the appropriate documentation will not be allowed ashore.**

If the vaccine cannot be given for health reasons, local health authorities usually accept a waiver, written in English or French, stating the medical reasons why immunization is contraindicated.

Surgery and blood transfusions
Cruise ships do no not carry blood products and the ship's medical staff do not have the resources to perform therapeutic endoscopy or invasive surgery. Patients with uncontrolled bleeding need to be disembarked for definitive treatment. Blood products have very occasionally been delivered by the Australian, UK, and US military to ships in mid-ocean.

The ship's medical staff can manage severe blood loss with fluid replacement (intravenous colloids and crystalloids), traditional surgical techniques (packing and tamponade), and specific medications e.g. oestrogens.

Kits that enable the bedside typing of blood have been used for type-specific blood transfusions from passenger or crew donors. Sensitive rapid HIV antibody tests are available for screening but the ship's medical staff cannot perform the other screening and routine tests that would be performed in a blood bank. (See p. 589)

Other medical considerations for cruise ship travellers

Some general advice follows, but please keep in mind that individual cruise lines have their own policies. For specific information, travellers should always contact the cruise line directly.

Cruise lines reserve the right to refuse or revoke passage to anyone who, in their opinion, might require treatment, care, or attention beyond that which the ship's facilities can provide.

The ship's master has the right, at any time, to disembark a passenger, who in his opinion, is a danger to themselves or to others.

Pregnancy

Most cruise lines will not accept passengers who will have reached the third trimester of pregnancy by the end of their cruise.

Cruise ships are not staffed by obstetricians or neonatologists and complications including miscarriage, ectopic pregnancy, or premature labour will normally require referral to a shore-side specialist. (See Medical disembarkation / evacuations, and Blood transfusions — above.)

Infants

Most cruise lines will not normally accept infants below the age of three to six months.

Impaired immunity

Individuals with impaired immunity are more susceptible to infectious diseases and they may require special investigations or treatments that are not available on board.

Travellers with special needs

Wheelchair accessibility

Getting around the ship

In older ships, access may be limited by narrow doorways, safety barriers, and thresholds. Newer vessels are more accessible and many have a few cabins specially designed for wheelchair access

Going ashore

The gangways may be very steep in some ports but assistive devices can make these transfers easier and safer.

When a ship anchors in a port rather than docking alongside a quay (tender or boating ports) transfers can be difficult and in some weather conditions impossible.

Port facilities

Many ports have not, as yet, made any accommodation for passengers with disabilities. It is vital to find out as much as you can, well in advance of the cruise.

Visually impaired
Audible lift announcements, Braille signs, and menus are available on some ships.

Hearing impaired
Many cruise lines can supply kits that include TTY/TTD text telephones, visual smoke detectors, and various visual alerts

Assistance animals
Assistance animals, from guide dogs to helping hands monkeys, have travelled on cruise ships, but they must comply with all of the applicable quarantine regulations.

Vaccination certificates, certificates of health, and microchip identification may be required.

Dietary restrictions
Food and beverage departments try to accommodate specific dietary requirements such as low sodium, low fat, etc. More sophisticated diets such as low phenylalanine must be provided by the traveller

Cruise lines *cannot* guarantee that meals are free of certain ingredients e.g peanut oil, nor should they be relied upon to do so. Sensitized individuals who have anaphylactic reactions to foods should contact the cruise line's medical department.

Conclusion
Cruise lines strive to maintain a healthy environment, and most large ships now have excellent medical facilities. Travellers and their healthcare providers must understand, however, that facilities on board cannot equate with those of shore-side hospitals.

8 Environmental and recreational hazards

Accidents

Accidents are the leading cause of death, injury, and serious ill health in travellers. Accidents abroad follow predictable patterns, and are not just random events: this means that travellers can do much to avoid them or reduce the risks.

Dr Richard Fairhurst is a Consultant in Accident and Emergency Medicine; Medical Director of Lancashire Ambulance Service and NHS Direct North West Coast. He was formerly the Chairman of the British Association for Immediate Care, Chairman of the British Aeromedical Practitioners Association, and Chief Medical Officer of Europ Assistance and Green Flag Travellers Medical Service. He has supervised the medical assistance rendered to more than 70 000 ill or injured travellers abroad, and has logged more than 5000 flying hours repatriating some of them.

Many travellers abroad think of exotic infections as perhaps the biggest danger to their health, but in fact these represent only a small proportion of medical problems involving travellers. In surveys by travel assistance companies (the companies that insurers use to deliver medical assistance and, if necessary, to carry out medical evacuation), trauma consistently accounts for about one third of all requests for help. By comparison, a little over 10 per cent are due to travellers' diarrhoea, while only half of 1 per cent involve the usually recognized tropical or exotic infections (Table 8.1). Such figures are hardly surprising when one considers that accidents are also the main cause of death in the UK between the ages of 2 and 45, and that most trips are to non-exotic destinations, close to home.

Table 8.1 Cases reported to Green Flag Travellers Medical Service from abroad between 1 June 1993 and 31 May 1994

Diagnosis	No.	%
Trauma	2454	30.93
Gastrointestinal	1148	14.47
Respiratory	909	11.46
Generalized infections	686	8.65
Heart and circulation	648	8.17
Curtailment*	555	7.00
Genito-urinary	379	4.78
Skin	377	4.75
Dental	240	3.02
Musculoskeletal	184	2.32
Nervous system	181	2.28
Mental	70	0.88
Blood	44	0.55
Hormonal	31	0.39
Cancers	28	0.35
Total	7934	100.00

* Request to return to UK due to unexpected insured event e.g. death of family member

Infectious diseases are important, of course. They are preventable, and a proper programme of vaccination, together with the general precautions described elsewhere in this book, are vital. However, travellers also need to employ similar strategies to protect themselves against injury, the foremost of these being simply *to avoid circumstances in which there is a risk of injury.*

Risk and the traveller

Travellers fall into different categories of risk: many have paid out a great deal of money in the expectation of enjoyment for themselves and their families, and are under pressure to have a good time regardless of inconvenient safety rules and common sense; others, alone perhaps, and travelling on business, are under pressure to complete their business objectives at any cost, to press on regardless with itineraries, and to use dangerous short cuts whenever necessary to achieve results.

The language of risk analysis is rich with value-laden words. Whether the risk is *avoidable* or *unavoidable* very much depends on your standpoint: the business executive driving at 120 m.p.h. on a motorway to make an important appointment often considers himself to be taking an unavoidable risk! We now have a classification based on probability (Table 8.2).

Because of these pressures, and the absence of the usual constraints of home, family, and work, most people behave differently abroad, sometimes in quite a reckless, uncharacteristic manner — exposing themselves to risks they would never dream of taking at home. Of course, a certain amount of risk-taking is all part of the excitement

Table 8.2 Description of risk in relation to adverse event (A) or death (D)

Probability	Risk range	Example	Estimate
High	>1:100	(A) Transmission to household contacts of measles and chickenpox	1:1–1:2
		(A) Transmission of HIV from mother to child (Europe)	1:6
		(A) Gastrointestinal effects of antibiotics	1:10–1:20
Moderate	1:100–1:1000	(D) Smoking 10 cigarettes a day	1:200
		(D) All natural causes age 40	1:850
Low	1:1000–1:10 000	(D) All kinds of violence and poisoning	1:3300
		(D) Influenza	1:5000
		(D) Road traffic accident	1:8000
Very low	1:10 000 –1:100 000	(D) Leukaemia	1:12 000
		(D) Playing soccer	1:25 000
		(D) Accident at home	1:26 000
		(D) Accident at work	1:43 000
		(D) Homicide	1:100 000
Minimal	1:100 000 –1:1 000 000	(D) Railway accident	1:500 000
		(A) Polio associated with vaccination	1:1 000 000
Negligible	<1:1 000 000	(D) Hit by lightning	1:10 000 000
		(D) Radiation from nuclear power station	1:10 000 000

and enjoyment of being on holiday — but if you are to avoid accident and injury, you must think carefully about the risks and decide whether these are really justified.

Everyday risks

First of all, travellers should realize that they face at least the same probability of everyday accidents abroad as they do at home. Travel does not suddenly remove these dangers; on the contrary, the enjoyment and carefree attitude that travel engenders can increase the hazards.

As a general rule, *you should continue to apply your usual safety standards even if the legal requirements in the country you are visiting are lax.* For example, most motorists in the UK comply with the seat-belt law in the knowledge that this markedly reduces the risk of serious injury; to stop wearing seat-belts abroad, just because there may be no legal requirement to do so, is inviting trouble. The same applies to wearing helmets on motorcycles and mopeds and observing traffic regulations. If you accept that driving at more than 70 m.p.h. is dangerous (and UK accident statistics clearly demonstrate that it is), then you should stick to 70 m.p.h. abroad, even in countries where speed limits do not exist or are not enforced.

The same reasoning applies to safety in the home. In the UK each year, there are approximately 6000 deaths and two million injuries in the home, with causes ranging from domestic poisoning to the misuse of electrical appliances; 70 per cent of them are due to accidental falls.

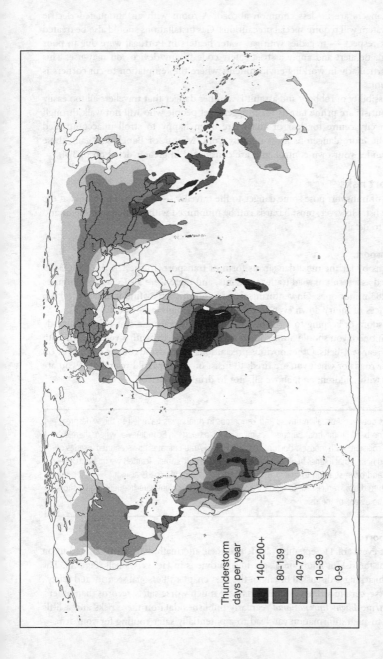

Map 8.1 Lightning strike regions in the world (average thunderstorm days/year). We tend to think of lightning as an extremely uncommon hazard, but for the past 30 years, an average of 73 people have been killed by lightning in the USA, and survivors may be severely disabled. Safety measures include: going indoors, and staying clear of trees, water, wire objects, and heavy equipment. (Source: National Lightning Safety Institute, USA; **www.lightningsafety.com**).

Thunderstorm days per year

140–200+
80–139
40–79
10–39
0–9

Such dangers are no less common abroad. A room with an antiquated electric lighting system will require special precautions. Gas installations should also be treated with great respect — tragedies with gas water-heaters in Portugal were due to poor ventilation. Be alert and apply a strict safety code to any device you may use. This applies particularly in working environments where the temptation to cut corners is ever present.

The possibility of robbery and assault is another danger that travellers all too easily forget. Tourists are prime targets for muggers, yet people who will not walk through their own city centre for fear of attack are often happy to stroll unaccompanied through the more dangerous areas of New York, Miami, or Bangkok. Again, these risks are under your own control, and are considered in greater detail on p. 304.

Transport risks

All forms of transport pose some danger to the traveller — with road transport at the top of the list. However, most hazards can be minimized with a little forethought and attention to detail.

Road transport

Motoring is by far the most dangerous form of transport. In the UK, in 2000, 3409 people died as a result of road traffic accidents, and there were 38 155 serious injuries and 320 283 minor ones. On venturing abroad, motorists may find it difficult to keep their chances of injury down even to this appallingly high level (see Table 8.3).

The wisdom of keeping to a reasonable speed and wearing a seat-belt has already been mentioned: you should always insist on being provided with a vehicle with both front and rear seat-belts. Other obvious precautions are to avoid driving at night or on unfamiliar roads or when you are tired; to insist on proper child restraints if you are travelling with children; and, above all, not to drink and drive.

Collisions between Australian drivers and kangaroos in rural areas have led to the widespread use of 'Roo bars' on the front bumper. A similar problem exists in Scandinavia, where there are frequent collisions with mooses. Doctors from the United Arab Emirates have reported a series of lethal and near-lethal injuries in drivers who have collided with camels (camels weigh from 300– 500 kg, and often stray on to roads). The greatest risk is on unlit roads at night — when the temperature drops, camels like to lie on the warm tarmac. Accidents are frequent, and visitors need to be aware of the risk.

Air transport

The tragic events of 11 September 2001, and their aftermath, have been referred to on p. 250, but the risk of injury on a scheduled airline is in fact very small (Fig 8.1). The threat of hijacking is discussed briefly in the next chapter, 'Personal security and safety'.

Of course, certain airlines and airports have much worse safety records than others. The magazine *Flight International* regularly publishes data on these risks and a little attention to such information can lead to a potentially safer routing for your trip.

Table 8.3 Safety of road travel in different countries*

	Fatalities per 100 million vehicle km	Road deaths per 100 000 population
Egypt	44	
Kenya	41	
Kyrgystan	24	
Sri Lanka	23	
Republic of Korea	21	22.7
Greece		20.9
Turkey	20	10.1
Morocco	17.8	
Yemen Arab Republic	14.4	
South Africa	10.4	
Albania	7.8	
Ecuador	7.5	
Portugal	6.1	22.4
Slovenia	5.6	
Spain	5.3	15.1
Czech Republic	4.9	13.2
Hungary	4.8	13.5
Slovakia	4.8	
Macedonia	4.2	
Oman	4.2	
Senegal	4	
Iran	3.9	
Zimbabwe	2.8	
Hong Kong	2.4	
Israel	1.8	
Poland		18.3
United States	1.1	15.3
France	1.8	15.1
Belgium		14.7
Luxembourg		13.4
New Zealand	1.9	13.3
Ireland	1.7	12.4
Austria		11.9
Italy		11.0
Iceland		9.8
Canada		9.7
Germany	1.6	9.5
Denmark	1.7	9.4
Australia	1.2	9.4
Japan	1.5	8.5
Switzerland	1.3	8.4
Norway		8.0
Finland	1	7.8
Netherlands	0.9	6.8
United Kingdom	0.9	6.1

Source: Association for Safe International Road Travel (ASIRT); International Road Traffic Accident Database (OECD)
* Detailed reports on individual countries are available from ASIRT (**www.asirt.org**)

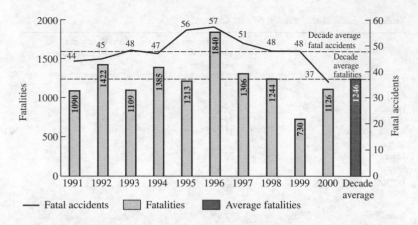

Fig. 8.1 Air travel: fatal accidents and fatalities 1990-2000. (Reproduced with permission from *Flight International*).

In 1991, a Lauda Air Boeing 767 was lost without survivors in Thailand. This was a very unusual accident in that the aircraft was at cruising height and the cause was malfunction of the thrust reversers of the engines. This case illustrates well the difficulty of trying to avoid a particular type of aircraft at risk: the Boeing 767 aircraft is available with various types of engine and thrust reverser combinations, only one of which caused the accident.

It is concerning that the official cause of the crash of a Transworld Airlines Boeing 747100 on 17 July 1996 has not been conclusively determined, though it is widely suspected that this was due to the explosion of vapour in the almost empty central wing tank.

Reassuringly, 1997 saw a series of incidents in which airliners landed safely despite one leg of the undercarriage being retracted. There were no passenger fatalities, and only a few minor injuries as a result of these. The most notable incident was the safe landing of a Virgin Atlantic Airbus 340 at London Heathrow Airport.

There have been two accidents in which cargo planes have hit buildings with loss of life to the occupants of the buildings: one at Schipol Airport, Amsterdam; and one in China.

Another factor that may influence your choice of airline is the type of on-board medical equipment carried and the training of cabin staff in its use. Defibrillators are the only way of treating fatal complications of heart attacks; automated electrical defibrillators (AEDs) are compact, safe, and simple to use with minimal training. For years, many airlines refused to carry them, but resistance has crumbled and many airlines have introduced them or announced plans to do so. They are becoming a legal requirement in the USA, which will increase pressure for universal introduction. Medical kits also vary considerably between airlines.

Part of your safety strategy should start at the airport. There have been several terrorist attacks in airport buildings — don't linger land side, but check in and go through customs and immigration to the much more secure air side.

Airlines are required by their regulating bodies to provide safety briefings on every flight. Listen carefully to the briefing and read the safety instruction card. Even though you may have travelled by air hundreds of times before, a particular airliner might have a different configuration and different safety equipment. Not all oxygen masks fall out of the cabin roof on depressurization (on DC10 aircraft they are in the head rest of the seat in front of you); and as a direct result of the British Midland M1 crash the 'brace position' has been changed to minimize injuries to the lower limbs. On flights with only short over-water sectors, the crew may not brief you on the location of life-vests; make sure you know where they are.

Turbulence occasionally causes injury and death (as in the case of a United Airlines B747 flying over the Pacific in early 1998), so move around the cabin as carefully as possible, and keep your seat-belt fastened at all times. Be particularly careful when hot drinks and meals are being served, because sudden movement can spill scalding fluid into your lap.

Baggage poses an additional hazard, both on and off the plane. Avoid travelling with more baggage than you can carry comfortably and beware of other travellers who cannot keep their luggage trolleys under control — this is a frequent cause of injury. On boarding the plane, try to restrict your hand luggage to one small item: the more the cabin is cluttered, the greater the risk in an accident. Overhead racks are getting larger and larger, but resist the temptation to put heavy items in these racks; in an accident they may fall on top of you and may even prevent your escape.

Duty-free alcohol is a particular problem. A fully laden Boeing 747 may be carrying up to 350 litres of inflammable alcohol in its cabin: this not only creates an obstruction but also constitutes a considerable fire risk. Things are beginning to improve in the UK, but the sooner customs authorities around the world rationalize the system and allow passengers to buy duty-free goods at the port of entry, the safer everyone will be.

Smoking on board aircraft is potentially hazardous — not only to your own health, but also to the safety of the aircraft. If you must smoke during a flight, be very careful to extinguish cigarettes and matches properly; use only the ashtrays provided. Above all, do not smoke when moving around on the aircraft, and never smoke in the washrooms. There is a recent example of a serious cabin fire caused by an unextinguished cigarette left in a washroom. Fortunately, this hazard is diminishing rapidly, as most airlines are adopting a no-smoking policy.

Once out of the realm of commercial airlines, the risks of accidents increase greatly, and there have been several recent accidents involving private aircraft (p. 261). If you are thinking of travelling in a private aircraft, try to form an impression of whether the operation is being run professionally; if it is not, it is probably dangerous, and you should make excuses and find another way of getting to your destination.

Sea transport (see also p. 304)

Accidents and injuries at sea to passengers on Western-owned carriers are unusual, though the tragic loss of a car and passenger ferry, the *Herald of Free Enterprise,* in 1987 highlighted problems with ferries all over the world. Sadly, lessons take a long time to be learned: on the 28 September 1994 *The Estonia* was lost in the Baltic with the loss of more than 900 lives, after inundation through a damaged bow door. There have been several horrific accidents in the Far East, mostly due to overloading. If a ferry is full, wait and catch the next one. On ships, always observe simple safety measures. Make sure you know how all the safety devices work, and where they are located. Where is your life-jacket? Where is your muster station for the life-boats? Where are the emergency exits, and what signals will be used in case of an emergency? Does someone at home know of your travel plans?

The loss of the *Oceanis* off South Africa in 1991 shows how observance of safety procedures, coupled with an efficient air-sea rescue service *can* avoid loss of life, even when the hull is a total loss.

The risks of injury are greater from rough seas than from the vessel foundering. Remain seated, make sure you are clear of any loose fittings that may crash around, and if possible lie on your bunk. If you have to move around, be very careful of wet floors and in particular of steep stairways. Do as any professional sailor would do and use both hands.

Finally, we cannot leave the subject of sea travel without mentioning the possibility of piracy (Map 8.1). In many areas of the world this is still commonplace. In general, pirates are interested in robbery and not in murder. If you are unfortunate enough to be the victim of piracy, remain calm, obey instructions, give up your possessions as required, and do not provoke an argument or a fight.

Rail travel

Rail travel is remarkably safe, but a succession of accidents in the UK, such as those in Clapham, Southall, Ladbroke Grove, Hatfield, and Selby, clearly demonstrates that there is no room for complacency. Rail safety standards in the UK are currently under close scrutiny, with attention focusing on signalling technology, escape systems, and the safety and structural strength of aging railway carriages. Safety standards in developing countries are unlikely to be better.

In a number of incidents, many injuries have been caused simply by the impact of one human frame upon another — the time when we will see safety belts and closed luggage bins in trains may not be far away. When travelling by train, sit down: passengers who are standing at the moment of impact are much more likely to be seriously hurt than passengers who are sitting down. In one crash that involved a commuter train travelling at a speed of just 10 m.p.h., 50 out of 59 passengers who were standing received injuries to the head and face; only 13 of 32 seated passengers who were taken to hospital had head injuries.

Most injuries are the result of being hit by an open carriage door or falling under the train on getting off. So keep well away from your train as it approaches the station and, at the end of your journey, refrain from opening the door and stepping off until the train has stopped.

One cannot leave the subject of trains without mentioning the habit of riding on carriage roofs, and walking on the outside of carriages, which is almost the rule in some developing countries. It may be picturesque, and tempting in the heat, but don't do it — it is extremely unsafe.

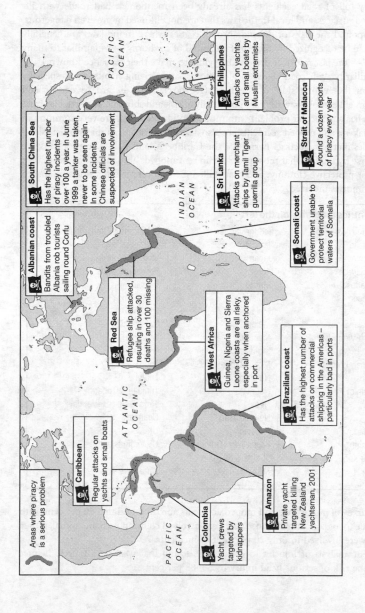

Areas where piracy
is a serious problem

Caribbean
Regular attacks on
yachts and small boats

Colombia
Yacht crews
targeted by kidnappers

Amazon
Private yacht
targeted killing
New Zealand
yachtsman, 2001

Brazilian coast
Has the highest number
of attacks on commercial
shipping in the Americas –
particularly bad in ports

West Africa
Guinea, Nigeria and Sierra
Leone coasts are all risky,
especially when anchored
in port

Red Sea
Refugee ship attacked,
resulting in over 30
deaths and 100 missing

Albanian coast
Bandits from troubled
Albania rob tourists
sailing round Corfu

South China Sea
Has the highest number
of piracy incidents –
over 100 a year. In June
1999 a tanker was taken,
never to be seen again.
In some incidents
Chinese officials are
suspected of involvement

Philippines
Attacks on yachts
and small boats by
Muslim extremists

Sri Lanka
Attacks on merchant
ships by Tamil Tiger
guerrilla group

Somali coast
Government unable to
protect territorial
waters of Somalia

Strait of Malacca
Around a dozen reports
of piracy every year

PACIFIC OCEAN

ATLANTIC OCEAN

INDIAN OCEAN

PACIFIC OCEAN

Map 8.2 Areas where piracy is a serious problem. Adapted from *Geographical*, May 2000, by kind permission

Risks at your destination

Road hazards

The heavy toll of road accidents has already been mentioned. Bad roads with ill-maintained surfaces, and local traffic laws that are not enforced or are even dangerous, may compound the risks of driving abroad. (Cities where traffic laws are generally ignored can be recognized by the constant sound of car horns — so familiar to many travellers — the last resort of drivers struggling to make their presence known.)

Unfamiliarity with road signs, local customs, and driving habits, and especially driving on the 'wrong side' of the road (see box), are a hazard to drivers and pedestrians alike: most travellers are potentially at risk and should take particular care.

Greece has a particular problem with moped accidents, which are very common in holidaymakers; and moped accidents are also a serious problem in many other island holiday destinations, such as Bermuda, the Caribbean, and Bali. The problems are made worse by the fact that most people who rent mopeds abroad do not wear crash helmets or protective clothing, and that skilled medical care is often not available to treat the injuries incurred.

Countries that drive on the left		
Antigua / Barbuda	Indonesia	St Vincent & Grenadines
Australia	Jamaica	Seychelles
Bahamas	Japan	Singapore
Bangladesh	Kenya	Solomon Islands
Barbados	Macau	Somalia
Bermuda	Malawi	South Africa
Bhutan	Malaysia	Sri Lanka
Botswana	Malta	Swaziland
British Virgin Islands	Mauritius	Tanzania
Brunei	Montserrat	Thailand
Cayman Islands	Mozambique	Togo
Cyprus	Namibia	Tonga
Dominica	Nauru	Trinidad & Tobago
Eire	Nepal	Turks & Caicos Islands
Fiji	New Zealand	Uganda
Grenada	Pakistan	UK
Guyana	Papua New Guinea	US Virgin Islands
Hong Kong	St Kitts & St Nevis	Zambia
India	St Lucia	Zimbabwe

One survey of motorcycle and moped accidents abroad found that 60 per cent were simply due to loss of control, and 20 per cent involved collision with an animal. Other vehicles were involved in only 20 per cent of incidents.

A recent analysis of injuries to cyclists has found that wearing a bicycle helmet reduces the risk of serious head injury by 63–88 per cent.

Political and cultural risks

Insurance policies exclude war risks and riots but, unfortunately, civil disturbances, bombings, or even invasion are liable to occur virtually anywhere nowadays. Politically unstable areas (which vary from time to time) are obviously best avoided, although this may not be possible for the business traveller.

Foreign ministries (such as the Foreign Office in the UK and the Department of State in the USA) publish country-by-country advice on their websites, with frequent updates, and will generally provide specific guidance for trouble spots on request. If you are unfortunate enough to be caught up in a riot, *coup d'état*, or invasion, keep in contact with your own country's consular or diplomatic representatives.

A more recent problem has been the specific targeting of tourists by fundamental terrorists, such as the killing of 71 people in Egypt in 1997 as a method of damaging the stability of the Government.

At a more personal level, most difficulties with the local population or authorities can be avoided by finding out how you are expected to behave at your destination. As a general rule avoid political discussions of any type, and avoid making political statements even in private. Don't use cameras or binoculars in aircraft, airports, government installations, or ports, however great the temptation to photograph an interesting item of local flora. In some societies, women still have a very sheltered status; visitors to such countries are well advised to comply strictly with local customs. Such issues are considered further in the next chapter.

Theft

The risk of theft while shopping can be reduced by being discreet with large amounts of cash, and shopping only in areas which are known to be safe for visitors. If a bag, briefcase, or handbag is snatched, particularly by a motorcyclist, let it go. More people are seriously injured by being pulled over in this situation than from any other type of robbery.

Hotel safety

Fires

Hotel fires are unfortunately all too common and smoke, reduced visibility, and panic are the most serious hazards. Some basic precautions include finding out where the fire escape is as soon as you arrive at a hotel, following it down to see exactly where it emerges, and, if possible, finding out what the fire alarms actually sound like. Keep a torch or flashlight handy in your hotel room in case of an alarm at night, and in the event of a fire, try above all to stay calm. Remember that smoke rises and that it is safest to crawl on the floor in a smoke-filled room. In the ski resort hotel fire in Bulgaria in 1988, there were no burn or smoke injuries — all the casualties sustained broken limbs while jumping out of windows to escape from the smoke.

Lifts

Hotel lifts are a potential source of danger. If the lift looks unsafe, it probably is; use the stairs instead. Lift cages with only three sides (the fourth side being the wall of the lift shaft) are common in Europe and pose a particular danger. Do not under any circumstances lean against the wall of the lift shaft as it slides by; sadly, people have lost limbs when their clothes were trapped between the lift cage and the shaft wall.

Balconies

Remember that hotel balconies and their balustrades are often designed to look nice rather than to be safe. Make sure the fixing of the balustrade is secure, and that the height of the balustrade is sufficient to stop you overbalancing and falling. There are at least 20 deaths in UK citizens resulting from falls from hotel balconies each year, often related to alcohol consumption.

Camp sites

Camp sites in all countries pose particular risks: lack of security, leading to robbery and assault; and vulnerability to natural disasters such as fires, floods, sandstorms, and avalanches. In some countries there is also the risk of being attacked by dangerous animals or bitten all over by insects. Tents should be in groups, with someone always on the watch. If you choose to camp alone in a remote area then you must accept that you are taking a serious risk.

Sports, hobbies, and special pursuits

Most sports and special pursuits involve a risk factor, which is often an important component of the sport's enjoyment and attraction. When accidents do occur, they can usually be traced to entirely avoidable factors — such as poorly maintained equipment, lack of training, or an inadequate level of fitness — rather than any intrinsic danger of the sport itself. Most serious skiing accidents, for example, are due either to inadequate mental and physical preparation or to badly adjusted ski bindings (see p. 381).

As a traveller intent on cramming the maximum amount of enjoyment into the time available, you may be tempted to cut corners, but this is unwise. Always make sure that the equipment you use is maintained to the highest standards (as the experts do), and if the sport you are interested in involves a high level of exertion, avoid 'overdoing things' until you have built up an appropriate level of fitness and stamina.

Certain pursuits — for example scuba-diving (p. 372) and hang-gliding — can be carried out safely only after a fairly long period of graduated instruction and training, including training in the avoidance of the specific risks involved. While abroad you may be offered an opportunity to indulge in such pursuits with only a minimal degree of instruction and supervision: offers of this type are best declined until you have undergone a proper training, and preferably obtained a certificate of competence.

If your pursuit carries you far away from human habitation, make sure that a responsible person knows where you are going and when you expect to return to base. If possible, take a radio, or a satellite phone. When you are injured on a crevasse on a mountain, or marooned in a boat at sea, nobody can help you unless they know where you are.

In our experience, however, it is not the esoteric pursuits on holiday that carry the biggest risk, but the simple ones. Fathers, unaccustomed to exercise, seem particularly prone to ligament and bone injuries, or even heart attacks, from playing cricket or football on the beach. Every year, there is a terrible toll from diving into shallow water, with serious neck and spinal injuries in young men leading to paralysis for life. This accounts for approximately one-tenth of all spinal cord injuries. *Do not under any circumstances dive into water of uncertain depth, or take running dives into the sea from a sloping beach.*

Accidents and injuries do not need to be serious in order to be inconvenient: make sure that you are prepared for the run-of-the-mill cuts, scrapes and grazes, stubbed toes, and sprains that are a common by-product of going on holiday, and that you have a sensible supply of antiseptic, dressings, painkillers, and basic essentials.

Legal problems abroad

In many countries, it is common practice for people involved in accidents resulting in injury to someone else to be imprisoned until the matter of liability is resolved. In 2000, a British woman was imprisoned in Dubai for five weeks and charged with manslaughter following a jet ski accident, in which another holidaymaker died. One of the contributors to this book was imprisoned in Turkey following a traffic accident.

At any moment, there are believed to be about 2500 British prisoners in overseas gaols, of whom 50-80 are believed to be innocent.

In addition to help provided by consular officials, Fair Trials Abroad and Prisoners Abroad are two British charities that may be able to provide help and advice. (**www.f-t-a.freeserve.co.uk** and **www.prisonersabroad.org.uk**).

Alcohol

Travellers may use alcohol as an adjunct to enjoyment or in consolation for loneliness; it increases all other risks of injury and should be treated with great care. Alcohol and swimming make a particularly bad mix: almost half of all drownings are associated with alcohol consumption (p. 370).

A recent study has shown that in road traffic accidents involving pedestrians, the pedestrian is more likely to be intoxicated with alcohol than the driver of the car that hits him. Unfortunately, travellers are under great pressure to consume alcohol in excess, most of all on the airlines, where it is given out with reckless abandon, particularly in the first-class cabin.

Consequences of injury abroad

The consequences of any injury abroad are often more serious than they would be if the same injury were sustained at home. In many areas of the world no organized emergency medical services are available to provide care at the site of an accident, or even an ambulance service to take the casualty to hospital. The more 'unspoilt' and picturesque the location, the greater the probability of the local 'hospital' being unworthy of such a title.

No medical help may be available at all. Small islands are always a risk. Usually, it requires a population of about a quarter of a million people to support a comprehensive medical service, and an island with a population smaller than this may well not have one (although better facilities may be available within reasonable range). If the island is many miles from the nearest mainland, even the simplest injury can cause problems. Similar risks apply to travellers, visiting small, isolated communities anywhere — desert oases, for example.

If you or any of your companions has suffered injury, and you cannot speak the local language, you may not be able to summon help even when it is available. Find out how the local system works, and what the emergency telephone number is. Remember that however good the local emergency services, you have problems if you cannot contact them or make yourself understood.

Summary of advice for travellers

- All life's activities involve a balance between risk and benefit: we take risks in order to obtain benefit. Travellers who wish to avoid injury must examine the risks they run and decide whether they are justified. Everyone should have a strategy for safety, and wherever they are, whatever they are doing, should know very clearly what their escape route will be and how to behave in an emergency. Above all, no one should expose themselves to avoidable risks that they would never take in their normal environment.

Personal security and safety

Personal security abroad is an issue that is intimately related to safety and health. Travellers can be extremely vulnerable, and must take precautions to reduce the risks.

Nicholas Cameron MC is a Research and Risk Management Consultant for AKE Ltd, UK, the leading specialists in hostile environment training and awareness for journalists and the media industry.

What is a hostile environment? Contrary to popular belief, it need not be a war zone. Hostile conditions may be encountered anywhere from modern sophisticated cities to the desperate conditions of a sub-Saharan African refugee camp, from conflict zones to the climatically challenging conditions of a Scottish hillside. For most people, the world has become a much smaller place, and the opportunity to travel has never been greater. More opportunities to travel, however, mean an increased likelihood of finding oneself in a hostile environment.

In today's high-tech, globalized community, we are bombarded with popular accounts of crime and conflict — almost as they happen — and we assume that we are aware of the risks within our own environment. We accept these risks as part of modern life, and within our daily routine have developed strategies for reducing or even eliminating risk completely. However, when travelling abroad we move away from the familiar, into an unfamiliar environment with unaccustomed risks. Abroad, whether at work or at play, actions that in our home environment might be considered innocuous can lead to anything from interruption and inconvenience to much more dire consequences.

Do your homework

In our everyday behaviour, appearance, and in everything that we say or do, we constantly reveal information about ourselves; in our home environment, this information is interpreted as more or less acceptable. In a foreign environment, the same information may be interpreted from a different perspective, provoking offence or even hostility that we may not be aware of. National origin, ethnic grouping, religion, language, gender, cultural emblems, and social class can arouse local passions that place the traveller at risk. Risk in this context is not constant; tensions may increase locally as a result of economic, political, or religious crises over which you have no control. It is essential, when travelling in a potentially hostile environment, to become familiar with the social and cultural standards of behaviour necessary to avoid offence.

Local cultural awareness is particularly important in highly religious societies such as in strictly Islamic countries. Illegal acts, such as drinking alcohol and possession of drugs, may result in significantly harsher penalties than might be expected at your home base. Drug smuggling is deemed so severe that the death sentence is considered the appropriate penalty. Women must accept that in certain Islamic societies they must conform to strict codes of behaviour — Western liberal attitudes to dress and open displays of affection may not be tolerated. For even minor transgressions the penalties can be harsh.

Tourism is a welcome source of revenue for most countries. However, there are areas where tourists may not be welcome; disputes over environmental issues or social conditions within the vicinity of hotel complexes can create resentment against tourists. Extremists intent on the destruction of a country's tourist industry have made a particular point of targeting tourist areas. Travellers need to be aware of local sensitivities.

Local, national, and international politics — concerning issues that we may not even be aware of — can lead to sudden tensions with unforeseen consequences for the individual traveller. Antipathy may be generated towards tourists in general, people of a particular national or ethnic origin, or employees of a specific company. Detention, confiscation of possessions or equipment, and expulsion may be the result. Travel for whatever reason now includes, to a greater or lesser extent, a certain element of adventure; today's tourists and business travellers need also be adept voyagers.

The important thing is to find out as much as possible (culturally, socially, and politically) about the country you are visiting, in advance of your trip, and to plan accordingly.

Trouble spots

At the start of 2002, there were in excess of 22 wars and serious terrorist insurgencies going on around the world. There are many other, less widely-publicized conflicts. While most are well-known trouble spots, some can come as a surprise. It can be quite a shock to arrive in a foreign country and find armed security forces on the streets — but this may be the first indication that all is not well. The list in Table 8.4 is not by any means exhaustive — sporadic terrorist attacks have also occurred in London, Madrid,

Paris, Athens, and Tokyo. Terrorist campaigns reach across international borders, and can disrupt travel without warning.

The fact that conflict exists within a country does not always mean that one should not go there. It is however prudent to take the necessary precautions in order to reduce the risks involved. It is helpful to understand the history of the conflict, and why hostilities have begun. It may also be advisable to obtain a report immediately prior to departure. Talk to people who have just visited the area, scan the Internet for recent reports, and phone the security officer at your embassy in the country concerned for advice. The circumstances within conflict zones can change quickly, and so can the risks.

Specific security risks

Travellers face an increasing range of risks, ranging from the simple disruption of travel arrangements to suicide bombings, politically motivated assaults, and criminal activity. In some parts of the world, the criminals may even be the police or the security forces themselves. The nature of risk to which one is exposed depends on individual circumstances and destinations. Some travellers have specific fears, which may or may not be justified.

Robbery, physical attacks, and street crime

Ostentatious displays of wealth can act as a magnet for crime. Business travellers and tourists carrying lap-top computers, camcorders, cameras, and cellular phones become tempting targets for local criminals. Remember that wealth is relative: tourists arriving in some popular destinations may have more cash in their pockets than a local person can hope to earn in a year — temptation indeed! Sophisticated scams and routine trickery are common tactics to trap the unwary traveller; however, plain violence is no less common.

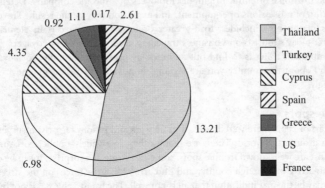

Fig. 8.2 Reported rapes per million British travellers.

Table 8.4 Some current trouble spots

Afghanistan	Civil war, War on terrorism
Algeria	FIS/GIA conflict
Angola	Second civil war
Burma	Karen insurrection
Colombia	FARC and ELN insurgencies
Congo (Congo Brazzaville)	Civil conflict
Democratic Republic of Congo	General war (DRC, Zimbabwe, Angola, Rwanda, Uganda, and Namibia)
Ethiopia	Eritrea war
Georgia	Civil war
India	Kashmiri and Naxalite uprisings
Indonesia	Civil disturbance — Aceh Province, Kalimantan Province (Borneo) Papua Province (West Irian Jaya)
Israel	Second Palestinian Intafada
Kosovo	Ethnic Albanian–Serb conflict
Laos	Civil disturbance
Liberia	Civil conflict
Macedonia	Ethnic Albanian insurgency
Nepal	Maoist attacks
Nigeria	Civil disturbances; religious conflict in the North
Philippines	Moro Islamic uprising
Russia	Second Chechen war
Sierra Leone	Civil war
Solomon Islands	Civil disturbances
Somalia	Civil conflict
Sri Lanka	Tamil war
Sudan	Second civil war
Uganda	Civil conflict

Theft is much more likely to be opportunist than a premeditated attack, which requires detailed planning.

The following precautions may be helpful:

- Leave your passport and tickets or valuable documents in your hotel safety-deposit box and carry only a photocopy.
- Whenever possible, walk in the middle of the pavement. Walking too close to buildings or to the kerb leaves you vulnerable to a would-be thief.
- Stand several feet back from kerbs while waiting to cross the street. Motorcyclists can readily grab handbags or briefcases while pedestrians wait for the light to change.
- Do not wear expensive or *expensive-looking* jewellery, especially anything of sentimental value, including wedding or engagement rings and dress watches.
- Carry two wallets, one containing out-of-date credit cards and small denominations of local currency. In the event of a robbery you can hand it over — it might be enough to get you out of trouble. Carry small denomination bills for normal purchases in one place and large denomination bills in another. This will prevent criminals from knowing how much money you have.
- Don't carry a large amount of cash, and don't carry credit cards you do not plan to use. Use travellers' cheques wherever possible and ensure that you have signed them

only once. Arrive in the country with enough cash for some days. Avoid changing large amounts of cash at the exchange bureau, as this will attract attention.

- For women, be especially careful with your purse or handbag. Carry it close to your body with the opening facing in or the zipper closed. Some women find that it is safest to carry their money and identification in a small purse that they can safely place in a pocket. If necessary, a bag for sunglasses, cosmetics, and other inexpensive items can be carried, that would be expendable in the event of a robbery. A money-belt worn under clothes is ideal.
- Men should carry their wallets in front pockets to combat the threat of pickpockets.
- Avoid walking or jogging alone, especially at night. Use well-illuminated streets and walk facing on-coming traffic. At night, carry a small torch.
- Take advice on any danger spots to avoid, and if necessary, obtain the services of a reputable guide from a trusted source.
- Obtain a simple street map, even if only a sketch from the staff at your hotel; but take care when consulting it, so as not to appear vulnerable.
- Make sure someone knows your plans and that you have access to some form of communication in case of delays or difficulties. In developing countries, cell phone coverage often does not operate beyond a certain radius from major cities.
- Trust your instinct — if you get that uncertain feeling about someone or something take action and don't leave it too late. If you are approached or followed by a suspicious person, cross the street or change direction. Try to look confident — muggers look for victims who seem like easy targets — but don't overdo it. Seek areas where the presence of others will discourage personal threats.
- Avoid predictable movements and activities; for example, don't take the same routes and visit the same places at the same times. Make things as difficult as possible for any would-be attacker to plan an attack against you.
- If a robbery does occur, don't resist. Street criminals are invariably armed. Your ego and any valuables you are carrying should not take precedence over your life and safety. Make as much noise as you can — it might be enough to scare the assailant away. Avoid excessive alcohol consumption if you expect to be out in a vulnerable area, even a small amount may dull your reflexes.

Hotel security

In the developing world, there is the largely true perception that only wealthy foreigners can afford to stay in exclusive hotels. Larger and reputable hotels are normally positioned in prominent city centre locations. Whilst they are generally safe enough, they can provide a focal point for the more undesirable elements of that particular city. The large hotel chains will have their own security staff and procedures and should be able to arrange guides and cars.

Hotels that are used exclusively by expatriate communities or are positioned in vulnerable areas should be frequented with caution. If possible, select a hotel room in or near the locality in which your business will be conducted, unless of course that area has a high crime rate or is near government buildings in a politically unstable country.

Arrange for a hotel representative to collect you from the airport, and use care when allowing porters to carry your baggage — even if they look authentic, they may be impostors. Displaying names or company logos may also attract unwanted attention. Use caution when answering telephone calls and be aware of offers that seem too good to be true. Elaborate scams involving many convincing people have been known to target visitors to certain hotels.

Most reputable hotels will have access to safety-deposit boxes, which should be used to store large amounts of cash or other valuables. There are various devices on the market that can increase hotel security; portable door locks, which slip between the door and door frame, will prevent unwanted access. Also ensure that you identify visitors before opening the door.

Be careful not to conduct sensitive or important discussions in your room, in areas where you can be overheard, or on hotel telephones. Maintain a low profile when the hotel is used for business meetings.

If you see evidence of poor security and fire hazards in the hotel lobby, consider moving to another hotel. Where are the fire exits? Could you find your way out in the dark?

Check your room for the following features:
- A sprinkler system or smoke detectors, and preferably both.
- An external staircase for fire escape.
- Door locks that close securely.
- Room windows that lock securely and that are not accessible by others.
- That it is between the third and sixth floors (out of reach of criminals, but within reach of fire ladders).

When leaving your room:
- Ask the maid to clean your room in person or by phone. Do not display the 'Please clean room' sign — criminals can read too.
- Display the 'Do not disturb' sign at all times; it suggests that you may be in.
- Leave the television or radio on; it also suggests that you are in.
- Do not tell the lobby clerk of your departure or the time of your expected return.
- Do not always hand the key in at the lobby desk.
- Do not leave important papers in your room that might generate the interest of others.

In case of a hotel fire:
- Respond to all fire alarms.
- Never use an elevator during a fire.
- If the fire is in your room, get out and close the door. Only then should you report the fire to hotel personnel.
- Leave your room if you can. Take your key with you.
- Feel the door — if it is cool, open it slowly and go to the nearest exit. Crawl on the floor if the hall is filled with smoke — there is more fresh air near the floor.
- If your door is hot, do not open it. Your room may be the safest place to be.
- Use the telephone to call for help, or signal from your room.
- Do not break a window. Open a window only if it can be closed again; an open window may draw smoke into your room.

- If you exit the floor during a fire and go down an emergency stairwell, ensure that you will be able to return to the floor — many exit doors to stairwells cannot be re-opened.
- If you cannot leave your room during a fire, fill the bath-tub with water, and seal all door cracks with wet towels, blankets, curtains, or clothing.

Airline security

The terrorist atrocities in New York on 11 September 2001 have resulted in a massive increase in airline security world-wide, both at the airport and on board during the flight; one can only hope that such extra security measures will be sustained and free of loopholes. Check carefully before you leave, to ensure that your hand luggage does not include any items you will not be allowed to carry. A current list of items banned from hand luggage in the USA can be found at **www.FAA.gov/apa/tipbroch.htm**.

Having the correct documentation, visa requirements, and vaccination certificates is essential. In certain countries, customs and immigration officials habitually extract money from travellers. If you fail to pay, the delays can be interminable. It is wise to travel with low denomination currency — the US dollar is the currency of choice.

Never leave your luggage unattended, the airport security may remove them or worse still, they could be stolen. Be perceptive of people around you prior to boarding the aircraft.

The actual selection of an airline will mostly be dictated by the destination; however, you should always consider the airline's security history. Has it been targeted in the past? The safety record of the airline is also a relevant factor. Especially since 11 September, most Western airlines have reasonable security and safety standards with which they have to comply, but there are other airlines with less stringent safety procedures. If possible, route yourself through airports known to have consistent, high-standard security procedures and screening. Avoid those that do not. Some other tips:

- Non-stop flights are preferable: fewer take-offs and landings reduce the potential for problems.
- Fly wide-bodied aircraft. Hijackers don't like planes with large numbers of passengers.
- Although first-class travel is a comfortable way of travelling if you can afford it, consider sitting in business or economy class when travelling on airlines or routes that have previously been targeted by hijackers, or during periods when a hijacking is possible. The first-class section usually becomes the 'command post' during a hijacking, and anyone sitting in that cabin will be viewed as potentially 'important'.
- Although most travellers select an aisle seat on aircraft for the convenience of being able to get up and move around on long flights, window or centre seats are preferable during a hijacking. Passengers in such seats will be less accessible to the questions and interests of hijackers, and during any attempt at rescue, those sitting in window and centre seats will be less vulnerable to gunfire along the aisle.

What to do in the event of a hijacking

Before the suicide hijackings of 11 September 2001, the conventional advice was never to confront people trying to hijack a plane, especially if they claimed to have a bomb; and to remain calm and obey the hijackers, keeping a low profile in the hope of avoiding being singled out. Comfort came from the knowledge that the survival rate from such a situation was 98 per cent, and passivity seemed the least risky option.

Since then, however, there is an overwhelming sense that the rules have changed. Will it ever be possible again, for a hijacker's demands to be taken purely at face value? Aircraft deviating from their scheduled routes risk being shot down, and anyone attempting to instigate a hijack must accept the likelihood of being killed, by passengers and crew if not by an air marshal or on-board security guard. In one incident following 11 September, a mentally disturbed passenger knocked his way into the cockpit during a flight from Los Angeles to Chicago: half the plane — men and women alike — rose to tackle him.

In a hijack situation, fear of death or injury is only natural. Recognizing this reaction may help you adapt to the incident more effectively. Try to regain composure as soon as possible after the hijacking occurs. Pause, take a deep breath, and attempt to organize your thoughts.

If you speak the hijackers' language, conceal it. Although it might be expected that using their language might enhance rapport, experience with previous hijackings indicates that travellers are better off speaking their native tongue, and acquiring what information they can by listening to the hijackers' conversation. This may provide you with vital information about what the hijackers plan to do next. Try to make notes about the physical make-up of the hijackers: mannerisms, type of weapons carried, conversation, any names that they use, etc. This may be of great importance to law enforcement after the incident is over.

If a hijack situation continues for longer than a few hours, attempt to do isometric exercises in your seat, to enhance your circulation, to reduce muscle stiffness, and to keep your mind off the incident. If you believe a rescue attempt is imminent, slide down in your seat. Cover your head using both of your arms and a pillow to avoid being injured if gunfire takes place.

If you are held hostage and you are wearing or carrying anything that could provoke or irritate the hijackers, discreetly remove it and get rid of it. Hijackers often collect passengers' passports in order to determine their nationalities, and having your passport protected in a leather passport case or cover may make its identity less obvious; this may be helpful if people from your country are likely to be singled out by hijackers from particular parts of the world. If you are asked questions by the hijackers, respond simply. Avoid saying or doing anything that might give the hijackers a basis for taking more than a casual interest in you. During the incident, attempt to seem uninterested in what is going on. Read a book, sleep, or do whatever is possible to avoid attracting attention. When occupied in this way, you will be less influenced by the events around you; hijackers leave people alone who are not a threat to them.

Kidnapping

In some parts of the world, kidnapping is a growth industry. Tourists and business travellers are normally not the target, but opportunist abductions have occurred when individuals have found themselves in vulnerable positions. The hazard is greater when continually visiting a risky area (thus setting predictable patterns of movement), and most importantly, standing out from the crowd. In South America, specifically Colombia, kidnapping for ransom is used by guerrilla organizations to fund terrorist campaigns. Kidnapping for political motives has also occurred in certain regions — militants may kidnap foreigners to gain political leverage during negotiations or to demand some other political concession.

For companies at special risk of being targeted, kidnap insurance may be worthwhile. Is there an alternative to visiting a risk area? If not, plan your travel arrangements with care, seek advice from one of the many specialist security companies, and keep a low profile: be the 'grey' man or woman.

Vehicle movement

Driving is statistically the most hazardous activity that a traveller will be involved in and yet it is the one that receives the least attention; 80 per cent of crime and political violence takes place while the target is in his or her car, or is in proximity to it.

Before you attempt to drive in a foreign environment, ensure that you are fully conversant with local road-safety regulations, if there are any, and have all necessary documentation with you, such as an international driving licence and insurance certificates. If possible, ensure that someone else does the driving. If there is an accident, let the local driver sort it out. A cursory check of any vehicle will inform you of its roadworthiness. Are the tyres bald? Is there a spare tyre and tool kit? Is there sufficient water in the radiator? Does the vehicle have sufficient oil and petrol? Is the driver reliable? If you are not happy with any of these, then change the vehicle.

When driving in hostile environments, or even in heavy traffic, ensure that the windows remain closed and the doors locked. Even as a passenger, you should know the routes and have a good map of the city. When getting into a vehicle, notice what is going on around you. Always fasten your seat belt, and keep doors locked and windows up. When travelling in a car as a passenger, always keep your valuables or briefcase on the floor, to make them less visible and less vulnerable. If possible, never stop in an unknown area and respond only to genuine security force instructions. Do not pick up hitchhikers or allow your driver to pick up so-called friends. Park the vehicle in a well-lit area and never leave any valuables visible in an unattended vehicle. Ensure that drivers do not leave the vehicle unattended at any time; if they must leave the vehicle, it should always be locked.

If travelling by taxi, always travel with a colleague and use authorized taxis. Do not hail a taxi in the street and if the cab is arranged by someone else, ask for the colour, make, number, and cab driver's name. When a pre-booked cab arrives, ask the driver for his details — not the other way around. Always take the back seat and ensure that the driver drops you off in a busy, well-illuminated place. Don't get into a vehicle if you have an uncomfortable feeling about the situation or if you were expecting a particular driver and another arrives whom you do not recognize. Attempt to establish rapport with your driver. Do not buy merchandise from street vendors; do not offer money to the poor when the vehicle is at a stop light; and do not pay to have the car's windows washed. All of these situations can escalate into serious crime and increase your risk.

If you are confronted with a 'car-jacking', keep your hands visible and surrender the car to the criminal. Do not argue with the criminal.

When using public transport, ensure that you have a travel plan and understand the system. Make sure that you know which bus or train route you should be on and which connecting routes are required. Travel in busy, illuminated buses or trains and try to sit near the emergency alarm. Be aware of displays of wealth and have your ticket to hand and not in your wallet. Do not appear ignorant or nervous, and always remain alert. Arrange for someone to meet you at the termination of your journey.

Summary of advice for travellers

- Most travellers have completely uneventful journeys.

- Security risks always exist in an unfamiliar environment.

- Be aware of how local people might interpret your appearance, behaviour, and presence.

- Plan your journey carefully. Use all available sources to obtain up-to-date information; consult recent visitors, travel guides, the Internet, travel information centres, the Foreign Office, etc.

- Keep a low profile. Don't draw attention to yourself by the way you dress, any display of wealth, behaviour, or manner — this might attract the interest of criminals or political radicals. In some countries, 'wealth' may be considerably less than you think. Be the 'grey' man or woman.

- Avoid being on your own: few travellers become victims when they are in the company of others.

- Be as unpredictable as possible in your daily routine: the plans of criminals and political extremists depend for success on being able to predict when their victim will be in a particular place at a particular time (hotel, office, walking/jogging route, etc.).

- If concerned about the security situation, ask yourself 'Is this journey really necessary?'

Altitude illness

Travellers are drawn to high-altitude places in ever-increasing numbers — Nepal alone now receives more than one hundred thousand trekkers from around the world every year. It can be easy to underestimate the dangers of altitude illness; deaths from these conditions are all the more tragic because they are entirely preventable.

Dr Buddha Basnyat is Medical Director of the Nepal International Clinic and of the Himalaya Rescue Association. He is Professor of Clinical Physiology at the Institute of Medicine in Kathmandu, and Consultant in Medicine at Patan Hospital.

Mountain climbers, serious trekkers, romantics sauntering through the foothills of the Himalayas, native porters, skiers in North America and Europe, pilgrims to high-altitude shrines, diplomats posted to La Paz or Lhasa, miners in South America, and Everest marathon runners have something in common: they are all exposed to the effects of high altitude and may be at risk from a potentially fatal but eminently preventable problem — acute mountain sickness, commonly referred to as AMS.

AMS consists of headache plus any one of the following symptoms to different degrees: nausea, tiredness, sleeplessness, or dizziness. It occurs at altitudes of around 8000 ft (2400 m) or higher, where pathophysiological changes due to lack of oxygen may manifest. Another term, 'altitude illness' is also widely used. This 'umbrella' term includes the benign AMS and its two life-threatening complications, water accumulation in the brain (high-altitude cerebral oedema or HACE) and water accumulation in the lungs (high-altitude pulmonary oedema or HAPE). These complications may follow AMS, especially when people continue to ascend in the face of increasing symptoms.

In keeping with the Jesuit tradition of painstaking documentation, Father Joseph de Acosta, a sixteenth-century Spanish Jesuit priest, is credited with having first described the effects of high altitude in humans. In vernacular Nepali, mountain sickness is called 'lake lagne'; in Sanskrit it is aptly called 'damgiri' ('dam' means breathlessness and 'giri' means mountain).

Those most at danger from complications are people who do not 'listen to their body' and heed the early warning signals of AMS. They can go on to suffer from HAPE and HACE, and may even die — a process that has been carefully documented in important autopsy studies performed by Walter Bond and John Dickinson during the 1970s in the old Shanta Bhawan Hospital in Nepal.

Chronic mountain sickness is an entirely different condition, recognized by Carlos Monge Medrano in high-altitude, long-term residents of South America during the 1920s. Such maladaptation is seldom found in the Sherpas or Tibetans, possibly due to thousands of years of exposure to high-altitude living. (South American populations are relative newcomers to high altitude.) The present discussion will be confined to acute exposure to altitude in short-term sojourners.

Acute mountain sickness (AMS)

If a participant on an Everest trek suffers from a mild headache and nausea at Namche Bazaar (12 300 ft, 3749 m), he might take an aspirin and wait for these symptoms to go

Table 8.5   Altitude of cities above 3000 feet

		Metres	Feet
Afghanistan	Herat	927	3042
Afghanistan	Kabul	1815	5955
Afghanistan	Kandahar	1055	3462
Algeria	Tamanrasset	1400	4593
Andorra	Andorra La Vella	1080	3543
Angola	Nova Lisboa	1700	5577
Angola	Sa da Bandeira	1786	5860
Antarctica	Byrd Station	1553	5095
Antarctica	South Pole Station	2800	9186
Argentina	Salta	1178	3865
Armenia	Gyumri	1529	5016
Austria	Badgastein	1086	3563
Austria	Seefeld, Tirol	1204	3950
Austria	St. Anton am Arlberg	1304	4278
Bolivia	Cochabamba	2550	8367
Bolivia	La Paz	3658	12 001
Botswana	Francistown	1004	3294
Botswana	Gaborone	993	3224
Botswana	Maun	942	3091
Brazil	Brasilia	1061	3481
Canada	Banff, Alta	1397	4583
Canada	Jasper, Alta	1061	3480
Canada	Lake Louise, Alta	1534	5032
China	Lhasa, Tibet	3685	12 090
Colombia	Bogota	2645	8678
Colombia	Medellin	1498	4916
Costa Rica	San Jose	1146	3760
Cuba	San Antonio de los Banos	2509	8230
Ecuador	Cuenca	2530	8301
Ecuador	Quito	2879	9446
Ethiopia	Addis Ababa	926	3038
Ethiopia	Asmara	2325	7628
Ethiopia	Diredawa	1162	3812
Guatemala	Coban	1306	4285
Guatemala	Guatemala	1480	4855
Honduras	Tegucigalpa	1004	3294
India	Bangalore	921	3021
India	Cherrapunji	1313	4309
India	Darjeeling	2265	7431
India	Leh	3506	11 503
India	Simla	2202	7224
India	Srinagar	1586	5205
Iran	Esfahan (Isfahan)	1773	5817
Iran	Kerman	1859	6100
Iran	Kermanshah	1320	4331
Iran	Mashad (Meshed)	946	3104
Iran	Shiraz	1505	4938
Iran	Tabriz	1366	4483
Iran	Tehran	1220	4002

Table 8.5 (*continued*)

		Metres	Feet
Kashmir	Gilgit	1490	4890
Kenya	Kisumu	1149	3769
Kenya	Kitale	1920	6299
Kenya	Makindu	998	3274
Kenya	Marsabit	1345	4413
Kenya	Nairobi	1820	5971
Kenya	Nanyuki	1947	6389
Kenya	Narok	1890	6200
Kenya	Tsavo	1462	4798
Lesotho	Maseru	1528	5013
Madagascar	Antananarivo	1372	4500
Madeira	Arieiro	1610	5282
Malawi	Lilongwe	1100	3610
Malawi	Zomba	957	3141
Mexico	Chihuahua	1423	4669
Mexico	Ciudad Juarez	1167	3830
Mexico	Cuernavaca	1560	5118
Mexico	Durango	1889	6198
Mexico	Guadalajara	1589	5213
Mexico	Guanajuato	2500	8202
Mexico	Mexico City	2308	7572
Mexico	Morella	1941	6368
Mexico	Oaxaca	1528	5012
Mexico	Pachuca	2426	7959
Mexico	Puebla	2162	7093
Mexico	Queretaro	1842	6043
Mexico	San Cristobal	2276	7467
Mexico	San Luis Potosi	1859	6100
Mexico	San Miguel de Allende	1852	6076
Mexico	Taxco	1171	3842
Mexico	Toluca	2680	8793
Mexico	Torreon	1143	3750
Mexico	Zacatecas	2446	8025
Mongolia	Ulan Bator	1325	4347
Morocco	Ifrane	1635	5364
Morocco	Ketama	1520	4987
Morocco	Ouarzazate	1135	3723
Mozambique	Lichinga	1365	4478
Namibia	Keetmanshoop	1004	3295
Namibia	Tsumeb	1311	4301
Namibia	Windhoek	1728	5669
Nepal	Kathmandu	1337	4388
Pakistan	Quetta	1673	5490
Peru	Cajamarca	2640	8662
Peru	Cuzco	3225	10 581
Rwanda	Cyangugu	1529	5015
Rwanda	Kigali	1472	4828
Saudi Arabia	At Ta'if	1471	4826
Saudi Arabia	Ha'il	971	3185

Table 8.5   (*continued*)

		Metres	Feet
Sikkim	Gangtok	1812	5945
Somalia	Hargeisa	1334	4377
South Africa	Bloemfontein	1422	4665
South Africa	Johannesburg	1665	5463
South Africa	Kimberley	1197	3927
South Africa	Newcastle	1199	3934
South Africa	Pretoria	1369	4491
Spain	Avila	1128	3701
Spain	Cuenca	944	3097
Sri Lanka	Nuwara Eliya	1880	6188
Swaziland	Mbabane	1163	3816
Switzerland	Arosa	1847	6059
Switzerland	Davos-Platz	1588	5210
Switzerland	Montana	1495	4905
Switzerland	St. Moritz	1833	6013
Tanzania	Arusha	1387	4550
Tanzania	Dodoma	1120	3675
Tanzania	Ifinga	1625	5330
Tanzania	Mwanza	1131	3709
Turkey	Erzurum	1951	6402
Uganda	Arua	1280	4200
Uganda	Fort Portal	1539	5049
Uganda	Gulu	1113	3650
Uganda	Jinja	1172	3845
Uganda	Kabale	1871	6138
Uganda	Kampala	1312	4304
Uganda	Lira	1085	3560
Uganda	Masindi	1148	3760
Uganda	Mbale	1220	4003
Uganda	Mbarara	1443	4734
USA	Albuquerque, NM	1620	5314
USA	Amarillo, TX	1099	3605
USA	Aspen, CO	2369	7773
USA	Baker, OR	1027	3369
USA	Billings, MT	1099	3606
USA	Bishop, CA	1253	4112
USA	Boulder, CO	1611	5288
USA	Butte, MT	1693	5554
USA	Carson City, NV	1448	4751
USA	Chadron, NE	1004	3295
USA	Cheyenne, WY	1876	6156
USA	Colorado Springs	1881	6172
USA	Denver, CO	1625	5331
USA	El Paso, TX	1206	3956
USA	Flagstaff, AZ	2137	7012
USA	Grand Canyon, AZ	2015	6611
USA	Grand Junction, CO	1481	4858
USA	Great Falls, MT	1119	3671
USA	Helena, MT	1180	3873

Table 8.5 (continued)

		Metres	Feet
USA	Hot Springs, SD	960	3148
USA	Laramie, WY	2217	7272
USA	Missoula, MT	976	3203
USA	Petrified Forest, AZ	1653	5425
USA	Rapid City, SD	970	3181
USA	Reno, NV	1344	4411
USA	Rock Springs, WY	2058	6752
USA	Roswell, NM	1117	3666
USA	Salt Lake City, UT	1288	4226
USA	Santa Fe, NM	1934	6344
USA	Scottsbluff, NE	1207	3961
USA	Sheridan, WY	1226	4021
USA	Twin Falls, ID	1264	4148
USA	West Yellowstone	2025	6644
USA	Yosemite NP, CA	1210	3970
Venezuela	Caracas	1042	3418
Venezuela	Merida	1635	5364
Yemen	San'a'	2377	7800
Zaire	Lubumbashi	1230	4035
Zambia	Livingstone	963	3161
Zambia	Lusaka	1260	4134
Zambia	Mbala (Abercom)	1658	5440
Zambia	Mongu	1054	3459
Zambia	Ndola	1269	4163
Zimbabwe	Bulawayo	1342	4405
Zimbabwe	Fort Victoria	1088	3571
Zimbabwe	Harare	1472	4831
Zimbabwe	Umtali	1119	3672

away. However, if the symptoms progress to vomiting and a splitting headache, he must assume that he is suffering from AMS and make plans to descend. It is amazing how many people in this situation ignore the dangers and continue to ascend with their friends, trying to blame their symptoms on poor fitness or 'flu. For some people, it's the high investment of time, effort, and money; for others, perhaps, it's peer pressure or reluctance to accept defeat. A further problem is that many in the burgeoning adventure travel industry are clueless about mountain sickness.

AMS may set in within hours to days of arrival at high altitude. The onset of symptoms is usually gradual, which is why it is so vital to watch out for early warnings. Does a person feel excessively tired? Is that person the last one to drag themselves back into camp?

What causes AMS?
AMS is caused by a lack of oxygen. Although the proportion of oxygen in the atmosphere always remains the same (21 per cent), as we go higher the 'driving pressure' decreases. The driving pressure depends directly on the barometric pressure, and forces oxygen from the atmosphere into the capillaries of the lungs. Reduced

driving pressure results in decreased saturation of oxygen in the blood and throughout the tissues.

Just what causes some people to suffer from AMS but not others is largely unknown, but there are clear-cut and important preventive factors that are now well established (see below). The exact mechanism (pathophysiology) of AMS has similarities to that of HACE.

High-altitude cerebral oedema (HACE)

Our trekker in the above example would probably go on to suffer from HACE if he continued to ascend despite the headache and vomiting; the symptoms of HACE are an extension of those of AMS. From fatigue, there is progression to lethargy and then to coma. Or there may be confusion and disorientation. A useful test is to see if the person can walk in a straight line. If he walks like a drunk or is unsteady, it has to be assumed that he has life-threatening HACE and needs to descend promptly with assistance. This situation is serious enough to justify immediate helicopter evacuation.

HACE is probably caused by shifts of fluid into the tissues of the brain. Reduced oxygen levels cause swelling within the confines of the bony skull. The resulting rise in pressure may *lead to lethargy and eventually coma.*

High-altitude pulmonary oedema (HAPE)

This disease may follow AMS, but often it may appear independently. The typical scenario would be a trekker who has no headache or nausea, but finds he has a harder time walking uphill, that he is out of breath on slight exertion compared with the initial days of the trek. There may be a nagging cough and he too may have ascribed these symptoms to a cold. He may be suffering from subclinical or early HAPE — a well-recognized entity. With further ascent this may progress to shortness of breath even at rest. Descent is now obligatory, or the outcome may be fatal.

Low oxygen causes the pulmonary artery to narrow and this results in exudation of blood near the smaller branches of the lungs (the alveoli). If the exudation continues, blood may escape into the alveoli leading to a cough with watery, blood-tinged phlegm. Such exudation, or 'water-logging' of the lung tissue interferes further with oxygenation. A popular, compact device called a pulse oximeter can measure the oxygen level in the blood simply and rapidly, using a sensor attached to the index finger. It can be very helpful in confirming if HAPE is present.

What is acclimatization?

Acclimatization is a state of physiological 'truce' between the body of a visitor and the hostile low-oxygen environment of high altitude. This truce permits the trekker to ascend gradually. (This is distinct from 'adaptation' — permanent change to the organism, perhaps over thousands of years, perhaps even at a genetic or evolutionary level, to facilitate survival at altitude. Scientists are trying to decipher if the Sherpas or Tibetans have made such an adaptation.)

For acclimatization to take place, the single most important step is *hyperventilation* — the trekker unconsciously breathes *faster* and *more deeply* than normal, even at rest, to make up for the lack of oxygen. However, hyperventilation also leads to loss of carbon dioxide from the blood, making the blood more alkaline and, in turn, depressing ventilation. However, 48 to 72 hours after exposure to high altitude, the kidney comes to the rescue and begins to excrete alkali from the blood to restore a more balanced environment in which hyperventilation can continue unabated.

Preventing altitude illness

There is little doubt that altitude illness is entirely a preventable illness: no one should die from it. For the past quarter of a century, one of the most important objectives of the Himalayan Rescue Association in Nepal has been to preach the gospel of prevention, from its aid posts in Pheriche, at around 14 000 ft (4250 m) in the Everest region, and Manang, at around 12 000 ft (3650 m) in the Annapurna region. There are four golden rules, plus some important general principles that should always be followed:

1. **Understand and recognize the symptoms of AMS.** Recent growth in adventure travel has made trekking at high altitude simpler and more accessible, with the result that more and more people who go trekking are ignorant of the basic facts of altitude illness.
2. **Never ascend with obvious symptoms.** Incredibly, I have known people who have hired a horse or a yak to go up higher when they were too sick to walk. This is courting disaster.
3. **Descend if symptoms increase.** It is amazing how striking and dramatic the relief may be with even a couple of hundred feet of descent. People with signs of HAPE or HACE have to descend.
4. **Group members need to look out for one another** (perhaps like the buddy system in scuba-diving). This rule gets broken with unfailing regularity every trekking season in the Himalayas, because people are just too determined to complete their trek, even if one of their party members is ill. A trekker with AMS, HAPE, or HACE will want nothing more than to be left alone, unbothered, at the same altitude — potentially a fatal option. There is no alternative but to bring the person down to a lower altitude, accompanied by a friend who speaks the same language.

Following a conservative rate of ascent

Going too high, too quickly, is the single most important cause of susceptibility to AMS. Beyond about 9000 ft (2750 m), the sleeping altitude should be no higher than about 1500 ft (450 m) from the previous night's altitude. The *sleeping* altitude, not the altitude achieved during the daytime, is what is important. Altitude sickness often manifests at night because during sleep the oxygen level in the blood may dip further. Many mountain climbers will have been to 14 000 ft (4250 m) or higher in the Alps or in North America, but few will have slept at that altitude. In the Himalayas, you do not have to be an experienced climber or use crampons to be able to 'hang out' at 15 000 ft (4550 m) or higher for days: easy accessibility to these altitudes makes exposure to AMS also much easier.

While ascending, every second or third day should be a rest day for acclimatization. 'Climb high and sleep low' is the dictum, but it is important not to exert oneself excessively in trying to fulfil this. The trekker should not be in a hurry in the mountains. The itinerary should be planned so that there are enough 'leeway days' in case more time is needed to acclimatize. Trying to do a high-altitude two-week trek in one week is always fraught with problems.

Avoiding excessive exertion in the initial days
Excessive physical exertion at high altitude makes one more susceptible to AMS. It is important to take it easy at high altitude, especially in the initial days.

People who are very fit, for example, marathon runners or those who carry very heavy backpacks, seem more vulnerable to AMS than others, probably because they push themselves harder. I once looked after a trekker who felt he could not break his morning jogging sessions despite a strenuous day of trekking ahead — even at 4000 m! The feeling of 'man against nature' may be greater in this fitter group.

Avoiding alcohol
Jim, a rock star, decided to 'whoop it up' with four bottles of beer, on arrival at 3500 m in the Everest region. He fell ill with severe AMS and needed to be helicoptered out two days later. He had been warned not to drink alcohol on the trek, especially while ascending. Alcohol may dehydrate the trekker but more importantly it depresses breathing or ventilation. Sleeping pills may have a similar effect.

Maintaining adequate hydration
Adequate amounts of fluid (about 3 litres a day) are necessary in the mountains — dehydration mimics altitude sickness and may even predispose to it. On the other hand, excessive water drinking should also be avoided as this may lead to electrolyte imbalances.

Maintaining a high-carbohydrate diet
A high-carbohydrate diet aids ventilation and efficient use of oxygen. The good news is that, in many high-altitude places, there is not much alternative: rice, potatoes, and other starch-laden foodstuffs tend to be the staple diet.

Drug prevention (prophylaxis)
Diamox (acetazolamide) may be necessary for people going on rescue missions at high altitude or flying in to high-altitude cities like La Paz or Lhasa. People with sulpha allergy should not take diamox, the primary drug for prevention, and further details are given below. A second drug, dexamethasone (see below) should also be carried, particularly if the destination is remote: this can be life-saving if HACE supervenes.

Treatment
Descent
Wherever possible, this has to be attempted. There is really no magic altitude to descend to, but the sick patient may suddenly feel something 'lift' and feel hungry.

This is the altitude to which the body is adjusted. Patients with HAPE need to descend slowly and with assistance: excessive exertion even during descent may increase the blood flow to the lungs and exacerbate the problem.

Oxygen

Lack of oxygen at altitude is the chief reason why people suffer from altitude sickness, so breathing supplemental oxygen is obviously going to make a difference. But oxygen is a hard commodity to come by in the mountains — cylinders of oxygen are not easily portable. When oxygen is available in cases of AMS, it should be used.

Drugs

Acetazolamide (Diamox)

This is the most tried and tested drug for altitude sickness prevention and treatment. Unlike dexamethasone (see below), this drug does not mask the symptoms but actually treats the problem. It seems to works by increasing the amount of alkali (bicarbonate) excreted in the urine, making the blood more acidic. Acidifying the blood drives the ventilation, which is the cornerstone of acclimatization.

For prevention, 125 mg twice daily, starting the evening before and continuing for three days once the highest altitude is reached, is effective. A recent article in the *British Medical Journal* suggested taking a higher dosage — 750 mg daily. Our experience in the Indian subcontinent has consistently been that 250 mg per day has been rewarding, while excessive dosage may increase the side-effects. However, the optimal dosage remains under debate.

Side-effects of Diamox are:
- An uncomfortable tingling of the fingers, toes, and face (called 'jhum jhum' in Nepali);
- Carbonated drinks tasting flat;
- Excessive urination;
- Rarely, blurring of vision.

In most of the treks in Nepal, gradual ascent is possible and prophylaxis tends to be discouraged. Certainly, if trekkers develop headache and nausea or the other symptoms of AMS, then treatment with Diamox is fine. The treatment dosage is 250 mg twice a day for about three days.

Dexamethasone

This steroid drug can be life-saving in people with HACE, and works by decreasing swelling and reducing the pressure in the bony skull. The dosage is 4 mg three times per day, and obvious improvement usually occurs within about six hours. Like the hyperbaric bag (see below), this drug 'buys time', especially at night when it may be problematic to descend. Descent should be carried out the next day. *It is unwise to ascend while taking dexamethasone.* Unlike Diamox, this drug only masks the symptoms.

Dexamethasone can be highly effective; many people who are lethargic or even in coma will improve significantly after tablets or an injection, and may even be able to descend with assistance. Many pilgrims at the annual festival at Gosainkunda Lake in

Nepal suffer from HACE following a rapid rate of ascent, and respond remarkably well to dexamethasone. Mountain climbers also sometimes carry this drug to prevent or treat AMS. It needs to be used cautiously, however, because it can cause stomach irritation, euphoria, or depression.

It may be wise to pack this drug for emergency usage in the event of HACE during a high-altitude trek. In people allergic to sulpha drugs (and therefore unable to take Diamox), dexamethasone can also be used for prevention: 4 mg twice a day for about three days may be sufficient.

Nifedipine

This drug is generally used to treat high blood pressure, but also seems to decrease the narrowing in the pulmonary artery caused by low oxygen levels, thereby improving oxygen transfer. It can therefore be used to treat HAPE; unfortunately, its effectiveness in treating HAPE is nowhere as dramatic as that of dexamethasone in treating HACE. The dosage is 20 mg of long-acting nifedipine, every six hours.

It can cause sudden lowering of blood pressure, so the patient has to be warned to get up slowly from a sitting or reclining position. It has also been used in the same dosage to prevent HAPE in people with a history of this disease.

The hyperbaric bag

This is a simple, effective device, made of airtight nylon; it is about 7 ft (2.10 m) long and looks like a long duffel bag. With the patient inside, the bag is inflated with a foot pump until it resembles a large, sausage-shaped balloon. There is a one-way valve to avoid carbon dioxide build-up inside, and it has transparent panels to assist communication with its occupant. (It is sometimes also called a Gamow bag).

The pressure inside the bag is 2 p.s.i., so the effect is about the same as bringing the patient down a couple of thousand feet. For both HACE and HAPE (but especially, in our experience, for HACE), the changes are usually dramatic within an hour. However, there may be a 'rebound' two or three hours after therapy and the patient may need to get in the bag again. Just like dexamethasone, this bag only helps to 'buy time': descent is still mandatory as soon as possible.

Other problems at altitude

Periodic breathing

An abnormal breathing pattern whilst asleep is a common occurrence at high altitude: short spells of an increased breathing rate alternate with brief periods when breathing slows down until it seems to stop (the medical term for this is 'Cheyne Stokes' respiration). It is a problem only if it makes the sufferer wake up repeatedly, breathless, anxious, and unable to sleep. An effective remedy is diamox, 125 mg before dinner, which counteracts the low oxygen dips during sleep that trigger the problem. Sleeping pills should be avoided.

Sleep disturbances
These are fairly common at high altitude but, in general, sleeping pills are best avoided. If one has to take them for some reason, they should be taken with diamox.

Upper respiratory tract infections and symptoms
Many people develop a persistent, bothersome cough and cold-like symptoms in the cold, dry air of high altitude. An anti-histamine at night (like Benadryl, 25 mg) may help suppress the cough. Antibiotics are sometimes useful, but keeping the head and face covered and breathing through a silk or wool scarf to humidify the air may also help. Many studies have shown that upper respiratory tract infections can predispose to AMS.

Peripheral oedema
There may be swelling around the eyes, fingers, and ankles at high altitude, but this may not indicate AMS *per se* unless accompanied by the symptoms of AMS. These symptoms without AMS usually require no treatment.

High-altitude syncope (fainting)
This is a well-known but harmless problem in which fainting occurs suddenly, usually shortly after arrival. Simple measures like keeping the individual in a reclining position and raising the legs are helpful.

Travellers with pre-existing health problems or conditions
High blood pressure: Blood pressure initially increases at high altitude due to the initial stress of low oxygen triggering neurohumoral changes. However, people who suffer from high blood pressure can go up to high altitude as long as this is well controlled and they continue to take their medication.

Coronary heart disease: People with a history of heart attack (myocardial infarction) and even those with coronary artery bypass grafts or angioplasty but with no angina, can trek up to high altitude provided they are fit and able to walk rigorously at low altitude. The high altitude does not seem to add any extra burden to the heart.

Epilepsy: Although seizures may be provoked by altitude, there is no convincing evidence that it is unsafe for well-controlled epileptics to travel to high altitude — though such people should always take their anti-seizure medications conscientiously.

Migraine: Sufferers may have more attacks in the mountains, and this may sometimes be difficult to distinguish from AMS. If in doubt, it is best to descend.

Lung disease: Also noteworthy is the limited observation that **bronchial asthma** is not exacerbated at high altitude due to the cold and exercise. However, it is prudent for asthmatics to carry inhalers and other medications. Obviously, people with **chronic obstructive lung disease** may be more short of breath, and travel at high altitude would be inadvisable.

Neck surgery and radiotherapy: People with **treated cancers** like lymphoma or tumours in the neck who have had extensive surgery or radiation treatment may be especially prone to AMS because of damage to the *carotid bodies* — tiny organs within the carotid arteries that sense oxygen and aid ventilation.

Diabetes: Diabetics on insulin should have a reliable glucometer to check their blood glucose regularly, but high altitude does not seem to cause additional risks.

Corneal surgery: People who have had non-laser surgery (radial keratotomy) to correct their short sightedness may run into problems at high altitude due to swelling of their cornea caused by the low oxygen. Such people tend to become more hyperopic (long-sighted) and should carry corrective lenses if travelling to high altitude.

Pregnancy: Pregnant women should not sleep higher than 12 000 ft (3650 m) as this may endanger the foetus. Additionally, high-altitude places are generally remote, making emergencies more difficult to deal with.

Children: Children do not suffer any more from the effects of altitude than adults. However, it is important that a child should be able to communicate any symptoms to a responsible adult, so that prompt descent can be arranged. It may therefore be dangerous to take to high altitude those children who are not yet old enough to do this.

Contraception: Oral contraceptive pills may predispose to abnormal blood clotting (thrombosis) at high altitude. The hypoxia (low oxygen), the excessive red blood cells (polycythaemia) in the blood, and the possible dehydration in this environment may already be other predisposing factors for thrombosis. Hence, it is best to use other forms of contraception at high altitude.

Other disease risks

Many high-altitude destinations are in developing countries, so it is important to be up to date with vaccinations against diseases like typhoid and hepatitis, to know about travellers' diarrhoea and its treatment, and to understand the other precautions described elsewhere in this book. Malaria is not a risk at altitude — transmission does not normally take place above 2000 m.

How long should you boil your drinking water? In one elegant series of experiments, it took 5 minutes to kill all of the bacteria under study at 60 °C, and at 70 °C the effect was instantaneous. Conclusion: heating your drinking water to a visible boil is adequate, at any altitude.

Conditions that mimic altitude sickness

Improving medical facilities in countries such as Nepal have made it much easier to distinguish between altitude illness and conditions that can produce similar symptoms, such as bleeding in the brain (subarachnoid haemorrhage), strokes, dehydration, and blood viscosity related problems like venous thrombosis.

Mountain porters

It is important to be aware that porters may be just as vulnerable to the effects of altitude as tourists. For your own safety, as well as concern for their welfare, it is essential to confirm with the trekking agency that your porter has been provided with proper clothing, boots, and equipment prior to the start of the trek. More information is available from the International Porter Protection Group, at **www.ippg.net**

Summary of advice for travellers

- Most of the problems of high altitude are totally preventable. With careful precautions, your experience in the mountains should be safe and rewarding.

Effects of climatic extremes

Tourism has now reached every corner of the globe, including those with the most inhospitable climates. Preparation, knowledge, and expertise are required to survive these visits. This following section is designed to give an overview for those with limited medical knowledge of medical problems encountered in extreme climatic conditions.

Dr Chris Johnson researched into the effects of cold on the human circulation while working for the British Antarctic Survey, and he currently surveys the medical problems that expeditions encounter world-wide.

By a mixture of physiological acclimatization and technological adaptation, native peoples have learnt to live in the harshest of environments on earth. Until recently, these remote areas were accessible only to dedicated travellers who generally had the training and experience to cope with the rugged conditions. Package tours can now, within a few hours, whisk any wealthy urbanite to the wastelands of Antarctica, the Amazon jungle, or the deserts of Mongolia. A healthy bank balance is no protection against the health, environmental, and zoological hazards that may then be encountered. One does not have to visit an exotic part of the globe, however, in order to encounter environmental hazards. The Scottish mountains and English fells annually claim victims of hypothermia, while heat stroke may affect long-distance runners anywhere in the world.

General considerations

Humans have been very effective at changing the world to suit their needs. An air-conditioned hotel provides the same environment anywhere in the world. This chapter assumes that you will want to travel beyond the limits of luxury. In extreme climates your life will then depend upon your knowledge and the equipment you use. Ensure that both are adequate. Carry appropriate first-aid, obtain medication such as anti-malarial tablets and sunscreen, and have a dental check before departure. Without transport, be it vehicle, skis, mule, or skidoo, you will be stranded, so make sure that they are in good condition. Take more food and water than you expect to use.

In a survey of expeditions, environmental hazards caused 14 per cent of all medical problems, while animals and insects caused another 8 per cent, but these two categories caused 40 per cent of the *serious* medical problems that travellers to remote areas encountered. Find out about the area that you are visiting, local knowledge is valuable, and you can be forewarned about specific hazards. Use guides in areas of high risk. Learn about the local wildlife. Insects are a serious problem both because they can cause skin problems and because they transmit malaria and dengue fever. Large animal attacks are relatively rare but can be fatal (p. 217); bites from smaller animals such as scorpions and snakes are common and can ruin a journey (p. 231). Dogs and bats may carry rabies. If you do have a serious medical problem you may need evacuation and this will be very expensive, so check that your insurance is adequate.

Environmental conditions

The weather conditions you encounter can be defined by four factors: temperature, humidity, wind-speed, and the amount of solar radiation.

Temperature

Humans regulate their body temperature very accurately, and even minor variations in the temperature of vital body organs cause a person to feel unwell. Serious variations may result in death. The thermoneutral zone for an adult — that is, the temperature at which an adult at rest lying on a hammock in the shade wearing scanty clothing, neither gains nor loses heat — is 28°C. Temperatures above 28°C, or any form of exertion at a temperature near to this value, mean that the body must actively lose heat to maintain a normal core temperature. At temperatures below this value, a resting adult will cool unless clothed or taking exercise. The lower the temperature, the more protection an individual needs. However, temperature by itself is a poor guide to environmental conditions.

Wind speed

Still air is a good insulator and body heat is retained. In hot climates air movement is beneficial as sweat can evaporate faster and the body can lose excess heat more easily. But in cold climates, if the wind blows away the insulating layer, body temperature falls. The combination of temperature and wind speed is described as the wind-chill factor (see Fig 8.3). High wind-chill conditions can cause very rapid heat loss from exposed parts of the skin and result in *frostnip* or *frostbite*, or chill the whole body, resulting in *hypothermia*.

Moisture

Water has approximately 30 times the thermal conductivity of air and moist air conducts heat much more rapidly than dry air. Humid environments are less

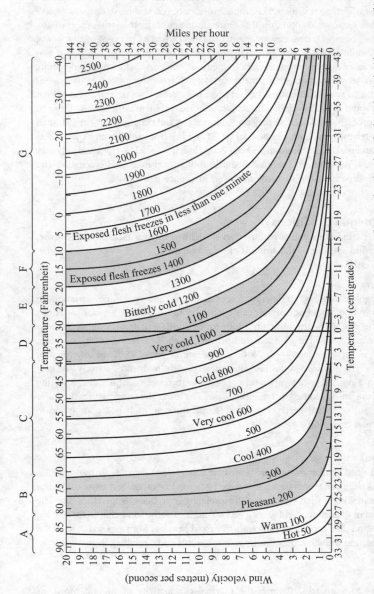

Fig. 8.3 Wind chill index. The Wind Chill Index is indicated by the point at which the air temperature (horizontal axis) and wind velocity (vertical axis) cross; record it at hourly intervals to monitor deteriorating conditions. Zone A: No danger. Zone B: little danger when wearing light clothing providing meals are regular and overexertion avoided. Beware of a sudden deterioration in the weather. Zone C: requires full clothing protection, waterproof shelter, hot food and drink, prevention of overexertion. In the UK, most deaths from hypothermia occur in this zone. Zone D: travel becomes dangerous on overcast days — sudden rain, sleet, hail, or snow can be hazardous. Zone E: Temporary shelter is dangerous to live in, travel should be contemplated only in heated vehicles. Zone F: Exposed flesh starts to freeze. Zone G: exposed flesh freezes in less than one minute, and survival efforts are required.

comfortable than dry conditions. In hot climates, high humidity results in sweat evaporating more slowly. Droplets often fall off rather than evaporating effectively on the skin surface. The cold dank conditions of a European coastal town in winter may be far more unpleasant to live in than the drier but colder environment of polar regions. Damp clothing loses its insulation and the wind cools quicker.

Radiation

There is always a difference between measured temperature in shade and sunlight. Radiant heat warms, but can also burn exposed skin. Near the equator, the effects of sunlight are obvious. Less obvious though are the effects of radiation at high altitude, where the atmosphere has less chance to attenuate the sunlight, and in snowfields, where much light is reflected off the snow. The glare of the sun in Antarctica can be four times that measured in an equatorial desert. Near the poles, the ozone hole magnifies the damaging effects of solar radiation, especially during the spring.

The Wet Bulb Globe Temperature (WBGT) heat index (see Fig 8.4) was developed to give an indication of the environmental hazards when the weather is hot, humid and sunny. It is calculated from measurements of dry bulb, wet bulb and black globe thermometers. Athletic event organizers and the military use the Index to judge how safe it is to exercise in hot conditions.

Climatic types

The combination of these four factors enables us to describe four extreme climates.

Hot and dry

Equatorial deserts have low humidity, little rain, scanty vegetation, cloudless skies, intense sunshine, and winds that vary from light breezes to violent storms able to stir up dust and sand. At night, clear skies allow rapid heat loss to space by radiation and convection, so there can be heavy dews and occasional frost. There is a wide variation in shade temperature with daytime highs of 55°C (130°F) and night time lows of – 5°C (23°F) in the western Sahara and – 42°C in the Gobi desert in winter.

Hot and wet

Tropical rain forest has shade temperatures typically in the region of 34°C (95°F). Abundant moisture, frequent cloud cover, and shade from the tree canopy combine to maintain the temperature at a fairly constant level throughout the year, with little variation between day and night. Humidity varies from 65 per cent during the day to 100 per cent at night, and breezes are rare.

Cold and wet

Large areas of the world, including most of western Europe north of the latitude of the Pyrenees are generally described as 'temperate', but this description can lead people to underestimate their hazards. Air temperatures between 15°C (59°F) and – 2°C (28°F) are comfortable in dry weather but may be very dangerous when high winds combine with rain, hail, sleet, or snow.

Wet bulb globe temperature (WBGT) heat index

$$WGBT = 0.7T_w + 0.2T_g + 0.1T_{amb}$$

where:
Tamb is the dry bulb temperature,
Tw is the wet bulb temperature,
Tg is the black globe temperature, made by ,measuring the temperature recorded from a thermometer surrounded by a 6-inch blackened sphere.

TEMPERATURE (°F)	EXAMPLE
Wet bulb × 0.7 =	78 × 0.7 = 54.6
Dry bulb × 0.1 =	80 × 0.1 = 8.0
Black globe × 0.2 =	100 × 0.2 = 20.0
Heat Index	82.6

Wet bulb reflects humidity. Dry bulb reflects ambient air temperature. Black globe reflects radiant heat load.

Modification of sports activity using wet bulb globe temperature

HEAT (°F)	LIMITATION
<50	Low risk for hyperthermia but possible risk for hypothermia
<65	Low risk for heat illness
65-73	Moderate risk toward end of workout
73-82	Those at high risk for heat injury should not continue to train; practice in shorts and T-shirts during the first week of training
82-84	Care should be taken by all athletes to maintain adequate hydration
85-87.9	Unacclimatized persons should stop training; all outdoor drills in heavy uniforms should be cancelled
88-89.9	Acclimated athletes should exercise caution and continue workouts only at a reduced intensity; light clothing only
90 or above	Stop all training

Fig. 8.4 Wet bulb globe temperature (WBGT) heat index and modification of sports activity using WBGT

Cold and dry

In these polar areas shade temperature rarely, if ever, rises above freezing (0°C or 32°F). Much of the land is covered with snow and ice. If the skies are clear there will be brilliant summer sunshine and a lot of radiant heat, but winds result in a sharp drop in apparent temperature and bring with them blizzards that can make travel impossible. Proximity to the geographical poles results in marked seasonal variation in day length.

Body temperature and its control

Human beings control the temperature of their main organs very precisely. The heat-regulating centre is in an important area at the base of the brain called the hypothalamus, which responds not only to the temperature of the blood reaching the brain but also to nerve impulses arising in the skin. Although the traditionally quoted value for normal human body temperature is 37°C (98.4°F) measurements of morning oral temperature in a large group of young adults gave a value of 36.7°C ± 0.2°C. There is a regular daily variation of 0.5°C to 0.7°C (about 1°F) and fertile women have an additional monthly cyclical temperature variation associated with their menstrual cycle. Usually the core temperature is kept constant by physiological and behavioural mechanisms, but it will rise if the body produces more heat than it can dissipate or if fever resets the brain thermostat. Core temperature falls when heat loss exceeds the ability of the body to generate heat. A shift of 1.5°C (3°F) in core temperature causes measurable disturbance to the ability of a human to function normally.

Surrounding the core heat-producing organs of the body — the heart, brain, liver, and kidneys — which are maintained at constant temperature, is a buffer zone or 'shell' consisting of limbs, fatty tissues, and skin. The temperature of this shell can vary considerably as can the rate of flow of blood from core to periphery and thus the rate at which heat is transferred. In a hot climate the shell will match core temperature, veins will be prominent, and the skin warm and flushed. In colder environments the temperature of the hands may drop to a few degrees above freezing, while the skin surface of the trunk may be 10–15°C (18–27°F) below core temperature. Peripheral blood vessels will be constricted with hands and feet pale and cool.

Heat production

The body continuously generates heat as a result of the normal metabolic processes of the body, with the rate of heat production increasing when a large meal is digested. Muscular activity, either voluntary exercise or involuntary shivering, generates substantial heat. Young children have an additional ability to generate heat in brown fat without needing to shiver, so called '*non-shivering thermogenesis*', and it is possible that some adults may retain this ability.

Heat transfer

Heat always travels from a hot object to a cooler one. Heat is transferred from the body to the environment, or vice versa, by radiation, conduction, convection, and evaporation.

All objects radiate some heat in the form of electromagnetic waves. If an object is very hot, this *radiation* will be visible and the object will glow. Most obvious is the radiant heat of the sun, but exposed skin will radiate heat to its surroundings. Our bodies are not hot enough to produce visible radiation, so we cannot see the heat loss from our bodies unless we use an infrared camera. But, in cold conditions up to half of all body heat will be lost by radiation.

Convection is the term given to the transport of heat by the motion of warmed gases or liquids. As a fluid is warmed it becomes lighter and so rises away from the heat source. Further fluid replaces that which has floated away and is in turn heated. As the heated fluid cools elsewhere it contracts, becomes denser, and sinks. In this way a convection current is established. Clothing will reduce convection from the skin.

Conduction is the transfer of heat from a warmer to a cooler object by direct contact. Metals conduct heat away quickly, water quite rapidly, while still air is a poor conductor.

Heat is required to turn a liquid to a vapour, the so-called latent heat of vaporization. If the skin surface is wet the *evaporation* of water will cool the skin. If body temperature is high and a person is sweating this heat loss is very desirable; if however a person is cold and wet after becoming drenched on a fell walk the same physical process will lead to hypothermia and is dangerous. The evaporation of a litre of sweat results in the loss of 2400 kilojoules of heat (equivalent to 325 calories per pint). High rates of sweating that lead to droplets of perspiration falling from the body are an ineffective cooling mechanism, only liquid in contact with the skin cools.

The amount of heat gained or lost by these four mechanisms can be modified by activity, clothing, shelter, and technological aids. In addition long-term exposure to extreme conditions can affect the way the body works, a process known as acclimatization.

Hot climates

Body temperature rises either if fever resets the central brain thermostat, or if metabolic heat production exceeds the body's ability to get rid of that heat. Body temperatures up to 40°C (104°F) can occur in fever and during exercise, but judgement and physiological functions are impaired above 39°C (102°F). When air temperature exceeds body temperature the body can no longer cool itself through radiation, convection, or conduction and must rely *solely* on the evaporation of sweat.

Body temperature usually rises if a person takes vigorous exercise. Long-distance runners in humid conditions may not be able to sweat enough to cool themselves and can then collapse from overheating. Accelerated metabolism with excessive heat production is also seen as a rare but dangerous result of sensitivity to certain drugs. The recreational drug MDMA or 'ecstasy' is best known for this effect, although other drugs including some general anaesthetic agents and strong tranquillizers can have similar effects.

Body temperature also rises if a person cannot sweat enough to cool themselves, for instance because of inappropriate clothing, dehydration, or salt deficiency. Heat stress initially causes a rise in both pulse rate and body temperature. More serious symptoms will develop unless the stress is lessened or muscular activity reduced.

Acclimatization

A person moving from a cool climate to a hotter area will develop alterations in body function that enable him or her to cope better with the heat. After acclimatization, a person sweats more readily. Changes to their circulation enable water to be absorbed in much larger quantities from the stomach and intestines, and transported more swiftly to the skin. The sweat glands produce more perspiration, are able to work longer without fatigue and retain more salt in the body. Depending upon the severity of the heat stress, and pre-existing fitness level, full acclimatization takes one to three weeks.

Most people adapt to a hot dry desert climate quicker than to a hot/wet jungle climate. This is because:

• The high humidity of the hot/wet environment is maintained by day and by night, and the higher this relative humidity the more difficult it becomes for sweat to evaporate from the body and cool it.

• Nights in the desert vary from cool to cold, so the body's sweating mechanism has some rest; this is not so in the jungle.

• Acclimatization in the jungle can be transferred to the desert, but someone used to the desert may need time to additionally acclimatize to a hot and humid climate.

Physical effort in the tropics is exhausting; the heart and circulation must both supply energy to the muscles and absorb and transport fluids around the body to allow sweating. Young, lean and physically fit people find it easier to adapt to heat and it is always worthwhile trying to improve physical fitness before an arduous trip. Thin people have a greater surface area to body weight ratio and so lose heat more easily, while fit people cope better probably because their sweat glands are used to getting rid of the heat associated with exercise.

Overweight people of any age suffer in hot conditions. A degree of acclimatization can be induced before travel by lying for an hour or so daily in a hot bath, or by taking regular lengthy saunas — adding steam to mimic the humidity of the destination. You should, however, subject your body to these heat stresses only if you are physically fit with no known cardiovascular disease. Many elderly people nowadays safely globetrot to remote destinations. If you have travelled before you will know your limits, but if you are not an experienced traveller, plan a gentle trip initially. Cruise ships, international hotels and air-conditioned coaches are relatively stress-free, but some guided tours that spend all day sightseeing using local transport can be physically taxing, and demand good stamina and general health.

Many larger buildings in the tropics are air-conditioned with moderate temperatures and low humidity. Air-conditioning significantly reduces overall heat-stress but will delay full acclimatization. Those working abroad should remember that a week working in an air-conditioned office does not acclimatize you to the conditions outside.

Thirst, salt, and water

People are bad at judging how much water they need to drink. Newcomers to a hot climate typically drink only three-quarters of the amount that they really need. You should drink water or watery drinks (beware of alcohol, which dehydrates) *beyond* the point of thirst-quenching. You are drinking enough if your urine is consistently pale in colour: dark urine or low urine output are signs of developing dehydration. If you do not drink enough, you may in the short term feel fatigued and develop a headache; while during a longer stay, you may form kidney stones, which are common amongst temperate climate visitors to the tropics. Children left to their own devices will become progressively dehydrated if they exercise in the heat; they must be encouraged to drink regularly.

Sweating causes loss of salt from the body, and these losses must be replaced. You can take salt tablets, but some people find these irritant, leading to vomiting or stomach upsets. It is preferable to take salt regularly both by adding it liberally to food and also by mixing it with drinks: the required salt concentration is one quarter of a level teaspoonful (about one gram) per pint or two level teaspoonfuls to each gallon. This concentration is below the taste threshold and must be accompanied by a mixed diet. Athletes planning long runs in unaccustomed heat need to learn about fluid and electrolyte replacement and drink adequate amounts of appropriate glucose/ electrolyte beverages before, during, and after the event. Sports drinks are a palatable way of replacing both energy and salts but, if you mix them yourself, never make the solutions too concentrated, as serious consequences can result.

A fit, acclimatized person can absorb and sweat up to 1 litre of fluid per hour, about twice the rate of an unacclimatized person. A traveller walking in a desert during the night should drink one gallon (5 litres) per 24 hours, while the unprotected daytime traveller needs about twice this amount.

Children

Children are generally quite happy to travel to the tropics, but are at risk of heat illnesses, particularly if their ability to sweat is affected. They should not spend too long in the sun and should not exercise vigorously for long periods until they have had time to acclimatize. They need to be encouraged to drink. Dehydration must be avoided and it is essential to give them an appropriate balanced electrolyte solution if they get an upset stomach. Use high factor sunscreens.

Clothing and shelter

Physiological acclimatization enables humans to live more effectively in hot climates, but the main reason that humans are so successful at colonizing a wide variety of environments is that they use technology in the form of food, shelters, and tools to help them survive.

Hot and humid climates

Buy lightweight clothing. Shorts and T-shirts are comfortable and appropriate in a resort hotel, but do not protect you from sunburn and may offend local cultural norms outside the hotel. Elsewhere, long-sleeved shirts and lightweight trousers are preferable. Select a material that you feel comfortable in: cotton garments have proved satisfactory for many years; nylon feels uncomfortable against the hot skin. Denim is totally unsuitable for tropical trekking, because it quickly becomes waterlogged and dries slowly. Travel clothing companies now offer cotton/synthetic combinations that suit some people and are easy to wash and pack. A hat protects you from radiant heat and, in the jungle, prevents bugs dropping onto you. However, up to 30 per cent of all body heat loss occurs from the forehead and scalp. Heavy or impermeable headgear will increase heat stress, so choose hats with care. In many equatorial countries the political situation is volatile, so avoid buying camouflage gear from army surplus stores; it could be dangerous to be mistaken for a guerrilla! Temperatures can drop at night, so pack a fleece pullover and a lightweight sleeping-bag as well as your mosquito net.

During rough travel, you should have two pairs of shoes: trail shoes suitable for coping with wet, slippery travelling conditions and camp boots suitable for work around camp and resting in the evenings. The trail shoes should be lightweight, have a protective toecap, and offer good traction both in mud and if crossing wet logs or river rocks. They should dry out quickly. Ankle protection, either with high boots or gaiters may reduce both the risk of snake bite and the number of animals getting into the footwear and settling on or in you. Properly soled, rubber wellington boots are useful around camp as your feet then stay dry. Thongs and open-toed sandals should not be used in the jungle because of the risk that parasites such as jigger fleas can settle and bore into your feet.

Shelters should keep off the rain and be designed to take advantage of any breath of air. Dig deep run-off drains around tents or shelters to ensure that heavy downpours do not flood the habitation. Bedding is best placed on some form of platform and surrounded by insecticide-impregnated mosquito netting.

Hot and dry climates
During the day, you should ensure that your skin is protected from the sun, using a combination of broad-brimmed hat, clothing, and sunscreen. Even apart from the long-term risk of skin cancer, tropical sunburn can be extremely painful and may hinder the working of sweat glands, thus causing serious illness. Choose materials light both in weight and in colour. While colour is not important for jungle clothing, in the desert a light colour will aid the body's heat balance by reflecting radiant heat away. The Arab head-dress, the khaffieh (a one-metre square of muslin) is very useful in a variety of ways: it can be wrapped around the face for protection in sand-storms or used as a neckerchief to prevent sunburn under the chin from reflected ultraviolet solar radiation. (See also Sun and the traveller, p. 331). Desert boots with thick crepe rubber soles and suede or canvas uppers are preferable. However, if you plan to clamber around the very sharp rocks found in some stony deserts you need much stouter boots. As in the jungle, desert footwear requires 'time off' to dry out. Shelter during the day should be designed to reflect heat; a double-layered construction with insulation between the walls minimizes the effect of solar radiation.

Heat illnesses

Over the years various terms have been used to describe heat related illnesses. Heat exhaustion, hyperpyrexia, heat-stroke, and sun-stroke all describe the range of symptoms associated with an excessively elevated body core temperature and a failure of the sweating mechanism to cool the body adequately. Investigations have looked at body temperature, fluid intake, and salt consumption. Despite much work, the fundamental reasons why a few people cross from the common malaise of heat exhaustion to the life-threatening condition of heat-stroke remains poorly defined.

Heat exhaustion

Heat exhaustion is the term used to describe exhaustion and malaise related to heat exposure in casualties with normal or mildly elevated core temperatures. Classically, heat exhaustion has been ascribed to one of three causes, water-deficiency, salt-deficiency, or anhidrotic heat exhaustion (anhidrotic = absent sweat), although these causes form a spectrum of physiological disturbance rather than different discrete illnesses.

Water-deficiency heat exhaustion occurs if you are unable to drink enough in a hot environment. Extreme examples occur in people stranded in a desert or adrift in tropical seas without water. The potential victim is thirsty and complains of vague discomforts such as lack of appetite, giddiness, restlessness, and tingling sensations. Very little urine is passed and it is deeply coloured. Lips, mouth, and tongue become so dry that speaking is hardly possible. Body temperature rises steadily, the pulse rate increases, breathing becomes faster, and the lips are blue. Hollow cheeks and sunken eyes complete the picture before the victim sinks into a coma and, if not treated, death.

Salt-deficiency heat exhaustion commonly occurs in an inexperienced newcomer two or three days after arrival in a hot climate. They will have been sweating a lot and may have had plenty to drink but taken inadequate salt supplements. Quite often, diarrhoea or vomiting hasten the onset. The body's salt reserves have diminished and the tissues that require it malfunction. Increasing fatigue is soon followed by lethargy, headache, giddiness, and extremely severe muscle cramps. The face and lips typically look very pale as the patient collapses, still soaked with sweat.

Anhidrotic heat exhaustion is a fairly rare disorder of sweating in people who have been in a hot climate for several months. The skin of the trunk and upper arms develops a rash of little blisters (called miliaria profunda) and the affected skin is dry when surrounding areas are sweating profusely. It is worst in the heat of the day — symptoms include fatigue, unpleasant sensations of warmth, giddiness on standing up, frightening palpitations, and rapid, sometimes gasping breathing. The face sweats profusely, and there is a frequent and insistent urge to pass urine, sometimes in larger quantities than usual. The disorder is often preceded by an attack of prickly heat (see p. 340). These seriously heat-intolerant individuals should avoid hot environments — either by travelling somewhere cooler, or remaining inside air-conditioned buildings — for at least a month, and then continue to exercise caution in very hot weather as another attack might progress to heat-stroke.

Treatment of heat exhaustion

Fully conscious victims of heat exhaustion must be cooled and rehydrated. Get them into shade, and if near civilization get them to take a cold bath. In remote areas, pour water over their clothes and fan them vigorously with anything handy. Give them plenty to drink, at a rate of a pint of water every 15 minutes. If it seems likely that the casualty is lacking salt, add salt to some of the drinks at a concentration of one level teaspoonful of salt per half litre fluid. Water, fruit juice or squash are preferable to carbonated drinks as too much fizzy fluid can cause abdominal distension and slow the replacement process. Continue giving them fluid until they pass urine. Subsequently they should not risk heat stress for the next two days and ensure that they continue to drink a lot.

If the casualty is confused or restless, they must be continuously nursed. Do not allow them to sit up or move as this may precipitate a fatal collapse. Try to cool them as fast as possible, using any available means. If they can drink, force them to take fluids even if they don't want them. If available, administer intravenous fluids. Ensure that they don't choke if they lose consciousness. Seek urgent medical assistance and try to arrange transport to the nearest hospital.

Heat-stroke

Heat exhaustion is common, but death from heat-stroke is rare. Most people, if they feel very hot will stop exercising, seek a cooler environment, and drink. If however physical circumstances, psychological pressures, drugs, or illness prevent this normal response, then a person is at risk of developing heat-stroke. Although they are variants of the same condition, two types of heat-stroke are recognized.

Classic heat-stroke affects elderly people subjected to prolonged heat stress. Continuously hot weather for several days gradually raises their body temperature until the victims lose their ability to compensate. Past heatwaves in large cities have claimed hundreds of lives from this cause. Babies or animals left in a sealed car on a hot day will suffer a similar fate, and the higher temperatures involved mean that death can occur in a matter of hours.

Exertional heat stress is a condition more commonly seen in young fit adults who exercise vigorously in the heat. Typically psychological factors — the excitement of a marathon race or the encouragement of an army drill sergeant — force them to continue exerting themselves beyond their normal endurance.

Numerous factors have been suggested to increase the likelihood of developing heat-stroke (Table 8.6).

Collapse is associated with:

- Lack of physical fitness, pregnancy, or obesity
- Continuous hot weather, both by day and night. In athletic events and during military training, the risk of heat-stroke appears to be related more to the climatic exposure of the victim on the preceding day, than to the prevailing conditions. Possibly people's poor ability to judge their fluid losses and the lingering effects of the previous days' biochemical changes associated with heat stress lead to this delayed effect

Table 8.6 Risk factors for exertional heat illness

Physiology	Conditions	Drugs
Age	Hot climate	Alcohol
Poor physical fitness	High humidity	Therapeutic or recreational drugs
Lack of acclimatization	Inappropriate clothing	**Psychological stress**
Obesity	Recent air travel	Peer pressure
Pregnancy		Overmotivation
Fever		

- Strenuous exercise (leading to excessive internal heat production) (Fig. 8.5)
- A fever
- Inappropriate clothing for the conditions — particularly windproof or waterproof garments
- A recent long air flight which may have lead to dehydration
- Use of prescription drugs, including cold remedies and diuretics. Overindulgence in alcohol or use of recreational drugs (MDMA 'ecstasy' or MDEA 'Eve')
- Premature return to activity after a previous episode of heat exhaustion, particularly in an unacclimatized person
- Any of the above in a person whose sweating ability is seriously impaired by a skin complaint or disorder.

In some studies it has been suggested that women are more likely to suffer heat-stroke, that some people may have a genetic predisposition to the condition, and that a person who has recovered from heat-stroke may be more susceptible to re-developing the condition in future. The evidence for these suggestions is not conclusive. Remember that if a person has a high temperature in the tropics, heat illness is not the only diagnosis. They may alternatively have an unrecognized fever-producing illness such as malaria, which needs appropriate treatment (see also p. 448).

Heat-stroke affects many body systems. The cardiovascular and respiratory systems will be stressed with a high pulse rate and rapid breathing. The victim will be confused, irrational, suffer memory defects, and their vision affected. They may develop a severe pounding headache and then lapse into coma. Unseen, their gut lining will be breaking down so that toxins from inside their intestines are released into their bloodstream, and there will be numerous biochemical abnormalities, most notably because their muscles also begin to break down. If they have drunk plenty they may still be sweating, but their skin may be hot and dry. Usually their core temperature, if measured by a rectal or tympanic membrane thermometer will be above 40°C, but a lower temperature does not exclude the diagnosis. Untreated, body temperature will continue to rise and death usually occurs once core temperature reaches 44°C, although survival from higher temperatures has been reported. Untreated heat-stroke kills at least 50 per cent of its victims, prompt and effective care reduces the mortality to 10 per cent, but it remains a highly dangerous condition.

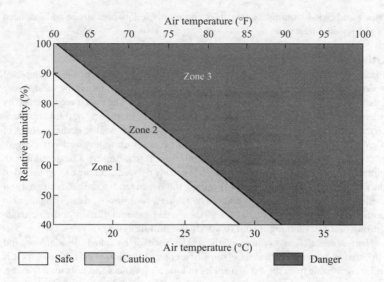

Fig. 8.5 Risk of exercise in hot humid weather

A key difficulty with heat-stroke is recognizing it. Victims are often confused and refuse help. They may even complain of feeling cold and shivering. Consider the circumstances; an athlete on a hot day is unlikely to be suffering from the cold, and it is more likely that they have a deranged temperature control mechanism.

Treatment

Rapid treatment is essential: this condition can result in death within two to four hours of the first symptoms. Victims require immediate cooling. The longer a person stays hot, the more damage their body suffers. As a first-aid measure, shelter the victim from the sun, remove all clothing, and cover with a wetted bedsheet, towel, or other lightweight material and start fanning to promote cooling by evaporation. Take water to the casualty, not the casualty to water! Drowning, infection, or a crocodile could all add to the victim's woes if immersed in a watercourse. Keep the coverings wet; fanning and wetting must continue all the way to hospital. In hospital, or at a base-camp or hotel more rapid cooling can be provided by electrical fans and cold water sprays. Where such facilities are available, for instance on army bases, immersion of the victim of exertional heat-stroke in an iced-water bath has been conclusively shown to be safe and effective. Rehydration is also essential. Fluids can be given by mouth if the patient is conscious or intravenously if the patient is comatose. The cooler these fluids are, the better. An unconscious person must either be nursed in the three-quarter-prone recovery position or, where facilities exist, have an endotracheal tube passed. Kidney failure and blood-clotting abnormalities commonly follow heat stroke and will need expert hospital treatment.

Other conditions caused by heat

Prickly heat or miliaria rubra (literally red millet seeds) consists of a vast number of vesicles or tiny blisters set in red, mildly inflamed skin, worst around the waist, upper trunk, armpits, front of the elbows, and even on the scalp. The rash is accompanied by intensely irritating prickling sensations. The cause is unknown, but an important factor is the constant wetting of the skin by un-evaporated sweat as occurs at times of high humidity in hot/wet climates. The skin becomes unhealthy and waterlogged, sweat ducts are blocked with debris, and infection starts, causing a large number of pimples. The itching prevents sleep, which is usually delayed until the coolest period of the night, around 4 to 5 a.m. Not surprisingly the victim tends to be bad tempered and inefficient. The prickling can be relieved by taking a cool shower, dab-drying the skin gently to prevent further damage, and then using calamine lotion and zinc oxide dusting powder. Clothing should be starch-free and fit loosely.

Heat oedema (heat swelling) of the ankles used to be called 'deck ankles' and appeared in passengers when their ships first entered tropical waters. Nowadays it is indistinguishable from the swollen ankles of long air journeys and lasts for a few days in the unacclimatized newcomer to extreme heat. The condition requires no treatment and will disappear as acclimatization progresses.

Heat cramps are common, especially amongst athletes. They are usually ascribed to sodium deficiency although other electrolytes may be involved. They are very painful, and occur at random intervals in whichever muscle group is being used most. Electrolyte replacement and rest will usually alleviate the problem.

Heat syncope (fainting) typically occurs when an unacclimatized person first arrives in a hot area. Initially their circulation is unstable, and they may faint if they stand still for a period, or if they standup suddenly. Sitting with their head between their knees or lying them flat will make them feel better. Rest followed by gentle exercise will prevent another faint.

Cold climates

People's idea of a 'cold' day varies and depends upon their activity, clothing, and previous experience. Any temperature below the thermoneutral zone of 28°C can result in a drop in body temperature if a person is injured, infirm, or elderly and the lower the temperature, the greater the risk of problems. Cold may cause either a fall in core temperature, which is defined as *hypothermia* when it drops below 35°C, or peripheral cold injuries such as frostnip, frostbite, immersion foot, or chilblains..

Humans who constantly expose their hands to very low temperatures develop circulatory changes that enable them to work more efficiently, but this mechanism apart, we have no physiological ability to acclimatize to low temperatures. Instead humans survive in the cold by dressing warmly and by the use of shelters — be they snow holes, huts, luxury hotels, or cars. The body burns food to generate heat and you must eat a lot to survive in the cold. The colder it is, the more you must eat and vigorous exercise such as cross-country skiing or manhauling a sledge in a polar climate means that you may need to eat two to three times your usual diet, say 5000–7000 calories (21 000–29 000 kJ) per day.

Wind is the greatest enemy in a cold dry climate. It strips away the thermal insulating layer of still air surrounding the body and from within clothes. The combined effect of temperature and wind is known as the wind-chill index and can be calculated from Fig 8.3. By assessing the present and possible trend of temperature and wind speed, a traveller can allocate the prevailing conditions to one of the zones on the graph, and then decide whether it is safe to travel away from shelter.

Moisture increases the rate of heat loss by conduction and evaporation from the skin surface while wind strips away the warm boundary layer of air that surrounds the body. In a cold wet climate accidental hypothermia may develop because clothing has been saturated by driving rain or by a fall into cold water. The wind-chill index takes no account of humidity but the approximate danger of wet clothing can be assessed by assuming that the perceived air temperature is 6°C lower than the indicated wind-chill temperature.

Clothing for cold conditions

Comfort and survival in the cold depend upon the clothes you wear and how well you look after them. Clothing should fit well and be built up on the 'layer' principle from the innermost air-trapping layers to the outermost windproof and/or waterproof coverings. Each layer must be larger than the one beneath it to prevent constriction and to preserve the cushion of insulating air. As many layers as possible should be made from materials that retain a high level of insulation even if they are damp. Synthetic materials such as polypropylene and fibrepile are superior to natural fabrics in this respect. Down jackets are superbly warm in cold dry environments, but provide little insulation once they become wet. Zipped garments, provided the zips are good quality, allow heat loss to be adjusted quickly and easily. Neck, armpit, and wrist openings are recommended as they permit ventilation by 'bellows action' so that water vapour from sweat can escape during hard work. Rucksacks can hinder the normal transmission of sweat through clothes and cause underlying garments to become saturated. Damp clothing must be regularly dried and aired.

Good outer 'shell' garments are vital. In cold wet climates they should prevent rain soaking into clothes, but allow sweat to escape. One technique is to use a waterproof poncho that prevents rain from reaching undergarments, but allows extensive ventilation around the body so that sweat can evaporate. A popular alternative is to buy clothing that includes semi-permeable materials such as Gore-Tex. Cheap fully waterproof PVC trousers and jackets are unsatisfactory as they prevent moisture escaping and undergarments become saturated. In cold dry environments the shell should be totally windproof, but allow sweat to escape easily. Clothing made from cotton Ventile or containing semi-permeable materials are effective.

In still air at 0°C a quarter of the body's heat production may be lost from the head, and this loss will rise substantially in colder conditions. The scalp and ears should be completely covered by a hat, while the neck and chin should be protected by a scarf.

Footwear must be chosen very carefully. Tight boots or socks impede the circulation and so increase the risk of cold injury.

In extreme conditions, mittens are more effective than gloves at keeping fingers warm but, whichever is chosen, ensure a good overlap of sleeves with the hand-wear, because a strip of frostbite on the inner side of the wrist is extremely painful. Always carry a spare hat and pair of gloves in case one pair is blown away. Below minus 15°C avoid wearing metal adornments such as earrings, studs, or metal rimmed spectacles. The metal can conduct heat away from the body and cause localized cold injury. Spectacles usually frost over in driving snow or if the temperature falls below minus 20°C and if you rely on lenses to see, you may find it preferable to use contact lenses. Goggles or glasses with protective side-flaps are necessary to prevent painful ultraviolet damage to the cornea — *snowblindness* (see p. 428).

Survival in cold conditions

In a polar climate, the contrast between the inside of a heated building or vehicle and its surroundings can be dramatic. A vehicle breakdown on a remote Scandinavian or Canadian road in winter may be life-threatening unless you have appropriate survival equipment. Adequate clothing, some food, and a snow shovel may make the difference between life and death. Skis or snow-shoes allow you to travel 20 times faster than you can walk on foot in deep soft snow. If staying in a mountain hut, rig a hand-line between buildings to ensure that you do not become lost if you need to visit an outside toilet at night.

Dehydration can be a problem in cold dry conditions, as newcomers may not notice that they are sweating a lot when they exercise. It is quite common for skiers to develop a mild form of heat exhaustion in the first few days after arrival in a cold area. As in hot climates, the symptoms are lethargy, headache, and cramps and the treatment is the same: keep drinking until one's urine becomes dilute. However, away from civilization, it can be difficult to obtain water in polar areas as most of it is in solid form. Melting snow or ice requires a lot of fuel. It takes double the energy to boil ice from minus 40°C as it does to boil water from 0°C. It is therefore tempting to drink water from a stream, but take care. Glacier outflow streams contain tiny ground-up particles of rock that can act as a powerful laxative, while many streams are home to beavers and other animals that carry giardiasis (see p. 46). Unless you know water is safe, it should be filtered and sterilized. In southern polar regions most animals are inquisitive and friendly; the same is not true in areas of the North, where some dogs may be rabid and bears may be hunting for a meal.

Children in cold climates

Children have a greater skin surface area relative to their body size than adults and can lose heat faster. They are prone to cold injury and are often not very good at looking after themselves. They enjoy rolling around in snow or snowballing, both of which lead to rapid heat loss. Inspect them regularly, ensure that they stay warm and that their boots are not full of snow. Take particular care when carrying small children in backpacks. You may be very warm carrying them up a hill, but the well-padded trussed-up babe may be silently slipping into a hypothermic state. In Scandinavia parents often tow toddlers in pulkas (sleds), but this practice is illegal in very cold weather (typically if air temperature is below $-10°C$ ($14°F$)) as there have been a number of tragedies.

Hypothermia

The most important harmful effect of cold is accidental hypothermia, defined as the generalized chilling of a person such that he or she has a core temperature of $35°C$ ($95°F$) or less. In the field, measuring the temperature of the mouth or armpit is useless. Placing a thermometer in the stream of urine is reliable, but requires a minimum of 200 ml of urine to be passed. Usually the only simple practicable method is to place a thermometer in a casualty's rectum. Special low-reading thermometers must be used as the usual clinical thermometer reads no lower than $34.5°C$ ($94°F$).

Hypothermia caused by falling in cold water will be *acute*, that is of sudden onset. *Chronic* accidental hypothermia typically occurs in cold/wet climates when a person is exposed to wet and windy conditions for several hours and runs out of energy to maintain body heat.

Acute accidental hypothermia

Falling into water colder than $5°C$ ($41°F$) is a great shock to the body. The victim gasps, shivers violently, curls up, inhales water, and may drown within five minutes. Some victims die immediately as a result of cardiac arrest brought about by the shock of freezing water on the skin and face. Others cannot swim because of intense muscle contractions and some simply inhale large amounts of water. If the subject is wearing plenty of insulative clothing, a life-jacket that keeps their head out of the water, has face protection to prevent cold water from splashing onto their face, and has been well enough trained to know to keep *perfectly still* in the water, survival rates improve. Approximate survival times for well-dressed and trained subjects are about an hour in freezing water; around three hours in water at $10°C$ ($50°F$); six hours at $15°C$ ($59°F$); and many hours at $20°C$ ($68°F$) (Fig. 8.6). Factors that accelerate the onset of hypothermia in water are increasing age; lack of fitness; liability to panic; lack of recent food intake for internal heat production; and the recent drinking of alcohol, which without food causes a severe fall in blood sugar, with immediate confusion and clumsiness.

If a casualty is rescued unconscious after 5–15 minutes in cold water, then it is probable they have inhaled water and drowned, and vigorous cardio-pulmonary resuscitation should begin. If he or she is conscious, but can talk only clumsily, or is incoherent and cannot answer questions, hypothermia is the probable diagnosis. Victims who have been in water for prolonged periods must be treated with great care as their circulation will have become disturbed by the hydrostatic squeeze on their body. Removal from the water can result in cardiovascular collapse and many cases of post-immersion sudden death have been reported. It is, however, vital to remove the victim from the water as soon as possible. Try to avoid constricting the chest with any harness and if possible keep the casualty horizontal. Once rescued keep the victim still, and protect them from further heat loss.

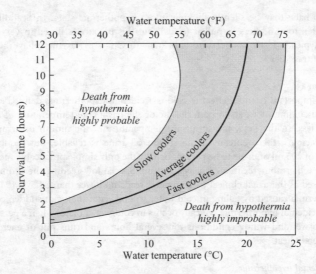

Fig. 8.6 Likelihood of death from hypothermia

Where possible, commence rapid re-warming in a bath (showers are dangerous as the casualty may faint and add a head injury to their woes) in which the water is kept at 40°C (104°F). Ideally resuscitation facilities should be available — collapse may occur at any time until the patient is out of danger. If rapid bath re-warming is not available the victim should be nursed in a warm tent or room in a bed with duvet, 'space blanket', or light blanket insulation only. A conscious victim will re-warm as a result of metabolic heat production if given food and fluids, but an unconscious victim must be provided with external warmth. Heat packs can assist re-warming, but must be carefully wrapped and positioned to avoid causing burns to a person with a poor skin blood supply. The supply of external heat by forced hot-air circulation systems, electric blankets, and the like requires hospital care, with intravenous fluids, oxygen, and injectable drug supplies available immediately.

Chronic accidental hypothermia
Chronic hypothermia affects otherwise fit adults walking or mountaineering in a cold and hostile environment. The direct cause is usually the combination of soaked garments with a high wind-chill, but associated factors include injury, over-exertion, and lack of food, spare clothing, tent or sleeping-bag. Mist, rain, sleet, hail, snow, and white-out may occur suddenly, and inadequate navigational skills, absence of map, compass, GPS, torch, and whistle help to compound the situation. It differs from acute immersion hypothermia only in its slower speed of onset and the fact that physiological derangement can be more severe.

Always be alert to the possibility of a member of a group developing hypothermia, as the victim is too exhausted to recognize that anything is wrong and may try to reject any help that is offered. In difficult conditions, a 'buddy system' — in which companions are paired off to watch one another — is desirable. Warning signs include complaints of feeling cold, tired, or listless; inability to maintain the pace, stumbling, and then repeated falls; unexpected, unreasonable, or uncharacteristic behaviour with unusual aggression; and failure to understand or respond to repeated questions or commands. Uncontrollable bouts of shivering which then cease, and disturbances of vision, herald collapse and unconsciousness with dilated pupils. The victim's pulse at wrist or neck may be irregular. In the unlikely event that 'body core' temperature measurement has been possible, it will have been about 35°C (95°F) at the start of the above list of signs and symptoms and about 32°C (90°F) by the time the shivering is diminishing. Death may occur suddenly at temperatures below 28°C (82°F). The sooner the following actions are taken, the better the outcome:

- Stop activity.
- Protect from wind, rain, etc., by rigging a tent, poncho, or other bivouac or shelter, laying the victim in the 'head-down' position if he is conscious, or the coma position if not, on a groundsheet, 'space blanket', or in a large polythene bag.
- Strip off wet clothing and insulate the victim with anything available. Ideally use sleeping-bags to cover the body and try to prevent further heat loss from neck, head, and face.
- If unconscious re-warm using the body heat of a companion — stripped and in bed or bag beside the casualty. If conscious, a hot sweet drink followed later by hot food will hasten recovery.
- Observe for cessation of breathing or pulse in which case mouth-to-mouth resuscitation and/or external cardiac massage must start.
- Send two people for help, but first give them fluid and food in case they too are affected by the cold conditions.
- Transport facilities should include an adequate number of helpers, and an effective method of keeping the victim warm and dry. If available, intravenous infusions and warm packs in the groin and armpits may improve the casualty's condition.

General comments
It can be extremely difficult to determine whether a hypothermic victim is dead or alive. They will look cold and blue and feel rigid, pulses will be very difficult or impossible to feel and the pupils may be fixed and dilated. The aphorism that death should be certified in a hypothermic patient only if they have started to fester is an exaggeration, but conveys the need to persist with appropriate resuscitation. Patients whose core temperatures has been as low as 9°C (48°F) have survived, as have the victims of prolonged immersion.

A person who has been even mildly hypothermic is likely to take several days to recover and will feel weak and exhausted during this time; they should rest. Profound hypothermia can result in serious damage to muscle and secondary damage to other body organs. Appropriate medical advice and early transport to hospital should be arranged.

Frostbite

In severe weather conditions, local chilling of exposed or poorly insulated tissues such as nose, cheeks, chin, ears, hands, or feet can result in the body-part freezing without the general chilling of hypothermia. The time required for the 'frost' to 'bite' depends on the degree of wind-chill and the amount of tissue at risk. If the air temperature is at –30°C (-22°F) and there is a wind, cold injury can develop in less than a minute. Downhill skiers and snowmobile drivers are at high risk of developing cold injuries on exposed parts of the head and neck. Frostbite of the hands and feet is more likely to occur if the blood supply to the periphery has been reduced either by general body cooling, dehydration, or tight clothing. Touching bare metal or spilling volatile fluids such as petrol onto bare skin can accelerate the process.

The initial stage of the process is *frostnip*, and experienced cold-weather travellers may notice its development as a transient burning 'ping'. More commonly, this warning sign is not noticed and a companion has to draw attention to the problem. The skin looks pale and waxy, becomes freezing cold, and feels hard. In the initial stages, affected facial skin can be re-warmed easily either by blowing exhaled warm air or placing a warm hand over it. The area should become painful and flush as the blood supply returns. Cold hands can be re-warmed by removing gloves and placing them in your own or a companion's armpits. Feet can be re-warmed by placing them on the belly of an altruistic companion. Never rub chilled areas with snow or massage them, because the delicate tissues will suffer more damage. If re-warming is successful, ensure that clothing is adjusted to try to prevent a recurrence and head for safe shelter as swiftly as possible.

If cold injury is not treated quickly, more serious damage will occur. Established frostbite is a very serious problem, particularly when it involves fingers and hands or feet and toes. Permanent and disabling damage may develop, although appropriate treatment can minimize this. A speedy but gentle journey to hospital is essential. Once frost-bitten tissue has thawed, up to three months of skilled medical care may be necessary; moreover, if tissue that has thawed is even slightly chilled again, it is liable to much more extensive damage.

If a foot becomes frozen in a wilderness area, there are three stages of treatment:

1. If the journey must be completed and no transport is available, it is possible to walk or ski to safety on a frozen foot, though NEVER on one that has thawed. Give hot food and drinks to maintain core temperature and correct any clothing defects. Give a painkiller, and, if available, an antibiotic such as a penicillin or tetracycline to prevent infection.

2. If you reach warm shelter from which it will be possible to evacuate the victim, remove the boot and sock as carefully as possible, cover the foot lightly with gauze, pad it with cotton wool, and wrap it up loosely. Make the casualty comfortable and warm, and immobilize the foot before setting off. Ensure that the patient remains warm during the transfer.

3. Once the casualty reaches civilization and medical help their limb should be re-warmed in water at 40°C (104°F); do not use hot tap water. The re-warming process will be intensely painful and a powerful painkiller such as morphine or

nalbuphine if available will be required to control the agony. Antibiotics, painkillers, and anti-tetanus toxoid should be given as soon as possible. Keep him or her in a room where a temperature of at least 21°C (70°F) can be maintained. Expose the injured foot to the warm air, wash it gently with a mild antiseptic solution such as warm 1 per cent cetrimide and dab it dry. Keep it elevated.

If the fingers and/or hand are frost-bitten, clean the skin area with the cetrimide solution and dab dry very gently. Separate the fingers with cotton wool after winding a sterile dressing around each, and place a thick sterile pad in the palm of the hand so that the fingers are in a 'glass-holding' position. Bandage the whole lightly and elevate the forearm in a sling. Commence a course of antibiotics and painkillers. Ibuprofen is recommended for pain relief as it both relieves discomfort and may reduce long-term tissue damage.

After re-warming the frost-bitten part will look dreadful, a mixture of black skin and pale- or blood-filled blisters. Any blisters that have burst will leak copious amounts of fluid and dressings will need to be changed frequently. Serious frostbite requires expert treatment, but if appropriately treated the end results of the injury are likely to look much less spectacular than its initial appearance. The patient should be encouraged and reassured.

Once a person has been frost-bitten the affected part of the body is always more likely to freeze again and special care must thereafter be taken to protect it against further injury.

Immersion foot (trench foot/pernio)
Immersion foot occurs when the lower limbs and feet remain in cold conditions for hours or days. Tight footwear increases the risk by impeding the circulation. The term 'trench foot' was given to this syndrome in the First World War and it remains commonest amongst military personnel who, under wartime conditions, are unable to dry their socks and feet regularly. White-water rafters have developed the condition after long trips on cold rivers. The foot remains chilled at between 0°C and 10°C (32–50°F) for several hours, and this causes damage to nerves and blood vessels but not actual freezing of the skin. After the first sensation of cold passes off, the feet feel numb, and this continues for the long period of immobility and restriction of blood that is a prerequisite of the disorder. The casualty may be unable to walk, or may walk with difficulty, complaining that it feels like walking on cotton wool. Inadequate food, general chilling, lack of sleep, and exhaustion complete the typical picture.

On examination, the skin is blotchy-white and the ankles are swollen and marked deeply with pressure ridges from boots and socks. As the patient warms up, and the affected area is dried gently, the feet become hot, red, and more swollen, and there is intense pain. The victim must be taken to hospital, and if this is likely to take time, should be treated with painkillers and antibiotics, as for frostbite. The legs must be elevated, protected from further damage, and exposed in a warm room. Blisters may form on the feet in the first two days or so and must be kept scrupulously (but gently) clean. Prolonged disability may result.

Chilblains

Chilblains are the mildest form of cold injury and are due to alternate exposure to wet/cold conditions and rapid re-warming. They occur more commonly in women and are characterized by changes in the colour of the skin and the formation of blisters or nodules on the surface of chilled parts of the body, which appear 12 to 14 hours after re-warming has occurred. These skin lesions may be very itchy or feel numb and tender. There is no specific treatment for the problems affected areas should be kept clean and dry and swollen areas elevated.

Other cold-associated conditions

Vigorous exercise in polar conditions (below –30°C (–22°F)) — for instance running, cross-country ski racing, or climbing at high altitude — can result in frosting of the lungs. Chest pain develops and blood may be coughed up. Tremendous exertion is required to overcome the extremely efficient heat exchange mechanisms in the upper air passages and this problem is likely only to affect athletes.

Sunburn and snowblindness

Solar radiation can be intense in polar areas, and its ability to burn the skin may be enhanced by thinning of the ozone layer. Radiation comes not only directly from the sun, but may be reflected upwards off the snow. The ultraviolet light can penetrate clouds and you may still be burnt on an overcast day. Always use high factor sun creams and ensure that the underside of your chin, nose, and cheeks are protected. Snowblindness is an ultraviolet burn to the cornea or front of the eye. After some hours outside the eye becomes initially itchy and then very painful. The lids become so swollen that you can no longer see and travel becomes impossible. The condition is very unpleasant, but can be prevented by using sunglasses that block ultra-violet light. (see also p. 350 and p. 428.)

Asthma

Very cold weather may precipitate asthma, and athletes in cold climates have been shown to be more prone to develop a wheeze. Those with known asthma should be cautious if suddenly going out into very cold air and may need to use more bronchodilators.

Infection

Very cold weather may increase the dangers of respiratory viruses. While the hazards are not at present fully understood, exertion during a viral illness is always potentially dangerous.

Cold urticaria
A widely distributed, itchy, pale rash covering parts of the skin that have become chilled is common as people re-warm after they come indoors from a day's skiing or walking on a cold day. The condition is harmless and generally does not require treatment.

Eye injuries
The cornea (front) of the eye can freeze in individuals such as skiers and snowmobilers who force their eyes to remain open in high wind-chill situations. The condition produces symptoms similar to those of 'snowblindness' caused by ultraviolet light. Re-warming and rest are the only treatments. Proper snow goggles prevent the problem and it is worth the effort of putting them on as severe injury may require a cornea transplant to prevent loss of sight.

Further reading
A superb summary of research information and treatment protocols for medical problems encountered in extreme climatic conditions can be found in 'Cold and Heat', pages 112–316 in *Wilderness Medicine*, fourth edition. ed Paul S Auerbach. Mosby 2001.

Acknowledgement
In previous editions of this book, this chapter was written by the late Col James M Adam and I acknowledge my debt to his writings.

Summary of advice for travellers

Hot climates

- Full acclimatization takes about three weeks.

- Thirst sensation is a poor guide to your true water requirements in a hot climate — always drink more than you think you need.

- Salt requirements are high — you should consider adding more salt than usual to your food and even adding salt to your drinks.

- Dress in lightweight, well ventilated, clothes, and ensure that your skin is protected from sunburn.

- Do not take prolonged vigorous exercise in the heat until you are acclimatized. Be especially cautious when exercising if the weather is humid.

Cold climates

- Weather conditions can change rapidly; make sure that you can reach shelter or have the knowledge to survive in the wilderness.

- Ensure that you are dressed warmly and have spare clothing in case of accidents.

- Victims of frostnip and hypothermia are usually unaware of their problem. Never travel alone and keep an eye on each other.

Sun and the traveller

A suntan can be considered both attractive and socially desirable, but obtaining one can have harmful effects on the skin, both in the short and long term. Understanding the circumstances likely to lead to painful sunburn, and to more permanent and serious damage — and avoiding them — can improve your trip.

Professor John Hawk is a Consultant Dermatologist at St John's Dermatology Centre, St Thomas' Hospital, London, and Head of the Photobiology Department at the St John's Institute of Dermatology. His research interests include the effects of sunlight upon all exposed skin, as well as the rarer abnormal skin conditions that may also follow exposure to sunlight.

The sun's rays have been this planet's energy source since its formation some four and a half thousand million years ago, since when they have initiated and maintained life, both by providing warmth and light, and by fuelling specific important biological processes such as photosynthesis in plants and the manufacture of vitamin D in human skin. The light and warmth the sun provides also improves the quality of life. Furthermore, despite the dangers described below, there is some, as yet unsubstantiated evidence, to suggest that mild ultraviolet radiation exposure can improve work performance.

Unfortunately, however, solar energy is not always useful to living tissues; in many circumstances it is also damaging. Well-recognized examples of this include sunburning, ageing, and cancer of human skin, and cataracts of the human eye; sunbed radiation can also have the same effects.

Other skin reactions, affecting only some exposed subjects, may also occur. As many as 15 per cent of UK inhabitants develop an irritating, spotty rash within a few hours of sun exposure, which may last for up to a week or so. This is **polymorphic light eruption** (often mistakenly called 'prickly heat'), and is usually a harmless condition, kept in check by avoiding strong sunlight and using high-protection factor sunscreens. Another relatively common, also abnormal reaction is an excessive sunburn-like response caused by the use of certain photosensitizing perfumes or cosmetics applied to the skin, or medications taken by mouth.

During man's evolution, skin responses have developed to protect to a greater or lesser extent against many of these phenomena, particularly the tanning and thickening reactions of exposed skin; these occur however only as a result of sun damage, and not before. Thus a tanned skin may give protection against the damage of further exposure, but unless already genetically present as in naturally dark-skinned people, its acquisition through sun exposure is always associated with injury, though less in those who tan easily.

If a tan, in spite of these negative factors, is still considered a social necessity, it should be acquired gradually, moderately, and carefully to minimize the inevitable accompanying damage and its unpleasant consequences, namely sunburn in the short term and skin ageing and cancer in the long term. Preferably, however, an artificial tanning preparation, perfectly safe although not protective against later sun exposure, should be used instead.

Effects of sunlight on the skin

The harmful rays

The damaging rays in sunlight are called ultraviolet radiation (UVR). Short-wavelength UVR, or UVC, is the most noxious to living matter but is completely absorbed by the oxygen and ozone in the atmosphere. Thus, if ozone should be sufficiently depleted by the effects of chlorofluorocarbons and similar chemicals from aerosols and other sources, as frequently pointed out as a possibility but not yet significantly occurring, some UVC (and more UVB as defined below) radiation may well penetrate to the earth's surface and lead to increased skin sunburning and cancer. Perhaps more important, it may also lead to the death also of much unicellular life with the likely consequent disruption of important ecosystems that help support our existence.

Middle-wavelength UVR (so-called UVB), strongest in midday midsummer and tropical sunlight, namely when the sun is high in the sky, also has a marked tendency to produce sunburn. This is generally followed by tanning in susceptible subjects and, less satisfactorily, by skin ageing and often cancer after chronically repeated exposure, especially in fairer subjects.

Long-wavelength UVR (so-called UVA) also burns, but at much higher radiation doses than UVB and UVC while tanning also tends to occur, conveniently just before the burning, although still with associated damaging effects. Thus, chronically repeated exposure to UVA also causes skin ageing, and may accelerate or even induce by itself the onset of skin cancer. UVA rays are the main component of UVR in sunlight but, because of their relatively poor absorption within skin, cause overall only about one tenth of the total UVR effect on skin around midday in summer and in the tropics; they are also a major component of sunbed radiation. However, since they are present for most of the day and year in sunlight, even when UVB is absent, they tend to cause continual moderate damage.

Circumstances leading to damage

The larger the UVR dose received from sunlight or sunbeds, the worse the skin damage induced. The amount of damage, at least from sunlight, thus depends on the time of day, season, locality, and duration and circumstances of the exposure.

The amount of UVR in sunlight, as stated above, is strongest when the sun is high in the sky, namely in the middle of the day in summer, particularly at low latitudes near the equator. If in addition one is at high altitude, or there are adjacent UVR-reflecting surfaces such as snow, shiny metals, white materials, or rippling water, or there is lots of blue sky visible, from which much of the arriving UVR is in fact scattered, the exposure dose will be increased further. Sunburning is therefore particularly likely on beaches, at sea, in desert areas, and on ski slopes, even in winter in the last instance.

Furthermore, the presence of cooling winds, haze, or light cloud, as well as swimming in cool water and the wearing of thin, close-fitting or loose-weave clothing, tend not to reduce UVR intensity significantly, if at all in some cases.

Individual susceptibility to skin damage

The damage caused by sunlight at times of high UVR intensity also depends on the type of exposed skin. Thus, genetically black-skinned people are well protected against most sunlight effects, while brown- and yellow-skinned individuals are several times better off than white people, though still burn if exposed for long enough. Most white individuals, on the other hand, burn relatively easily, particularly those with red hair and freckles, although some of course also tan fairly readily, if often with prior burning.

Most people know from experience how they react in summer sunlight and should protect themselves accordingly. So, if your skin is completely unable to tan (as is the case with albinos) or unable in patches (as in the disease vitiligo), special care is needed — although some protection still develops from superficial skin thickening. Nevertheless, no harm comes from careful protection in all cases, even in relatively darker individuals.

While the short-term effects of sunlight are most often a problem for fair-skinned sunbathers, as well as watersports, skiing, and other outdoor enthusiasts, its chronic effects, such as skin ageing and cancer, particularly the former, may occur in any white-skinned person, and many also with darker complexions, who indulge in regular outdoor activities or live in or near the tropics.

The effects of UVR exposure

UVR penetrates skin well, probably better when the skin is wet or oily, and damages the contained cellular DNA and membranes. Tissue may die as a result, while debris and chemicals produced during the process may also damage surrounding tissues, leading to the following short-term and long-term changes.

Early changes
1. Sunburn i.e. redness, soreness, and in severe cases swelling, blistering, and weeping of the exposed skin within hours of exposure.
2. Tanning i.e. formation of the protective brown pigment, melanin, in the skin over the days to weeks following exposure.
3. Hyperplasia i.e. thickening, also over days to weeks following exposure, of all the skin layers by cellular division, but particularly of the superficial, protective, dead horny layer.

Late changes
1. Photoageing i.e. degenerative changes in chronically exposed skin, apparent as a loss of substance and firmness, along with dryness, coarseness, irregular brown blotchiness, yellowing, and wrinkling; large blackheads, whiteheads, and small dilated superficial blood vessels may also be present.
2. Precancers and cancers i.e. persistent rough patches or irregular, steadily enlarging moles, lumps, or sores in chronically damaged skin; usually blackish, brownish, or reddish.

All these changes are responses to UVR-induced injury, but the tanning and hyperplasia are to some extent useful protection against the other damage reactions.

Thus, subsequent UVR from sunlight is partly absorbed before it reaches vulnerable skin targets, although the acquisition and maintenance of a tan and hyperplasia always result in at least some permanent injury, but less in those who tan easily.

The only other substantiated, potentially beneficial result of skin UV exposure is the production of vitamin D in the skin, but since adequate amounts are also available in the diet, and from minimal sun exposure in any case, UVR exposure for this reason alone is not justifiable. It has, however, been further claimed, as stated previously, that UVR exposure may improve work rate and indeed mood. However, any such change seems most likely to result from the visible portion of sunlight acting through the eye, and skin UVR exposure for this purpose is thus also inappropriate.

A final purported benefit of UVR exposure is, of course, the purely cosmetic, subjective, and psychological one of having a tan. It should be understood, however, that this has no known direct health-giving effect.

Preparation for a sunny holiday

You need do very little, apart from remembering the advice in this chapter and obtaining an adequate supply of high-protection sunbarrier cream (sun protection factor (SPF) of 15–25 times or so) of a type that suits you cosmetically. Check the label that such a preparation also offers good UVA protection.

Courses of sunbed treatment have ill-advisedly been advocated to give a prior tan and consequent protection against later sun exposure. Such protection though is at best mild, and is associated with the occurrence of some permanent ageing and pre-cancerous skin damage especially in the fair-skinned; in addition, there are other often annoying side effects of sunbed treatment such as itching skin, dryness, redness, and freckling, and occasionally, drug-associated rash, polymorphic light eruption, and a tendency to skin blistering, and lessened skin resistance to minor injury. The only reason for tanning of this type is therefore cosmetic, and the use of over-the-counter artificial tanning preparations on the skin, which are totally safe, is far preferable.

If, in spite of this advice, you are still desperate for a pre-holiday sunbed tan, exposures three times weekly (e.g. on Mondays, Wednesdays, and Fridays) for two to three weeks before the holiday should give your skin some colour if it is capable but regular use of a sunscreen when you arrive at your destination is still necessary because of the minimal protection usually offered by this type of tan. In addition, you should not undertake such a course any more than twice a year.

Effects of sunbeds

As stated above, most sunbeds have emitted principally UVA radiation in the past, although many recent models now produce much more UVB. Previously, as a result, they induced good tanning without burning in people who could tan well, but with relatively little hyperplasia from the UVA, such that the overall protection from any tan achieved was generally minimal, and other protection remained necessary. The output of modern sunbeds, however, more closely resembling that of sunlight, is likely to give better protection, but this cannot be guaranteed and other precautions are thus still needed. Nevertheless, whichever radiation they emit, all sunbeds lead to long-term ageing and a tendency to cancerous changes with constant use over the years, especially in the fair-skinned.

> If you use a sunbed, use proper eye protection and be careful when you stand up. A 31-year old woman died recently in the UK after a 20-minute tanning session; she hadn't worn goggles, missed her footing and stumbled down stone steps.

On holiday

Your intention on holiday in sunny climates or in snow should be to take full advantage of the enjoyable aspects of the presence of sunlight while avoiding the harmful ones. So, if you don't care about a tan, and preferably even if you do, aim for exposure more towards the ends of the day, when the UVR intensity, even in hot weather, is low. Otherwise, wear loose-fitting but tightly woven clothing, preferably cotton or similar, and a hat where possible; apply fairly liberally a highly protective sun-barrier cream to the exposed areas every hour or so when outside.

If however you insist on a non-artificial tan, and your skin is capable of producing one, you should start for the first day or two by exposing your unacclimatized skin to no more than about 10–20 minutes' sunlight per day when the UVR intensity is strong (namely when the sun is high in the sky), whatever the weather; in addition, you should apply relatively freely a moderately protective sun-barrier cream (say SPF 5–10) every hour or so, particularly after swimming or exercise. Over the next few days you can gradually increase your exposure, and if you must, and your skin feels comfortable, apply the sunscreen a little less frequently or change to a preparation with a slightly lower protection factor. At the end of a day in the sun, it is also worth using a moisturizing cream to help minimize any skin dryness or irritation. Nevertheless, this is not generally the optimal way to treat your skin if you really wish to look after it; for the best approach, the rules in the previous paragraph about taking care apply.

If you tan readily, however, and decide to do so, you should be fairly brown after about a week to 10 days, although increasing tanning may gradually continue for some weeks. Since most people initially burn easily on sensitive areas of the body such as the nose, lips, and very white areas, you should take extra care at these sites. Conventional high-protection sunscreens are generally effective for these regions, particularly as ever more effective filters are steadily developed, but thicker, over-the-counter creams and pastes containing zinc oxide or titanium dioxide are particularly good. Modern, cosmetically more acceptable, preparations of these are now widely available; they contain very fine (micronized) titanium dioxide particles and frequently offer maximal protection.

If you decide to wear very little, you will need to be especially careful with the pale, previously unexposed areas of skin, particularly again when UVR intensity is high. Once more, use a high-protection factor cream, most reliably one containing micronized titanium dioxide. If you ever start feeling uncomfortable and weather-beaten, however, cover up before it is too late and a severe burn ensues that could spoil your holiday, your tan, and your skin!

In general, with a little thought and care, you should have no major problems, especially if you expose mostly towards the ends of the day and cover up, or else carefully and regularly use today's strong sun-barrier preparations. If you must have your tan, you should acquire it using the relatively careful approach outlined above. On the other hand, carelessness and overdoing it during the first few days, perhaps inadvertently if the weather seems poor, will very likely lead to painful burning, swelling, blistering and peeling, a poor or patchy tan, and permanently damaged skin to increase your chances of later wrinkling, dryness, itchiness, and even skin cancer.

Sunscreens and tanning lotions

The regular, careful use of sun-barrier preparations (also variously known as sunscreens, suncreams, and suntan creams, oils, or lotions), as already discussed above, is a very effective way of protecting against many of the effects of UVR in sunlight, particularly since very high-protection factor preparations are now available. There are two main types of these preparations, namely absorbent and reflectant, as well as combinations of the two.

Absorbent sunscreens

These are the well-known, conspicuously packaged, and pleasantly perfumed oils, creams, and lotions available at pharmacists and other retail outlets. They act by absorbing much potentially harmful UVR before it reaches the skin surface and then dissipating it as relatively innocuous minor amounts of heat. Advantages are their cosmetic acceptability and efficacy in protecting against UVB, but negative points are the ease with which some dry or wash off (thus needing repeated applications), their occasional tendency to produce allergic rashes or to irritate the skin immediately after application, and their relative inefficiency against UVA rays, although many recently developed preparations now also give excellent UVA protection.

Reflectant sunscreens

These contain zinc oxide or titanium dioxide and reflect incident UVR back from the skin. Until relatively recently they were reserved mainly for medical use, although, being relatively effective against UVA, they were also available over-the-counter for thick application to areas such as the lips and nose, which are particularly liable to sunburning. Recent preparations, however, have been markedly improved by the incorporation of very small (micronized) particles of titanium dioxide; they are thus now suitable for most people. Nevertheless, they are still a little messier than many of the purely absorbent products.

The many sunscreens that are combined absorbent/reflectant preparations generally work very well and are probably the best choice for most people looking for effective high protection. Choose one with a sun protection factor (SPF) of 15–25 or more that suits you cosmetically. However, the one or two high SPF absorbent screens which themselves offer high UVA protection may suit you better if you can find one.

The efficacy of sunscreens can be gauged to a large extent by their experimentally estimated SPF; this value tells you by how much any skin damage is reduced during your stay in the sun if you apply the product regularly, carefully, and relatively freely every hour or so throughout the day. For example, a product of SPF 12 means your skin suffers one-twelfth the injury it would have received without the preparation in place. Attempts have also been made to give an indication of the UVA protection provided by a sunscreen, but no universally reliable method has yet been found; some approximate indication, however, is given on most product packs.

All SPF values are, however, approximate, so do not assume that a preparation of SPF 15 is necessarily much different from one of 13 or 17. In addition, cost is no guide whatsoever, so choose the cheapest product that suits you. You should preferably always use a preparation of SPF 15–20 or more, giving good UVA protection, whatever your skin type, but particularly if you burn easily. If you tan easily or are brown-skinned, you will certainly manage with lower values, but maximal protection of the skin is still achieved with the higher levels, particularly as far as the risk of long- term adverse effects is concerned.

Finally, it should be reiterated that sunscreens work only if applied liberally before exposure and frequently thereafter, especially after swimming or exercise, so remember this or they will prove useless in practice.

Tablets to protect against the sun, for example those containing beta-carotene or other vitamin A derivatives, have also been advocated at times, but have never been shown to work effectively. The added, very slight possibility of adverse eye effects with high doses means you should probably best avoid them.

So-called pretanning agents (more in vogue some years ago) are of little value, although the over-the-counter artificial or fake tanning preparations (referred to earlier) which stain the skin brownish for a few days, are harmless and usually provide a very reasonable colour. However, they provide no protection at all against later sun exposure, and the precautionary measures referred to elsewhere in this chapter must therefore still be used.

If you happen to get a spotty red, itchy rash when using your sunscreen, it is usually not because of the screen but because of so-called polymorphic light eruption (often colloquially called prickly heat), the annoying but harmless condition mentioned earlier. Cover up for a few days and use a higher SPF screen with good UVA protection when things have settled; if the trouble persists or recurs, you may need to see a doctor, perhaps a dermatologist, on your return home.

Cold sores may also worsen on sun exposure, so use a strong sunscreen on any susceptible sites. Melasma — a fairly persistent, blotchy, brown discoloration, most common on the cheeks — may occur too, particularly in women who use perfumed preparations on the exposed skin or are on the pill or pregnant; a very high SPF sunscreen giving good UVA protection will best reduce the chances of this.

Treatment

The short-term effects of sun exposure can usually be partially reversed; they also resolve spontaneously within hours to days unless extraordinarily severe. However, simple calamine creams or lotions may sometimes soothe burnt areas, and mild analgesics such as aspirin, paracetamol, or ibuprofen tablets, taken as soon as possible after exposure, may further relieve pain and inflammation. Steroid creams (obtainable only on a doctor's prescription, except for the mildest types) used frequently and early after exposure can be slightly helpful. Ibuprofen gel or mousse preparations may also be worth trying.

In addition, to minimize damage, do not sunbathe for two or three days after any burn, thereby allowing relatively full healing to take place. If you are unfortunate enough, however, to develop a patch of severe burning, treat it in the same way as an ordinary heat burn — keep it clean and dress it regularly to avoid infection. Widespread severe sunburn may, on the other hand, require plentiful oral fluids and bed-rest with painkillers, perhaps steroid tablets, and antibiotics; if very severe, hospital admission with intravenous fluids and other intensive care measures may be necessary. Some people have even died as a result of overdoing sunbathing as, for example, during a day out on a boat with a cooling breeze and soothing alcohol as distractions.

The delayed effects of constant sun exposure, once present, cannot be satisfactorily treated, except to some extent by aggressive dermatological surgery (particularly laser techniques) and, to a much lesser extent, by the regular use of moisturizers. In addition, the long-term application of preparations such as tretinoin (Retin-A) and so-called alphahydroxyacids have been advocated to improve skin photoageing changes, but the effects of these are at best mild, slow, and continue only as long as the preparations are used. Further, they frequently irritate the skin early on, while long-term adverse effects, although unlikely, have not been fully evaluated as yet.

Summary of advice for travellers

- Too much sun exposure, whether in acute or repeated lesser episodes over many years, is harmful to the skin.

- In the short term, too much sun exposure can cause pain, redness, swelling, blistering, and, occasionally scarring of the skin. Very rarely, extreme exposure can produce fever, coma, or even death. In the long term, dryness, itchiness, thinning, yellowing, wrinkling, coarseness, looseness, freckling, dilated blood vessels, and cancers of the skin are all possible.

- The best way of minimizing such problems is to avoid or protect against excessive exposure in the first place, rather than trying to treat resultant conditions once they have developed.

- UVR intensity in sunlight is highest in the middle of the day in summer, whatever the weather, and particularly near the equator or at altitude. Stay out of the sun at those times of the day, where possible, or wear a hat and cover up, using loose, tightly-woven fabrics. Use waterproof high-factor sunscreens, rated for both UVA and UVB, in ample quantity applied frequently; also wear good-quality protective sunglasses. And, if you have blue eyes, fair skin, and a tendency to burn easily, take extra special care — your eyes and skin are then at much higher risk of damage.

Hay fever seasons world-wide

Between 10 and 15 per cent of people suffer from hay fever — an allergy to air-borne pollen and spores. For sufferers, one pollen season a year is bad enough, but a repeat performance on your travels may not be an attractive option. Peak seasons vary between countries: a badly planned trip through Europe could take in the worst times for pollen at each stopping point, whereas a similar itinerary in reverse might be entirely problem-free.

Professor Jean Emberlin is Director of the National Pollen Research Unit, University College, Worcester. She is a geographer turned botanist turned meteorologist who has made a life-long study of patterns of pollen dispersal and has helped thousands of sufferers from all over the world plan their travels to avoid trouble.

The plants that cause hay fever have wide distributions, so if you suffer from hay fever in your home country, it is likely that the same or very similar plants that cause your symptoms will be growing at your destination.

In most of Europe, grass pollen is the main culprit in hay fever and pollen-related asthma. Grasses are almost ubiquitous, growing in virtually every habitat; individual types are often found throughout continents or even hemispheres. For example, a common grass in Britain, *Holcus lanatus* (which we know as 'Yorkshire fog'), also grows in Jamaica and Hawaii. As a group, grasses are closely related, so cross-reactions occur between the pollen of the different types. If you are allergic to one type of grass pollen, you will react to most of the others.

If you want to avoid having hay fever on holiday, the best advice is to either choose a venue which has low pollen counts all year round, or to time your holiday to miss the peak pollen seasons. The timing and severity of pollen seasons do vary in different climates and vegetation zones, so it is important to be aware of when the peak seasons occur in different places (see Appendix 9). In general, places that usually have low pollen counts through the summer are exposed coastal resorts with onshore winds, such as the Algarve and the west coasts of Britain and France. There can be problems with some central and eastern Mediterranean coasts such as the Adriatic, when local air circulations (like sea/land breezes) carry pollen from inland sources.

Grass pollen seasons start and finish earlier at lower latitudes in Europe. Typically, seasons in southern Mediterranean areas (e.g. south of Spain, Balearic Islands, South Italy, southern Greece) start in late April or early May. Easter holidaymakers in these locations can meet with grass pollen concentrations high enough to cause problems. The peak season comes in late May and June, several weeks earlier than in Britain. By July, the grass pollen counts are going down but may still be high enough in the first half of the month to induce symptoms. The second half of July sees lower counts in most of these areas.

The Mediterranean island venues are especially favourable because of sparse grasslands and more mixing of air from the sea. In contrast, inland areas can have very high pollen counts for grass during the peak season: the Po Valley, including Milan (May/June) and central southern France (May/June) can have severe grass pollen seasons. Conversely, Scandinavia has a later grass pollen season than the UK, with peak counts in July in many areas. Again, however, concentrations are lower near western coasts.

Tree pollen causes hay fever in about 25 per cent of sufferers. The amounts of tree pollen produced often vary a lot from year to year. Many sufferers do not realize what is causing their symptoms since they do not get them every year, as in the case of grass hay fever. Birch pollen is the second most important allergenic pollen type in the UK. In Scandinavia, Germany, Austria, and Switzerland, the concentrations of birch pollen can be very high. Birch ranks as the top allergenic pollen in Finland, Sweden, and Norway, where concentrations can reach several thousand per cubic metre (in the UK they rarely exceed 750). In Scandinavia, the season typically starts suddenly in late April and lasts only a few weeks — so it is worth trying to avoid it.

Cross-reactions

People who are prone to develop allergies may become sensitized to new types of pollen when abroad. For instance, olive pollen can cause symptoms of hay fever. If a person visits the Mediterranean area during the olive pollen season (May–June), they may become sensitized to it. No symptoms will be apparent on the first exposure, but on subsequent visits the person would have hay fever. Olive is closely related to ash and privet; the latter two do not usually cause problems on their own, but if a person has become sensitized to olive pollen (by being exposed to very high concentrations), they are likely to also develop reactions to ash and privet. Privet pollen counts are not very high generally, but hedge-cutting can create problems.

Tropical areas

Tropical areas have some pollen in the air all year round, but there are peak times, which can be avoided. For instance, peak times in Florida are April–October for grass, January–May for trees, and May–November for weeds. In the Caribbean, avoid October–March and June and July, as this is when grass pollen counts are high; tree pollen counts peak May–October; and weeds flower mostly between December and August.

General advice

If you are planning to go to a destination during the pollen season it is best to seek advice from your GP or pharmacist before you go and to take your medication with you. Availability of remedies varies a lot in different countries. Products may be marketed under unfamiliar names and it may be difficult to find (and explain in the local language) what you want. Also, take the usual precautions to avoid exposure to pollen that you would at home e.g. counts are usually highest early in the mornings and in the evenings, so do not do strenuous things at these times; wear sunglasses to keep pollen out of the eyes; change your clothes after being out of doors.

Although general guidelines to the timing of pollen seasons can be given (see Appendix 9), they do vary annually because of weather and local conditions. If the timing of your holiday is close to a pollen season, go prepared, and then check local information. Many European countries and the USA now issue local pollen reports and forecasts via radio, newspapers, TV, etc. There are also several useful web-sites (particularly for Europe and the USA) that give pollen forecasts:

- **www.pollenforecast.org** provides regional pollen forecasts for the UK from mid-May to August.
- **www.pollenuk.worc.ac** provides general information on pollen and hay fever.
- **www.cat.at/pollen/** gives current forecasts for the main allergenic types in individual European countries plus general maps of average seasons on a continental scale.
- **www.pollen.com/** provides current pollen forecasts for the main allergenic pollens in all areas of the USA.

Summary of pollen seasons in main destinations

Pollen seasons vary with climate, local vegetation, and topography. The information given in Appendix 9 can be used as a guide to good places for pollen-free holidays. There may be slight differences in the timing of pollen seasons from year to year, depending on the weather, but the main seasons are unlikely to differ much from the 'averages'.

Symptoms of seasonal allergic rhinitis may be due to pollen from various different types of plants and fungi. Grass is the main culprit in most areas but trees, weeds, and crops can cause problems. In order to identify a suitable pollen-free or spore-free area, it is important to know which pollen types a person is allergic to. The information given in Appendix 9 is intended as a general guide. Abnormal weather, local conditions, or other factors can cause deviations from the anticipated pollen seasons, so total freedom from pollen and spores cannot be guaranteed.

If you suffer from other allergies

DO

- Travel with anti-histamines and an allergy kit
- Carry a note of the local names of anything you might be allergic to
- Stick to simple foods without sauces or dressings, if you suffer from food allergies
- Find out when the local hay fever season is
- Make sure your travelling companion knows how to help you

DON'T

- Assume you are immune if you have never had problems
- Touch strange plants when you travel
- Carry on taking any medication that might be causing a photosensitive reaction (pp. 416–18)

Summary of advice for travellers

- Choose your destination wisely e.g. a beach where the breeze comes in from the sea; the windward side of an island. Alpine resorts are also suitable — they have very short pollen seasons

- Many tropical areas have vegetation that does not rely on wind pollination (e.g. jungle vegetation is insect-pollinated); that is why many tropical destinations are problem-free

- For temperate climates, avoid late spring and early summer; for the tropics, the worst time of year tends to be immediately after the rainy season

- Avoid countryside with open meadows and well-developed agriculture

- Shower and change your clothes after going outdoors; your clothes and hair can trap pollen which will give trouble later

- The pollen count tends to be highest late mornings and evenings on warm, dry days; avoid parks, gardens, and open spaces at these times

- Keep the windows closed when driving

Yachting and sailing: 'nautical tourism'

Increasing numbers of people choose to spend their leisure time at sea — an isolated environment with limited options for medical care. Careful preparation, an understanding of preventive measures and basic medical skills, and an extensive knowledge of safety procedures on board are essential requirements for safety and success.

Dr Nebojša Nikolić is the author of the *Adriatic Nautical Academy Medical Manual* and Lecturer in Maritime Medicine at the College of Maritime Studies, Rijeka, Croatia. He is an experienced sailor, official physician of the Croatian national sailing teams, and a member of the International Society of Travel Medicine, the International Maritime Health Association, the Royal Institute of Public Health and Hygiene, and the Society of Public Health.

All over the world, the popularity of sailing is increasing. Some regions of the world like the Caribbean islands, Australia, New Zealand, the North American coast, and Europe (particularly the Mediterranean basin), are especially popular sailing areas, and the number of 'nautical tourists' world-wide now runs into millions (there are an estimated two million in the Mediterranean alone, every year).

Sailing is one of the most beautiful experiences that nature can offer, but for some people, the cost has been high: injury, illness, and loss of life. Almost always, the problems are foreseeable and preventable.

Background

People usually sail cruising or racing yachts, 7–12 metres long and with between four and eight people on board. Although basic sailing manoeuvres are simple, sailing can be a demanding and complicated task that requires prompt and precise actions in many situations. It also requires a good knowledge of navigation, meteorology, and safety procedures on the sea.

Nautical tourists sailing their own boats are usually better trained in the full range of sailing procedures, but the majority of sailing tourists nowadays rent their boats from chartering companies. They tend to be much less experienced — perhaps not surprising considering that they may spend only 7–10 days at sea every year. Another serious problem is the quality of their training: the only proof of their competence when renting a boat is the licence they bring with them, but to get a licence for a sailing boat, you don't even have to know how to sail! The licence for a small motor boat is the same as the one for a 12-metre sailing boat; in most countries, licensing authorities do not require any demonstration of sailing capabilities before issuing one. Many charter companies make no checks on qualifications and sailing skills.

Competent or not, the majority of nautical tourists sail mainly in coastal waters (and sometimes also under ocean traffic conditions); it is this that distinguishes their medical problems from those of other tourists — though of course, the medical needs of the sailing tourist, whilst ashore, are the same as for the rest of the tourist population.

Environmental problems and other stress factors

Sudden temperature changes and the effects of humidity, wind, rain, fog, strong solar radiation, and other macroclimatic factors, have a greater effect on board seagoing vessels than elsewhere, and heavy storms during sailing easily endanger the life of the whole crew.

Hot climates

Most nautical tourists go cruising in the summer months, when temperatures are high. This can become a problem, especially for those coming from cooler areas. Acclimatization to a hot climate takes time, but many tourists charter their boats only for 7–14 days. With incomplete acclimatization, physical and mental performance suffers, which can be extremely dangerous under sailing conditions. Under conditions of heat or cold, extreme overstressing of the circulatory system can lead to heart failure. Obesity, lack of fitness, lack of exercise, difficulty adapting to an enclosed space, lack of sleep, stress, psychological instability, and, finally, abuse of alcohol, nicotine, and drugs, are factors that may complicate the situation.

The skin problems associated with hot, moist conditions (like 'prickly heat'), are well-known to sailors (p. 340); and sea water itself can cause problems — 'sea water boils' appear when permanent wetness allows bacteria that normally inhabit the skin surface to penetrate to deeper layers. 'Immersion foot' not only results from war conditions in the trenches but can also be a problem for unlucky sailors who are forced to spend a long time in wet shoes, under bad weather conditions.

Cold climates

Sailing in a cool or cold environment is also popular. With modern sailing gear, heavy weather conditions pose no problem — though charter tourists are not always prepared to pay the cost of such equipment.

On the water, a foolhardy approach to the cold decreases comfort and impairs performance. Though this may not directly place life in peril, impaired performance can certainly contribute to injury or inability to perform some vital tasks aboard.

At sea, one is constantly engaged in a real battle for survival. Even in waters at a pleasant temperature for recreational swimming, like 28°C, human life can be endangered with prolonged immersion. Sailors should have no excuse for not knowing how to keep themselves warm and must anticipate that in cold weather their efficiency will suffer. See also p. 343.

Submersion incidents

Drowning and near-drowning from falling overboard are a major risk for every sailor. It is not an easy and simple task to stop the boat when sailing or to perform complicated manoeuvres that will return the sailing boat into a position from which the victim can be lifted back on board. At night or in rough seas there is a high possibility that any victim may not be found at all.

Falling overboard a lurching boat in rough seas or being tossed over the side by a jibing boom or giant wave can happen easily. One can trip over gear strewn on the deck, lose balance on a slick deck, or be yanked off the foredeck if the leg is caught in a bight in the anchor rode. The unlucky sailor can fall off the boat while relieving himself over the transom — most overboard victims are found with their flies open!

Workload aboard

Sailing is probably the most pleasant and relaxing way of spending a holiday, but in bad weather, things can suddenly change, and heavy physical work can become unavoidable. Inability to shorten the sails in the storm because of physically inadequate crew can be disastrous, and what was a pleasant vacation can turn to tragedy in a few minutes.

The ship's movement can also cause problems. It not only induces motion sickness in sensitive persons but also reduces the depth of sleep, because of the unavoidable muscular compensatory movements. Probably 90 per cent of seafarers suffer once, or even several times, from motion sickness. This incidence is lower on small ships, but having a member of the crew suffering from sea-sickness in a storm and literally not caring that the ship may be capsizing, is just one of the horror stories that 'weekend captains' relate.

A further stress factor for crew members on long-distance sailing is the need to keep watch. Limited numbers of crew, or a habit of sailing only with family members, means that this problem can turn a pleasant holiday into an exhausting experience.

Nutrition aboard

Nutrition on board and problems connected with it are a significant part of the world's nautical heritage. Nutrition aboard cruising vessels is usually good, but if the weather is bad and distances are longer, food preparation can become almost impossible and the crew forced to eat only uncooked, cold meals.

Hot weather creates problems for food storage. Refrigerators aboard are typically small, and due to the need to save battery power, usually operate only when the motor is on (it is usually off when sailing). On a hot summer's day, food taken aboard can be easily spoiled and become dangerous to eat. Common problems also include abuses of alcohol, coffee, and tobacco. Excessive consumption of cold drinks can have an adverse effect on the gastrointestinal tract too.

Sailors often combine their sport with fishing, but even fresh fish can sometimes be dangerous to eat. Although there are numerous types of marine poisonings, the nautical tourist needs to be aware of three major types of fish poisoning (scombroid poisoning, ciguatera, and puffer-fish poisoning), and of course shellfish poisoning (especially paralytic shellfish poisoning).

Scombroid poisoning is the commonest type of food poisoning in sailing. The easiest fishing method in sailing is trolley fishing, usually catching blue fish. Unfortunately, people often leave the fish overboard in a sack in the water, to avoid unpleasant smells, preparing the fish only in the evening when the boat is anchored or moored. If the fish is not refrigerated, histamine is produced in the tissues, causing the symptoms of scombroid poisoning (see p. 68).

Ciguatera is another common type of marine poisoning and is confined to a circum-global belt (35°N to 35°S latitude), which includes some of the most popular cruising areas like the Caribbean (see p. 66).

Even when cooked, tropical *puffer-fish* can cause one of the most violent biointoxications (see p. 66). This fish can be found from 47°N to 47°S latitude and approximately 10 deaths occur each year following puffer-fish consumption. The best advice regarding them can be found in Judaic dietary laws (Deut. 14:910): *'These ye shall eat of all that are in the water; all that have fins and scales shall ye eat; and whatsoever hath not fins and scales ye may not eat; it is unclean unto you.'*

Socio-psychological factors

Socio-psychological factors can have a profound influence on the health of the crew. Everyone going to sea has his or her own set of goals and expectations. For some it is the personal challenge, while others are attracted by the sense of solitude. Everybody also carries aboard their own mental and emotional 'baggage'; their own style of decision making, of dealing with discomfort, of interacting with others, and of simply amusing themselves. Since we are all unique, it is difficult to predict how each of us would respond to the variety of stressful situations that can be encountered at sea.

When someone goes sailing with their family, they bring their home problems aboard. Under sailing conditions and with limited space, every problem soon comes to the surface. Everybody agrees that a two-man crew can be a disaster, unless the individuals are known to be well suited. With larger crews, things are easier, but they are not without their own stresses and choosing the crew is one of the most important decisions. Very often, the boat functions like some kind of group therapy with every conceivable problem becoming visible, but on board, this can happen fast, unexpectedly, and without any control.

Medical care at sea

The isolated marine environment poses difficulties for medical care; these are at their most complicated in off-shore sailing, but even in coastal sailing can be difficult.

Sudden illness or injury on board without the presence of a doctor can become a very serious problem. Chronic diseases brought to sea can become a problem too. Nautical tourists do not have to pass a pre-embarkation medical examination, like seafarers in the merchant navy; many of them are entering a stressful environment that can worsen their condition and endanger their life.

There is no doubt that coastal sailing makes cruising safer, but even under ideal conditions it usually takes more than a few hours to reach the nearest medical facility ashore. Weather conditions and distances can limit air rescue by helicopter, while rescue by boat arriving from the coast sometimes needs almost the same amount of time. Sailing under off-shore ocean conditions is, of course, incomparably more hazardous because of the long sailing distances and extreme weather conditions.

Radio medical advice

Although medical science has made significant advances during the last decade, there has been relatively little change in the approach to illness aboard an isolated vessel far out to sea.

On merchant ships, where there is no possibility of a medical doctor on board, medical help is provided by the captain or second officer of the deck, who has undergone some preliminary training, with the assistance of radio medical advice (from doctors ashore, who advise and guide seafarers through medical procedures). More than 300 coastal radio stations throughout the world provide that service. Modern satellite communications (INMARSAT) make this accessible virtually in every corner of the world where people sail (from 70°N to 70°S). It is free of charge and organized and co-ordinated within international conventions.

Similarly, the health skills required from the nautical tourist exceed the scope of simple first aid: preliminary training, a suitable handbook and medicine chest, and access to radio medical advice are necessary. The aim is to reach a level where the sailor can perform those tasks necessary to stabilize an injured or ill person, until professional help can be reached on the shore or can come from the coast. In off-shore sailing, the aim is higher: the sailor has to be capable of treating the injured or sick person for longer periods of time.

Medical training is not compulsory for getting a licence, but good sailing schools now offer special medical courses for sailors. There are a few medical manuals on the market, but the most comprehensive is still the official WHO/IMO manual, *International Medical Guide for Ships.* (see Further Reading) It is written for merchant marine seafarers and exceeds the level of sailing tourists' medical knowledge and equipment aboard — but it is still the best bet for any sailor.

International standards require every vessel to be equipped with a quality radio transmitter, vital for the security of the voyage, safety of life at sea, and the quality of medical help aboard. Under the new world-wide Global Maritime Distress and Safety System (GMDSS), the channel for automatic digitalized calls for help (DSC — Digital Selective Calling) is channel 70. If medical attention or advice is needed, the sailor is automatically connected by radio to a centre on shore with a designated doctor. After giving appropriate details and familiarizing the doctor with the contents of the medical chest on board, the sailor receives detailed and precise instructions on further treatment.

Telemedicine and remote diagnosis
New technology is making it easier for electrocardiograms, blood pressure readings, oxygen levels, and other important medical information to be recorded and transmitted by satellite to specialist centres anywhere in the world. Using this equipment is easy for unskilled people to operate, and is becoming gradually more affordable. Such systems make it much easier to distinguish a genuine emergency from a false alarm. An example of this technology can be found at **www.telemedicsystems.com**.

Medical chest
There are various standards for medical kits aboard and different countries have their own regulations, but the principal rule should be that it has to be co-ordinated with the manual and medical training of the person giving help. Again, regarding its contents, the best advice would be to follow the recommendations given in the *International Medical Guide for Ships*.

The medical chest itself has to be made of plastic, blow-resistant, and resistant to corrosion. The drugs in the kit should be divided into two groups — one to be used exclusively under radio medical advice (with no other instructions for use), and the other to be covered by instructions in the manual.

Injuries
The large amount of activity that has to take place in a confined space not only makes injuries more likely, but contributes to the difficulty of dealing with them.

Injuries inflicted by sailing gear
There are several routine tasks and pieces of equipment on board that can cause injury. Without a doubt, this includes windlassing, where improper handling of the ropes can easily lead to fractures of the fingers. Forces on the winches can be measured in hundreds of kilograms. Jib stays and cabin openings, especially the front cabin opening, are typical causes of injuries. Due to the heavy weight load liable to occur on sails, it is possible for the sail pulley to give way. The most dangerous injury in sailing is caused by the boom, from which a blow to the head could be fatal. This kind of injury usually happens when the boat is changing direction during sailing down the wind. Ropes can cause abrasions on the hands or, when manoeuvring the front sail, on the legs, when the sheet is pulled carelessly. A slippery deck can result in dangerous falls; and the chain, anchor, and 'travellers' on the deck can inflict injuries to the feet.

Even the inside of the boat has its dangers. As a rule, lighting below deck is poor and stairs can cause falls and injuries. The kitchen on a sailing boat is anything but a safe place, and cooking during sailing demands the highest attention and caution. Fire on board can occur all too easily, and there is simply no escape from it. Butane gas leaks and motor exhausts are constant hazards below deck.

Injuries caused by environmental factors

One of the commonest causes of disability — especially in places like the Caribbean — is sunburn. The risk is generally compounded by the cool breeze on the deck of the moving sailing boat, which removes the usual sensation of warmth — nature's warning system.

Injuries caused by low temperatures are rare in nautical tourism, but with the recent fashion of sailing to more extreme places like Cape Horn or even Antarctica, they are likely to become more common.

The open sea is one of the most dangerous places to be during a thunderstorm. Lightning is attracted to the highest object, and at sea this is the boat. It will strike the mast, the fly bridge, a metal antenna, or the sailor, and take the path of least resistance to the water. It can not only seriously damage the boat's electrical equipment, endangering further navigation, but can also injure the sailor. Lightning kills 30 per cent of its victims and maims two-thirds of the survivors. (see also p. 281)

Sea accidents

Sea accidents happen, and are usually caused by collision with objects floating on or below the surface of the sea or with rocks, by running aground, or — and this is every sailor's worst nightmare — by colliding with another ship.

Piracy

Sadly, private yachts are often targeted, and some of the worst trouble spots are shown in Map 8.2 (p. 299).

Injuries inflicted by dangerous sea animals

Swimming and fishing are part of yachting tourism; the nautical tourist can come into contact with marine life. Although most marine life is harmless, some can injure or endanger life.

The most threatening of these — a *shark* attack — is actually rare, but caution should always be taken. Fish such as *barracudas, dusky serranus, cog* or *conger eels, sting rays*, and *moray eels* can also cause uncomfortable injuries. *Single-celled organisms*, of which many are toxic, present a problem only when they appear in large numbers. Stings made by some marine life, like *sea urchins*, are dangerous because of secondary infections and can cause allergic and/or irritant dermatitis. *Starfish* and *bristle worms* can also injure with their venomous spines.

Of all the injuries caused by poisonous marine life, the most widespread are the ones caused by *cnidarians* (jellyfish and corals). *Fish* with their own poisonous thorns can produce serious poisoning. Some of them, particularly in tropical seas — like *scorpion fish, lionfish,* or *stonefish* — can cause death. In the Mediterranean and east Atlantic the most poisonous is the *Weeverfish* group. *Sea snakes, cone shells,* and *blue ring octopus* are also dangerous sea animals and their poison can kill (see pp. 231–41).

Before embarkation

The boat and the crew have to be in the best possible condition. Boats (the engine, tanks, rigging, safety equipment, radio, and electric and gas installations) have to be checked regularly before every trip. Aboard, the skipper is the one who is responsible for the boat and the crew, and so is the one who has to take necessary precautions.

1. *Determine the risk* Every skipper should determine the risk of the trip taking into account the sailing competence and experience of the crew, current health of each member of the crew, length of time before embarkation, destination, itinerary, length of stay, purpose (cruise or race), food, and water sources.

2. *Record keeping* It is important to keep records of any illness and injury aboard, especially medicine given, in the log. Also any pre-existing medical conditions should be noted and a general medical examination should precede all planned off-shore voyages of long duration. The medical background of every member of the crew should be made available to the skipper. Any member of the crew who is taking medication should bring sufficient supplies aboard, and this should be checked by the skipper.

3. *Immunizations* Immunizations and anti-malarial protection should be taken according to travel health advice from a skilled source, dependent on any possible ports that the boat will visit. Documentation of all immunizations should be brought aboard.

4. *Medical training* At least one member of the crew should have medical training according to *Model Course 2* recommended by the WHO (for coastal sailing) or *Model Course 3* (for off-shore sailing). The rest of the crew should have medical training to *Model Course 1* (corresponding to a standard first-aid course).

5. *Medical manual and medical chest* A good-quality medical manual and a proper medical chest must be kept on the boat. The chest has to be checked before sailing and its contents selected according to the level of training, number of the crew, and type of voyage.

6. *Physical condition and sailing competence* The skipper has to be sure that the crew is in good health and is physically competent to carry out all tasks that can become necessary during voyage.

7. *Proper rest* Before sailing off, ample rest is necessary. During the voyage, when organizing work-shifts, the skipper has to ensure that each member of the crew has enough rest and sleep.

8. *Food and water supply* Nutrition has to be planned carefully taking into account any weather delays that might make it impossible to replenish food and water supplies. Alcohol should be avoided.

9. *Minimizing the effects of the environment* Sun protection of the skin is necessary, especially for the first days of the voyage, as well as eye protection with sunglasses. Clothes should be of the highest quality to protect the body from cold and water. Sailing clothes today are made of hi-tech materials like 'Gore-Tex' or 'Polartec' which give needed heat and water protection, but allow perspiration of the body and free movement.

10. *Safety gear* A life vest and/or safety lines must be worn in every risky situation, such as during a storm or when a sailor is alone on deck, especially if automatic pilot is used. There have been many instances where boats have been found, running on automatic pilot, but with no sailor still on board. If children are on the boat, a net should be used on the railing.
11. *Electronic equipment* Radio and GPS should be checked regularly; a hand-held GPS running on batteries should be carried in addition to one connected to the main electrical supply. A magnetic compass in addition to an electronic one is a must. Radar is also strongly advised.
12. *Weather forecasts* These should be monitored regularly.

There is no doubt that sailing includes not only an element of adventure, but the possibility of considerable risk to life — perhaps this is part of its allure. For a growing number of enthusiasts, sailing offers the ultimate pleasure that nature can give; careful attention to the health and safety considerations outlined in this chapter can contribute greatly to its enjoyment.

Summary of advice to travellers

- Be confident in your sailing skills and experience.
- Be confident in the competence of your crew.
- Ensure that your boat is in perfect condition.
- Check that all safety equipment is on board and working.
- Ensure that you are competent in procedures of medical care at sea.
- Keep a medical manual and medical chest aboard.
- Ensure that you have a good-quality radio aboard.

Water and watersports

Travellers should prescribe themselves a large dose of caution to go with their sea and lakeside adventures on vacation — and should make sure that activities like scuba diving take place only in a safe, well-supervised setting.

Surgeon Commander Simon Ridout was formerly Principal Medical Officer at Royal Naval Air Station Culdrose, UK. He is an experienced diver, both for the Royal Navy and for sport.

Dr Jules Eden is a Medical Examiner of Divers, and also runs **www.e-med.co.uk**, a website that helps the traveller and diver with medical problems when away. He runs one of the busiest recompression chambers in the UK, which is based in London, and so has great experience in prevention and treatment of decompression sickness.

Many people consider water and watersports an essential part of their vacation, but unfortunately most activities involving water — from swimming to snorkelling, scuba diving, sailing, wind-surfing, and water-skiing — also involve some element of risk. Water in any form, from hotel swimming pool to river, lake, lagoon, or open sea, demands respect.

The old adage not to swim with a full stomach is correct, and alcohol is its most dangerous filling: as many as half of all drownings in the 20- to 30-year-old age group take place after drinking. People drink more when on holiday, but should bear in mind that mixing alcohol with watersports too often results in tragedy.

Swimming

Swimming pools, whether fresh-water or salt-water, require filtration and cleansing unless the water is frequently changed. If this is not done, eye and ear infections are a hazard. If the general cleanliness and hygiene standards of a hotel are satisfactory, its swimming pool is likely to be safe from disease.

However, swimming pools may hold other hazards. Poor supervision, inadequate depth markings, unmarked and steep transitions from the shallow end to the deep end, slippery surrounds, and diving boards too close to the shallow end, pool bars serving drinks in glasses, and inadequate procedures for responding to an emergency, are just some of the safety pitfalls that crop up repeatedly. *Holiday Which?* periodically investigates pool safety at popular European resorts, usually with alarming results.

In a review of 58 people with diving injuries sustained in the USA, 45 had dived into a swimming pool, eight into a river, four into a creek, and one into a lake; 41 had major spinal injuries. 46 of the victims were male, and only in 15 patients was alcohol not present in the blood. Misjudging the water's depth, in pools and at the beach, is by far the most common problem, and takes a terrible toll every year.

Fresh-water lakes, dams, and slow-flowing rivers are all infected in countries where schistosomiasis (bilharzia) is endemic (p. 104). Do not be influenced by the attitude of local kids. They frequently have a low-grade chronic infection that gives rise to a partial immunity.

Seawater is safe from schistosomiasis. Other aspects of seawater and disease are discussed on p. 84. The open sea does pose the danger of tidal streams and currents: local advice should be sought if in doubt as to the strength of the tide. Few people can

Leptospirosis

Leptospirosis (also sometimes referred to as Weil's disease) is a disease hazard for people who swim in fresh and brackish water. It is a zoonosis — an infection that can spread naturally between vertebrate animals and man. Although it is found in virtually all areas of the world, it occurs most frequently in tropical and sub-tropical regions (including popular travel destinations such as Hawaii and the Caribbean islands) since leptospires — the spiral-shaped bacteria that cause the infection — survive best in a warm and moist environment.

A well-publicized outbreak occurred in 2000, involving participants in the Eco Challenge expedition race that took place in Sabah, Malaysian Borneo — a series of endurance events including sea canoeing, mountain biking, jungle trekking, canyoning, kayaking, and caving. It attracted 312 athletes from 26 countries including the United States, Canada, Australia, the Netherlands, China, Malaysia, and the UK. As many as half of the participants are believed to have been affected (see Map 14.1 p. 604).

The leptospires are carried in the kidneys of many species of animal, especially rodents, which act as 'maintenance hosts' and form a reservoir of infection; they shed leptospires into the environment when they pass urine. Humans can acquire infection through occupational (e.g. dairy farming, sugar-cane harvesting) or recreational exposure (e.g. canoeing, rafting, wind-surfing, pot-holing and caving) which results in direct or indirect contact with infected urine. The micro-organisms generally gain entry through small cuts or abrasions of the skin although they can also pass through the intact mucous membranes which cover the eye and mouth.

In man, the usual incubation period before symptoms develop, is 7–12 days. Most patients develop only a mild illness, and severe disease, associated with jaundice and kidney failure, is fortunately rare. Early symptoms resemble an influenza-like illness with headache, muscle pains, particularly in the lower back and thighs, and fever. There may also be some nausea and vomiting. Most cases are self-limiting and resolve without the development of significant liver or kidney involvement but a few patients will require temporary dialysis whilst their kidneys recover. Provided adequate medical care is available, the mortality associated with leptospirosis is less than 5%. Where such care is lacking, especially if dialysis is not available, higher mortality rates are seen. Antibiotics may aid recovery if given within the first 72 hours or so of the onset of symptoms. Penicillin by injection is the drug of choice (benzylpenicillin, 1.2 g iv or im every 4–6 hours) for severe cases, whilst amoxycillin or doxycycline can be prescribed orally in mild cases. Erythromycin can be used for patients who are allergic to penicillin.

Simple measures can significantly reduce the risk of acquiring infection. Covering cuts and abrasions with waterproof plasters and wearing footwear, to reduce the risk of cuts to the feet, before occupational or recreational exposure is effective. Measures such as removal of food waste will deter rodents, and other animals that might be carriers of leptospires, from areas of human habitation.

If you become unwell, it is important to make sure that any doctor looking after you is told about any possible risk of exposure to leptospirosis.

Prophylaxis with doxycycline may be of value in a small number of high-risk situations but expert medical advice should be sought beforehand. (A dose of 200 mg of doxycycline would be taken on the first day of exposure, and then once weekly through the period of potential risk.)

Dr Tim Coleman, Leptospira Reference Unit, Hereford Public Health Laboratory, UK.

swim against a current of one knot (one nautical mile per hour) and even the strongest swimmer cannot swim against half a knot for very long. Swimming along the shore rather than out to sea is always safer, and reduces the danger of overestimating how far one can swim.

Sharks, sea snakes, and other dangerous marine animals are another reason for caution. Local advice and custom should be sought: for example, some areas are safe by day but not by night. (See section on animal bites and stings, p. 217.)

Snorkelling

Snorkelling is an easy, cheap, and pleasant method of bridging the gap between the sea surface and its floor. It enables the swimmer to see the underwater world of fish and coral reefs. Snorkelling is safe provided a few simple rules are obeyed.

First, the right sort of equipment should be used. A mask is essential because, unlike fish, our eyes are not designed for use underwater: we require air in contact with the eyes in order to see clearly. As well as the eyes, the mask *must cover the nose*: during descent, the increasing pressure pushes the mask painfully against the face, but this can be counteracted by blowing some air through the nose into the interior of the mask. Snorkellers who use goggles without a nosepiece are liable to end up with black or bloodshot eyes: goggles should therefore be avoided.

The snorkel should be a simple 'J' or 'L'-shaped tube about 2 cm in diameter and 35 cm long. Too long or too narrow a snorkel should be avoided, as it will increase breathing resistance. Modern snorkels have purge valves that make them easier to use.

Do not take more than one deep breath prior to a dive. The urge to surface for another breath derives from the build-up of waste carbon dioxide in the blood rather than from the falling level of oxygen. Taking several deep breaths, or 'hyperventilating' before a dive, delays the build-up of carbon dioxide, so that the snorkeller may use up all his oxygen and lose consciousness before the urge to surface and breathe again is felt. Hyperventilating prior to a dive in an attempt to stay underwater longer has led to many deaths by drowning.

Beware of sunburn: use a water-resistant sunscreen on your back, or wear a T-shirt, when the sun is strong.

Scuba diving

Scuba diving is an acronym for Self-Contained Underwater Breathing Apparatus — also known as an aqualung. Scuba diving can be a fascinating pastime, but it is also potentially dangerous unless carried out with proper training beforehand and an appreciation of the risks involved and methods of avoidance. Some of the main medical and physiological hazards are described below, but newcomers to the sport should realize that these are not the *only* hazards (or necessarily the most common ones) and must undergo a full training course before attempting to dive in open water.

Medical fitness

Anyone intending to take up scuba diving should have a medical check-up if there is any doubt about fitness; dive centres in some countries such as Malta and Australia require a medical certificate, sometimes including a chest X-ray report — check before you go, because obtaining a certificate abroad can be difficult and expensive.

Some medical problems are known as 'absolute contraindications to diving'. This means that if you have such a problem you must never dive. Examples of these are epilepsy that is still being treated, lung conditions like emphysema, and heart problems that may lead to fainting underwater (heart block, Wolff–Parkinson–White syndrome).

Other medical problems are called 'relative contraindications to diving' and this means that there may be instances where the person can dive but only after a thorough examination by a doctor who specializes in diving medicine. Example, such problems are asthma, diabetes, obesity, and recovery from heart attacks or operations.

When you sign up for a course you will have to fill in a self-declaration form for your health status; any YES box which is ticked then means you have to contact a diving doctor for medical clearance, so always make sure you are fit to dive before handing over any money or booking trips or courses.

A number of physical handicaps do not, however, cause much difficulty under water, and scuba diving is growing in popularity with handicapped people (see p. 522) but always check and get passed as fit with a doctor first.

Effects of pressure

On land, our bodies are subject to atmospheric pressure — the pressure exerted by the column of air that extends for ten miles or so above our heads. Underwater, pressure increases rapidly: in fact, with every 30 feet or 10 metres of depth, the pressure increases by an additional one atmosphere (14.7 p.s.i.). Thus at 30 feet depth, the total pressure is twice the surface pressure, and at 90 feet it is four times the surface pressure.

Fluid-filled parts of the body are not affected by the increase in pressure but air-filled parts, such as lungs, middle ears, and sinuses, are noticeably affected. Unless the pressures inside and outside the body are equalized, the higher pressure squeezes the lower pressure and causes tissue damage and pain.

Lungs

Charged aqualung cylinders contain air at high pressure (up to 200–250 bars); the aqualung regulator (which delivers the air to the diver's mouth) is designed to reduce this pressure and supply air to the diver at the same pressure as that being exerted externally on his chest, irrespective of his depth. Thus at 10 metres, air is supplied to the diver at a pressure of two bars, and at 30 metres at a pressure of four bars. In this way, the pressure of air in the diver's mouth is equalized to the external pressure, and breathing is just as easy as at the surface, apart from a slight resistance to the airflow caused by the regulator. During ascent, however, the air in the lungs expands as the external pressure drops *and if the diver makes the mistake of holding his or her breath, the lungs will over inflate with the risk of a 'burst lung'* (see below).

Ears and sinuses

During descent, some discomfort or pain is usually experienced in the region of the eardrums and less obviously over the forehead, due to the difference between the external pressure of air in the ears and the sinuses. This discomfort is easily relieved by pinching the nose and (by means of a little expiratory effort as though you were sneezing) forcing some additional air up into the sinuses and middle ear, via natural passages connecting these structures to the back of the nose (see also pp. 256–7).

During ascent, this additional air escapes back out again without any action on the part of the diver. Problems are rarely encountered except when injury or illness has caused damage to the air passages, or during a heavy cold when the passages may be blocked by mucus: diving with a heavy or even moderate cold is inadvisable.

Scuba diving abroad

A basic diving training course should include instruction and practice in the use of diving equipment (including buoyancy control); safety and emergency procedures including life-saving; lectures on the theory and practice of diving, the various hazards involved and their avoidance; and the supervised acquisition of experience, beginning in a swimming pool or shallow water and gradually progressing to deeper dives in open water. A full-time course covering the above could be expected to take around three to four days.

In addition to physiological hazards caused by pressure changes, divers have to learn to deal with all sorts of other stresses, which range from mask-flooding to air-supply failure, from buoyancy problems to zero underwater visibility. While a trained diver will be able to cope with such eventualities, a succession of such mishaps can rapidly reduce the novice to a state of helplessness or panic, with disastrous results.

Travellers thinking of taking up diving on vacation should undergo some basic training — for example, at any dive school run by instructors certified by the Professional Association of Diving Instructors (PADI) or National Association of Underwater Instructors (NAUI).

Most diving centres abroad apply stringent safety procedures and will not hire out equipment or organize dives except for those who can produce a recognized certificate of competence (such as the PADI 'open water diver' qualification) or have undergone the centre's own training course. In some places, however, a beginner may be offered a 'try-out' dive with little or no instruction or supervision, while at the same time being asked to sign an insurance disclaimer absolving the dive centre of any responsibility in the event of an accident. *This arrangement is best avoided unless you are unconcerned about your safety. Beginners should insist on several hours' instruction in the basic techniques and, on their first few dives, the accompaniment and undivided attention of an experienced instructor.*

Diving illnesses

Decompression sickness (DCS), also known as the 'bends'

Causes

Under pressure, more nitrogen is dissolved in the body tissues. The amount dissolved depends upon the depth (pressure) and time spent under pressure. If the pressure is released quickly, bubbles of nitrogen come out of solution into the body tissues (just like gas bubbles appearing in a bottle of lemonade when the top is released) and cause the symptoms of decompression sickness.

Types of DCS
The symptoms depend upon where and to what extent the bubbles are released. Joint pains are the most common, but more serious symptoms are caused if the bubbles affect either the spinal cord or the brain. Weakness or numbness of the limbs, difficulty in passing urine, and disturbance of vision or balance are all symptoms of decompression sickness. Decompression sickness symptoms usually appear within three hours of a dive but may be delayed for up to 24 hours. It is helpful to consider DCS in three categories:

- Type I (mild),
- Type II (serious), and
- Arterial gas embolization (AGE).

Type I DCS
Type I DCS is characterized by

- Mild pains that begin to resolve within 10 minutes of onset (niggles);
- 'Skin bends' that cause itching or burning sensations of the skin; or
- Skin rash, which generally is a mottled rash causing marbling of the skin or a violet coloured rash that is most often seen on the chest and shoulders. On rare occasions, skin has an orange peel appearance. It is important that this is not confused with other causes of a rash whilst diving. A suit squeeze will generally have a different pattern and look more like bruising, whilst a neoprene contact dermatitis will be in areas where a suit rubs, such as the neck or cuffs.
- Lymphatic involvement is uncommon and usually is signalled by painless pitting oedema — that is, a swelling of the lower limbs in which a thumb when pressed in will leave an impression. The mildest cases involve the skin or the lymphatics. Some authorities consider anorexia and excessive fatigue after a dive as manifestations of Type I DCS.
- Pain (the 'bends') occurs in the majority (70–85 per cent) of patients with DCS. Pain is the most common symptom of DCS and is often described as a dull, deep, throbbing, toothache-type pain, usually in a joint or tendon area but also in tissue. The shoulder is the most commonly affected joint in most divers after a shallower than 40 metre dive, whereas the knees are affected more in deep divers. The pain is initially mild and slowly becomes more intense. Because of this, many divers attribute early DCS symptoms to overexertion or a pulled muscle.
- Upper limbs are affected about three times as often as lower limbs. The pain of Type I DCS may mask neurological signs that are hallmarks of the more serious Type II DCS.

Type II DCS
Type II DCS is characterized by nervous system involvement, lung symptoms, and circulatory problems. Pain is reported in only about 30 per cent of cases. Because of the anatomical complexity of the central and peripheral nervous systems, signs and symptoms are variable and diverse. Symptom onset is usually immediate but may be delayed as long as 36 hours.

Nervous system

The spinal cord is the most common site for Type II DCS; symptoms mimic spinal cord trauma. Low back pain may start within a few minutes to hours after the dive and may progress to paresis (weakness), paralysis, paraesthesia (tingling, 'pins and needles', altered sensation), loss of sphincter control, and girdle pain of the lower trunk.

DCS can be dynamic and does not follow typical peripheral nerve distribution patterns. This strange shifting of symptoms confuses the diagnosis, differentiating DCS from traumatic nerve injuries.

Other common symptoms include headaches or visual disturbances, dizziness, tunnel vision, and changes in mental status. Labyrinthine or inner ear DCS ('the staggers') causes a combination of nausea, vomiting, vertigo, and nystagmus in addition to tinnitus and partial deafness.

Lungs

Pulmonary DCS ('the chokes') is characterized by:

• Inspiratory burning and discomfort behind the sternum (breastbone)
• Dry coughing that can become paroxysmal like a coughing fit, and
• Severe shortness of breath and respiratory distress. This occurs in about 2 per cent of all DCS cases and can end in death. Symptoms can start up to 12 hours after a dive and persist for 12–48 hours.

Circulatory system

Complex movements of fluid result in hypovolaemic shock, which is commonly associated with other symptoms. For reasons not yet fully understood, fluid shifts from intravascular to extravascular spaces. The problems of tachycardia (rapid heart beat) and postural hypotension (dizziness when you suddenly sit or stand up) are treated by oral rehydration, if the patient is conscious, or intravenously if unconscious. The treatment of DCS is less effective if dehydration is not corrected.

Thrombi or clots may form from activation of the early phases of blood coagulation and the release of vasoactive substances from cells lining the blood vessels. The blood-bubble interface may act as a foreign surface causing this effect.

Arterial gas embolization (AGE)

While ascending from a dive, the air in the lungs expands as the pressure reduces. Normal breathing allows this excess air to be dispersed. If, however, divers either hold their breath, or have a pre-existing lung disease that causes air to be trapped in the lungs, problems can occur. As trapped air expands it can cause the lung to burst. The medical term for this is pulmonary barotrauma, sometimes also called 'burst lung'. The air escapes from the lungs and may enter the bloodstream. This is known as arterial gas embolism.

Gas emboli can lodge in coronary, cerebral, and other systemic arterioles. These gas bubbles continue to expand as ascending pressure decreases, thus increasing the severity of obstruction and clinical signs, according to their location. In the heart, coronary artery embolization can lead to myocardial infarction (a 'heart attack') or abnormal rhythms. Cerebral artery emboli can cause stroke or seizures.

Differentiating cerebral AGE from Type II neurological DCS is usually based upon the suddenness of symptoms.

AGE symptoms typically occur within 10–20 minutes after surfacing. Multiple systems may be involved. Clinical features may occur suddenly or gradually, beginning with dizziness, headache, and profound anxiety. More dramatic symptoms of coughing up blood, chest pain, shortness of breath, confusion, visual disturbances, weakness or paralysis, convulsions, or unresponsiveness, shock, and seizures can occur quickly. Neurological symptoms vary, and death can result. Central nervous system DCS is clinically similar to AGE; since the treatment of either requires urgent recompression, differentiating between them is not of great importance.

Burst lung is unlikely with correct training, which teaches divers to avoid holding their breath while ascending, and thorough medical screening, which prevents those with past or present chest disease from diving.

Treatment

Treatment of decompression sickness requires recompression of the diver in a recompression chamber (commonly but mistakenly called a decompression chamber) to force the offending bubbles of nitrogen back into solution. Oxygen is also breathed to speed the elimination of nitrogen from the body. The chamber operator then follows a schedule, called a therapeutic table, for bringing the recompressed diver safely back to the surface pressure.

In the absence of a recompression chamber the diver should be given oxygen to breathe while transport is arranged to the nearest chamber, if necessary by low-level flight in an aircraft or helicopter. (Water and aspirin are also a useful emergency treatment to reduce blood viscosity.) Never try to treat decompression sickness by diving again. This will make the diver worse rather than better.

Pre hospital treatment of DCS

- Extricate the diver from water, and immobilize if trauma is suspected.
- Administer 100 per cent oxygen, intubate if necessary, and administer IV saline.
- If the diver is conscious, rehydrate with non-alcoholic fluids at a rate of 1 litre each hour.
- Perform CPR and advanced cardiac life support (ACLS) if required as well as needle decompression of the chest if tension pneumothorax is suspected.
- Keep the patient lying flat, and DO NOT put them in the head down position as this can worsen brain swelling.
- Transport to nearest emergency department and hyperbaric facility, if feasible, and try to keep all diving gear with diver. Diving gear may provide clues as to why the diver had trouble (e.g., faulty air regulator, hose leak, carbon monoxide contamination of compressed air).

Prevention

DCS can always be avoided by diving within the rules of well-tried diving tables.

Always ascend slowly (no faster than 15 m/min), and only dive within the rules of a set of diving tables. These indicate what 'stops', if any, the diver should carry out during the ascent to release the nitrogen safely from the body tissues.

Any aqualung training course should include instruction in the use of diving tables, which cannot be described in detail here. Remember always to err on the side of safety when calculating safe dive times, depths, and decompression stops. If diving in a locality remote from a recompression chamber, it is wise to add a safety factor to further reduce the risk of decompression sickness.

Decompression computers are now widely used in many diving areas. They appear attractive because divers are given greater time under water when diving a variable depth profile in which there is gradual ascent throughout the dive, compared to traditional dive tables which assume a rectangular dive profile. While diving computers are based on the same mathematical algorithms as dive tables, they have not been tested on human dives to the same extent. A safety factor should always be added, rather than diving to get every possible minute under water. Problems can occur if only one diver of a pair has a computer, for example if the other goes deeper (even by two to three feet, for one or two minutes) or if partners are swapped for a second dive. Possibly because of such reasons, the introduction of dive computers in the UK was associated with a marked increase in the prevalence of decompression sickness. While this has now reduced, it is still not known if the return to previous levels is due to improved familiarity with dive computers, or to a fall in the number of dives taking place on account of other factors.

Nitrogen narcosis

A further important physiological hazard of diving is nitrogen narcosis. Although also caused by the presence of nitrogen in the body, this is quite different from decompression sickness in that the symptoms appear at depth rather than during or after the ascent.

Below a depth of around 30–40 metres, nitrogen builds up in the bloodstream to a level at which it may have toxic effects on the brain quite similar to the effects of alcohol or drug intoxication. Although nitrogen narcosis has been described as 'rapture of the depths', the symptoms are not necessarily pleasant, with a feeling of detachment from reality, possibly fear or apprehension, and most dangerously a loss of concentration and slowing of thought processes. The symptoms become more acute the deeper the diver descends below 40 metres. Fortunately, nitrogen narcosis is fairly easily dealt with by ascending 5–10 metres, when the symptoms will clear.

On occasions, nitrogen narcosis combined with apprehension may induce a state of panic. This is particularly dangerous under water as it may lead either to drowning or a pulmonary barotrauma if the response is to initiate a rapid ascent, for instance by inflating the life preserver. Diving in pairs, with each member of a team alert to the possibility of nitrogen narcosis in the other and ready to step in with pre-taught emergency drills, is the only solution. The dangers of nitrogen narcosis can be reduced if the maximum depth of the dive is built up gradually over a series of dives, e.g. 25, 30, 35, 40 metres on successive days.

Fifty metres should be considered as the absolute maximum depth for sports diving, below which it becomes unacceptably dangerous. This is for three reasons. First, mental co-ordination and thought processes are slowed due to nitrogen narcosis, limiting the diver's ability to act correctly in an emergency. Secondly, the high density of the air that is being breathed under pressure increases the diver's work of breathing, limiting physical performance. And finally, decompression tables have not been well tested and are less reliable below this depth.

Other diving problems

Other problems are more minor but far more frequent.

Ear infections

The ears are a frequent cause of trouble. In either polluted or warm tropical water, infection of the outer ear canal (*otitis externa*) may occur. This leads to a painful ear. As a preventive measure, otic Domeboro or 8 per cent aluminium acetate ear drops may be used. The drops should be instilled 2–3 times a day after diving or washing. Other measures include showering in fresh water after the dive, and drying the ear canal by shaking the head. Do not try to dry the ear canal with a towel, cotton wool, or a finger.

Antibiotic eardrops should only be used to treat established infections and should preferably include an antifungal drug, because fungal infection is a frequent cause of otitis externa. Eardrops containing alcohol should not be used, because this dissolves part of the cerumen (ear wax), reducing its naturally protective effect.

Infection of the middle ear (*otitis media*) is caused by bacteria from the nose or throat entering the ear while diving. This is another reason for not diving with a cold, sore throat, or chest infection.

Cuts and grazes sustained while diving in tropical waters may take up to three months to heal if nematocysts (p. 243) or other micro-organisms have entered the wound. Wounds are easily prevented by wearing a wetsuit, or a Lycra or Darlexx 'skin' if the water is very warm. Underwater photographers are particularly at risk, as they concentrate on looking through their camera viewfinders and may miss seeing a coral outcrop.

Diving and air travel

Finally, at the end of a diving vacation, it is not safe to fly home immediately after a dive. The decreased pressure, even in a pressurized aircraft, can bring on an attack of the bends. No diving should be undertaken in the 24 hours prior to a flight.

Insurance and medical support

Divers' Alert Network provides a 24-hour emergency telephone advice service for divers with medical problems, and is based at Duke University Medical Centre, USA. Tel. +1 919 684 8111. DAN also sells inexpensive insurance coverage.

In the UK, the Undersea Medicine Division of the Royal Navy provides a 24-hour, 365 days a year, physician-based advice and treatment service open to all. In the event of a diving emergency the Duty Diving Medical Officer can be contacted by Cellphone on 07831 151523 (International: +44 7831 151523) or on +44 23 92 584255.

Sailing and wind-surfing

Sailing and wind-surfing pose few medical problems. A sense of balance is needed for wind-surfing. Always sail upwind first, not downwind, or along a coast rather than out to sea. This lessens the dangers if the wind strength increases while sailing. Wind-surfers can quickly tire in a strong wind and become exhausted, particularly in cold water. There are many types of protective clothing available. These are either wetsuits or drysuits, both of which if correctly fitted will retain body heat without causing overheating during the often strenuous activity. Do not overestimate your abilities and sail into dangerous waters. Wearing a life-preserver or other buoyancy device is always advisable, however experienced you are.

Water-skiing

Water-skiing is quickly learnt by anyone with a sense of balance and timing. Unless high-speed or competition water-skiing is tried, the risks are few. Always wear a life-preserver in case you are stunned when falling into the water. Women should prevent a high-speed vaginal douche by wearing an adequate bikini or swimsuit that provides protection. For competition or high-speed water-skiing, a wetsuit should be used to help cushion the blow when falling onto water at high speed.

Surfing

The developing world offers some of the best waves for surfers, but with their remoteness from good medical care can come the obvious risks

• It is always wise to take a first-aid kit as the waves can break onto shallow rocky reefs and cuts and grazes can soon ulcerate without prompt care
• When surfing a new break always take time to find out what the waves break on to and where the rip currents are found
• Never attempt to go too far out if you are not a strong swimmer and always observe any safety flags put up by the local lifeguards
• Local surfers can be fiercely protective of 'their' breaks so it can be a good idea to mix in before going out.

Skiing

Most ski injuries can be prevented by preparation, instruction, care on the slopes and awareness of the potential hazards.

Mr Basil Helal was formerly a Consultant Orthopaedic Surgeon at the London Hospital and the Royal National Orthopaedic Hospital and a medical adviser to the British Olympic Association.
Dr Ernst Philipp is a Consulting Physician to the Centre for Health in Employment and the Environment (CHEE), Bristol Royal Infirmary.

Skiing is an exhilarating experience, and provides exercise in majestic surroundings. It remains a rapidly growing sport, and many people travel overseas to ski, often to continental Europe and North America.

There are several forms: downhill skiing; Nordic (cross-country) skiing; and ski mountaineering. 'Hot-dogging' is a form of acrobatics on skis, and ski jumping or 'flying' is for the few who dare. 'Figling' is done on boot-length Figl skis and generally used to ski over fresh avalanched snow. For the very expert, there is also the monoski, with platforms for both feet, and now especially popular, the snowboard.

Fashions change, and each form has its advocates. Perhaps ski mountaineering provides the purist with the most attractive elements that this form of sport can offer. However, unless skiers are aware of the possible hazards they face, and take careful steps to protect themselves, skiing can also be a most dangerous pastime. An added complication is that medical treatment abroad carries many pitfalls in terms of communication problems, the problems of a different medical system, and perhaps different approaches to treatment.

Preparation

Choose your ski resort with the advice of friends, brochures, or travel agents to ensure that it is suitable for your ability level and the range in the group you are going with. Suitable facilities for learners include easy slopes, proximity of lifts to accommodation, instructors who are fluent in the same languages, rest and restaurant facilities on the ski field, and a choice of other leisure activities at or near the resort. Runs should be marked on a field map for different ability levels. Remember too, that if a field has only a few lifts or trails, then long lift queues and crowded fields can occur at peak times of the year such as school and public holidays. Lessons from ski schools help to avoid queues and are worth considering, especially at weekends.

Prior to your arrival, listen to radio and TV reports on weather and skiing conditions.

Clothing

Ski wear should be warm, waterproof, and windproof. The ski outfit should in addition be easily visible against the snow and should not be so smooth as to allow frictionless descent down a mountain after a fall. A gap at the waist should be avoided.

Head gear When the head is uncovered, heat loss through the head can be as high as 90 per cent if full protective, insulated clothing is otherwise worn, so an adequate, warm, waterproof head covering that will also protect the ears is essential. Children can easily damage the skull in falls and collisions; a child's skull is not as hard as an adult's and well-fitting helmets are strongly advised.

A *facemask* to protect from high wind and driving snow is also a valuable asset.

Goggles or glasses should either have photosensitive lenses or have exchangeable lenses for varying conditions. They should protect against driving snow and high wind, and against strong sunlight. They should also provide side cover for the eyes, and this is especially important for ski mountaineering.

Mittens are warmer than gloves. A thin pair of warm gloves, cotton or silk, worn inside mittens allows one to handle metal bindings without getting a 'cold burn' in very low temperatures.

Socks A dry spare pair is always worth carrying especially if ski mountaineering or touring are envisaged.

Ski leggings should be worn by anyone planning to ski in deep snow, to prevent snow from entering the boots.

Undergarments should be light and allow freedom of movement. Two thin layers provide more insulation than one thick layer.

A small backpack does not interfere with skiing and can be used to carry clothes that are not needed — weather conditions change rapidly, and in any case it is much cooler towards the end of the day — as well as any extra items that may prove useful, such as bandages and a screwdriver or toolkit for running repairs.

Selection of skis, boots, bindings, and poles
Ski boots should be comfortable and allow some toe movement. Boots that are adjustable for heel grip and mid-foot grip as well as for ankle grip are preferred.

A different, softer boot is required for climbing on skis; and for Nordic skiing, a special shoe with a toe extension is necessary.

Bindings anchor the boot to the ski and are designed to release if an undue force is applied in a rotational or forward pitch direction. They should be adjusted according to the weight, bone thickness, and strength of the subject, and this is best done by an expert. The bindings require some momentum to release easily, so the most dangerous fall is a 'slow' one.

Special bindings which allow the heel to rise when climbing but anchor for skiing are necessary for the ski mountaineer; and quite different bindings, which provide only a toe grip, are used in Nordic or cross-country skiing.

Skis should be selected with care. They should not be too long, as this makes turning more difficult. The short, wide, 'Scorpian' ski or 'Compact' ski is ideal for the beginner, who can graduate to longer skis with experience. Longer skis increase leverage on the leg in a fall (see below).

Ski poles These should be of correct length, and the loops should break away on a strong tug.

Special equipment
Ski mountaineers need other special equipment, such as avalanche detectors, harnesses (e.g. Whillan's), and rope, and extra clothing protection.

General fitness
A graded exercise programme lasting at least six weeks is an essential part of preparation: skiing is an energetic pastime and is carried out at altitudes where the pressure of oxygen may be lower than most skiers are accustomed to in their home environment.

Running is most suitable for those who are accustomed to it, but can cause stress injuries in people who take it up suddenly and intensively in a last-minute attempt to get fit for a skiing vacation. It should preferably be carried out on grass or forest floor rather than on concrete or asphalt.

Cycling is much less traumatic and besides improving fitness, will also serve to strengthen the muscles that are used in skiing.

Leg strength Exercise specifically intended to strengthen the quadriceps muscles should be dynamic and not static, otherwise patellar chondromalacia (softening of the articular surfaces of the knee cap) may ensue.

Practising ski skills on artificial slopes
Artificial slopes are sensible places for beginners to become familiar with ski equipment and basic skills, but dry-slope skiing carries its own hazards. Most dry ski surfaces consist of nylon brush squares; falls can be abrasive, and if the thumb is caught in this surface its ligaments are easily torn. Protective clothing, including mittens, is essential.

Environmental hazards

Altitude (see also pp. 314–26)
Skiing generally involves ascent to altitudes of 8000–12 000 feet or over, where the atmospheric pressure is lower and the air is drier. Oxygen transfer to the lungs is less easy.

Altitude or mountain sickness can be very dangerous, and can cause both pulmonary and cerebral oedema; diuretic treatment and oxygen may be of some help, but descent to a higher pressure zone is the safest answer if there is no response to other forms of treatment. An early diuresis (passage of a large volume of urine) on ascent seems to indicate good adaptation to altitude. Minor symptoms, including sleep disturbances, are relatively common especially at some of the higher ski resorts.

More evaporation occurs at altitude, and the nasal passages dry more easily, especially during sleep, when this is often exacerbated by central heating. It is best to increase fluid intake — have an extra drink of water before you go to bed, even if you don't feel especially thirsty. Try also to keep the humidity in the bedroom high — a bowl of water or wet towels on the radiators can be very helpful in preventing a dry, sore throat.

Cold (see also pp. 340–9)

Skiing requires snow — except on dry artificial surfaces, of course. Unless you're unlucky with conditions, you are likely to be skiing at temperatures around 0°C or lower.

Skiing also requires muscular effort, and this is optimal at body temperature or slightly above (40°C). Getting yourself chilled increases muscle stiffness and slows reaction times, and at worst can be fatal, so it is wise to be prepared.

People with certain medical conditions should take particular care to avoid chilling or placing themselves at this risk: they include sufferers from previous heart attacks, chronic bronchitics, people with poor circulation, and some people in whom low temperature causes their red blood cells to break down (this is a form of allergy to cold).

Insulation Several layers of clothing will trap air at body temperature efficiently (p. 340). Generally speaking, clothes made from cellular materials, especially natural fibres, are best, and animal fur is the warmest. As mentioned previously, the outermost layer should be windproof and not too slippery.

Wind The chill factor in wind can lower the effective air temperature rapidly and substantially. Thus with a wind speed of 20 m/sec, 0°C will feel the same as –50°C on a windless day (p. 341).

Damp Insulation is rapidly degraded if clothing becomes wet. Cotton clothing such as denim is particularly unsuitable as the wind-chill factor with wet clothing easily leads to hypothermia. It may be sensible to carry a spare, dry pair of socks in a plastic bag when skiing in deep powder snow, for feet can easily get wet.

Heat conservation If cooled, the body tries to preserve its central core temperature. Heat loss is reduced by reflex constriction of the skin blood vessels. Heat is produced by muscle activity and this is the reason for the shivering reaction. Anything that reduces activity such as being stranded on a chair lift or on a drag lift can result in a rapid fall in temperature, and it is best to try to maintain some movement of the limbs under these circumstances. Similarly, concussion or any injury that results in immobilization will cause a rapid fall in temperature

Food You will require extra calories to combat the cold and to ensure that you enjoy strenuous activities at high altitudes. A porridge and toast (carbohydrate) breakfast is more quickly converted into energy than a fried breakfast. Carry hi-energy snacks like chocolate, and avoid strenuous skiing for more than two hours without food (see Fatigue, p. 391).

Alcohol Heat loss is increased by dilatation of the blood vessels of the skin; alcohol is a vasodilator — so beware. Like drinking and driving, drinking and skiing do not mix; drinking increases the risk of an accident on the slopes.

Some 25 per cent of skiing accidents requiring hospitalization are associated with alcohol consumption within two hours of the accident. It is also not a good idea to drink alcohol at the end of day to replace fluid, because it can inhibit interest in eating sufficient carbohydrate to replace the energy required for the next day of skiing and lead to a muscle glycogen deficit.

Cold injury The skin itself is at risk from injury, and the skier should carry a face mask to protect the nose and cheeks, and warm head gear that can come over the ears. The lips are also vulnerable. Frost 'nips' — white, numb patches on the skin — should have external warmth applied rapidly. Rubbing is dangerous, however, and can further damage the skin. Frostbite involves freezing of the deeper tissues and starts at the tips of the fingers and toes. Rapid and careful re-warming is essential.

Hand protection In practice, the hands are better protected by a mitten than a glove, for this allows better movement of the fingers. Remember that for handling of metal portions of equipment at very low temperatures a light cotton glove worn inside the mitten will protect against a cold burn. On no account should metal at temperatures below 10°C be handled, even with warm hands, as skin will blister or adhere to the metal. Chemical 'hand-warmers' are sometimes useful.

Children Children are particularly susceptible to cold injury and even frost nipped hands and feet can suffer permanent damage with subsequent distortion or stunting of growth. Make sure that children stay warm, and inspect them repeatedly if they are playing in snow, snowballing, etc.

Cigarettes Among the many harmful effects of cigarettes is vasoconstriction, or clamping down of blood vessels at the extremities. This has been well established by thermographic and doppler tests. So please do not give injured skiers a 'steadying' smoke — it may quite literally result in loss of their fingertips and toes.

Cold collapse is a response to a falling core temperature and to a reduction in the blood sugar level. Brain function fails if the core temperature falls below 35°C. Early signs include weakness with frequent falls, followed by a stage of aggressive behaviour which goes on to apathy, and then collapse and loss of consciousness.

Re-warming Rapid warming is essential and a fit person's body heat is perhaps the best emergency solution. If both victim and rescuer huddle together in a thermal blanket (which is made of light foil, can fold to the size of a handkerchief, and can be carried in a skier's pocket) or a sleeping bag, if one is available, there is an excellent chance of raising core temperature to a safe level — particularly if the partner is of the opposite sex!

If the limbs are frostbitten do not thaw them if there is a likelihood of refreezing and do not rub the frozen part, as this will further damage the skin.

Back in civilization, the accepted method of restoring the core temperature is by immersion in a warm bath (40–44°C) until flushing of fingertips occurs. Blisters should be kept intact if possible and antibiotics given to prevent infection of any damaged tissue; use open dressings to allow easy inspection.

Survival Failing visibility, perhaps due to mist or fog, may cause a delayed return. At nightfall, there is usually a marked drop in temperature. If there is no hope or even some doubt of reaching shelter, construct an igloo or a substantial snow hole and huddle up together if there are a number of you, or curl up tight to reduce the surface area from which heat loss can occur if you are alone. This will give you the best chance of survival.

Sun

Sunburn is a real hazard in the clear mountain atmosphere and barrier creams should always be worn, particularly by the fair skinned (see p. 352). Use lipsalve to prevent chapped lips. Reflected glare from expanses of white snow can cause severe eye damage conjunctival burns, and even *uveitis* leading to so-called snowblindness (see also p. 428). This is best prevented by wearing adequate sunglasses, possibly with side protectors.

Visibility and weather conditions

Unfavourable snow conditions (such as patches of deep snow, wet snow, or ice) contribute to accidents.

Firm, crisp, granular snow accompanied by good weather gives ideal skiing conditions. In contrast, ice or wet, sticky snow can catch you unawares and requires greater caution, slower speeds, and waxing of ski soles to give a smoother glide. Cold and windy weather can also produce bare patches of ice, ice-hard tracks in the snow, and lumpy, icy snow. In deep or heavy snow your weight should be further back over your skis to lift the tips and encourage a rearward fall that is less likely to cause injury. The presence of fog, mist, hail, sleet, or falling snow, often combined with wind or low cloud, produces poor skiing conditions. At such times the light is diffuse and there are no shadows. It therefore becomes very difficult to see contours, humps, and hollows on the ski run. The sensation of movement is also reduced because you cannot see landmarks as you pass them. When you stop there is also often a weird feeling that you are still moving. In such conditions the skiing is much easier and more pleasant if there are dark objects such as trees, rocks, pylons, or lift towers to break up the whiteness of the foreground and give you some idea of the whereabouts and steepness of the fall line of the slope. The fall line is the steepest and shortest line down the slope from where you are standing — a snowball would roll straight down it. You should reduce your speed to match the prevailing conditions.

Beware of ice, especially in the early morning before the air temperature warms up and in the late afternoon when the air temperature drops and freezes the superficial layers of compacted snow. Even during the day, the chill effect of wind blowing over the snow can form patches of snow crust, and ice and sunshine can cause patches of wet or slushy snow — all hazardous for the unwary skier.

Do not hesitate to leave the ski field early if the weather deteriorates. Weather can change very rapidly in the mountains and with little warning. These changes also alter the ice or snow surfaces and can create wind, blizzard, or white-out conditions that are all dangerous. Visibility of distance is also affected by flat light, cloud, and blowing snow.

Terrain

Cliffs are especially dangerous in poor visibility. Crevasses are fissures in the earth that are often concealed by a bridge of snow. Some are large and deep, and there is danger of injury or death from the fall. Others are narrower and a skier may be trapped a few feet down, be unable to move, and die from hypothermia if rescue is not rapidly to hand.

Collision can produce serious injury; obstacles include trees, buried rocks, and other skiers. If a skier wishes to stop, he or she should do so off the piste or track, and away from the bottom of a run.

Avalanches

Avalanches kill about 150 skiers and outdoor adventurers in Europe, and 50 in North America, every year. In heavily populated mountain regions such as Austria, the annual toll is around 40. The danger of avalanches exists whenever a poor bond between snow layers causes one layer to slide on another or where the snow becomes so lacking in cohesion that it cannot support itself on the slope. Known avalanche dangers on patrolled ski fields are often marked with a black and yellow chequered flag. The greatest obstacles to definitive and effective safety measures are the changes that occur during any winter season to the degree of risk and also changes in the areas of a snow field at risk.

- Avalanches are possible on most ski fields because steep slopes that are attractive to skiers are also prone to avalanching, and because many popular runs are in a basin surrounded by hills. They can occur on any slopes at an angle greater than 30°, especially during and immediately after storms, before the snow stabilizes, or after a moderate snowfall during windy conditions.
- Avalanches may cause some parts of a field to be placed 'out of bounds' — DO NOT walk or ski there.
- If an avalanche occurs, try to ski out of a valley or get to a ridge.
- If caught in an avalanche, get rid of skis, poles, and any pack you are wearing. Try to 'swim' on the surface, with your mouth closed, and move to the side of the slide.
- If buried in an avalanche, make an air space in front of your mouth as the avalanche slows.
- Skiers cause most avalanches they get caught in. Therefore the ability to recognize potential avalanche starting zones and avalanche paths, and to assess the likelihood of them sliding, is essential for anyone ski touring.
- Good places to travel that are less likely to avalanche are ridges and valley floors.

Places to avoid: likely avalanche areas
- Lee slopes and gullies (where wind-blown snow builds up).
- Slopes always in the shade (where cold temperatures help unstable crystals to grow deep in the snowpack).
- Slopes with cliffs or narrow gullies below them (where even a small avalanche may push you over the cliff or pile up on top of you in a gully).
- Cornices (which can break off well back from the edge).
- Sunlit slopes in spring (which are especially dangerous just after a fresh snowfall).

If you have to travel across a slope which you suspect is unstable, think what would happen if it did slide. If the consequences would be dangerous, turn back. If you cross a suspect slope, ski one at a time and quickly from one safe point to the next; even after one person has crossed safely, do not assume the slope is stable. Each skier should disturb the slope as little as possible.

The remainder of the party should stay in a safe place and watch the person skiing. When skiing suspect slopes, try to keep to the edge of them rather than travelling across the centre. Hands should be taken out of wrist loops, safety straps undone, and all clothing done up securely to prevent snow getting inside.

If you are really unsure of a particular slope, dig a snow pit, 1.5–2.0 metres deep, in a safe position. Look for the danger signs: these are soft snow under hard layers, loose snow layers, and obvious sliding layers.

Avalanche danger warning signs
- More than 30 cm of snowfall or 25 mm of rain in 24 hours.
- Rapid rises in temperature.
- Prolonged cold temperatures with strong winds.
- Wind-transported snow.
- Foot penetration of 60 cm or more.
- Settlement of new snow by less than 15 per cent in 24 hours i.e. before the snow stabilizes.
- A hollow feeling or sound under the snow when probed with ski poles.
- Small snow fractures which spread out from your skis.
- Snow which gives a 'whoomph' sound when you cross it.
- Sun, rain, or warm winds on new snowfalls.

Avalanche survival
Survivors should be aware of further avalanche danger, but a buried person's chance of survival depends on the speed of being found — 40 per cent survive being buried between one and two metres under an avalanche, but after three hours chances of survival are very small.

Avalanche transceivers
Avalanche transceivers are small, battery-operated radio sets worn close to the body in potential avalanche situations. They transmit a bleep signal received by another set which enables rapid location of a buried person. All sets should be set to 'transmit' if an avalanche threatens; survivors then turn their sets to receive in order to locate buried victims. To assist the search, survivors should note the position of a lost party member when the avalanche started and the position at which last seen.

Hazards from lift equipment

Cable cars Cable cars have been known to crash from a height, but such accidents are exceptionally uncommon.

Chair lifts Poor co-ordination when joining or leaving a chair lift can result in injury. The chair can give the unwary skier a sharp knock. People have also been injured by

---

New safety devices

A recent study has shown that a new safety device, the Avalung, can dramatically extend survival time. The device is like a waistcoat with a breathing tube; avalanche victims are often surrounded by trapped air, which quickly becomes contaminated with exhaled carbon dioxide; the device filters and traps exhaled carbon dioxide, preserving the air supply for an hour or more. Further information: **www.avalung.com**.

---

falling out of chairs and by having articles of their clothing hooked or trapped by the chair as they alight. Failure of the lift system, leaving the unfortunate skier trapped, suspended, and very cold, can provide a powerful temptation to try to jump off. Don't — even mild frostbite is preferable to severe injury or death.

Drag lifts T-bars and tow bars can entangle with clothing, or if released at the wrong moment can recoil against other skiers and cause injury.

Acclimatization and orientation

On arrival at the ski resort, allow yourself time to acclimatize. The higher the resort, the longer this may take.

Check that your clothing and equipment are suitable and in good order. Obtain a map of the ski area and select runs that are appropriate for your experience and ability.

It is important to obtain adequate insurance for yourself and your equipment as well as third party insurance (see p. 567). In isolated mountain resorts, medical costs are high and facilities and standards are sometimes poor; medical insurance should be sufficient to cover the cost of bringing you home by air ambulance, if necessary.

Ski injuries

The average overall injury rate is 4 per 1000 'skier days'. In 2000, 11 000 British skiers were injured in France alone.

In one survey, 58 per cent of injuries were in beginners, with 36 per cent in intermediate skiers and 6 per cent in expert skiers.

Not surprisingly, leg injuries are most common and, in another survey, accounted for 86 per cent of all injuries. Of these, 45 per cent were knee injuries and 43 per cent were tibial (shin) fractures; 8 per cent of injuries involved the arms — mainly wrist fractures; and 4 per cent were shoulder dislocations. Ski surfing tends to produce knee contusions and effusions (fluid in the joint) from falling forwards on to the knee.

Equipment factors

There are three important ways that the ski itself can produce injury. Firstly, it acts as a lever on the leg; a torque of as little as 7 kg at the tip of a ski can produce a fracture of the tibia (shin bone). Modern rigid ski boots protect the foot, ankle, and lower tibia from this kind of injury, but in doing so inevitably transfer stress to the knee, making ligamentous injuries at the knee joint an increasingly common hazard.

Secondly, if the bindings release a ski during a fall, and the ski is tethered to the ankle by a safety strap, the tethered ski may recoil against its owner; ski edges are sharp, and can produce severe lacerations. 'Ski stoppers' — a pair of prongs which project below the under-surface of the ski when the boot has been released from the binding — are preferable to safety straps. (Some skiers reduce the risk of losing skis without safety straps in deep snow by trailing ribbons from their bindings when skiing in deep powder.)

Thirdly, a 'rogue' ski — released during a fall — can become a dangerous projectile if it accelerates unchecked down a slope. It may strike or impale other skiers in its path. Ski stoppers reduce the likelihood of this occurrence.

Of the equipment-related injuries, 38 per cent are thought to be caused by boots, 46 per cent by poles, and the remainder by skis; 70 per cent of all lower-leg fractures could be prevented by correct binding tension. Check that your bindings release under reasonable force. They should have been adjusted professionally according to the size of your bones, your general muscularity, and experience, but you should always test them yourself. Do not handle the bindings or any other metal with your bare hands when temperatures are below freezing, or a cold burn will result.

Boots must be comfortable and hold the foot firmly so that movement is transmitted instantly to the ski, thereby protecting the ankle from injury.

Ski poles can cause injury, especially to the thumb; the strap and ski-pole handle should never be held in such a way that the thumb may become trapped. You should always be able to see both hands in front of you when you are skiing. Holding the poles close in to one's side can be dangerous, especially upon reaching the bottom of a slope, where a sudden rise uphill can drive the pole handle up and into the eye; I have seen an eye enucleated by this form of accident.

One other important point about the ski pole is that its loop should break loose with a strong tug. If its basket catches, on trees or brush, for instance, a severe injury to the shoulder can occur if the loop does not release. Such an injury can commonly result in a dislocation of the shoulder, but can also cause a less common but more serious injury — a traction injury on the *brachial plexus*, damaging the main nerves that enter the arm from the neck to supply the muscles and sensation of the upper limb; permanent paralysis may ensue.

On drag lifts, long hair must be tied back and loose clothing avoided. People have been scalped when hair has been caught in drag lifts.

If 'bum bags' are worn in front, the bag and its contents (especially cameras) can cause severe internal abdominal injuries in a fall: rupture of the spleen, liver, and small intestine have all occurred. When skiing, the correct position for the pouch is behind.

Other contributory factors

Many important factors that contribute to the risk of injury are under a considerable degree of individual control:

Inexperience and poor technique Beginners account for 70 per cent of skiing injuries: there is no substitute for skilled, *professional* ski instruction, so don't try to get by without lessons. Having attained a basic level of proficiency, don't become complacent about the need to improve your technique further. Lessons are not just for beginners.

Excessive speed This is especially dangerous on crowded slopes, often resulting in collisions with other skiers. It accounts for up to 10 per cent of accidents. In a recent case in the USA, a skier involved in a fatal accident was successfully prosecuted for involuntary manslaughter on the grounds of excessive speed. In some US resorts there are now well-marked speed restrictions and speed traps. Abusers risk losing their ski pass.

Alcohol 25 per cent of skiing accidents requiring hospitalization are associated with alcohol consumption within two hours of the accident.

Fatigue The majority of ski injuries occur on the first day of a ski holiday, especially towards the end of the morning or afternoon session. Make sure you stop skiing well before the stage when you are feeling tired and your legs ache.

Tired skiers are accident-prone because of glycogen depletion in their muscles. Give yourself plenty of opportunities for food, drink, and rest. Cumulative depletion of muscle glycogen can occur with time such that after three or four days of downhill skiing the reserves are almost totally exhausted; so it is advisable to mix light and heavy skiing days and consume a high carbohydrate diet to keep glycogen levels high. It is also important not to become dehydrated.

If you need to rest, do this off a run. The worst possible places to stop are near the bottom of a run and in the centre of the trail. This invites a collision.

Poor surface and conditions Rocky, icy, and slushy surfaces can be extremely treacherous, and should be avoided. They greatly increase the risk of injury. There are concerns that climate change could add to the dangers of skiing in some of the lower altitude resorts in years to come.

Snowboarding

Knee injuries are less likely than in skiers, but snowboarders are more likely to injure their arms — with wrist fractures, shoulder injuries and dislocations at the top of the list. Newcomers to the sport are said to be at greatest risk on their third day, decreasing subsequently with growing skill and experience.

Avoiding accidents

A lot of accidents occur at the start of the day when muscles are still cold and stiff after a long trip in the lift. Warm muscles work more easily and are therefore less easily injured, so it is worth doing a few warm-up exercises in the snow at the start of the day and after breaks for lunch or snacks or following long waits for and on lifts.

Always tell someone where you are going to ski that day and do not ski in an isolated area by yourself or ski alone in a white-out. Carry a cellular phone; keep in touch with your party, and know how to call for help in an emergency.

Watch for warning notices, safety fences, danger signs, marker stakes, ropes, red flagging, bluffs, and crossed poles or skis. They all mean 'danger'. In some countries, ignoring warning signs is a serious offence for which you may be prosecuted. In some resorts there are also signs to show where tracks or a road cross the path, where a run narrows, or where there is a ski lift crossing, a sudden sharp curve, a piste that is closed, a first-aid post, S.O.S., a telephone, an unpatrolled ski area beyond the sign, or changes in direction of the piste or trail.

The basic safety rules of the slopes are:

S ki in control
K eep clear of others
I F stopping — get out of the way
S top before you reach the lift line
A lways use ski brakes or straps
F ollow warning signs
E nter runs with care

The acronym for these rules is 'SKI SAFE'.

Ligaments

Whilst skiing, the body's weight is borne by one or other leg unless one is travelling directly downhill. Unlike the straight knee, the *flexed* knee permits a degree of rotation without damage to ligaments. An important principle to remember is that in an unstable or uncontrolled situation, totally unloading the inactive ski (usually the uphill one) and further flexing the knee bearing your weight will protect the ligaments from damage; sitting down may be undignified on skis, but ignominy is preferable to any sort of injury.

First-aid

In the event of an injury, first-aid treatment is most important in order to avoid compounding any damage that may have occurred. No skier who feels even moderate pain or the least instability on standing should ever attempt to continue skiing. A further fall may result in a much more serious injury. Any doubt about the integrity of joints, ligaments, or bone must be treated seriously and the part protected by splinting until an expert opinion can be obtained. The vast majority of doctors practising in ski resorts are very experienced and generally give wise counsel. Local orthopaedic surgeons usually give an extremely good service. There is, however, certainly in some European resorts, a tendency to resort to surgery when perhaps a conservative line of treatment would suffice. An injured skier can always request immobilization of the injured part in a cast and return home for treatment by a surgeon of his or her choice.

The 2001/2002 ski season saw a record number of deaths in Colorado: 14 skiers and 1 snowboarder. There was no discernible pattern to the deaths, but they did include a 5-year old who hit a tree during a private lesson, and who was not wearing a helmet. Following this accident, most ski resorts in the state now require children under 12 to wear a helmet.

Conclusion

Despite its many hazards, skiing is an enjoyable and popular activity. With care and attention to simple safety precautions, the small risk of injury can be reduced even further.

'Après ski' activity has its pleasures and its hazards — but that is another story.

Landmines

Landmines maim and kill long after wars are over. The victims are not just the dead or mutilated, but the impoverished communities that are left behind to starve, with only minefields to farm. Travellers to countries with former conflicts are also at risk, and need to be aware of the potential dangers.

Laura Bedford is a registered nurse. She has worked with VSO in rural Tanzania; and with Médecins sans Frontières in rural Angola, looking after victims of the on-going conflict and malnourished children, and co-ordinating medical activities in the field. At the other end of the scale, she has also advised and looked after a wide mix of travellers from Central London, at the Fleet Street Clinic.

Introduction

Landmines cost between $3 and $30 each: armies like them because they are a cheap and simple way to achieve short-term military objectives. But they cannot discriminate between a soldier, a terrorist, and a child, or a domestic animal. As mines are not visible in any way from the surface, it is impossible to tell where the danger lies, and even when mines are unearthed, children unaware of the danger of the device may pick them up and play with them.

There are many different types of mine, ranging from sensitive anti-personnel devices, designed for humans, to larger anti-tank or anti-vehicle types that require much weight to detonate them. The extent of the damage, and chances of survival, depend on the size of the mine. Victims of mine accidents most often have a leg blown off, and the majority of the victims I have seen have had the lower leg removed around mid-calf.

In the remote communities where landmine blasts most commonly occur, the prospects for survival are slim: there's little hope of surgery, or even a blood transfusion, let alone any prospect of support and rehabilitation.

The size of the problem

The statistics are grim. More than 50 mine-producing countries (including the US, Russia, China, and many developing countries) have manufactured more than 200 million anti-personnel mines over the past 25 years, and there are now believed to be at least 100 million unexploded landmines in more than 60 countries (see Table 8.7). Even if no more mines are ever laid, they will continue to be a hazard for many decades to come.

Afghanistan, Angola, Bosnia, Cambodia, Chechnya, Croatia, Iraq, Mozambique, Nicaragua, and Somalia are among the many countries with current conflicts where mine blasts are a daily routine. In Cambodia alone there are over 35 000 amputees, while in Angola, there are probably around 70 000. There are believed to be between one and two unexploded landmines for every man, woman, and child in Angola. (The population is around 11 million and there are 10–20 million mines.) According to Human Rights Watch, landmines kill as many as 120 people there per month. The global toll may be as high as 20 000 deaths per year (Map 8.3).

In Mozambique, recent floods have made the situation much worse: landmines are simply washed away, leaving no means of predicting where the danger lies. There are more floods to come.

At the beginning of 2002, India announced a plan to mine its entire border with Pakistan in Kashmir.

What is being done

Political measures

Achieving a global ban on landmines is a high priority, but there still does not seem to be the necessary political will to achieve this. Angola signed the Convention on the Prohibition of the Use, Stockpiling, Production, and Transfer of Anti-Personnel Mines and on their Destruction on 4 December 1997, but has yet to ratify it. Meanwhile, the Angolan government claims only to be mining strategic points such as dams and electricity pylons, and that these are mapped and will later be cleared. UNITA is said to be mining farmland and roads, and these mines are not marked. Either way, Angola, and many similar countries, remain strewn with landmines old and new, and other war debris and ordnance that are a danger to the public, prohibit development, restrict movement, and destroy communities.

De-mining

In some countries, there is an effort to clear landmines, though this is a very slow and costly procedure, requiring highly skilled teams and equipment that is not readily available in developing countries. (Organizations involved in de-mining in Angola include: Norwegian Peoples Aid (NPA) and World Vision, both of which were present in Malanje, and Care International.) The process is painstakingly slow. One small field I saw de-mined in Malanje took about six weeks to complete. It was being de-mined as it was behind a recently opened orphanage and there were fears that kids would run across it. There are two methods of de-mining: manual (hands and knees, metre by metre, with various metal detectors and prodders) and mechanical (using a huge sort of flailing machine that takes up the top layers of soil and explodes any ordnance in mid-air).

Rehabilitation

There are some organizations helping to fit prostheses (ICRC), though this is just the tip of a large iceberg. Again, this is a time-consuming and costly procedure. For example, there was a long waiting list for amputees in Malanje to register with ICRC. Once registered they would be taken to Luanda by plane (as road travel in Angola is so very unpredictable), and housed there for up to eight weeks while the fitting of and practice with a false limb took place. Then, they were sent back to Malanje. One thing that I will always remember about Angola is the large numbers of amputees you see getting around on crutches; they are amazingly resourceful. Because of poor medical attention and facilities, the stump remaining after amputation is often badly patched up with skin; it is an unsightly and difficult stump on which to mould and wear a prosthesis.

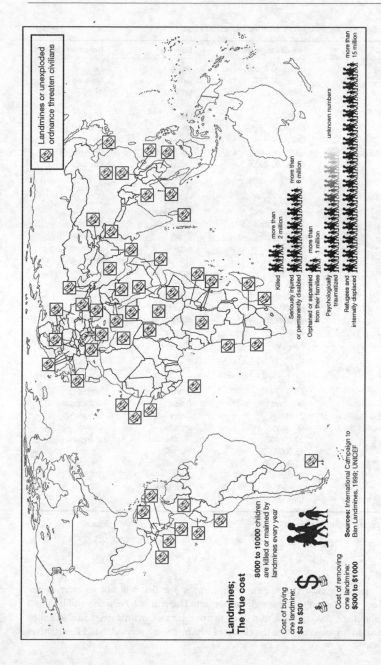

Map 8.3 Conflict and disaster: landmines

Table 8.7 Landmines: countries with the highest burdens

Country	No. of landmines	Country	No. of landmines
Afghanistan	over 10 000 000	Kuwait	Unknown
Angola	9–15 000 000	Laos	Unknown
Armenia	Unknown	Latvia	17 000
Austria	Unknown	Lebanon	9000
Azerbaijan	50 000	Liberia	18 250
Belarus	Unknown	Libya	Unknown
Belgium	Unknown	Luxembourg	Unknown
Bosnia–Herzegovina	6 000 000	Mauritania	Unknown
Cambodia	8–10 000 000	Mexico	Unknown
Chad	70 000	Moldova	Unknown
Chechnya	Unknown	Mongolia	Unknown
China	10 000 000	Myanmar	Unknown
Colombia	Unknown	Netherlands	Unknown
Costa Rica	1–2000	Nicaragua	108 000
Croatia	2 000 000	Oman	Unknown
Cuba	Unknown	Peru	Unknown
Cyprus	17 000	Philippines	Unknown
Czech Republic	Unknown	Russian Federation	Unknown
Denmark	9900	Rwanda	60 000
Djibouti	Unknown	Senegal	Unknown
Ecuador	60 000	Sierra Leone	Unknown
Egypt	23 000 000	Slovenia	Unknown
El Salvador	10 000	Somalia	1 000 000
Eritrea	1 000 000	Sri Lanka	Unknown
Ethiopia	500 000	Sudan	1 000 000
Falkland Islands/Malvinas	25 000	Syria	Unknown
Georgia	75–150 000	Tajikistan	Unknown
Germany	1300	Thailand	Unknown
Greece	Unknown	Tunisia	Unknown
Guatemala	2–4000	Turkey	Unknown
Guinea-Bissau	Unknown	Uganda	Unknown
Honduras	30–35 000	Ukraine	Unknown
Iran	16 000 000	Vietnam	Unknown
Iraq	10 000 000	Western Sahara	Unknown
Israel	Unknown	Yemen	100 000
Jordan	207 000	Yugoslavia	500 000
Republic of Korea	Unknown	Zimbabwe	Unknown

Source: Warchild, UN, US Department of State

Education

Finally, since it is clear that the mine problem is one that will not go away, 'mine awareness' is becoming increasingly important. The aim is to educate children and adults about the dangers, and to reduce the numbers of victims needlessly killed or mutilated. In Angola, thanks to the efforts of organizations such as UNICEF, initiatives involving theatre groups, posters, and radio broadcasts have done much to raise awareness of the potential dangers.

Landmines and travel

When peace returns, so does tourism. Many of the countries listed in Table 8.7 have growing tourist industries, and it is inevitable that travellers to these countries will be at risk. The number of travellers killed by landmines is not known, but includes the son of one of the contributors to this book, who lost a leg and died 24 hours later, after a promised helicopter evacuation had failed to arrive.

In areas where you don't know the risk, DO NOT go off the beaten track. Stick to well-defined and preferably well-used tracks that you see people walking on. Sometimes, minefields are indicated by the use of DANGER signs, but more often, they are not. Travel by road and by train, in an area of recent conflict, can be equally dangerous; roads, and particularly bridges, are often strategic points.

Local authorities often do not know, and are often scared of telling what they do know about mined land, so it is frequently hard to get any useful or trustworthy information. It is worth trying to enlist the help of a guide with good local knowledge. Local people sometimes know the places that should most carefully be avoided, but this is not always the case: I have come across villagers who have unknowingly built houses in minefields, with tragic results. I have also found that local people can often be complacent and would laugh in response to my question, 'Não tens minhas aqui?' You can sometimes see that certain areas of land are not used, either for habitation or for cultivation, and this may indicate a mined area, or it could simply be an unmarked or locally designated graveyard.

Things to be wary of include: vehicles and houses that have been blown up and abandoned; fields with visible remains of dead animals; and deserted villages (they are usually deserted for a reason). Minefields are often temporarily marked out with sticks and brush, so if you see something unusual, avoid it and tell someone what you saw. Most importantly, trust your own instinct and if you feel that things are not safe, then don't go.

Above all, anyone travelling for pleasure in an area where there is war or serious civil unrest should carefully weigh up the risks before going. It is neither heroic, nor exciting, to live, work, or travel in areas of serious conflict.

Sources of further information

www.icbl.org/
www.mag.org.uk/
www.icrc.org/
www.msf.org/
www.landminesurvivors.org
www.angola.npaid.org/

Further reading

Hargarten, S. and Cortes, L. (2001). Landmines: Not just another travel risk. *Journal of Travel Medicine*, **8**, 229–31.

Angolan diary
3 April 2000

Last week, a food truck blew up on a landmine (anti-tank) just off the road to Cangandala (i.e. just off the remains of the tarmac). The army informed us that the rest of the road was also mined; since that day we have been unable to go back to Cangandala. The whole incident was horrific and frightening — we had been driving up and down that road for months, and it is just luck that none of us were in the vehicle that detonated it. The whole community here is currently unable to go to Cangandala, which is disastrous for the people there. Our feeding centre has had to close as we have not been able to get food supplies down there, and for sure many children will die in the meantime. The driver was killed, and the other two passengers seriously injured (I think they too both died later in hospital). A population of approximately 8000 'internally displaced persons', mostly new arrivals, became cut off from all aid; even WFP food rations were suspended. Needless to say, the level of disease and death rose dramatically, and our main feeding centre in Malanje was inundated with really very sick and severely malnourished children and, later, adults too from Cangandala. All because of one mine.

23 October 2000

Last week there were three UNITA attacks on roads leading into Malanje, including the road to Cangandala. It has meant again that we were not able to visit Cangandala as much as normal last week, and on the day we went back, we saw the army de-mining the road: not too reassuring as you are driving along it!

30 October 2000

A truck was blown up on an anti-tank mine in Malanje, close to where we have been going with our (MSF) truck to get water. A good lesson why not to become complacent here. The driver lost both his legs and had serious head injuries; he ended up in hospital here, where I saw him by chance; he died later on the plane to Luanda. This really is such a mad place; have to keep reminding myself we are in a country at war.

Psychotropic drugs

The use and acceptability of mind-altering drugs varies from one country to another. Travellers who use such drugs do so at their own risk, but should realize that locally produced substances may have unexpectedly potent and possibly dangerous effects, and that the penalties for illegal possession are frequently severe.

Dr Martin Mitcheson was the Clinical Director of the South West Regional Drug Advisory Service and practises in the field of drug abuse.
Roger Lewis† was a research specialist in international drug traffic and the author of a number of studies of illicit drug markets in Britain, Italy, and elsewhere. He sadly died after a short illness in 2000.

In almost every society in the world, mind-altering or psychotropic substances are used for recreational, ritual, and medical purposes. Just as different cultures around the world favour different pharmaceutical, homeopathic, and folk preparations, they also display preferences for different types of social and recreational drug use. These preferences are influenced by such factors as the plant life indigenous to the region, traditional familiarity with particular drug effects, the impact of aggressive colonial marketing, and the solace and oblivion that some drugs may provide for individuals suffering from boredom, poverty, and privation, or ethnic groups threatened with extinction or assimilation.

Patterns of psychotropic drug use world-wide

Tobacco and alcohol
Tobacco and alcohol are, broadly speaking, available throughout the world, although some Islamic countries such as Saudi Arabia impose severe penalties upon individuals who consume, or traffic in, the latter.

Cannabis
Cannabis, known in its various preparations as hashish, ganja, marijuana, bush, grass, and countless other names, grows or can be cultivated in most parts of the world. Since the 1960s one of the attractions of countries such as India, Pakistan, and (until recently) Afghanistan to young European travellers has been the quality and quantity of cannabis preparations readily available to them. In Africa and the Americas the drug usually comes in herbal form and, despite the denials of many governments who view alcohol as 'civilized' and cannabis as 'primitive', cannabis is consumed in a controlled and considered fashion by large sections of the world's population.

The opium poppy
The opium poppy, from which morphine and heroin are derived, grows within a geographical band running from Vietnam's Gulf of Tonkin to Turkey's Anatolian plain. Some tribal peoples have successfully integrated the poppy into their daily lives, although addiction has emerged as a problem in Iran, Pakistan, and parts of Southeast Asia.

Once refined and converted into heroin, opiates present a particular threat to the young, semi-Westernized populations of Bangkok, Karachi, Tehran, and Singapore —

as well as an increasing problem of addiction, with associated severe physical and psychological difficulty, among young people in developed countries.

Cocaine

Cocaine is derived from the coca leaf, which originates in Latin America. The Indian peoples of Colombia, Bolivia, and Peru chew the leaf or drink an infusion as a source of nutrition and energy for work and relaxation. Problems have arisen associated with 'gringo' entrepreneurs intent on profiting from the sale of the plant's chemical derivative, cocaine, to North America and Europe. Like 'crack' in North America, cocaine-base smoking has become an increasing problem in South America.

Other drugs

Apart from the major psychotropics, travellers may come across other drugs that create legal, medical, and psychological problems. The peyote cactus, for example, may be found in the south-western USA and northern Mexico; the psilocybin mushroom in western Europe and North and Central America; and 'fly-agaric', the white-spotted mushroom of fairy-tale, in North America, northern Europe, and northern Asia. They all have strong hallucinogenic properties and are treated with respect by those folk cultures that employ them for such properties.

In recent years there has been an increase in the recreational use of minor tranquillizers, especially in developing countries with lax controls on pharmacy sales. There is a risk that they may be used to facilitate unwelcome sexual advances as they may induce a temporary memory loss. Substituted amphetamines have become a frequently consumed drug at dance venues; they are usually sold illicitly as 'ecstasy' (methylenedioxymethamphetamine) which can cause severe reactions even in small doses; these include hyperpyrexia (p. 338), delirium, and cardiac and respiratory distress, which have resulted in a significant number of deaths.

Drug problems involving travellers

Travellers may experience unforeseen physical problems from the consumption of psychotropic drugs abroad; and legal problems with the possibility of arrest and imprisonment, as a result of illegal possession (including inadvertent possession).

Physical problems

If drugs are used in situations where there is uncertainty about the strength of preparations, and if drugs are injected when sterile equipment is not available, the potential hazards of drug taking are increased considerably (see p. 588).

Problems include: overdose of drugs, either accidental or deliberate; intoxication produced by sedative tranquillizers; panic reactions resulting from consumption of a variety of drugs, including potent preparations of cannabis and psychedelic drugs such as lysergide or mescaline; and acute paranoid states from cocaine and amphetamines. Regular daily consumption of drugs of the sedative tranquillizer group, or of the opioid group, followed by abrupt cessation, can produce an unpleasant and potentially dangerous withdrawal illness, particularly when coinciding with physical illness of the type that may easily occur abroad. Physical complications may arise as a result of the mode of administration, particularly injection, or where a drug-centred existence leads to the neglect of nutrition and personal hygiene.

Overdose
The distinction between overdose and other acute reactions is partly dependent on the type of drug consumed and partly on the relative dose level. Broadly, opioids and sedative tranquillizers depress cerebral function and decrease the sensitivity of the brain's respiratory centre. When sedation is profound, reflexes that normally protect the airway by coughing when foreign material is present, are suppressed. A sedated person may be lying in a position where simple mechanical obstruction to an airway can occur.

When someone is believed to have taken an overdose of this kind of drug, hospital treatment is always recommended; while waiting for assistance, turn the affected person into the semi-prone 'recovery' position. This is achieved by laying them on their side, with the upper leg bent, their face at an angle towards the floor, and their neck gently extended, with the lower jaw pulled forward to maintain an airway. In this position, regurgitated food from the stomach is much less likely to be inhaled into the lungs. If breathing is so depressed that mouth-to-mouth ventilation is necessary, it is important to remember to clean any food debris from the mouth before inflating the lungs. These techniques are clearly explained and demonstrated in first-aid books. The specific medical antidote for opioid overdose is an injection of the pure antagonist, nalorphine.

Other acute reactions
Acute anxiety or fleeting hallucinatory experiences can occur under the influence of alcohol, other sedative tranquillizers and volatile inhalants, as well as psychedelic drugs. Acute panic reactions popularly referred to as 'bad trips', occur most frequently amongst novice consumers, those taking the drug in anxiety-provoking situations, older people experimenting with an unusual experience, and any consumer who unexpectedly encounters an unaccustomedly large dose. These factors are more likely to occur in a foreign country.

Reactions to ectasy require immediate medical treatment. Adequate consumption of non-alcoholic fluids protects to some extent but paradoxically if too much fluid is consumed there is a risk of over hydration.

Adverse reactions are uncommon from the relatively weak psychedelic drug cannabis, particularly when this is consumed with some care by inhalation; but they are more likely to occur when cannabis is consumed by mouth with less control over the dose. The predominant symptom and sign of an adverse reaction is acute anxiety that may be related to subjective perceptual disturbance, or to external anxiety-provoking events. In a severe reaction, true hallucinations may be experienced. These perceptions may lead the sufferer to believe they are experiencing a severe psychiatric illness and a simultaneous increased heart rate may lead to fears of imminent death. The management of these acute reactions is reassurance, which will need to be repeated often since short-term memory is usually also affected. A companion should endeavour to relate the sufferer's current experience to the fact that they have consumed a drug. The use of tranquillizers plays a small part in the management of acute reactions. Admission to a psychiatric institution is generally counter-productive.

Persecutory delusions (paranoia) are the principal serious adverse reaction to both amphetamines and cocaine. Individual dose response can vary widely. The acute episode is indistinguishable from acute schizophrenia. Disorder is generally self-limiting within a period of two or three days if the person ceases drug use. Administration of major (phenothiazine) tranquillizers may confuse the diagnosis.

Drug withdrawal reactions

Withdrawal from the sedative tranquillizer group of drugs is potentially medically hazardous since epileptic convulsions and a confused state with hallucinations can occur (the syndrome known as delirium tremens – DTs – in alcohol withdrawal). The immediate management of severe withdrawal is to administer any convenient drug of this group such as alcohol, phenobarbital, or benzodiazepines such as diazepam (Valium). It is highly probable that the alcohol withdrawal syndrome is exacerbated by poor nutrition, which is common in chronic alcoholics, and it is important to ensure adequate vitamin supplements, particularly B_6, to avoid the risk of permanent brain damage.

Disease in drug users

Hepatitis occurs commonly amongst heavy drug users and is broadly of two types: hepatitis A, otherwise known as infectious hepatitis, occurs in association with poor hygiene, and is common where food products may be contaminated by excreta used as fertilizer or infection carried by flies from latrines to food preparation areas. The onset usually occurs within four weeks following infection. Hepatitis B, C, and D, otherwise referred to as serum hepatitis, are usually transmitted by blood products or other body fluids (see pp. 57–8). In relation to drug use, this occurs as a result of using a needle or syringe contaminated by blood from an infected person. It should be noted that it is extremely difficult to adequately re-sterilize the disposable syringes now almost invariably used in industrialized societies. In an emergency, when sterile syringes and needles are not available, it is of some benefit to use the following cleaning method: draw up clean (boiled but cool) water, and flush the equipment twice; discard the water and repeat twice with fresh household bleach (not disinfectant); rinse twice with clean water. The relative poverty of medical services in developing countries often results in needles and syringes being reused, with a high risk of infection as a result of any injection. Serum hepatitis has a longer incubation period than hepatitis A, of the order of two to three months from the time of infection.

HIV, though less contagious then hepatitis B, is transmitted in a similar way and is particularly common in Central and East Africa and areas where intravenous drug use is common or which are frequented for commercialized sex, including Thailand and India. It should be noted that in some areas blood transfusion is one means by which impoverished people can raise money and therefore blood transfusion products are more likely to be a source of infection.

Any form of hepatitis can be a debilitating and potentially serious illness requiring medical care and in severe cases medical repatriation is needed. Active immunization is available to protect against hepatitis A and B; but not as yet to confer protection against C and D hepatitis, nor against HIV infection. Hepatitis is discussed in greater detail on p. 54 and HIV on p. 468.

Legal problems

Young travellers in particular may be offered psychotropic drugs in foreign countries. Such drugs may be widely used by the local population, but are formally illegal. Some countries like Turkey and Thailand conduct the specific policy of applying the full force of their laws against foreign nationals, who are highly visible as well as being more vulnerable. This particularly applies to countries that have reputations as centres of illicit traffic and have attracted the censure of importing countries.

It always pays to do one's homework about the countries one intends to visit. Travellers in sunny places tend to forget that things are rarely as easy-going as they seem. A single cannabis cigarette in Greece means prison for one year plus one day, minimum. In some countries second-class passengers often ask first-class passengers to assist with their luggage allowance. There may be no ulterior motive to such a request, but even inadvertent smuggling still means severe penalties.

If taken into custody, never sign anything unless it can be read and understood. Remember this even under intense physical and psychological pressure. The only friend left in such circumstances may be your Consul. Consular officials may not be able to do a great deal but should be able to recommend a local English-speaking lawyer (fellow prisoners may also have some ideas). Different countries have different regulations regarding legal aid, if it exists at all. It makes sense to discover the details as soon as possible.

Your Consulate will inform your family about your situation unless you wish otherwise. Generally, the Consul is expected to visit you as soon as possible after your arrest, to ensure you are legally represented and to make sure that your treatment is *no worse* than that of the local population.

Prescribed drugs

Many drugs such as heroin and other opioids, cocaine, and cannabis, are subject to international treaty agreements governing the international trade in these substances. At present the majority of stimulants and sedative tranquillizers, including barbiturates, are not so strictly controlled but may be restricted under local regulations. In many countries the importation of any potential drug of abuse may be regarded as a criminal offence.

Patients who need to take regular medication for the treatment of physical or psychological disease should of course have consulted their usual physician before undertaking foreign travel. Because of the laws regarding importation of psychoactive drugs, anyone requiring a continued supply should arrange with their physician to receive a local legal prescription from a doctor in the country they intend to visit.

Note that an open letter to 'any doctor whom it might concern' will usually be insufficient to obtain immediate treatment because (a) any drug mentioned in the letter may not be legally available in the destination country and, (b) even if it is, many doctors are not prepared to take on patients at short notice, nor are they prepared to take on nationals of another country.

However, specialists working in the field of drug dependence often do have knowledge of similar colleagues in other countries and may be able to organize medical care by prior arrangement, particularly if it is only to cover a short visit or to attend to family affairs, and in particular, bereavements. These particular precautions refer primarily to opiate drugs and amphetamines.

Minor tranquillizers and barbiturate sedatives prescribed in small amounts should be declared to customs officials and may or may not be accepted for importation. Major tranquillizers (phenothiazines such as chlorpromazine) and tricyclic anti-depressants are almost always permitted, although problems could arise if a customs official was uncertain of the status or content of the tablets: in some cases, tablets may be confiscated for analysis.

Summary of information for travellers

- Consumption of psychotropic drugs in a situation without the support of friends or in unfamiliar surroundings is more likely to result in an anxiety reaction.

- The strength of preparations available in producing countries is likely to be greater than that of preparations which are available at home, where the product may have been diluted to increase the seller's profit margin and where the active principle may have been reduced in potency due to the time taken in transit.

- The consumption of unaccustomed powerful drugs increases the risk of adverse reactions.

- The risk of physical complications from self-injection of drugs is considerably higher in countries where injecting equipment is expensive and imported.

---

9 Some common troubles

Skin problems

Skin problems typically account for one third of all health problems in travellers. This chapter explains how to recognize, treat, or prevent the most likely problems.

Dr Francisco Vega–López is a Consultant Dermatologist at University College London Hospitals NHS Trust, UK, where he has established a specialized clinic in Tropical Dermatology and Skin in the Traveller at the Hospital for Tropical Diseases. Previously, he practised internal medicine and dermatology in rural and urban Mexico for more than 15 years, and dermatology in South London for two years.

Introduction

Diseases of the skin are amongst the commonest causes of medical consultation. It has been estimated that more than half of the global human population suffers or will develop a skin complaint at some stage in their lives. In Britain and other European countries, up to 20 per cent of all patients who consult a GP do so because of skin disease or symptoms. A similar picture has been recorded in tropical developing countries. Despite their frequent presentation, fortunately most skin diseases have a very low mortality rate. However, the main problems linked to several skin conditions are the high costs in psychological and emotional terms, as well as the degree of resulting disability.

Ideally, a traveller requires a healthy skin. Itchiness, a burning sensation, a painful and nasty-looking spot or abscess, and the need to apply frequent medicated creams and ointments are just a few of the ways in which the ideal holiday or business trip can turn into an unforgettable nightmare.

This chapter presents a brief description of the commonest skin disorders and symptoms relevant for travellers of all ages. Particular emphasis is given to practical aspects of diagnosis, prevention, and treatment of skin problems during travel. (Certain skin diseases occurring in specific areas of the world are presented by geographical region in other chapters of this book.) Finally, a few simple but essential recommendations to prevent skin problems are provided.

The traveller with previous skin disease

Psoriasis

This is a very common skin disease world-wide, particularly affecting young individuals of both sexes. The main clinical signs and symptoms include the presence of raised plaques, pink or red, with white scaling. The inflammatory plaques are usually located on the extensor surfaces of the body, but the scalp and nails can also be affected. Less common clinical presentations occur in the skin folds, such as under the breasts, between the buttocks, the armpits, the groins, and external genitalia.

Psoriasis commonly adopts a chronic, unpredictable course with alternating periods of activity and remission. It may cause itchiness or a burning sensation on the affected areas of the skin, but more often it is without symptoms. Although there are a number of successful treatments to improve the condition, there is currently no definitive cure. In general, psoriasis tends to improve on holidays in sunny climates; but sunburn is known to trigger its development. Bathing in sea waters in tropical countries seems to have a beneficial effect in many people with psoriasis. Travellers with psoriasis taking certain medications for other medical conditions may experience a flare up shortly after the start of the treatment. Caution should be taken by those requiring beta-blockers, ACE inhibitors, lithium, and anti-malarials.

Atopic eczema

This frequent skin condition tends to affect more than one member in the family, and often coexists with asthma and/or allergic rhinitis (hay fever). Commonly, it appears in early childhood and the inflammatory activity tends to subside after a few years. Atopic eczema manifests as patches or raised plaques of inflamed skin causing severe itchiness. These plaques may be thickened and suffer from fissuring which predisposes to infections. This form of eczema commonly affects the face and flexural areas of the body surface, such as the neck, forearms, and behind the knees.

Many young individuals tend to improve while on holiday, but very hot and humid countries may not be tolerated and can cause a flare up. Frequent moisturising of the skin is essential to control the itchiness, protect the barrier function of the skin, and prevent infection. Toddlers and school children with atopic eczema are particularly susceptible to acquiring superficial bacterial, fungal, and viral infections. These respectively include impetigo, ringworm, and molluscum contagiosum.

Contact eczema

Irritating chemicals, water, and a vast number of allergenic substances (compounds that induce allergy) can cause this form of acute or chronic eczema. Common allergens include nickel, cobalt salts, cosmetics, perfumes, textiles, rubber, inks, and food proteins. Young individuals of both sexes are commonly affected, but all age groups can develop this problem when the skin surface is in direct contact with the offending agent. In many cases, contact eczema represents an occupational disease for persons involved in the handling of animal proteins, latex gloves, dentistry materials, nursing activities, and hairdressing — to mention but a few.

The palms of the hands are most usually affected, since these are one of the most exposed areas of our body. However, the hands can subsequently spread contact with the chemical in question by touching the face and other parts of the body. Caustic substances will cause a severe burn, but milder irritants can induce itchiness, burning sensation, redness of the skin, pain, and blistering. The best measure to prevent contact eczema is the avoidance of irritating substances.

The traveller with contact eczema in hot and humid climates may develop symptoms on areas of skin subjected to pressure from tight clothing, shoes, money-belts, and straps from heavy backpacks causing severe friction on the skin surface. Medicated adhesive tape and bandages used to treat wounds in the traveller may also cause acute contact eczema. Hotel soaps and toiletries can sometimes cause similiar problems.

Simple measures to treat most forms of mild acute contact eczema include the use of a mild antiseptic applied in soaks three times daily, moisturising of the skin, and 1 per cent hydrocortisone cream to provide anti-inflammatory action. Tests to accurately diagnose troublesome allergic forms of contact eczema have to be carried out in a dermatology department.

Travellers at particular risk

Individuals with previous medical conditions are at a higher risk of developing skin problems, particularly those that are infectious in origin. Most travellers at increased risk of skin infection are aware of this and already know how best to avoid trouble or, if unlucky, the best ways to deal with it.

All medical conditions that interfere with the proper functioning of our immune system or tissue repair mechanisms increase the risk for infectious skin diseases. In particular, individuals suffering from one or more of the following conditions — diabetes mellitus, chronic alcoholism, intravenous drug use, a variety of cancers, and AIDS — should take careful advice from doctors, nurses, and travel specialists before embarking on a holiday or business trip. Chronic liver and kidney diseases as well as long-term treatment with corticosteroids and immunosuppressive medicines may also predispose travellers to acquiring skin infections. Patients with high blood pressure and other cardiovascular problems taking specific medication must be aware of the possibility of developing skin reactions when exposed to direct or indirect sunshine (see below).

Skin wounds

Minor abrasions, wounds, and injuries to the skin occur commonly in travellers. Fortunately, only a few of these result in serious localized or even systemic life-threatening infections. Following an accident, the open wound should be thoroughly washed with clean water and mild soap. A sterile, non-allergenic (does not cause allergy) dressing should be used to protect the wound from dirt and prevent the entry of unwanted microbes. Resting of the affected body part should help trigger the protective mechanisms of tissue repair to complete healing successfully. Particular attention should be paid to wounds occurring on the hands and feet while scuba-diving, snorkelling, or trekking in the tropics. Nasty bacteria and fungi can be directly deposited into the skin following an injury from coral reefs, tree bark, soil, vegetation, and rusty metal or wood debris.

Voluntary service or aid workers in developing countries must be aware that personal health is a priority. Minor skin wounds have to be readily treated, and strong protective shoe-wear as well as proper clothing should be the norm. Particular protection with mask and gloves is recommended in tree-planting projects, farming, building, and activities involving contact with livestock in the tropics. These measures are valuable in the prevention of fungal and bacterial infections that can be acquired through direct skin contact or by inhalation of the infective organisms.

Other common minor skin wounds, such as those from scorpions, spiders, and snakes, require immediate attention. Specific anti-serum to inactivate the poison will be required as well as treatment of the skin wound with water and soap, antiseptics, anti-microbial cream, and, in some cases, systemic antibiotics. The same applies to bites inflicted by small vertebrates such as racoons, otters, rats, squirrels, armadillos, and dogs. (See Chapter 6, 'Animal bites' for more information on snakes, scorpions, and spiders, as well as rabies.)

Skin diseases by pathogenic organisms

Viruses

Molluscum contagiosum infection consists of small, discrete, whitish millimetric pimples, acquired by direct contact with an infected person. The condition is common world-wide in healthy children and particularly represents a nuisance to individuals with deficient immunity such as those with organ transplants or HIV. Also, young travellers with atopic eczema can be more susceptible to acquiring this viral infection.

The lesions are usually asymptomatic but some children experience moderate itchiness. Scratching of the lesions may result in self-spreading of the infection to nearby sites on the skin. Most commonly, the disease affects the face, neck, and trunk, but any part of the skin can be affected. Superimposed secondary superficial skin infections may be the result of scratching and picking of the pimples. Avoidance of direct skin contact with infected persons is the best preventive measure. Individual pimples can be removed by a variety of topical and minor surgical procedures, but very young children are reluctant to accept this approach. Often the best strategy is to leave the lesions untreated in order to allow the normal immune system to eventually eliminate the infection; this may take 18 months or more.

Common warts are caused by a papilloma virus. Although strictly not a traveller's disease, their appearance may coincide with a journey overseas. People with deficient skin immunity show a marked predisposition to developing warts, and young individuals with atopic eczema are frequently troubled by them. A number of preparations to treat common warts can be purchased over the counter, but severe cases require the attention of a doctor or nurse. Common warts require treatment by a dermatologist only in certain individuals, such as those recovering from a transplant, under immunosuppressive therapy, or with a previous history of skin cancer.

Infections by **Herpes simplex** (cold sores (p. 426), genital herpes) can be acquired through direct skin contact, kissing, and sexual contact. Most commonly, localized infection on the lips or oral mucosa manifests after febrile illness or prolonged sun exposure and intense physical exertion during a beach holiday. In the exhausted traveller, a primary infection by herpes virus inside the mouth and upper pharynx may present with fever, painful ulcers, odorous breath, and lymph node enlargement on the upper neck. Severe cases make eating and drinking impossible, requiring specific intravenous medication and bed rest following the accurate diagnosis by a doctor.

Bacteria

Many travellers suffer from superficial skin infections following injury with luggage, whilst actually travelling, during some physical activity, and so on. Bacteria such as staphylococci and streptococci can penetrate the skin and cause red patches, a localized boil, or even superficial ulceration. Sweating around the warmer parts of the body and skin folds subjected to friction from unusual physical activity may in some cases predispose to these infections. Clinical diseases in this group include **impetigo, folliculitis, boils, abscess**, and **cellulitis**.

Minor injuries at home or in the garden usually heal satisfactorily within a few days. The picture can be modified, however by deficient hygiene, change of diet, excessive drinking, and 'roughing it' while travelling. Washing of the skin in antiseptic soaking water, twice or three times daily, will resolve most superficial skin infections. Some infections, however, will require medical attention and systemic antibiotics. This also applies to travellers developing an allergic reaction to common insect or mosquito bites and subsequently suffering a superimposed bacterial infection.

Uncommon, but more severe skin infections may result from practising sports in polluted estuaries or tropical oceans during the hot summer months. Skin infections acquired through injuries while fishing, snorkelling, and scuba-diving, or following ingestion of raw seafood (oysters in particular) usually require immediate medical attention. Serious skin infections in this group present with a high fever, painful skin, dark red/violaceous lesions, and general malaise. The skin becomes red and shiny from inflammation.

Proper menstrual hygiene, with a frequent change of tampons, is the best preventive measure for a potentially lethal bacterial condition named **toxic shock syndrome** which requires treatment in hospital. This simple measure also prevents mild but very uncomfortable irritation from 'nappy-type' **vulval dermatitis,** caused by friction and frequently complicated by yeast or bacterial infection. If you are travelling in remote areas and medical services are not available, initial antiseptic treatment of superficial **vulvo-vaginitis** can be carried out by vulval bathing in 50–80 ml of vinegar (any locally available brand) diluted in 5–8 litres of water, twice daily for 10–15 minutes each time, and for two or three days. Improvement of symptoms such as irritation, burning sensation, and itchiness should be expected following the very first or second treatment. This mildly acidic solution changes the superficial chemical balance and most common yeasts as well as bacteria are successfully eliminated. Soothing of irritated broken skin and vestibular mucosa of external genitalia can also be achieved by using a barrier cream such as zinc oxide (Lassar paste).

Finally, travellers must be aware that tampons and sanitary towels may not be readily available in rural regions of the tropics (see p. 440). A definite diagnosis and proper treatment of most vulvar skin conditions require a physician and often a dermatologist.

Fungi

A number of common fungal infections occur world-wide, both at home and during travel. Frequent examples include superficial infections such as **ringworm**, **athlete's foot**, and **thrush**. Proper hygiene, including a daily shower and change of clothes, may prevent skin colonization by fungi. Compounds such as those contained in 'over-the-counter' creams like Canesten and Daktarin, applied for 6 to 8 weeks, are sufficient to cure superficial fungal infections. Pessaries for single–dose vaginal treatment are also readily available.

However, a number of other deeper fungal infections (subcutaneous and systemic) are not only more severe in clinical terms, but also more difficult to diagnose and treat, as many of them occur only in particular regions of the world. Most of these rather serious diseases are caused by direct inoculation of the fungus into the skin, but they can also be acquired through inhalation of infecting spores during normal breathing. This occurs during trekking excursions where the walker is exposed to soil, vegetation, tree bark, and decomposing organic debris, where fungi have their natural habitat. Desert regions, tropical rainforests, and jungles, in particular, and also archaeological sites and caves are renowned sites for acquiring respiratory and/or skin diseases by fungi. Some of these fungal infections (known as mycosis) include uncommon diseases such as **sporotrichosis**, **chromoblastomycosis**, **mycetoma**, **histoplasmosis**, and **coccidioidomycosis**. These represent only a few and there are many others posing a risk for the most adventurous traveller exploring remote regions in deserts or the tropics.

Avoidance of infection can best be achieved by wearing strong shoes and proper clothing at all times. Sandals (no matter how expensive, comfortable, or trendy) would represent a health hazard when walking in rural Africa, southern USA, Latin America, or Southeast Asia. Tourists in sandals climbing pyramids, walking in the jungle, or kicking scorpions off their path must be desperate to catch a skin infection! Walkers, archaeologists, and explorers venturing inside caves (mountainous, ground level, or underground) and grottoes must be familiar with specific environmental hazards and wear masks in order to avoid inhaling infecting spores which may result in fungal disease of the lungs. Avoid especially those areas covered in droppings from bats and a variety of birds to prevent catching **histoplasmosis**.

Safety standards established by qualified national tourist operators should be followed when planning holidays to the jungle, to caves, or, even more so, to partially unexplored remote regions of the world.

The treatment of all deep fungal infections is highly specialized and can be offered only by local physicians who are familiar with particular diseases or by medical centres in capital cities in the developed world. Unfortunately, there is no cure for several of these severe fungal diseases of the skin.

Parasites

Unlike fungal diseases, infections caused by parasites are commonly seen in the returning traveller. Such parasites include simple microscopic organisms of only one cell, as well as complex worms with a very sophisticated anatomy and physiology. Some parasitic diseases are transmitted by insect bite, as in the case of **leishmaniasis** and **onchocerciasis**; others, like **schistosomiasis** (bilharzia), are acquired through the skin by swimming in polluted waters; and others, as in the case of **cutaneous larva migrans,** by walking or laying down on infested beaches. Unfortunately, most travellers like to visit nature, or swim in a lake, or walk bare-footed in the sand.

The term **leishmaniases** (see also p. 179) refers to a group of skin conditions which, on rare occasions, causes a potentially lethal organic disease of the liver and spleen. These conditions represent a public health problem to local indigenous communities in certain areas of the world. Of more relevance to the traveller are those skin leishmaniases acquired through the bite of sandflies carrying particular species of the parasite *Leishmania*. Correspondingly, different skin diseases result from different species of parasites.

Cutaneous leishmaniasis can be acquired in all the countries of the Mediterranean basin, Afghanistan, North Africa, Middle East, and Latin America. In general, skin leishmaniasis from the Old World is less severe than that originating in Central and South America.

A few weeks after the sandfly bite, a red nodule or an ulcer are the first signs of illness. The initial skin lesion appears on the site of the bite (usually face, ears, hands, forearms, ankles) but, in aggressive forms, new lesions can appear and spread to nearby sites within a few weeks. Unless infected by bacteria, the nodules and ulcers may not be symptomatic at all, and this can be a determining factor in delaying seeking medical advice. Some lesions acquired in the Middle East may heal spontaneously after a few months, without treatment, but if the diagnosis is suspected, referral to a specialized centre is compulsory. Certain forms of Central and South American leishmaniasis can produce fast disfiguring ulceration of the face, tissue destruction, and scarring. Investigations for diagnosis and treatment are available only in specialized hospitals.

Onchocerciasis (also called **river blindness**) is transmitted by the bite of a blackfly in specific regions of Africa and Latin America that are near to fast-flowing streams or rivers where the blackflies breed (see also p 173). As happens with other insect bites, these bites occur on exposed parts of the body such as the face and upper and lower limbs. Several weeks after the bite, the adult worm (*Onchocerca volvolus*) reaches maturity inside the human body and reproduces periodically to yield generations of young worms causing skin symptoms. Such periodic reproductive activity can last for many years, in spite of treatment.

The main symptoms of disease include severe itchiness and eczema-like lesions on the limbs, back, and buttocks. Firm nodules on the skin of the scalp, neck, and buttocks can also be found. In some cases, generalized itchiness all over the body can be desperate. One of the most severe complications of this disease occurs in the eye, resulting in blindness.

Tests for the diagnosis and specific treatment are available only in specialized centres. Protection from insect bites and avoidance of travelling in endemic areas of the world are the best preventive measures against onchocerciasis.

Schistosomiasis (also called **swimmers' itch** or **bilharziasis**) is acquired by swimming or bathing in contaminated waters (see also p. 104). Young parasites penetrate the skin leaving a minute, usually unnoticeable, wound. The parasite matures within the human body and causes acute as well as chronic disease of the skin, respiratory system, liver, and bladder. Common skin symptoms are allergic reactions such as urticaria, swelling of the face (eyelids, cheeks, and lips) and severe itchiness. Specific tests for diagnosis and treatment are available only in specialized centres. Prevention includes strict avoidance of bathing or swimming in contaminated waters of Africa and the Far East.

Cutaneous larva migrans results from acquiring the dog or cat hookworm parasite which is found in beaches or soil contaminated by faecal matter passed by infested pets (see also p. 117). Parasitic larvae readily penetrate the human skin on buttocks, back, abdomen, or feet. Potentially, any site of the human body resting on the infested sand or soil may become the port of entry for these parasites. Once in the skin, the parasite migrates within this tissue and does not cause symptoms in other organs. After a few days or weeks in the skin, symptoms and signs of disease manifest as an intensely itchy rash with burning sensation, spots, and the characteristic red, angry-looking larval track left by the serpiginous movements of the parasite. Scratching and breaking of the skin results very often in superimposed superficial bacterial infection. The infection by this parasite may last several months if left untreated. Specific treatment with anti-helminthic drugs has to be provided by a qualified physician. The outcome is complete cure in most cases.

Ectoparasites

This group of infestations are caused by a number of mites, lice, bugs, fleas, and ticks which induce disease not only in humans but, in some cases, in many other living animals. In most cases, disease remains confined to the skin but in others, these ectoparasites may transmit serious illness such as typhus (by ticks, body louse, and fleas) and other fevers.

Scabies is caused by a microscopic organism, *Sarcoptes scabiei*, and is usually acquired from another person by direct skin contact (see also pp. 202–3). In the right context it may be transmitted sexually. Very itchy small papules (spots, pimples) affect the trunk, upper limbs (often hands), external genitalia (particularly in males), and thighs a few days following transmission. Infants and immunosuppressed individuals may, however, present with a severely itchy disseminated or generalized rash.

Left untreated, scabies may persist for months, and regular hygienic measures that help to prevent the disease are no use as a cure. Also, it is well recognized that even very clean individuals may acquire the infestation. Diagnosis and treatment require a physician. Cure is achieved with one treatment applied topically in most cases. Few individuals may require a second course of topical treatment, but most cases still complain of itchiness for several weeks after effective treatment. Complicated cases and outbreaks of scabies in institutions require treatment with tablets.

Pediculosis (*lice, nits, crabs, ladillas*) of the scalp and hair, body, and pubic area are caused by organisms respectively called *Pediculus capitis, Pediculus corporis*, and *Phthirus pubis* (see also p. 200). Nits and head lice are a common experience in school children all over the world, and most teachers and parents are familiar with the diagnosis and treatment. Over-the-counter anti-nit combs and preparations resolve the problem satisfactorily with one or two treatments. Re-infestations can be a problem in deprived or overcrowded communities.

In contrast, the **body louse** can be acquired during travel as these millimetric insects are transmitted by direct contact with persons or their infested hair and clothes, including bed linen. Camping sites, refugee camps, and other overcrowded environments are renowned for outbreaks involving dozens of individuals. In the past, severely affected regions of the world included those with temperate climates where the peak incidence was observed during the coldest months of the year. These small insects suck blood from the human skin and inject irritating substances that may cause not only the common symptoms of severe itchiness and burning sensation, but, less commonly, allergies and superimposed bacterial infection. Even worse they can transmit serious fevers such as typhus.

The **pubic louse** or **crab** cements its eggs to the pubic or perineal hair but, in cases with heavy infestation, eggs can also be found on the eyebrows, eyelashes, moustache and beard, arm pits, and body hair. Again, itchiness and burning sensation are the main symptoms. Lice can be seen by the naked eye, and the search has to include all the suspected body regions. Effective treatment includes the use of one topical preparation such as malathion, carbaryl, or permethrin lotions. Twice-daily moisturising of the skin, 24 hours after the treatment, may result in symptomatic relief. Superficial infections from scratching have to be treated accordingly.

Bed-bugs occur world-wide and bite humans, particularly at night, in order to obtain a blood meal. During the day they hide in wall or bed cracks, folds of old wallpaper, mattresses, carpets, and floor boards (see also pp. 201–2). These wingless insects measure a few millimetres and the commonest species is *Cimex lectularius*. Characteristically, the bites will be in clusters on those parts of the body that have come into contact with the mattress, such as the buttocks, back, abdominal skin, and thighs. Travellers must be particularly aware of them in 'budget' hostels with low standards of hygiene. Heavy biting causes disturbed sleep; in some uncommon chronic cases in babies it has resulted in iron deficiency.

The main symptom is severe itchiness and red, angry-looking bites measuring up to 1 centimetre or sometimes more. Measures for control include the spraying of all suspected furniture and run-down buildings with 5 per cent DDT. Soothing calamine cream or 1 per cent hydrocortisone cream provide symptomatic relief. The bites will heal without treatment within a few days unless they are complicated by secondary bacterial infection.

A high number of **flea** species are found world-wide and cause skin irritation and nuisance by biting humans in order to obtain a blood meal. These small insects can also transmit severe diseases such as typhus, tularemia, and plague. The commonest flea causing bites in humans is *Pulex irritans*. However, in the tropics another species, *Tunga penetrans,* will bite humans and pigs, inducing a disease named chigoe or 'jigger'. Female fleas of this type burrow into the soft skin of toes, toe-webs, groins, or genitals causing severe itchiness, irritation, and nearly always a superimposed bacterial infection produced by scratching. Chigoe fleas may attach to the skin and increase their body size up to 1 centimetre following a few days of blood feeding. If the engorged flea body is removed, the small head part may remain buried in the skin of the patient. Advice from a physician should be sought in these cases.

Strong and comfortable shoes and socks prevent the acquisition of these types of fleas, that are poor jumpers. Avoidance of walking on bare feet and insecticide spraying are effective measures of control and prevention. Symptomatic relief from common flea bite can be provided by 1 per cent hydrocortisone cream applied four times daily for a few days.

Soft and hard **ticks** belong to a subclass of arthropods and can be found world-wide in nature and also in other vertebrates acting as reservoirs. Trekking in woodlands and areas with rough vegetation represent the main risk for tick bites. Aid workers in farms and horse-riding travellers can also acquire ticks from cattle and horses. A number of species not only cause limited skin disease following a blood-sucking bite but also act as agents of serious systemic illness such as typhus, relapsing fever (borreliosis), and Q fever (see also p. 195).

Ticks are very resilient organisms and they can survive in nature for several months and even years after a single blood meal. The bite is quite painful and as the efforts to remove the tick from the skin can be unsuccessful, secondary bacterial infection represents a common problem. Careful attention must be paid to ensure that the whole body and mouth parts of the tick are removed from the skin as soon as possible. Application of vaseline to cover the tick and surrounding skin interferes with their respiration and the organism drops off the skin after a few minutes. Measures of prevention include strong shoe-wear, trousers tucked into the socks, and regular examination of the skin on lower legs, ankles, and feet in order to search for attached ectoparasites. Spraying of insecticide on suspected areas is also recommended. In unfortunate cases of Lyme disease or typhus, a reddish/brownish circular lesion can be found on the skin around the tick bite at the same time that fever and a skin rash develop. Immediate medical advice is necessary should fever and a rash on the trunk develop several days after a trekking, farming, or horse-riding holiday.

Skin diseases from sun exposure

Acute damage
Direct irradiation of the skin from acute exposure to sunlight, even if only for a few minutes, may result in severe burns in the susceptible individual (see also p. 350).

Persons with very pale skin, red hair, light-coloured eyes, and freckles represent the population at highest risk. However, most white individuals experience sunburn following sustained exposure to direct sunlight during the peak hours of sun irradiation (11.00 a.m. to 4.00 p.m.). All travellers to the tropics and to mountainous resorts are targets for developing problems from sun exposure.

Ultra-violet irradiation is only one of the components of sunlight causing inflammation of the skin and tissue destruction. These clinically manifest as **sunburn,** with redness of the skin, pain, burning sensation, and blistering. **Prickly heat** refers to an acute condition presenting with itchiness and small blistering of the neck and trunk following sun exposure in hot and humid environments. The small vesicles/blisters appear as the result of blockage of the sweat glands. Symptomatic relief can be achieved by moisturizing the skin with 'cold cream'.

Severe cases of sunburn can be complicated by dehydration with symptoms of sunstroke and by superimposed infection of the skin after rupture of the blisters. Oral re-hydration with 3 to 4 litres of water for an adult is recommended once the problem has occurred. Sunburn can be prevented by the use of protective clothing (hat, T-shirt), parasols, sunblock cream or lotion, and above all, by avoidance of intense and acute exposure to direct or indirect sunlight. Persons with very pale skin, who tend to burn, are advised to use sunblock factor 25 or higher. For all white individuals, sunblock (factor 20 or above) should be applied every 3 to 4 hours during daylight time. Following a swim in the pool or ocean, sunblock cream or lotion needs to be re-applied.

Long-term damage

Premature ageing and **cancer of the skin** result from overexposure to sunlight, particularly in individuals with fair skin, freckles, red hair, and blue eyes. However, all white individuals are at a higher risk than those with darker skin, and we now know that cancer of the skin manifests in individuals with particular genes. It is clear, however, that not only genes play a part in the developing of skin cancer. Environmental factors, such as intense and episodic exposure to sunlight, are most important for the traveller.

Malignant skin tumours include **basal cell carcinoma** (often presenting as rodent ulcer), **squamous cell carcinoma**, and **malignant melanoma**. Skin cancers are uncommon in children and young individuals (indeed, they are commonly diagnosed in persons above the age of 20); and the risk increases with age. Persons with many dark moles on the body (nevi), and particularly large nevi of 5 or more millimetres in diameter, have been found to have an increased risk for the development of malignant melanoma. Suspicious-looking nevi, skin cancers, and malignant melanoma require immediate consultation with a dermatologist.

Uncommon problems

A number of complicated sun-related conditions are familiar mainly to doctors and dermatologists practising in the tropics. However, certain travellers from temperate latitudes may develop these rarer diseases as a result of exposure during a holiday. Such diseases include the following: solar urticaria, actinic prurigo, actinic dermatitis, and polymorphic light eruption. Diagnosis and treatment of these conditions is highly specialized.

Sun exposure and travellers at special risk

Individuals with certain skin or general diseases may particularly suffer from sun exposure. Usually, such patients are aware of the risks and succesfully avoid sunny environments. Some of the commonest problems are found in persons with the following conditions: lupus erythematosus, rosacea, cutaneous or liver porphyria, seborrheic dermatitis, atopic eczema, herpes simplex, and dermatomyositis.

Skin diseases from cold exposure

Prolonged exposure to very cold or freezing environment results in damage to the skin and other soft tissues, particularly in those individuals who have an increased susceptibility. Cold exposure can result in **frostbite** or a condition named **trench foot**; those with increased susceptibility manifest with **chilblains** and a number of other less common conditions (see also p. 348). In all cases, the symptoms start following exposure to cold, with or without other aggravating factors such as wind and immersion in water. The main symptoms are pain or numbness, followed in severe cases by blistering and gangrene of body areas with poor circulation in the fingers, nose tip, cheeks, ears, and toes. A pale and bluish discoloration of the affected region or limb indicates such poor circulation. Protective clothing and avoidance of immersion in freezing waters are the best measures to prevent these conditions.

Once any of the above problems have developed, immediate warming of the affected region is indicated, but may not result in full recovery. Medical advice may be necessary in determining whether other forms of treatment or surgery are indicated in severe cases.

Skin diseases from drug reactions

Most medicines taken by mouth or injection can induce allergic reactions in normal individuals. Persons taking several medicines at the same time and/or those above the age of 60 represent the population at higher risk for the development of drug reactions. It is advisable for the traveller to take a medical kit with safe drugs previously known to be effective and well tolerated. This should include painkillers, anti-inflammatory drugs, anti-histamines, and, in certain cases, antibiotics.

Redness of the skin and urticaria

Allergic reactions to medicines usually appear within minutes or a few hours after taking the suspected drug. Most commonly they present with redness of the skin on the face and neck, but the upper trunk, buttocks, and rest of the body can be affected as well. Very itchy and raised urticarial wheals (hives) may also be observed on the same sites; they usually last minutes or a few hours and disappear without leaving a scar. More severe cases involve swelling of the face (particularly of the eyelids and lips) and of the upper respiratory tract, causing difficulty in breathing and requiring obvious emergency diagnosis and treatment by a hospital doctor.

Future attacks of drug allergy can be avoided by stopping the medication. In the absence of medical help, an anti-histamine tablet (chlorpheniramine, diphenhydramine, or aminopiridine, three to four times daily; cetirizine, once or twice daily) may result in symptomatic improvement. Moisturizing of the skin with any available cold cream or milk cream may also soothe the itchiness and burning sensation. Although any medicine can induce an allergic reaction, most rashes result from **antibiotics** (penicillins, gentamicin, tetracyclines, sulphonamides), **anti-epileptic drugs** (carbamazepine, barbiturates, phenytoin), **beta-blockers** to treat blood hypertension (propranolol, atenolol), **anti-inflammatory drugs** (ibuprofen, naproxen) and **anti-malarials** (chloroquine).

Medicines reacting with sunlight

Travellers in the tropics or sunny skiing resorts must be aware that certain medicines can induce very uncomfortable, and potentially very dangerous, skin conditions following sun exposure. These can manifest as acute dermatitis with redness, itchiness, stinging sensation, and blistering of the skin exposed to sunlight. The clinical range of presentation on the skin is quite variable and can be life-threatening in cases accompanied by fever, general malaise, or severe blistering with superficial ulceration and complicated by secondary infections.

If you are taking any of the treatments listed in the box on p. 418, ask your doctor for advice before exposing your skin to strong sunlight. Remember that you *must not stop* taking your regular medication without your doctor's advice. Extra care and protection from direct or indirect sunlight represents a simple answer for most travellers. Contact with plants and plant saps can have a similar sensitivity effect–see Box below.

Some plants that can cause photosensitivity

Agrimony	Figs
Angelica	Giant hogweed
Bergamot	Mangoes (sap from skin of fruit)
Bind weed	Milfoil
Buttercup	Parsnip
Celery	Persian lime
Citrus plants	Red quebracho
Cow parsley, wild chervil	St. John's wort
Dill	Wild carrot
Fennel	

Drugs and medicines that can cause photosensitivity

Amiodarone,	Oral contraceptives
Anti-histamines	PABA
Beta-blockers	Piroxicam
Chlorpromazine (Largactil)	Promethazine (Phenergan)
Ciprofloxacin (and related antibiotics)	Psoralens
Coal tar	Retinoids
Frusemide	Sulphonamides
Hexachlorophene	Tetracyclines (including doxycycline)
Nalidixic acid (Negram)	Thiazide diuretics (like bendrofluazide)
Non-steroidal anti-inflammatory drugs	

Seek medical attention in case of tropical skin disease

If you suspect a travel-associated condition, consult a prestigious local doctor overseas, or request medical attention in the emergency department of a health centre or hospital as soon as possible. Early signs and symptoms of most tropical diseases afflicting the traveller can be easily recognized and treated by local physicians. However, if signs of disease or symptoms develop upon return to your home country, you should seek medical advice from your family GP or specialist in travel health.

Most cities in developed regions of the world offer specialist treatment for the traveller, and many capital cities (in both the developed as well as developing world) have centres of excellence in medical care and research in the field of tropical diseases. Please refer to Appendix 8 in this book for details.

Once you are home, remember that a skin rash, a non-healing insect bite, a skin ulcer, a fever, general malaise, irritability, tiredness, and diarrhoea, all require medical attention.

Summary of advice for travellers

There are a few simple measures to help the traveller avoid serious skin disease:

- **Basic hygiene:** daily shower and hand-washing before meals protects against bacterial skin infections and diarrhoeal diseases. This will also prevent minor skin cuts and abrasions, as well as mosquito bites, from turning into serious bacterial skin infections.

- **Proper menstrual hygiene:** prevents vulval acute contact dermatitis ('nappy-like' inflammation), vulvo-vaginitis, chronic eczema, and toxic shock syndrome.

- **Foot-wear:** strong and comfortable shoes prevent blistering from friction and superficial infections, and protect against infection. Strong, good-quality swimmers' fins protect against cuts and wounds from sea urchins, coral reefs, and poisonous marine flora and fauna. Avoid sandals during trekking and visits to archaeological sites; they expose your toes to scorpions as well as fungal and bacterial infections. Use them on the beach, however, to avoid cutaneous larva migrans.

- **Clothing:** protects against direct sunshine and, for trekkers, against minor skin cuts and abrasions which may be the port of entry for unwanted fungi and bacteria. Beware of bed linen in budget hostels or pensiones. Avoid wearing clothes belonging to others with uncertain personal hygiene. All these measures will prevent superficial infestations by ectoparasites.

- **Insect repellents:** repellents applied directly to the skin in the form of an oily lotion or spray, such as 20–50 per cent DEET, can be very effective. Use permethrin solution to impregnate clothes while trekking, farming, or horse-riding in order to avoid bites from mosquitoes, ticks, and other insect species that may transmit serious illness.

- **Mosquito nets:** very useful in preventing minor skin lesions from insect bites and reducing the risk of serious illnesses like malaria and dengue fever.

- **Sun protection:** light, cotton tops are the best protection in hot sunny weather. Apply sunblock (SPF 20+) to all exposed skin, every three hours. This is particularly important for those with white skin. Avoidance of direct sun irradiation between 11.00 a.m. and 4.00 p.m, and using parasols, hats, and sunglasses, are the most effective measures to prevent acute burns, sunstroke and long-term effects of intense, sporadic exposure, such as skin cancers.

- **Protection from cold weather:** proper winter clothing and adequate indoor heating will prevent frostbite, chilblains, and hypothermia. Persons with an exaggerated response to cold (Raynaud's phenomenon, vascular lability) may need to avoid cold environments.

- **Protected sexual activity:** condoms are the main protection against most sexually transmitted infections and unwanted pregnancy. Kissing and oral sex, however, play a role in acquiring conditions such as herpes simplex and syphilis. Scabies and other ectoparasitic infestations may be acquired through sexual activities.

- **Moisturizing of your skin:** restoration of the skin barrier protects against a number of minor events. After showering or swimming, moisturizing of the skin and re-application of sunblock prevent flare-ups of eczema and ensure protection against sunlight.

- **First-aid and medical kit:** your medical kit should include insect repellents, skin moisturizer, painkillers, anti-histamines, and mild antiseptics, plus any regular medication (see also p. 573). Freshly brewed black tea (without milk or sugar) is a cheap and effective antiseptic to use in soaks or in the bathing of superficial skin infections.

Dental problems

A relatively trivial dental problem can give rise to a totally disproportionate amount of pain, discomfort, and inconvenience, and finding skilled dental care can be very difficult. A thorough check-up prior to departure, and adequate arrangements to cover the possible expense of emergency treatment are the main precautions to consider.

Andrew Dawood is a specialist in prosthodontics and periodontics in private dental practice in Central London. He shares a family passion for travel, and has worked in the jungles of South America and in teaching hospitals in South America and Asia.
Professor Gordon Seward is Emeritus Professor of Oral and Maxillo-Facial Surgery in the University of London. His profession has taken him to Europe, Africa, Australia, and the USA, and he has acted as an examiner in Nigeria, Malaysia, and Singapore.

Dental problems arising while travelling abroad are, in general, given little thought and consideration both by prospective travellers and by those responsible for emergency treatment. If a dental emergency occurs, travellers may have more difficulty finding help, and are more likely to have to pay for it out of their own pocket, than if they have a medical problem.

Before departure

Travellers on short visits or holidays abroad are unlikely to face a dental emergency (other than an accidental one) if they have had a careful examination by their own dentist, including 'bitewing' radiographs, within a few months of their journey, and any necessary treatment has been completed. However, the examination is not a guessing game, and the dentist should be told about current symptoms or problems. Furthermore, the initial appointment should be booked long enough before departure to permit treatment to be completed without haste. People with heavily restored mouths, or large, complex restorations should seek advice from their dentist on how to cope with any particular problems that might arise.

Travellers intending to spend a long time abroad should consider treatment for any conditions likely to cause trouble in the future — for example, currently symptomless impacted teeth or the replacement of a just adequate but ancient denture. Dental problems in long-term expatriates are surprisingly common. In American Peace Corps Volunteers (who each spend two years overseas), they consistently represent the third or fourth most frequently reported of all health problems.

The cost of specialist dental care can vary considerably in different countries around the world, and can come as a shock to people who have only ever used the National Health Service in the UK. In general, it is always best to have any routine dental work carried out in your home environment rather than abroad.

Dental problems associated with travel

Few dental problems are directly a hazard of travelling. Seasick passengers, if they vomit over the side of the ship, may lose their dentures! Swimmers also may lose dentures or orthodontic plates. Ex-aircrew members from World War II may recall that pressure changes could produce pain in filled teeth (a similar phenomenon may also occur with deep sea divers), but as modern aircraft are fully pressurized, this does not happen to civilian passengers. Some people suffer pain and locking of the jaw joints, and an awkward posture on a long flight that induces lateral pressure on the jaw has been known to exacerbate this complaint. An unaccustomed indulgence in alcoholic drinks can precipitate an attack of 'periodic facial migraine' (Horton's syndrome) — an uncommon cause of a recurrent severe throbbing pain in one cheek. For various reasons some people may drink more wine and spirits than usual on a flight, and sufferers may come to associate such attacks with flying.

Dental emergencies

Emergencies tend to fall into three categories: pain; lost or broken fillings and other restorations; and more serious emergencies (infection or traumatic injury).

Toothache

Extreme sensitivity to hot and cold may be the first sign of trouble. If treated at this stage, the tooth may settle down. If left untreated, the pain may become spontaneous and long lasting; the nerve in the tooth may eventually die, and act as a focus for infection and abscess formation.

A dental abscess can cause severe persistent pain, exacerbated by pressure on the tooth. In all cases, a swollen face should be taken seriously; it is wise to seek treatment early as there is a small but significant risk of life-threatening spread of infection if this is neglected.

The usual treatment for an abscessed tooth in many countries would be extraction; however, if the abscess is caused by death of the nerve, it is often possible to perform root canal treatment to save the tooth — the nerve chamber is opened with a drill, and the infection drained. Later, the nerve chamber is filled with an inert or antiseptic material. Where a high standard of dental treatment is available, baby teeth may be treated in a similar fashion; otherwise it may well be more sensible to accept loss of a milk tooth, rather than risk a spreading infection.

If treatment is unavailable antibiotics should be taken, although every effort must be made to see a dentist as soon as possible. Once an abscess develops, extraction with a local anaesthetic may prove more difficult, and the patient may have to take antibiotics for some days in the hope that the infection may subside sufficiently for the extraction to be performed.

Another type of abscess may develop where teeth are badly affected by gum disease. Such an abscess may sometimes be treated by deep cleaning of the tooth to remove infected deposits under the gum. However, once again, the only treatment offered in some countries may be extraction of the tooth. A similar abscess may develop around the crown of an impacted tooth, usually a lower wisdom tooth, and this is quite common in young adults, especially in smokers or if 'run down'. Extraction of the impacted tooth will eventually be necessary, although antibiotics, hot saline mouth washes, and good tooth brushing may help control the infection until the traveller returns home.

It is sensible for individuals who have suffered any kind of dental abscess in the past to discuss the management of such problems with their own dentist, who may well recommend travelling with a supply of appropriate antibiotics.

Occasionally, two to three days after a tooth has been extracted, the clot may liquefy and be lost from the socket exposing bone. This allows food debris to accumulate in the socket, which may become infected. Warm water pumped by the cheeks in and out of the socket may be sufficient to keep it clean and relieve pain, but in more severe cases expert irrigation and a medicated dressing may be needed.

Fillings, crowns, bridges, and dentures

Though often a source of great inconvenience, the loss or breakage of a dental restoration cannot be considered to be a true emergency. The freshly exposed tooth surface is often sensitive to hot or cold, and jagged edges may irritate the soft tissues of the mouth. It is not, however, absolutely essential to seek immediate treatment unless there is considerable discomfort. The survival and fate of a tooth are unlikely to be affected by a delay even of a few weeks; this means that it is almost always possible to wait until you can see your own dentist, or can find a dentist on personal recommendation. Be careful not to damage the tooth with hard food as it may have been weakened by loss of the restoration.

If extreme sensitivity or a toothless smile necessitate treatment in the absence of adequate facilities, it is wise to seek provisional treatment only. It is often a simple matter for a dentist to insert a temporary filling, or temporarily re-cement a crown or bridge, but in many countries even the most basic dental materials may prove to be unobtainable.

Repair kits

'Do-it-yourself' repairs and temporary repair kits are not to be recommended unless you are reasonably dextrous or have a handy friend or travelling companion who can help. Even then, dental restorations are usually lost only as a result of underlying problems such as decay, breakage, or poor dentistry. Typically, kits may contain a dental mirror, a mixing spatula, a cleaning and plugging instrument, and tubes of a dental dressing and temporary cement. One tube contains the paste, the other the catalyst to make it set. The cement will form a temporary filling for a tooth cavity, or can be used to re-cement a crown or bridge until expert help is available.

A 'first-aid kit for teeth', which also contains a sealed sterile needle for a dental cartridge syringe, can be obtained from the suppliers listed in Appendix 8 or from a good pharmacy. It is essential that any debris inside the crown or bridge, which may prevent it from seating fully, is completely removed before the restoration is temporarily cemented in place. It is a good idea to check that the cleaned restoration can be properly inserted before mixing the cement. If the cemented restoration is loose, it should be removed as there is a risk that it may be inhaled or swallowed.

Dental implants

Dental implants are titanium fixtures inserted into the jawbone in order to replace missing teeth. These types of restorations have become common, and often represent the best approach to tooth replacement. There are hundreds of different varieties produced by countless manufacturers, and each system has its own instrumentation and protocols. Travellers with dental implant-based restorations should note the manufacturer of their particular system, and discuss potential problems with their dentist prior to departure.

More serious emergencies

Fractured jaws and spreading infections need hospital dental treatment by an appropriate dentist (an oral and maxillo-facial surgeon). Standards of skill in treating jaw and facial bone fractures probably vary more from country to country than for any other injury. If it becomes clear that skilled treatment is not available locally, and if after emergency care the patient is deemed fit enough to travel and is not at risk from obstruction of the airway, it may be best to return home for further treatment.

A front tooth that has been broken as a result of a blow — particularly in a child — may not always seem to need urgent care: in fact, however, expert treatment within a matter of hours can make all the difference between conserving the tooth or losing it.

If a permanent front tooth is knocked out, it may be possible to reimplant it as a temporary measure. The roots of many reimplanted teeth are subsequently eaten away by the body, like those of baby teeth, and the tooth is lost again; but some survive and give good service. If there is to be a chance of success, the tooth must be reasonably clean when picked up and it must be washed in cold water or milk. Hold the tooth only by the crown, and do not touch, rub, or scrub the root. The root must be kept moist, so put the tooth in a clean container, in cold drinking water to which salt has been added (one teaspoon to a glass), or some milk. If the tooth has been thoroughly washed, it should be pushed back fully into its socket straight away. Be sure that the crown is the right way round! The procedure will not be too painful. The patient should bite on a handkerchief to retain the tooth in place, and get to a dentist as soon as possible. Milk teeth should not be reimplanted.

Reimplanted teeth, or teeth loosened by a heavy blow, should be splinted to their neighbours for a period of about a week. A dentist may also give antibiotics and arrange for a tetanus booster injection. If a dentist is not immediately available, a temporary splint may be improvised using softened chewing gum (preferably sugar-free), pressed around the tooth and its neighbours, and covered with aluminium foil. It is best not to reimplant a tooth that has fallen on to pasture grazed by animals, because of the increased risk of tetanus infection.

Teeth successfully replaced within 20 minutes are most likely to reattach normally. If the tooth is kept moist there is a reasonable chance of success for up to two hours. Beyond two hours the results are poor. In all cases, the tooth should be checked by a dentist upon returning home, and subsequently at regular intervals. Root canal treatment is frequently necessary, and if the tooth fails, it may be replaced by means of a temporary denture, bridge, or ideally a dental implant.

Choosing a dentist abroad

Non-sterile instruments and needles may be a source of hepatitis B (see pp. 56) and HIV infection (see pp. 448). You should satisfy yourself that any dentist you consult uses instruments that have been adequately cleaned and sterilized. Instruments contaminated with traces of blood or injection syringes used on more than one patient are dangerous.

'Cartridge' syringes are the safest for giving local anaesthetic. These are made of metal, and a fresh glass tube, closed with a bung at each end and filled with sterile local anaesthetic solution by the manufacturer, slides into the barrel for each patient. A fresh needle from an intact plastic capsule should be used for each patient. The syringe itself should be washed and sterilized between patients — autoclaving is preferable by far, but boiling of the cleaned metal part is acceptable. Absolute sterility of the metal part is less critical than with syringes in which the solution has to be drawn up into the barrel itself. 'Push-on' needles and plastic syringes should come from intact original packages, and should be discarded after each patient.

Beware of needles re-sterilized by soaking in antiseptics or by boiling. Beware particularly of plastic syringes that have been 're-sterilized' by soaking in antiseptic. Watch out for bottles of solution from which doses for other patients have been withdrawn. If needles which have been used on other patients are used to withdraw a further dose they can easily contaminate the contents.

The dentist should wear rubber gloves. Ideally, a fresh pair of gloves should be worn for each patient, although this may simply not be possible in some parts of the world. Gloves protect the hands and are more easily washed clean than bare hands. The dentist should wash them before and after touching the patient's mouth.

Bear in mind that high-speed drills use water as a coolant, and this water (and any other water used in your mouth) is likely to be only as clean as the local supply.

Personal recommendation is usually the best basis for choosing a dentist. Make it clear that you are prepared to pay for those items that so many of us regard as 'disposable' in the West, but which are not so readily available in less privileged parts of the world.

Important points to mention

If you have had rheumatic fever, St Vitus' dance (chorea), have a heart valve defect or disease, or a hole in the heart, a heart murmur, or have had heart valve surgery, then you should have antibiotic cover for nearly all dental procedures and should make this plain to any dentist you see. Antibiotic cover is also advisable if you have an artificial joint or a heart pacemaker and you should consult your cardiologist for further advice if you are in any doubt, since life-threatening infection may ensue. It is wise to carry a suitable antibiotic with you.

You should also tell the dentist about any steroid treatment that you have had, even many months before, as it may be necessary for you to have additional steroid treatment at the time of a tooth extraction or similar surgery.

Patients who are taking anticoagulant drugs or who have had trouble with excessive bleeding from cuts etc. or who suffer from haemophilia should make sure that the dentist understands the situation.

Naturally, you should tell the dentist about any serious illnesses you have had and any medicines, injections, or tablets that you take as a routine. If you are allergic to any drugs (e.g. penicillin or aspirin) or dressings, it is essential that the dentist or pharmacist knows about this. Language problems may make this difficult.

Remember also that not all cultures attach a great deal of importance to saving teeth. You must make your own feelings on this subject quite clear!

Financial matters

A few travel insurance policies include a specific section on emergency dental treatment, either as part of the package or as an optional extra. Many do not. If there is such a section, enquire beforehand about what it covers. While a spreading dental infection may need urgent hospital admission, insurance companies may not consider this to be included under the heading of emergency hospital treatment (perhaps because treatment is given by a dental specialist). Travellers at special risk of accidental injury (e.g. on skiing holidays) are advised to ensure that they are fully covered by appropriate insurance. The cost of such emergency treatment may be very high and so will be the cost of any crown, bridge, or denture work.

Reciprocal arrangements for British travellers

There are reciprocal agreements for emergency medical treatment with a number of countries, particularly within the EEC. In many countries, however, emergency dental care is not included, or may be obtained only from certain clinics or hospitals. Leaflet T2 gives details of entitlement and contains the E111 form, which you will need in EU countries (see p. 572). Details about acceptance of the E111 for dental emergencies within the EU can be found at **www.doh.gov.uk/traveladvice/eeachecklist.htm**, and reciprocal arrangements with non-EU countries can be found at **www.doh.gov.uk/traveladvice/hcagreements.htm**.

Looking after your teeth

When travelling in a hot country, it is sometimes tempting, and often necessary — when safe drinking water is unobtainable — to drink large amounts of canned or bottled soft drinks. In some countries it may also be customary to serve guests with heavily sweetened tea or coffee. Frequent consumption of sugary food or drink is especially damaging to the teeth. It may take only a few months for early decay to develop in a previously unaffected tooth; small quiescent or reversing lesions may become active and irreversible.

Tooth cleaning becomes even more important when sugar consumption is high or frequent. Using dental floss or an interdental brush every day will help to prevent decay on otherwise inaccessible surfaces. Dental floss has been found to be a versatile and indispensable travelling companion by one of the authors, who has had cause to use it on occasion as a clothes line, for repairing a tent, and for hanging a hammock. The possibilities are limitless!

Chewable, disposable toothbrushes may be an option for travellers living for short periods under extremely unhygienic conditions.

Children of above six years of age and adults can also use a mouthwash of triclosan 0.03 per cent and sodium fluoride 0.025 per cent twice a day after breakfast and after the final toothbrushing at night. Rinse for one minute or more.

Fluoride and living abroad

A small amount of fluoride (one part per million in temperate climates) in drinking water undoubtedly reduces the likelihood of tooth decay, particularly in children; however, an excessive fluoride intake (greater than two parts per million in a temperate climate) can lead to mottling and discoloration of developing teeth. In countries that have a well-developed mains drinking supply, the fluoride content is carefully controlled to the proper level. Not only is the appropriate small amount added where it is required, but a natural excess of fluoride is removed.

Cold sores

The herpes virus that causes cold sores predominantly affects the inside of the mouth, lips, and the areas of skin around the mouth, nose, and eyes. Initial infection usually passes unnoticed, though it can occasionally cause malaise, sore throat, enlarged lymph glands, and widespread ulceration of the mouth — the whole of the oral mucosa may be bright red and sore; this is most commonly seen in children and is called herpetic stomatitis. A slow recovery takes place over a period of about 10 days. However, the virus is not completely eliminated from the body, and remains in a latent form which, when reactivated, is responsible for the production of cold sores.

Cold sores are caused by a complex reaction involving herpes simplex virus Type I and the body's own defence system. Some individuals find that the condition may be triggered by exposure of the face to strong sunlight, although other factors such as cold temperatures, stress, menstruation, and any debilitating condition may also be important. The most common location for a cold sore is on the lip.

If an association between sunlight and cold sores has been observed, then the most sensible precaution is to keep out of the sun and to wear a hat or sun shade; sun-blocking preparations on the lips and face are essential.

Typically, arrival of the lesion is preceded by a period of itching and irritation over the affected area. Within a few hours, blisters appear and these then burst and form a scab. Healing takes place over a period of about 10 days.

Be particularly careful not to touch the cold sore with the fingers and then rub the eyes. An infection of the finger end around the nails is possible, or worse, a serious infection of the surface of the eye. Do not kiss while you have a cold sore and especially avoid kissing children, who may as a result develop herpetic stomatitis (see above). Obviously, it is antisocial to go to the dentist with an active cold sore, except in an emergency! Expect the dentist to protect himself and other patients by wearing rubber gloves.

Frequent sufferers should obtain a supply of the anti-viral agent acyclovir (Zovirax) to take away with them. The cream should be applied to the affected area, and can shorten the duration of an outbreak considerably, especially when used immediately the first symptoms are recognized.

Unless it is known for certain that fluoride is absent from the local water supply or is present only in a very low concentration (much less than one part per million), the use of fluoride supplements for children is unwise. In any case, supplements should be used only when prescribed by a knowledgeable dentist or doctor. Where fluoride levels are high, it may be wise to use bottled water for babies and small children, bearing in mind that water intake and thus total fluoride intake is higher in hot countries. The fluoride content of bottled water is frequently stated on the label.

Young children often swallow a significant amount of toothpaste when they brush their teeth. If the toothpaste contains fluoride, and fluoride levels in the drinking water are already on the high side, this may result in an excessive total fluoride intake. Only under these circumstances is it better for babies and young children to use a fluoride-free toothpaste.

Eye problems

Exposure to strong sunlight, dust, dry or polluted atmospheres, and infection, are the main difficulties that travellers face, compounded by the fact that there may be only limited access to skilled care if problems occur.

Timothy ffytche is a Consultant Ophthalmologist at Moorfields Eye Hospital and at the Hospital for Tropical Diseases, London.

Because we rely constantly on our eyesight to orientate ourselves in our surroundings, as travellers we need take particular care of our eyes. We take our eyesight so much for granted that it is only when things go wrong that we realize quite how much we depend on them. Fortunately, serious eye problems are unusual. A little commonsense and some simple precautions will ensure that most eye problems can be anticipated and avoided.

A particular problem for travellers to many parts of the world is that it is extremely difficult to find eye care of an acceptable standard when it is needed. Standards and methods of treatment vary considerably, and in many developing countries the number of trained ophthalmologists is very small; in several African states, for example, there is not even one trained ophthalmologist per million population. Some local doctors and pharmacists may have considerable skill in diagnosing and treating eye problems, particularly where specific diseases are common, but the traveller must not rely on this, and should beware of the risks of inappropriate therapy, harmful patent medicines, and folk cures.

Our aim is to provide information about the most likely hazards, especially in places where good health care is not readily available.

Sunlight

The effects of strong sunlight range from acute damage to the front surface of the eye (conjunctiva and cornea) by ultra-violet (UV) rays, to the more long-term effects of various wavelengths on the skin of the eyelids and on the internal structures of the eye, particularly the lens and the retina.

Short-term effects

The eyebrows and eyelashes throw a shadow across our eyes, filtering the light, and a reflex action usually makes us screw up our eyes in strong sunlight. This reduces the amount of light reaching the two particularly sensitive areas, the cornea and the conjunctiva. Acute over-exposure of the eye to UV light can temporarily damage the cornea. In mild doses, this causes discomfort, redness, inflammation, and excessive lacrimation (tear formation); when it is more severe, the pain becomes intense with extreme sensitivity to light, spasm of the lids, and blurred vision. This type of situation is most likely to occur at high altitude, over water, and particularly over snow, where the condition is often referred to as 'snow-blindness'. The excessive radiation causes swelling and loss of epithelial cells on the surface of the cornea, which is extremely painful. As with all UV over-exposure, the ocular effects have a delayed response time of several hours.

Treatment consists of applying an eye ointment to lubricate the corneal surface and keeping the eyes closed using an eye pad. This is usually sufficient to provide relief within a few hours from all but the severest episodes. Milder conditions can be treated with simple lubricant eye drops, such as artificial tears. The best approach, however, is to avoid trouble in the first place — by wearing the appropriate protection such as sunglasses that screen UV light, ski goggles, or a sun hat.

While sunglasses are effective under most conditions, skiers and mountaineers will know from bitter experience that goggles are often necessary. At higher altitudes the concentration of UV light is greater, because the atmosphere has not filtered it out. Goggles are also helpful if weather conditions change, since they help prevent the reflex watering of the eyes induced by cold wind and snow that may blur your vision and endanger your safety. Remember too that harmful UV rays can penetrate even seemingly dense cloud cover at high altitude; cloudy conditions are often deceptive (see also p. 352).

Long-term effects

Although everyone is susceptible to acute damage from UV exposure, it is the fair-skinned, blue-eyed individual who is most at risk from long-term exposure. Skin cancers are more common in people with a history of long-term exposure to sunlight. Cancers may occur on the eyelids and can be particularly difficult to deal with at this site. Protection with sunglasses and sunscreens are the sensible way to avoid problems.

There is a possible link between long-term exposure to UV light and effects on the lens and retina — it may increase the likelihood of developing cataracts and retinal degeneration. Retinal degeneration is a common cause of poor vision in elderly people; other factors that predispose to it are known existing macular disease, a family history of the condition, and having fair skin and blue eyes. People who have had cataract surgery are also at risk — their lens, a valuable natural filter to the damaging wavelengths, is no longer able to provide protection. Even if this has been replaced with an intra-ocular lens implant containing UV screens, this may not be sufficient.

To prevent these complications, always protect your eyes when the sun is strong, use good-quality sunglasses, and wear a hat. Don't forget that babies and small children also need good protection — whether they like it or not!

Environmental conditions and pollution

Our eyes have efficient mechanisms for protection. These include both the voluntary and involuntary blink reflexes, the tear film over the corneal surface of the eye, and the extreme sensitivity of the cornea. Stimulation of the cornea by something like a particle of grit provokes violent reflexes of watering and blinking in order to wash away the foreign body; where the stimulus is less intense, the eyes may just become red and feel sore and uncomfortable, particularly if the condition persists. Tears contain enzymes (lysozyme) that function as an anti-bacterial agent.

There are many irritants in the atmosphere. Dust, pollen, smoke, chemicals, pollutants, and many more can all cause chronic discomfort, and there are many parts of the world where these may be excessive. A further common source of discomfort is the drying effect that modern air-conditioning or central heating in buildings, the aircraft cabin, and cars may have on eyes and contact lenses.

All these things conspire to upset the natural lubrication of the eyes and can give rise to considerable discomfort, and sometimes cause long-term problems. Certain individuals are more susceptible than others, including those with known histories of allergies and those with naturally dry eyes. Many widely used types of medication (including diuretic drugs and HRT) can cause dry eyes, and added effects of travel can make things worse.

Treatment includes avoidance, if possible, of provocative atmospheres, and the liberal use of lubricating eye drops or anti-allergic medication if appropriate. Simple artificial tear drops, comfort drops, or proprietary eye lotion is usually all that is necessary to help wash out the irritants or replace deficient tear secretion. Drops that whiten eyes should not be used since they act by temporarily constricting superficial blood vessels in the conjunctiva. This can reduce the eyes' response to the irritation and when the effects of the drops wear off there may be a rebound effect leading to a return of the redness: they mask the symptoms rather than treating the cause.

In the very long term, the combined effect of continued exposure to heat, dust, and wind in desert conditions may give rise to permanent changes in the eye. A condition known as pterygium can occur. A slowly growing wedge of white, fatty tissue can extend from the conjunctiva across the cornea in the exposed part of the eye. Although benign, it may need to be surgically removed if it becomes cosmetically unacceptable or causes visual problems by growing into the pupillary zone. Its exact cause is unknown but it is heavily associated with exposure to UV light and occurs commonly in residents of developing countries; appropriate use of sunglasses may help prevent this condition.

Infection

Eye infections occur more frequently in hot climates, where a wide variety of germs may be present in the atmosphere, rivers, lakes, swimming pools, and the sea.

Conjunctivitis ('pink eye')

Bacterial conjunctivitis is the commonest infection, often producing a crust or sticky discharge that is likely to gum your eyelids together when you sleep. The affected eye is usually red, and feels gritty or itchy. Although rubbing provides temporary relief, it can make the situation worse and cause the infection to be transferred from one eye to the other. The risk is considerably greater in people who wear contact lenses, which are more likely to compromise corneal integrity.

Bacterial infection usually responds within a few days to treatment with antibiotics, such as gentamicin, sulphacetamide, or neomycin eye drops every two hours. Avoid using antibiotic preparations that also contain steroids; steroids may be widely available without a prescription in many developing countries, but may harm your eyes in the presence of a virus infection, which has identical symptoms.

Viral conjunctivitis does not respond to simple antibiotics; more specific treatment may be necessary. It should be suspected in any conjunctivitis that does not settle in a few days with antibiotics, and expert attention should be obtained. Patients with a history of eye infections with herpes should be aware that attacks can be provoked by exposure to strong sunlight, and should therefore wear protective sunglasses. If possible, travel with appropriate medication that could be used at the first sign of a fresh attack.

During an infection, the eyes can be kept clean by frequent warm saline washes with an eye bath or by wiping the lids with moistened cotton wool. A simple irrigating solution can be easily made by adding a teaspoon of ordinary salt to a pint of *boiled* water and allowing it to cool before applying it to the eye.

Remember that many forms of conjunctivitis are very infectious and can be easily transmitted to others. Make sure that such items as handkerchiefs, towels, face-cloths, eye baths, and eye drops are not shared, and it is probably best to avoid swimming until the infection has subsided.

Trachoma

One infection that gives rise to particular anxiety is trachoma. In hot, dry countries where this disease is endemic, it can lead to progressive blindness. However, travellers who contract trachoma conjunctivitis experience only mild symptoms of redness and irritation, with a sticky but rather watery discharge from the eyes. Blindness occurs only with recurrent infections over many years among people who are already debilitated through chronic malnutrition, primitive sanitary conditions, and over-crowding. The infective agent is spread by close contact with infected individuals, their fingers and their clothes, and by flies. Trachoma of the eye is caused by the same organism as the sexually transmitted disease, chlamydia (see p. 454), and it is possible to have both infections at the same time.

If you think you have trachomatous conjunctivitis, a three-week course of tetracycline eye drops, with ointment at night, will cure the condition. Antibiotics (tetracycline or erythromycin) should also be taken orally to ensure complete eradication of the infection. If you remain in an area where trachoma is endemic, re-infection may occur, and a further course of treatment would then be necessary.

There are several forms of more severe eye infection that may occur in certain parts of the world; they may be transmitted sexually or by flies and other insects, and include parasites and worm infestations such as onchocerciasis, filariasis, and some rarer conditions. If there is any suspicion of such a condition, such as any eye problem that fails to respond readily to treatment, an expert opinion should be sought as soon as possible. Antibiotic drops and ointment, although unlikely to cure the condition, will at least prevent secondary infection until the correct therapy can be commenced.

Trauma and foreign bodies

Major or even moderate trauma to the eye and lids requires speedy medical or ophthalmic attention. When chemicals or sprays get into the eyes, the immediate treatment consists of trying to wash out the irritant by copious irrigation either with an eye bath or under a running tap, or even, in extreme circumstances, by immersing the head in a bucket of water with the eyes open! No attempt need be made in this type of emergency to find an antidote to the chemical since this may waste valuable time.

Minor trauma consists mainly of abrasions caused by foreign bodies that sometimes become embedded in the eye. When this occurs the cause is usually obvious and if the reflex watering or the simple manoeuvre of pulling the upper lid down over the lower lid does not seem to wash away or dislodge the particles, then the likelihood is that there is a residual scratch, or that something is embedded on the cornea or under the upper lid. Impacted corneal foreign bodies are often visible and need to be removed by an expert in order to avoid damage, and antibiotic ointment should be instilled until the proper attention can be obtained. This may make the eye more comfortable and will help prevent secondary infection and allow an abrasion to heal.

Dust particles under the eyelid

In dusty conditions, whether you wear contact lenses or not, particles of grit may get stuck under the top eyelid. There are some fairly obvious ways to avoid this. Do not put your head out of the window while travelling. Keep your eyes closed in dust storms. Use protective spectacles or sunglasses whenever necessary. Dust particles under the eyelid are quite common, and should be suspected if nothing can be seen on the surface of the eye but the eye still feels as though a foreign body is present.

Removing a foreign body from under someone else's upper eyelid is a simple procedure (Fig. 9.1), and gives immediate relief from severe discomfort. Sit down in front of the affected person (who should also be seated), and ask him or her to look down, and keep looking down. Gently pull the eyelid away from the eye by holding the lashes firmly between the index finger and thumb of your left hand. While your patient continues to look down (this relaxes the muscles of the lid), gently press the centre of the eyelid about 5 mm from the lid margin, where you can see a shallow groove in the skin. Press downwards and slightly backwards, using a cotton bud. This gentle pressure will flip the lid inside out, and if you adjust your pull on the eyelashes slightly upwards, the eyelid will remain everted. Now wipe the inside of the eyelid gently with a clean tissue or the tip of a cotton bud (moistened so that you do not leave residual fibres) to remove the offending piece of grit, which is often so small that you cannot

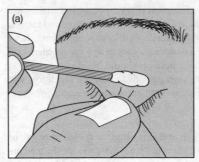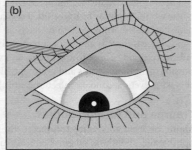

Fig. 9.1 Removing foreign body from under someone else's upper eyelid

see it. Finally, pull the eyelashes gently outwards and down so that the lid returns to its normal position.

Although it may sound complicated, this manoeuvre is actually quite simple, provided that both you and the affected person stay relaxed and avoid sudden movements, and that you perform each step without force. A pad to protect the eye for 24 hours will usually allow any scratch on the corneal surface to heal, but if symptoms persist an expert opinion should be sought.

Working abroad
Safety standards may be different abroad. If you intend to work abroad, or to take part in any activity involving a risk of injury to your eyes, make sure that you take along any protective or other safety equipment that may be needed — and be sure to use it.

Pre-existing eye problems
It almost goes without saying that anyone on regular ophthalmic medication for conditions such as glaucoma and ocular inflammations should make sure that they have an adequate supply of medication for their trip, carried in hand luggage for safe-keeping. Many ophthalmic preparations that are readily available at home may be scarce or unobtainable abroad, and drugs may often be dispensed in a different form or dosage. Patients with complicated medical conditions should also therefore carry a note with them explaining their diagnosis and current treatment.

Previous eye surgery
Certain types of surgery for retinal detachment may involve injecting gas into the eye (to maintain the volume of the eye after vitrectomy). The reduced cabin air pressure will cause this gas to expand; this will not only cause severe pain, but will reduce blood flow through the eye, with devastating consequences. Anyone who has had recent surgery for retinal detachment should consult their ophthalmologist before flying, and should avoid all air travel for at least three weeks.

People who have had previous corneal surgery, particularly radial keratotomy, should take note of the problems that may occur at high altitude (see p. 325).

Spectacles

Losing eyeglasses or having them stolen (an increasingly common experience) may be a great annoyance and, for some people, a calamity. The most sensible precaution is to have a spare pair available or to carry a recent prescription, since in many parts of the world new glasses can be made up very quickly without a great deal of expense.

Some travel insurance policies categorize spectacles and prescription sunglasses as 'valuables', and exclude or restrict cover for them. Read your insurance policy carefully.

Contact lenses

Everyone who wears contact lenses knows that their eyes can tolerate so much and no more. Rigid gas-permeable lens wearers who have overworn their lenses know how intensely painful this mistake can be. Lens wearers can develop irritable eyes with infection or allergy from cleaning, soaking, and rinsing solutions.

Discuss your trip with your contact lens practitioner before you leave. Travellers who normally wear contact lenses should take a spare pair, and also an up-to-date pair of eyeglasses as well in case of trouble, as well as a pair of sunglasses for protection from dust, wind, and sunlight. At the earliest sign of irritation or discomfort, leave the lenses out for as long as necessary. The commonest problems for rigid lens wearers are overwear and dust particles trapped under the lens. Remind yourself to keep blinking to circulate fresh tears under the lens. In overwear, the cornea, which has high oxygen demands, suffers from oedema (corneal swelling). This can be extremely uncomfortable — symptoms are very similar to over-exposure to UV light. Treatment involves removing the lens and resting with your eyes closed — there may be too much discomfort to do anything else! Mild pain-killing tablets will help a little.

A scratch on the cornea from a dust particle trapped under the contact lens may feel much the same. A gritty sensation when you blink, a feeling that the particle is still in there, and excessive watering, will usually make you keep your eyes closed. After removing the lens, a soft pad fixed by adhesive tape will rest the eye; but keep the eye closed under the pad. If you keep both eyes closed they move less, allowing the scratch on the cornea to heal more quickly.

An additional problem on long flights is that contact lenses tend to dry out. Humidity aboard an aircraft can be as low as 2 per cent, because the air supply is drawn from the rarefied outside air by compressors in the engine, and it circulates continuously. Always keep a lens case and lens solutions with you in your hand luggage when you fly; on most long-haul flights, it is safer and more comfortable to wear glasses.

Aerosol insecticide sprays are sometimes used on board aircraft, in accordance with international regulations, to clear the cabin of unwelcome stray insects. In a confined space, these aerosols may be absorbed by soft contact lenses and irritate the eyes, so it is sensible to keep your eyes closed during spraying and for a minute or so afterwards.

The painful condition of keratitis is an inflammation of the cornea, caused by bacteria (usually staphylococci) and viruses (either *Herpes simplex*, which also causes herpes blisters, or *adenovirus*, responsible for the common cold). It is not uncommon, whether you wear contact lenses or not. This sort of keratitis is treated with either antibiotic drops (such as gentamicin or neomycin) or anti-viral ointment (acyclovir).

Particular interest has centred on a rare but serious cause of keratitis called *Acanthamoeba*, which most frequently occurs in contact lens wearers, though it has also been found in corneal ulcers following minor trauma. *Acanthamoeba* is a protozoal organism that lives freely in the soil and in water, and does not normally cause infections in man. Because contact lenses cause the cornea to become more vulnerable, the organism is able to gain access to the corneal substance and establish a colony. All contact lens wearers should therefore be particularly careful to remove their lenses before bathing in swimming pools, hot tubs, and even in fresh water, and they should never moisten their contact lenses by licking them, since *Acanthamoeba* has even been isolated from normal saliva. It has also been found in contact lens solutions that have been left open for a while, but not in unopened bottles of sterile distilled water.

If you should develop an intensely painful red eye, with blurred vision and acute sensitivity to light, the chances are that you may well have a form of keratitis. If the degree of pain is out of all proportion to the apparent inflammation, particularly if you are a contact lens wearer, it is just possible that you may have this rather unusual corneal ulcer caused by *Acanthamoeba*. Whatever the cause, you should stop wearing your contact lenses and you should seek professional help immediately.

Do not rely on being able to obtain supplies of your usual cleaning, rinsing, and soaking solutions at your destination; take along an ample supply. Do not attempt to concoct your own solutions under any circumstances.

Contact lenses: some travel tips

- Don't wear contact lenses on any flight lasting longer than four hours.

- Daily-wear lenses are generally preferable to extended-wear ('sleep-in') lenses as they are less likely to cause long-term physiological changes to the eye and reduce the potential for bacterial infections and ulcers.

- If you will be travelling under extreme conditions of poor hygiene, it may be best to keep your lenses in for longer: this can mean anything from an occasional night, to a regimen of six nights' wear followed by one night's rest, or for longer than a week at a time. Not all types of lens are suitable for this, and you should consult your contact lens specialist before you travel. Alternatively, you may have to consider reverting to spectacles.

- Disposable lenses are very useful for travel: they allow a large number of spare lenses to be carried in case of loss, damage, or poor cleaning facilities, and are rapidly becoming the first choice of all contact-lens wearers for whom they are suitable.

- Disposable lenses and single–step solutions have greatly reduced many of the problems that used to be common among lens–wearing travellers.

Gillian Whitby, Optometrist, Whitby & Co, London

Many problems when travelling under conditions of poor hygiene can be avoided by using disposable contact lenses that do not require daily removal and cleaning.

Eye-care items to pack

Depending on where you are going, and how long you will be away, it is wise to take certain simple medications and equipment as part of an eye kit:

- sunglasses that screen blue and ultra-violet light (UVA and UVB)
- spare spectacles or contact lenses, a copy of your current prescription, and your optometrist's telephone number or e-mail address
- a spectacle screwdriver
- eye pads
- lubricant eye drops (artificial tears, comfort drops or gel)
- antibiotic eye drops and ointment
- an adequate supply of any regular medication and supplies (such as contact lens solutions), as well as written details of existing eye problems and any treatment.
- Keep any essential items in your hand luggage or on your person.

Note that in countries with no restrictions on the sale of medicines to the public, you may be offered eye drops and ointment containing steroids; these may be dangerous and should be used only on specialist advice.

Foot care

Most people spend more time on their feet when they travel than when they are at home, and problems with feet are among the commonest types faced by travellers of all kinds. Blisters and fungal infections are the most likely causes of trouble, but other types of problems can arise.

Paula Dudley is a podiatrist at the Fleet Street Clinic, London, and formerly a Senior Lecturer at University of Westminster School of Podiatric Medicine, London.

Footwear and blisters

Travellers and holidaymakers are likely to spend much more time on their feet than usual, particularly where mountain walking, hiking, or climbing activities are undertaken. Choice of footwear appropriate to these activities therefore needs careful consideration to obtain maximum benefit and enjoyment from the trip. Where new footwear is to be purchased, sufficient time should be allowed before the trip to look around for suitable styles and fit. Many adventure and travel equipment stores will have staff who can offer good advice on choice of suitable types.

In general, footwear, even sandals, should have soft upper parts, while the sole should provide good shock absorption and surface grip, especially in wet conditions. Many types of modern footwear will have soles constructed of synthetic material, which is usually superior to leather in flexibility and is more hard wearing. Footwear should be worn in gradually and well in advance, especially if it is new and rigid. A well worn pair should be examined for any worn areas exposing nails or rivets, or where the lining has become rucked up and may cause local irritation (a lining insole of cork or thin thermoplastic material can provide a smooth covering to such imperfections). Local friction, especially on thin-skinned sites, can cause the layers of the skin to shear and separate, and a blister will form, sometimes several centimetres in diameter. If these rupture, the underlying thin skin is left raw and painful, and highly vulnerable to secondary infection. Such blisters may arise from footwear that is too loose, allowing too much movement e.g. between the back of the shoe and the back of the foot. The style should fit snugly but be adjustable to allow for any swelling.

Prevention

As a sensible precaution, it is advisable to take a spare pair of comfortable, well-worn shoes, which can be alternated with any newer footwear. In the period prior to the journey, new shoes should be worn for increasingly long periods so that they are well softened up. It is also wise to ensure that all footwear is reasonably waterproof. Latest innovations in footwear design include 'breathable' upper materials that allow water vapour to pass through while resisting water intake. These and the lining material of the shoe are often quick drying. Proprietary leather softeners will help to make the leather uppers well fitting and suitably supple, reducing the need for a long breaking-in period. A similar effect can be achieved by applying castor oil to the leather. This is rubbed in with a cloth and left overnight to allow it to be absorbed. The leather is softened and its water repellent properties improved. Friction is greatest on damp skin and feet and footwear should always be ventilated as often as possible, especially in warm conditions. Surgical spirit, applied liberally to the skin, helps make it more resistant to blistering. This can usefully be done in advance of a trek as well as during it. Hydrocolloid dressings such as Compeed are very useful in both prevention of blisters on vulnerable skin, and in their treatment. They are waterproof and adhere well to awkward sites such as heels. Bear in mind that feet swell in hot conditions and during flights, so socks and lacing may need to be adjusted.

Treatment

Healing takes longer on the feet than anywhere else on the body, so stopping a small problem from getting worse is vital. As soon as discomfort or areas of abnormal redness are observed on any area of the skin, take action. Blister dressings or a layer of hypoallergenic first-aid tape applied direct to the skin can protect unbroken skin. These dressings and tapes need not be removed — just left until they fall off. Allergy even to this type of dressing or tape is still possible, so a vapour permeable clear film dressing (e.g. Tegaderm, Opsite) is a good alternative on sensitive skin although requiring more careful application, especially around curved areas such as heels. Such dressings have the advantage that they can be left in place for several days, while leaving the blister visible and drainable by inserting a sterile needle or scalpel blade through the film. Blood blisters (where tiny blood vessels within the skin have ruptured) are treated in the same way.

Blisters that are still intact should not be de-roofed, since this will leave a painful, raw area, open to infection. The roof of the intact blister should be pierced with a sterile needle. After puncture, gentle pressure should be applied to drain off the fluid, and then a low-adherent gauze dressing such as Melolin should be applied to the whole blister and be firmly strapped on by a flexible adhesive dressing. Some dressings, e.g., Primapore, Cutiplast, usefully incorporate a protective pad on an adhesive tape base. Care should be taken if the same footwear has to be replaced, as swelling may have occurred on the injured site — if it was too tight before it will certainly be too tight afterwards!

If the roof of the blister has already rubbed off, the raw surface should be carefully washed with warm water and soap and a thin layer of a suitable antiseptic cream applied. Jelonet or Bactigras tulle dressings are soothing/healing on large raw areas such as the back of the heel, applied directly to the skin with a thin adhesive dressing over the top. Different footwear should be worn until the skin has healed. The guilty boot should be examined for any obvious roughness before it is put back to work.

Fungal infections (see also pages 410–11)

Socks should be worn with any type of footwear, except sandals, and should contain a high percentage of a natural fibre, cotton, silk, or wool. However, synthetic fibres like nylon are often added to make them more hard-wearing and, more importantly, help 'wick' away moisture from the skin and keep it drier.

Footwear should be changed whenever possible, for example, flip-flops worn during the long mid-day break of the tropical forest trek, or trainers worn at the end of the day's trek in temperate or polar conditions. Double plastic boots (as worn in extreme cold conditions) seem to carry a greater risk of fungal infections than leather boots, though not if feet are allowed a boot-free period every day. Plastic boots, in conjunction with Yeti gaiters, have the advantage of keeping feet warm, dry, comfortable, and reducing the risk of trench or immersion foot (see p. 347).

Socks and feet should be carefully washed, dried and sprinkled with an anti-fungal powder such as zinc undeconoate 20 per cent (e.g. Mycota) or miconazole nitrate 2 per cent (e.g. Daktarin) every day. For established infection, or prevention in particularly susceptible individuals, an anti-fungal cream such as clotrimazole 1 per cent (e.g. Canesten) should be applied sparingly to the affected areas. If fungal infections are not detected and treated early, secondary bacterial infection can also become established or fungal infection can spread to nails. Even without these complications, untreated fungal infections can become disabling out of all proportion to the area affected.

Other soft tissue injuries

A sprain results from over-stretching and/or tearing of the soft tissues that support joints and may produce swelling, bruising, and pain in the affected area — most commonly, the outer ankle. It is usually caused by a sudden wrench to the foot when walking over uneven terrain. The sooner treatment is begun, the better, as the subsequent swelling can be disabling, and can render footwear tight and difficult to remove. The prompt application of cold in the form of a compress or one of the 'instant' ice-packs available in first-aid kits, can do much to reduce the damage. Arnica ointment can also be helpful in minimizing bruising of the area. Support to the affected joint can be provided by elastic, tubular bandage e.g. Tubigrip. This should feel comfortably firm rather than tight and care should be taken in the event of further swelling. Rest is also important where possible, preferably with the foot elevated. Pain relief can be obtained with anti-inflammatory medication.

More serious soft tissue tears are likely to incapacitate the sufferer and complete rest may be required. Where weight-bearing is unavoidable, firm elastic strapping should be applied to minimize harmful movement, but this is best done by a trained professional or first-aider.

Another common problem area is the back of the heel. As well as blistering, it may be subject to constant shearing from a firm edge of a boot or shoe, causing a painful, localized inflammation (bursitis) and/or irritation of the adjacent tendon. The principles of treatment are the same — to reduce inflammation — and it can be helpful to cover the offending portion of the shoe with a softer lining material to reduce chafing.

More severe or persistent aching, tenderness, or fatigue in soft tissues and joints may be associated with unaccustomed levels of activity, but may also indicate faulty foot mechanics. A good quality 'off-the-shelf' supportive insole, or a similar device properly prescribed, can significantly reduce symptoms and should be considered whenever prolonged treks are planned.

Cuts, abrasions, and insect bites

The skin of the foot and lower leg can be slow to heal compared with other body sites, as the blood supply is less efficient. For this reason it is important to clean even small wounds as thoroughly as possible to reduce the risk of infection, before applying any dressing. Travellers should also ensure that they have up-to-date cover against tetanus infection.

Cuts and abrasions should be thoroughly irrigated with clean, running water where possible, which will help clean the wound of physical debris and micro-organisms; and then gently dried with clean tissue or gauze. Small wounds can be simply covered with an adhesive dressing, but larger wounds may require additional protection using a suitable antiseptic e.g. Savlon dry powder spray, and a sterile gauze wound dressing secured with tape.

Foreign bodies sometimes enter the skin of the foot during barefoot activity. They may penetrate deeply and are not dislodged in wound cleansing, but may need to be removed with forceps, tweezers, or a sterile needle (often included in first-aid kits). More deeply embedded particles may require specialist treatment, but meanwhile the area should be protected with an improvised dressing to prevent pressure on the site.

Insect bites, usually occurring on the thin skin of the toes or top of the foot, can also become infected. The irritation they cause is likely to make the sufferer scratch the overlying skin, compounding the problem. Infected bites around the ankle can readily result in more serious infection, resulting in ulcers that can take weeks or even months to heal. Proprietary creams can relieve the itchiness, but where the bite becomes infected it should be treated as any other wound and observed for any spread of infection. Pure oil of *Melaleuca alternifolia* (tea-tree oil), can be dabbed directly on to fresh bites as necessary, helping to prevent infection and encourage healing.

Some foot care items to pack

- Individual sachets of pre-moistened, astringent (alcohol-impregnated) skin-wipes provide a quick, cooling clean-up for hot, tired, and sweaty feet. These are readily available in high street pharmacies.
- Blister dressings, e.g. Compeed for treatment and prevention.
- Astringent/anti-fungal foot powders e.g. Daktarin, Mycota. These act as dry lubricants to reduce chafing and their active ingredients help prevent and treat minor fungal infections and sweat rash.
- Anti-fungal cream, preferably containing the same active ingredients as the powders, to treat more acute infections.
- An antiseptic, dry powder spray e.g. Savlon, for treating skin splits and minor abrasions — especially useful for moist sites such as between the toes. A small bottle of pure tea tree oil for bites and small cuts.
- Moisturizing preparations for dry skin sites such as around the heel — creams and lotions containing *Melaleuca alternifolia* 5 per cent (tea-tree oil) are useful inclusions. As well as hydrating the skin the oil has antiseptic and anti-fungal properties.
- 'Instant' ice packs e.g. Koolpak, a useful first-aid measure in the event of injuries such as sprains.
- Elasticated tubular bandage, e.g. Tubigrip, can provide gentle support for minor sprains but is also a good way of keeping other first-aid dressings in place without the need for adhesive plasters.
- A selection of dressings e.g. Melolin, Jelonet, and tape for covering abrasions, open blisters etc, and some sterile needles for draining blisters.

Gynaecological problems

Gynaecological problems are common in women travellers. Most problems are not serious, but even a supposedly minor problem can ruin a trip.

Dr John Naponick is a public health physician with specialist training in gynaecology, obstetrics, and tropical medicine. He has worked in North America, West Africa, Central America, South and Southeast Asia.
Ellen Poage is a registered nurse and a health educator. She has travelled and worked in Central America, Africa, and Asia, and now lives in Fort Myers, Florida.

Women travellers who plan a long trip abroad, or who plan to live in a country where good medical facilities may not be easily accessible, are well advised to have a gynaecological check-up before they leave home — preferably six weeks or so before departure; it is always a good idea to begin a trip with a clean bill of health. Those with previous gynaecological problems should have a clear understanding of their medical history, or should carry a written note of any problems.

Menstrual problems

Personal supplies

Women should make a careful estimate of their likely requirements for personal hygiene. Although women throughout the world menstruate, not all of them take the same approach to feminine hygiene. So if you will be travelling to a remote area and you don't feel sufficiently adventurous to experiment with the only facilities that may be available locally — such as balls of cotton wool, cloths and towels tied on with strings, or even handfuls of leaves — be certain to ensure an uninterrupted supply of your own preferred variety of tampon, sanitary napkin, or pad.

In developing countries, locally made menstrual supplies are usually available in most major cities, although the standard varies. In relatively more advanced countries such as Thailand and Malaysia they may be of high quality. In poorer countries such as Bangladesh, napkins are beginning to replace the more traditional towel and string methods in the wealthier sections of the community; those made locally, however, tend to look (and feel) more like a mattress than the kind of slim-line designer product with which most women living in developed countries are familiar (see also p. 409, and **www.mum.org**).

Menstruation

Some women travellers prefer not to have periods at all while travelling; this can be accomplished by taking the Pill continuously, without a break between packets (see p. 478).

Women who travel to game parks should consider this option or should avoid close proximity to predatory animals (bears, lions, tigers, etc.) while menstruating. There have been a number of reported attacks on menstruating women. Likewise, if they swim or dive in shark-infested waters, they may possibly be at increased risk of attack by sharks.

In some parts of Southeast Asia, such as Indonesia, women may be asked not to enter local temples if they are menstruating.

Irregular bleeding

Periods may stop completely in travellers. Often, the cause of this proves to be pregnancy. However, an irregular cycle is usually the result of the hormonal changes that follow any disruption of normal routines, and may even be partly psychological in origin. One example of this phenomenon has been studied extensively: nursing students who leave home and move into shared accommodation almost always experience some disturbance of menstruation; after a while, a normal cycle returns, with the students menstruating in synchrony.

Heavy bleeding

A detailed discussion of causes of heavy vaginal bleeding is outside the scope of this book. Suffice it to say that certain types of frequent bleeding may be due to a serious underlying condition requiring surgical treatment, and expert medical advice should always be obtained.

In many cases, this kind of irregular bleeding may be due to a hormonal disturbance, and will respond to hormonal treatment. If you are bleeding heavily and are in a remote area where no skilled medical advice can be obtained, it is worth trying the following treatment *provided that* you have had a recent check-up, you are otherwise healthy, and you *are certain that you are not pregnant.* Take one combined oral contraceptive pill (for example, Norinyl 1 or Eugynon 30), four times a day for five days. These pills contain standard doses of progesterone and oestrogen hormones, and are readily available world-wide.

I call this a medical or hormonal curettage. Bleeding should stop during treatment, and you should have a period by the seventh day after the last day of treatment. If bleeding does not stop during treatment, the problem will require a skilled assessment and probably surgery or curettage. If you do not have a period within five to seven days of stopping treatment, you may be pregnant.

Remember that even if this treatment is successful, there may still be an underlying problem, so specialist advice should be obtained at the earliest opportunity.

Unintended pregnancy

Emergency contraception (the 'morning-after' Pill) is discussed on p. 481.

Some women become pregnant while travelling, and others begin their trip in the earliest stages of pregnancy. Those who choose not to allow the pregnancy to continue are advised to be very careful. A termination of pregnancy in a developed country, where technical facilities and specialist skills are widely available, is generally a safe procedure; a termination of pregnancy performed without these facilities, and under unhygienic conditions, can cause life-threatening complications and may have serious implications for the mother's future health and fertility. Remember that it is your responsibility to ensure that the facilities you choose are clean and safe — even if this means travelling on to a country where better facilities are available, or returning home.

Also remember that in most cases, time is on your side. Up to six weeks from the last menstrual period, a simple menstrual regulation procedure can be performed. In countries where it is available, RU 486 can be used up to nine weeks from the last period (see p. 482). Up to 12 weeks from the last period, the termination procedure is safe, although you should definitely avoid delaying any further than this. In exceptional circumstances, action can be taken at up to 20 or 24 weeks, depending upon local laws (see p. 482).

Those who are happy to continue with their pregnancy should make sure that they have access to adequate medical care (p. 484).

Genital and urinary tract infection

Thrush

Thrush or vaginal candidiasis is one of the most common gynaecological problems encountered by travellers in hot, humid, tropical conditions. Thrush is caused by overgrowth of a yeast normally found in the female genital area. Several factors promote growth of this organism: heat, humidity, the oral contraceptive pill, certain antibiotics, and diabetes. Doxycycline is one of the drugs that can trigger thrush; it is used increasingly as an anti-malarial drug, so any woman taking it should also ensure that they have sufficient medication with them if problems arise. The best way to prevent the problem is to keep the genital area dry and cool; cotton underwear which absorbs perspiration is strongly recommended, and synthetic fabrics should be avoided. See also p. 409.

A yeast infection is characterized by a red rash, itching, and a thick, white 'cottage cheese' vaginal discharge.

Treatment

Daily vinegar douches (one tablespoon (30 ml) vinegar per litre of water) may be sufficient to relieve the itching and return the vagina to its correct pH (acidity). If nothing else is available, yoghurt may also provide relief. When stronger treatment is required, clotrimazole (Canesten) 100 mg intravaginally, daily for seven days, or 500 mg intravaginally as a single dose (Canesten 1, Myceler) or nystatin (Nystan) 100 000 units intravaginally for 14 days may be used. An effective single-dose treatment is available without prescription in many countries — fluconazole 150 mg (Diflucan 150) by mouth. Despite treatment, the condition may recur if the predisposing factors mentioned above have not been rectified.

Cystitis

Cystitis, also called urinary tract infection or the 'urethral syndrome', is a common condition in women — it affects 10–15 per cent of healthy, non–pregnant women each year — and may be a particularly distressing and inconvenient problem in travellers. It often follows an unaccustomed increase in sexual activity. Symptoms usually consist of frequent urination. The infection is usually due to contamination of the urinary passage with bacteria from the patient's own anal area, but may occasionally be the result of a sexually transmitted disease. If laboratory facilities are available, cultures should be performed.

Pain on urination without frequency may be due to vaginal infection or to genital herpes. A thorough examination should be obtained.

Treatment

If symptoms of cystitis appear, drink plenty of fluids, particularly cranberry juice if available, because it alters the acidity of the urine and may provide some symptomatic relief. (In a recent study of sufferers from frequent urinary infection cranberry juice reduced the likelihood of subsequent attacks by 20 per cent).

Self-treatment with antibiotics is usually inadvisable. If there is no prospect of skilled medical care, and if symptoms persist, tetracycline 500 mg by mouth, four times a day for seven days (total dose 14 g) or doxycyline 100 mg by mouth, twice daily for seven days, may be taken. These drugs will cover the important possible causes of urinary symptoms, but may not treat antibiotic-resistant gonorrhoea, which should always be considered. (Please refer to p. 00 in the chapter 'Sexually transmitted diseases' for more information.) **These treatments are not recommended for pregnant/lactating women or those under 15 years old.** It is essential to complete the full course. Milk products interfere with absorption of these drugs.

Only if there is no possibility of a sexually transmitted disease would I advise using more conventional antibiotic treatment for a urinary infection — such as trimethoprim 200 mg twice daily for three to five days, or cotrimoxazole (Septrin, Bactrim, etc), two tablets 12–hourly for five days — without a laboratory diagnosis.

Self-treatment should be resorted to only if there is really no other option, and advice from a qualified medical practitioner should be obtained as soon as possible.

Choosing a doctor abroad

Unfortunately, it is not safe to assume that the high standard of medical ethics and professional behaviour you may be accustomed to in your home country will automatically apply to all doctors in every country you visit. For obvious reasons, when dealing with gynaecological problems in a strange country it is important to choose your doctor with care. Your embassy or consulate (or staff who speak your language from another embassy or consulate), expatriates, and local residents may be able to recommend a suitable physician; often, the most reliable recommendations are those from satisfied patients. If you can find a female doctor so much the better.

Always insist on a chaperone when being examined; use your commonsense, but be prepared to refuse if you are asked to submit to what seems to you to be an unreasonable procedure.

Other hazards

Female travellers appear to be at slightly *less* risk of malaria infection than male travellers; one possible explanation is that they take greater care to observe the necessary precautions!

Living abroad

Screening procedures normally taken for granted at home may not be offered as routine to long-term residents abroad. All women should request screening for cervical cancer and be familiar with the technique of breast self-examination. The American Cancer Society now advises mammography (to detect breast cancer at an early stage) annually in women over 40. The British Government recommendation is that women aged between 50 and 64 should be screened every three years (and above

64, on request). In developing countries, good-quality tests of this type are not always readily available. A gynaecological examination on return home is a sensible precaution; be sure to tell your doctor where you have been.

Psychological disorders

Travel can be stressful! Psychological aspects of travel receive insufficient attention, but are crucial to success and enjoyment.

Dr Michael Phelan is Consultant Psychiatrist at Charing Cross Hospital in London; and Honorary Senior Lecturer at Imperial College School of Medicine. He is a general psychiatrist who has a particular interest in the difficulties related to expeditions and travelling.

Introduction

Holidays and travelling are associated with relaxation, excitement, and fun. When going away, we expect a well-deserved rest and a break from everyday life. If travelling alone, we hope to meet people and make friends; if we are with others, we assume that previous disagreements and tensions will be forgotten, and that going away will help relationships flourish. Such high expectations of holidays are encouraged by brochures and guide books. However, holidays do not always live up to these high hopes. Stress arises from travel delays, discomfort, unfamiliar climate, strange food, and language difficulties — all of which are harder to cope with when feeling isolated and homesick. The end result can be misery, arguments with your companions, and, in extreme cases, serious psychological disorders.

As with many of the physical conditions described in this book, sensible preparations and an awareness of the risks reduce the likelihood of psychological problems. This section describes what you can do before setting off to lessen the chances of serious problems and highlights a variety of conditions that can affect the traveller abroad. Some advice is also offered for people with a psychiatric disorder who are planning to travel.

Preventing problems

Having decided where you are going, the most important decision with any trip is who to go with. If alone, you have complete freedom to decide where to go, how to get there, and what to do when you arrive. Lone travellers often describe an intensity of experience which is missing when accompanied. They relish the fact that they have met others easily. However, the downside of solo travelling can be loneliness and the lack of anyone with whom to share experiences.

Travelling with others has its difficulties. In everyday life it is unusual to spend all day, every day, with another person, but this is often the situation on holiday. The stresses of such intense closeness are compounded by the other tensions of travelling. Even the happiest relationships are put under pressure, and less secure partnerships can be destroyed. For some, the answer is to go on holiday with a group of friends, but this can make things more difficult: there is a continual need for compromise. The larger the group, the more likely that someone will not be happy and that conflict and tension will develop.

For the more sociable, an organized group holiday can work well, but for others, the idea of being with a group of comparative strangers 24 hours a day is unbearable. Before setting off with a group, couples need to consider that they may find themselves ostracized in a group of single people. Alternatively, there may be tension if one person fits in well with the others in the group, and their partner is isolated.

Whether travelling alone or with others, do everything you can to reduce the inevitable stress of the trip. Money is a common source of worry and conflict. It is easy to underestimate how much you will need, and it is vital to keep some in reserve for emergencies and unforeseen expenses. Agree beforehand how much you can afford to spend, but be prepared to spend more! Check all your travel arrangements, take out insurance, and ensure that you have the right luggage and clothes. Nevertheless, the best made plans go astray. Try to expect and accept that there will be disruptions, delays, and changes to your arrangements. Predict that your plane will be delayed — and be delighted and surprised if it arrives on time.

The days immediately prior to holidays are usually particularly busy. Packing and last–minute arrangements have to be fitted around work and domestic responsibilities, and you can end up departing in an exhausted and irritable state. Jet lag can exacerbate the situation (see p. 263). The first few days of any trip are usually the most stressful — recognize this and plan things so that you do not attempt too much to begin with.

Reduce stress on holiday

- pick your companions carefully
- recognize when you are tired
- have realistic expectations
- stay healthy
- have enough money and insurance
- expect delays, frustrations, and changes
- keep your sense of humour

Extended trips, lasting more than a month, require particular strategies. After a while the lack of structure can become unsettling, especially in unfamiliar environments. Travelling every day soon becomes exhausting, so try to arrange to stay in one place for a few days each week. If possible, establish a routine to each day. It can be helpful to write a daily diary — this allows a period of peaceful reflection, as well as a chance to ventilate any frustrations. The longer you are away the more important it becomes to have contact with friends and family at home; E-mail, the Internet, and cellular phones have transformed the possibilities for keeping in touch. Arrange to have post sent to you and, if possible, speak on the telephone as well. Reading newspapers from home (paper or digital versions) can also be a comfort and can help to tackle any feelings of being homesick.

Travelling for work can be seen as a glamorous perk, but for those who have to do it on a regular basis it quickly loses its charm and can be an exhausting and resented chore. All the stresses of travelling are compounded by having to spend time with work colleagues, with whom you may have little in common. It can also have a profound and damaging effect on family life, if frequent and long term. Think very carefully before accepting a job entailing extensive travelling. If you have to do it, negotiate time off after trips to rest and spend time at home.

Specific psychiatric disorders

Mental illness is common: one in four people will suffer from a psychiatric disorder during their lives, and some conditions may become apparent for the first time on holiday.

Panic attacks

These can occur spontaneously but will usually be precipitated by a feared situation, such as being in an enclosed space. The sufferer will rapidly develop a sense of extreme fear, and may believe that he or she is about to die. This fear will be accompanied by a number of physical symptoms including dizziness, chest pain, breathlessness, and tingling in the extremities. Associated hyperventilation (overbreathing) can exacerbate the physical symptoms, which in turn will convince the sufferer that he or she has a catastrophic and possibly fatal condition. Alarmed bystanders, who do not understand what is happening, will increase the person's anxiety through their own panic.

The immediate treatment for a panic attack is calm reassurance, and encouragement to breath in and out of a paper or plastic bag held over the mouth and nose (if a plastic bag is used do not put it over the person's head!). After the initial attack, further episodes are likely, but they are usually less severe. In the longer term, medication and specific psychological therapies are sometimes required to reduce the frequency and severity of panic attacks.

Depression

It is not uncommon to feel rather miserable or sad at times on any holiday, especially if things have not worked out as hoped or if there is tension with companions. Occasionally such feelings can develop into a depressive illness. Serious depression can also spontaneously occur. It can be exacerbated by excessive use of alcohol or illicit drugs. The affected person will be persistently depressed, may struggle to complete straightforward tasks, and may have little energy or interest. Other characteristic features are:

- Loss of appetite
- Poor concentration
- Disturbed sleep — usually early morning waking
- Frequent tearful episodes
- Preoccupation with worry and guilt
- Thoughts of suicide.

Severe depression must be taken seriously, especially if suicidal thoughts are present. Specialist help should be sought without delay. Anti-depressant treatment is usually effective, but will take at least two weeks to work; it is therefore sensible for the person to return home.

Acute psychotic states

These are rare, but extremely alarming for all concerned and occur when psychotic people lose their sense of reality and have strange, and usually, frightening experiences. They will often be preoccupied with persecutory ideas, feel that they cannot fully control their thoughts, and have auditory and visual hallucinations. They may be disorientated in time, place, and person. Their behaviour is often bizarre and inexplicable. They may be seen sitting naked staring up at the night sky, and talking aloud to God. Such experiences may be the beginnings of a serious mental illness such as schizophrenia, but this is unlikely. It is far more likely that the cause is illicit drugs, and that the effects will quickly wear off. Other causes of such states include severe heat stroke, malaria, and head injuries. In the case of head injuries, the onset may be delayed for many hours, and should be treated as a medical emergency.

Prescribed medication can also be the cause for a number of psychiatric symptoms. There have been reports of the anti-malarial drug mefloquine (Lariam) causing a range of different symptoms, including anxiety, depression, vivid dreams, paranoia, and hallucinations. The risk of developing such symptoms may be as high as 1 in 200. There are now a number of alternatives to mefloquine that still afford a high degree of protection from malaria. Mefloquine should not be used by people with a history of psychological or psychiatric problems.

Travelling with a psychiatric disorder

Having a stable, long-standing psychiatric disorder should not stop you going abroad, but there are some sensible precautions to take. Following a serious mental breakdown which has required hospital admission, you should usually not travel abroad for at least six months. If in doubt seek advice from a psychiatrist.

Certain psychiatric drugs may be affected by travel. For instance, some anti-psychotic drugs (especially chlorpromazine and trifluperazine) can increase susceptibility to sunburn (p. 418). Lithium levels can be increased by hot weather and inadequate fluid intake. Some drugs that can be bought over the counter in some countries may interfere with your regular medication. If you are on any psychiatric medication it is important that you discuss your travel plans with a psychiatrist, and take adequate supplies of medication in well-labelled bottles.

Coming home

Returning home is usually associated with a mixture of emotions — sadness that the holiday is over, but some pleasure at seeing friends and family again. Even long trips quickly become distant memories once the routine of everyday life returns. Your keenness to talk about your experiences is often met with a disappointing lack of enthusiasm from others. The best policy is to start thinking about your next trip!

Fever

Although fever can be harmless, it may be an early feature of serious illness, especially malaria, where a delay in treatment can result in death. Telling the difference may not be easy, and fever in anyone who has visited the tropics must always be taken seriously.

Professor Geoffrey Pasvol is Professor of Infection and Tropical Medicine at the Lister Unit of the Imperial College School of Medicine, Northwick Park and St Mark's Hospital, Harrow, UK.

Fever is a non-specific indicator of disease and for most travellers, as for patients at home, the most common causes are viral infections of the upper respiratory tract. However, in any visitor who is in, or has recently visited an endemic area, the diagnosis of malaria must be taken seriously because of the severe complications and even death which may ensue. Most cases (over 90 per cent) of *Plasmodium falciparum* malaria (the species of malaria that can kill) occur within six weeks of a visit to a malarious area and usually 7–12 days after an infected mosquito bite.

Fever in itself is non-specific and a definitive diagnosis in the absence of medical help and investigations is difficult. The early symptoms of malaria are frequently misleading, and often include diarrhoea, cough, or mild jaundice, which must not be mistaken for infectious diarrhoea, upper respiratory tract infection, or hepatitis. There are numerous possible causes of fever in the traveller abroad, and some examples of these are listed in Table 9.1.

Table 9.1 Some causes of fever in the traveller

Bacterial infections
> Pharyngitis / sinusitis / middle-ear infection / lower respiratory tract infections
> Typhoid and paratyphoid
> *Shigella* / *Campylobacter*
> Lyme disease

Viral infections
> Dengue
> Influenza / enteroviral infection
> Hepatitis A, B and E
> Glandular fever
> HIV infection

Rickettsial infections
> Scrub typhus

Protozoal diseases
> Malaria
> Leishmaniasis
> Amoebiasis (Liver abscess)

Helminths (worms)
> Acute bilharzia (known as Katayama fever)

Others
> e.g. skin infections, urinary tract infections

Simple clues to cause of fever in the traveller

- **Malaria:** the fever can sometimes be intermittent and very high, often over 40°C. Enlargement of the lymph glands or rashes are rarely due to malaria alone.
- **Dengue fever** can present with high fever, severe headache, and bone pain; hence the name 'breakbone fever'. A bright red rash over the whole body is sometimes seen.
- **Typhoid and paratyphoid** can present with mild fever increasing over days. Symptoms are mainly gastroenterological with abdominal pain, but a cough, slight confusion, and inattentiveness, sometimes with constipation, can occur. Red spots, 1–2 mm in size ('rose spots') which come and go are sometimes seen on the lower abdomen.
- **Infectious gastroenteritis** may start with vomiting, leading on to diarrhoea, sometimes with blood or mucus in the stool (when it is called *dysentery*). The fever may be only mild.
- **Viral hepatitis:** the symptoms are often non-specific. There may be a mild fever, dark urine, and light-coloured stools, which only after some time lead on to visible jaundice. Sometimes there is pain in the right upper part of the abdomen and this needs to be distinguished from the pain of gallstones, which is more often an acute cramping pain.
- **Trypanosomiasis** (sleeping sickness) may occur especially in people who have visited the game parks of Africa; it is spread by the bite of the tsetse fly, which is extremely painful. A severe swelling at the site of the bite with local lymph gland enlargement is seen.
- **Typhus** is most frequently seen in visitors who have been to the game parks and there may be a dark scab at the site of the bite (called an eschar) with a red rash on the trunk, enlarged glands, and a high fever.
- **Amoebiasis** is a cause of dysentery (blood and mucus in the stools). An abscess in the liver might occur weeks after a visit to an endemic area and presents with extremely high fever and pain in the right upper abdomen, as with hepatitis.

Less 'exotic' infections that may produce fever

- **Upper respiratory tract infections**: apart from gastroenteritis, the commonest infection in travellers. The cause is more than often viral, but bacterial sore throats, sinusitis, and middle-ear infections can occur which may require antibiotic treatment.
- **Urinary tract infection**: usually starting with increased frequency and burning when passing urine.
- **Pelvic inflammatory disease in women**: usually manifesting with pelvic pain and vaginal discharge.
- **Meningitis**: characterized by a fever with headache, stiff neck, intolerance of bright lights, nausea, vomiting, and, sometimes, a non-blanching rash.

Deciding what to do

In the absence of medical help, and in remote areas, it can be difficult to decide what to do when you develop a fever. Initially, there is no harm in symptomatic treatment with aspirin and/or paracetamol, but obviously after a period of time (say 48 hours) with no improvement one would need to seek medical advice.

In a malarial area, if no doctor is available, the most important step is to exclude and/or treat malaria. A number of dipstick tests can be used to confirm the diagnosis, and are a possible option for travellers. The best-known of these tests are the *Para*Sight F test (Becton Dickinson) and the ICT Malaria Pf test (ICT Diagnostics, Sydney, Australia) for falciparum malaria. A positive test is a good indication that the individual has falciparum malaria. These tests do not diagnose the other, less aggressive forms of malaria. Blood-film diagnosis of malaria (the 'gold standard') is not feasible where there is no access to a microscope or the necessary expertise.

If the test is positive, or if there are no tests available, standby treatment of malaria should be considered (see Table 9.2; also p. 149). Options for treatment include mefloquine (Lariam), and atovaquone + proguanil (Malarone). Quinine may also be used, but has a number of side effects.

If malaria has been excluded, and it is considered that the major symptoms are due to an upper or lower respiratory tract infection, the antibiotic co-amoxiclav (Augmentin) can be given. Patients allergic to penicillins (and co-amoxiclav is one)

Table 9.2 Possible fever remedies for a traveller's medical kit

Suspected diagnosis	Drug	Adult dose
All fevers	aspirin (300 mg) *or* paracetamol (500 mg)	Two tablets up to four times a day
Malaria	mefloquine (Lariam) *or*	Three tablets, followed by a further three, 6 hours later (each tablet 250 mg)
	atovaquone + proguanil (Malarone) *or*	Four tablets daily for three days (each tablet contains 250 mg atovaquone and 100 mg proguanil)
	quinine	Two tablets three times a day (each tablet 300 mg)
Gastroenteritis	ciprofloxacin (Ciproxin)	Two tablets twice a day (each tablet 250–500 mg) for 3–5 days
Respiratory tract infections	co-amoxiclav (Augmentin) *or*	One tablet three times a day (each tablet 625 mg), for 5 days
	clarithromycin (Klaricid)	Two tablets twice a day (each tablet 250 mg), for 5 days
Gastroenteritis where amoebiasis is suspected	metronidazole (Flagyl) *or*	One tablet three times a day (each tablet 400 mg), for 5 days
	tinidazole (Fasigyn)	Two tablets twice a day (each tablet 500 mg), for 5 days

may use clarithromycin (Klaricid). If gastrointestinal symptoms predominate, then ciprofloxacin (Ciproxin) might be the drug of first choice. Where amoebiasis or giardiasis is suspected, metronidazole (Flagyl) or tinidazole (Fasigyn) may be given in addition (see Table 9.2).

Without access to medical expertise, blind treatment of fever is subject to many pitfalls. Up to 50 per cent of cases with fever where anti-malarials have been used on a standby basis, have been shown not to be malaria; but it is better to over-treat the problem than to risk missing the diagnosis.

Indicators of serious disease in patients with fever

Obviously, there are many circumstances when fever in the traveller does not necessitate medical care. A decision when to take additional steps is a difficult one but *the following manifestations should alert one to a serious problem*:

- Any change in the level of consciousness
- Any degree of prostration (inability to sit up, stand, or drink), particularly where there is repeated vomiting and inability to take drugs by mouth
- In the case of respiratory tract infections, where there is respiratory distress with shortness of breath and an increased rate of breathing, say over 20 respirations per minute
- In gastrointestinal illnesses, when there is any clear evidence of major dehydration such as an extremely dry mouth with loss of skin turgor, sunken eyes, decreased urine output, or severe dizziness on standing up from the lying position
- Where a high fever persists for more than 48 hours
- Where there is any evidence of neck stiffness
- Where there is a rash which does not blanch with pressure.

10 Sex and contraception abroad

Sexually transmitted diseases

Travellers are at increased risk of acquiring sexually transmitted diseases. All travellers should know how to reduce the risks if they do not intend to avoid them.

Dr John Naponick is a public health physician with specialist training in gynaecology, obstetrics, and tropical medicine. He has worked in North America, West Africa, Central America, South and Southeast Asia.

When Christopher Columbus returned from his voyage of discovery to the New World, an epidemic of syphilis swept Europe. Ever since, historians have debated whether or not Columbus and his sailors were to blame. One thing that *is* certain, however, is that today's traveller is at as great a risk as ever of acquiring a sexually transmitted disease.

Sexually transmitted disease (STD), still popularly known as VD (venereal disease), has reached epidemic proportions in many countries and is a major problem world-wide, encompassing a wide range of infections. **STDs are nearly as common as malaria: there are more than 250 million new cases each year.** Everyone has heard of gonorrhoea and syphilis, but more recently recognized diseases such as chlamydia infection — often harder to document — may be twice as common. Herpes, once the subject of much public interest, has been eclipsed by the spectre of HIV and AIDS. Although HIV infection may be transmitted by contaminated needles, blood products, and from mother to fetus, (and is discussed in greater detail on pp. 468–76), it is still above all else an STD. Changing attitudes to sexual behaviour, as well as promiscuity and prostitution, have each contributed to the present pattern of STD.

As far as the individual traveller is concerned, however, the public health aspects of sexually transmitted infections are less important than their immediate implications.

Risk factors

All STD risk factors depend on individual behaviour. If you do not intend to place yourself at risk, you do not need to read this chapter. The only absolute ways of avoiding STD are abstinence or sexual intercourse with a partner who is known to be disease-free and is completely faithful. Any other type of behaviour will place you at risk of infection. Risk factors include:

Travel People behave differently when they travel. Tourists travel to seek adventure and new experiences, and to make new friends. Sex is certainly part of the attraction. Travellers separated from their families, for example business travellers, the military, long-term expatriates seafarers, and immigrants, are all at particular risk. In a recent study, one in ten British travellers reported sex with a new partner whilst abroad; only 75 per cent used condoms on all occasions. Sex is sometimes even the sole purpose of travel, as evidenced by the continuing growth of the 'sex tourism' industry to certain parts of Asia. The usual norms of the home environment no longer control behaviour. In addition to the risk of STD, there is also the risk of prosecution and imprisonment, as several Asian countries have started to crack down on 'sex tourists'.

Number of sexual partners The more sexual partners a person has, the greater the risk of acquiring — and passing on — an STD. Prostitutes in some Asian and African cities have infection rates reaching 100 per cent. Even if you have only one contact with a prostitute you are at high risk of contracting an STD.

Frequency of sexual contact The greater the frequency of sexual contact, the greater the risk of acquiring an STD. For example, men have a 20–35 per cent chance of acquiring gonorrhoea from each contact with an infected partner. Two exposures would obviously increase the risk.

Age The highest incidence of STD is found in the 15–30-year-old age group. The incidence declines as age increases. Theoretically one could reduce the risk by choosing a more mature partner.

Choice of partner Certain groups of people are known to be at high risk. They include intravenous drug users, homosexuals, prostitutes, young people with multiple sex partners, and bisexual men; special categories of high-risk groups for HIV infection include people who have received multiple blood transfusions, haemophiliacs, or anyone who has had regular sexual intercourse with individuals in the above categories.

Blood products and inadequately sterilized instruments Blood transfusion carries a risk of HIV, hepatitis B and C, syphilis, and malaria. Developed countries have instituted screening measures to reduce the risk, but developing countries lag behind. Avoid unnecessary blood transfusions and injections, unless the blood has been adequately screened and the equipment is known to be sterile (see p. 588 and pp. 589–94).

In addition to an increased risk of acquiring an STD, travellers face many other difficulties. They may be going from an area of modern medical care to an area with less sophisticated medical facilities. The medical professionals may or may not be as well trained, and the laboratory back-up services may be non-existent. Language barriers may pose an obstacle to communication.

Diseases

A wide variety of diseases can be transmitted sexually, and some are considered in Table 10.1. It is beyond the scope of this book to give exhaustive information about each disease; medical texts and lay publications are available for that purpose.

Bacteria, viruses, protozoa, and arthropods may all be transmitted by sexual contact. Sexual intercourse is the usual mode of transmission, but any close contact that allows transfer of infected materials or secretions can transmit disease. The disease can establish itself wherever it finds a suitable environment — usually those areas of the body that are warm, moist, dark, and lined with a mucous membrane, such as the genital area, the mouth, the rectum, etc.

The spectrum of diseases that can be contracted is immense and there is no limit to the number with which one may be afflicted at any one time. Furthermore, there is no such thing as immunity towards most of these diseases, so reinfection is likely unless precautions are taken. Infection with one disease may make it easier to transmit another: infection with chancroid, chlamydia, gonorrhoea, syphilis, or trichomoniasis may increase the risk of HIV infection by two to nine times.

Some sexually transmitted infections, such as crab lice, are merely a nuisance. Herpes may recur and be particularly troublesome. Human papilloma virus infection is linked to cancer of the cervix. Gonorrhoea and chlamydia can cause infertility and painful, incapacitating pelvic infection. Lymphogranuloma venereum can result in genital deformity. Syphilis can lead to insanity and damage to the nervous system, the heart, and major blood vessels. HIV infection is not a 'gay plague', it is a hazard that every sexually active male or female traveller must take seriously; HIV infection kills. These complications are presented not to scare you, but merely to make you aware of the far-reaching consequences that these diseases have.

Geographical distribution

While some places certainly have a higher incidence of STD than others, it is important to bear in mind that risk depends on behaviour, not geography.

STDs are a major public health problem in both developed and developing countries, but rates are higher in developing countries where STD treatment is less accessible. In developing countries, rates of syphilis may be 10–100 times higher, gonorrhoea 10–15 times higher, chlamydia 2–3 times higher. In large African cities, gonorrhoea may infect 3000–10 000 per 100 000 population, or as many as 1 in 10 people. This compares to rates of 233 per 100 000 in the USA and 30 per 100 000 in Sweden. Incidence rates of 310 per 100 000, and rising, have been reported for syphilis in St Petersberg compared with a rate of 2 per 100 000 in Finland. STDs appear to be more common in Africa than in Asia or Latin America.

HIV infection has been reported from almost every country in the world. The highest incidence is in the USA (New York and California); the Central African countries of Zaire, Rwanda, Burundi, Central African Republic, Congo, Zambia, Tanzania, and Uganda; and Haiti. In the UK and the USA, it has been mainly a disease of homosexual and bisexual men, but the rate of heterosexual transmission is rising and in the UK the number of new heterosexual cases has now overtaken that for homosexuals. In the UK, of 1746 cases in heterosexuals diagnosed during 2000, 1371 (78 per cent) were the result of sexual contact abroad — in travellers and migrants. Heterosexual transmission of HIV appears to be most common in Central Africa, but

Table 10.1 Sexually transmitted diseases

Disease	Causal agent	Occurence	Incubation	Likely symptoms	Complications
Gonorrhoea	*Neisseria gonorrhoeae*	world-wide (250 million people affected at any one time)	2–7 days	Burning on urination, penile and vaginal discharge	Infertility; arthritis; pelvic abscess
Chlamydia	*Chlamydia trachomatis*	world-wide	5–7 days	Same as gonorrhoea but may be milder	Infertility
Syphilis	*Treponema pallidum*	world-wide (50 million cases each year)	10 days–10 weeks	Painless ulcer, rash	Occur late; cardio-vascular problems or mental charges
Chancroid	*Haemophilus ducreyi*	subtropical and tropical	3–14 days	Painful necrotizing ulcers, painful swelling of lymph nodes	Localized
Lymphogranu-loma venereum	*Chlamydia trachomatis*	subtropical and tropical	3–30 days	Small painless ulcer	Stricture of rectum; genital elephantiasis
Herpes	Herpes simplex virus	world-wide	2–12 days	Painful multiple ulcers	Recurrence; cancer of cervix (possible)
Trichomoniasis	*Trichomonas vaginalis*, (a protozoan)	world-wide	4–20 days	Vaginal discharge and irritation	Local only
Non-specific vaginitis	*Gardnerella vaginalis*	world-wide	7 days	Odoriferous vaginal discharge	Local only
Anogenital warts	human wart virus	world-wide	1–20 months	Cauliflower-like growths	Localized

Table 10.1 Sexually transmitted diseases (continued)

Disease	Causal agent	Occurence	Incubation	Likely symptoms	Complications
Scabies	Sarcoptes scabiei (a mite)	world-wide	2–6 weeks	Itching; skin eruptions	Local infection
Pubic lice	Phthirus pubis (the crab louse)	world-wide	1–2 weeks	Itching	Local infection
Intestinal infections	Campylobacter jejuni Shigella species Non-typhoidal salmonella Entamoeba histolytica (amoebic dysentery) Giardia lamblia (giardiasis)	world-wide in those who practise anal–oral sex as well as by non-venereal transmission	Varies	Diarrhoea; jaundice; etc.	Depend on disease
AIDS	HIV	world-wide	2 weeks–12 years (or more)	Fever; weight loss; etc.	Opportunistic infection; death
Hepatitis B	Hepatitis B virus	world-wide	2–6 months	Jaundice	Carrier state; chronic liver disease

is growing world-wide. HIV transmission by contaminated blood products, from mother to fetus, and in injecting drug users is found in Africa, Asia, the Middle East, and eastern Europe.

Hepatitis B is spread by the same route, occurs all over the world, and is more easily transmitted. Hepatitis C is also transmissible by intimate contact.

Lymphogranuloma venereum (LGV) and granuloma inguinale (GI) are diseases of the tropics and subtropics. LGV is sporadic in the developed countries and endemic in East and West Africa, India, Southeast Asia, South America, and the Caribbean. GI is unusual in that it occurs mainly in the tropics and subtropics, but small outbreaks do occur elsewhere.

Most other STDs occur world-wide. Gonorrhoea and syphilis in particular are found more often in urban settings, sea-ports, and trading centres; the young (15–35 years) are most often infected; males outnumber females.

Prevention

Public health measures

STD prevention/control is based on four concepts: education about risk reduction; detection of asymptomatically infected individuals and those with symptoms who are unlikely to seek treatment; effective diagnosis and treatment of infected people; and evaluation, treatment, and counselling of sex partners.

Several countries have managed successful STD programmes. In Sweden, the rates of gonorrhoea and chlamydia have been reduced. In other countries, programmes have been successful within limited small populations. In Nairobi, the rate of genital ulcers among prostitutes in a low-income area has been reduced from three episodes per woman per year to one episode per woman per year. The Lusaka Hospital in Zambia has seen a decline in new STD cases.

The good news is that STD programmes can be successful; the bad news is that for the person at risk, the risk may be reduced in some countries or in limited geographical areas, but not eliminated.

Personal protection

The only sure way to avoid STD is to avoid sexual contact altogether, or to keep to a mutually faithful relationship with one partner known to be disease-free. Anyone not willing or able to do either should know how to minimize the risks and maximize protection.

It is important to acknowledge the risk factors already described, and to avoid sexual contact with individuals who are at highest risk. In the USA the usual advice on

---

The ABC of safe sex

'A' is for abstinence. If you can't abstain, 'B' faithful, and if you can't be faithful, then use 'C' for condoms.

Juan Flavier, former Philippine Health Secretary

avoiding STD/HIV infection includes avoiding sexual intercourse with an infected partner; if the partner is infected or the infection status is unknown, use a new latex condom with each act of intercourse; and when a male condom cannot be used, consider using a female condom.

In attempting to choose a partner belonging to a low-risk category, bear in mind that surveys have shown many people are prepared to lie in order to have sex; one survey of young, sexually active Californians showed that 47 per cent of the men and 60 per cent of the women claimed that they had been lied to for the purposes of sex; 34 per cent of the men and 10 per cent of the women admitted that they themselves would also be prepared to lie; 20 per cent of the men said that they would lie about having a negative HIV-antibody test; and nearly half of both men and women said that they would understate their number of previous partners. Of those who had been sexually involved with more than one person at a time, more than half said their partners did not know.

Clearly prostitutes constitute a high-risk category, and in many Asian countries up to 90 per cent of all sexually transmitted infections result from contact with prostitutes. Brothels, massage parlours, and singles bars offer a high probability of infection.

While it is worth trying to examine a prospective partner for sores, ulcers, pus, or other signs of disease, remember that patients with a wide variety of infectious conditions, including HIV infection, often look and feel healthy. It is more important to try to find out about their sexual history.

Safe sex
STDs (including HIV infection) are transmitted by body fluids such as blood, semen, vaginal secretions, urine, and saliva. The term 'safe sex' is used to describe sexual acts that do not allow exchange of body fluids. Examples of safe sex are mutual or simultaneous masturbation, and consistent and correct condom use from start to finish of sexual contact (vaginal, anal, or oral). This approach should be the rule in all casual encounters.

Contraceptive measures
Male condom (sheath) When used consistently and correctly, condoms are very effective in preventing a variety of STDs including HIV. Condom failure usually results from inconsistent or incorrect use of condoms rather than condom breakage. Condoms are regulated medical devices in the USA and subject to rigorous testing. Condoms available from other sources may not be so reliable. Correct condom use includes:
- Use a new condom with each act of intercourse.
- Carefully handle the condom to avoid damaging it with fingernails, teeth, or other sharp objects.
- Put the condom on after the penis is erect and before any genital contact with the partner.
- Ensure that no air is trapped in the tip of the condom.
- Ensure that there is adequate lubrication during intercourse, possibly requiring the use of exogenous lubricants.

- Use only water-based lubricants (e.g. K-Y Jelly or glycerine) with latex condoms; oil-based lubricants (e.g. petroleum jelly, shortening, mineral oil, massage oils, body lotions, or cooking oil) that can weaken latex should never be used.
- Hold the condom firmly against the base of the penis during withdrawal, and withdraw while the penis is still erect to prevent slippage.
- The effectiveness of spermicide in preventing HIV transmission is unknown. No data exist to show condoms lubricated with spermicides are more effective than other lubricated condoms. Therefore, latex condoms with or without spermicides are recommended.

Female condoms Laboratory studies indicate the female condom ('Reality') — a lubricated polyurethane sheath with a ring on each end, that is inserted into the vagina — is an effective mechanical barrier to viruses, including HIV. Clinical studies are ongoing.

Vaginal spermicides, sponges, diaphragms Several studies have demonstrated vaginal spermicides (i.e. film, gel, suppositories; contraceptive foam has not been studied) used alone without condoms reduce the risk for cervical gonorrhoea and chlamydia, but protection against HIV has not been established in human studies. The vaginal contraceptive sponge protects against cervical gonorrhoea and chlamydia, but increases the risk of candidiasis. Diaphragm use protects against cervical gonorrhoea, chlamydia, and trichomoniasis.

Non-barrier contraception, surgical sterilization, hysterectomy Women not at risk of pregnancy may still be at risk for STDs. Women using oral Pills, Norplant, Depo Provera, other hormonal injections, or who have been surgically sterilized or had hysterectomies are not protected from STD/HIV infection.

Intrauterine contraceptive device (IUCD or IUD) The IUCD does not protect against STD/ HIV. The risk of pelvic inflammatory disease (PID) is higher in women who wear an IUCD, especially just after IUCD insertion.

Vasectomy Vasectomy does *not* protect against STD/HIV.

Other time-honoured methods of STD prevention include washing the genital area and urinating immediately after the sex act. These are sensible measures (**although not scientifically proven**), although keeping a full bladder during the sex act is a prerequisite for the latter, and is not always comfortable or possible. Avoiding transfer of body fluids is much more reliable.

When consulting your doctor prior to travel for advice on the most suitable contraceptive method (pp. 476–83), it is worth taking into account the possible need for protection against STD. As shown in the preceding section, most contraceptives offer no protection against STD/HIV.

In case of infection
If you think you have caught an STD, or even if you just suspect you have been exposed, you should seek examination by a fully qualified medical practitioner. Early

prompt treatment is essential if the disease process is to be arrested and permanent complications are to be avoided. Incorrect, inadequate, or inappropriate treatment may mask the symptoms and allow the disease process to advance. Some diseases, such as syphilis, disappear for long periods of time after the initial symptoms, as if cured, only to reappear again in a more serious form at a later date. There is no effective cure for HIV infection.

Travellers sometimes face a problem in obtaining correct diagnosis and treatment. Some sexually transmitted infections take weeks to appear, and by then the traveller may have moved on to a different country, where the disease may be unfamiliar: several infections favour hot climates, but unfortunately many physicians know only about locally occurring diseases. It is always advisable to tell the physician exactly when and where exposure took place.

You should try to locate the best possible medical facilities: expatriates, diplomats, medical associations, and local businesses may be helpful in directing you to qualified practitioners. In areas where STDs are common, STD clinics can be found more easily. You should not be reluctant to attend a clinic if you think you have a disease: we all think it will never happen to us, but it can.

Diagnosis

Some diagnoses can be made on simple inspection, some require microscopes and cultures, and some a serological examination (blood test). The more reliably a diagnosis can be documented, the greater the likelihood that treatment will be effective. I would recommend keeping detailed records of any symptoms you have had, any diagnoses that have been made, any laboratory examinations done, and all treatment. This information may be valuable to your physician upon your return home should you fail to get better.

Dangers of self-diagnosis and treatment

I would discourage you from attempting either self-diagnosis or self-treatment. If you found yourself alone on a desert island you would have to decide for yourself what to do in those circumstances, but such situations are rare, and you should usually be able to obtain some sort of medical advice. Drugs are available in some countries without prescription, but you may do yourself much harm by making the wrong diagnosis and giving yourself the wrong treatment.

There are several reasons for this. First, there is no one drug that will treat all sexually transmitted infections, and use of the wrong drug may not cure the infection or may not *completely* cure it.

Second, no drug is free from side effects, and if you use the wrong drug you may expose yourself to undesirable effects without obtaining any benefits.

Third, there is the problem of *resistance* to certain antibiotics and other drugs. Diseases unfortunately appear capable of keeping one step ahead of medical science. When penicillin first became available in the 1940s, small doses of the drug were capable of killing a wide range of microbes. Since then, certain strains of organism have become resistant to penicillin — i.e. they are able to escape the lethal effects of the antibiotics. This has happened to some strains of gonorrhoea, and *especially those found in many parts of Asia.*

Indiscriminate, inappropriate, or incorrect use of a drug against bacteria that have developed resistance to that drug may mean that (i) the infection is not cured (at least using normal doses) and (ii) drug resistance is further encouraged, thus increasing the public health problem. Few buttocks are large enough to receive injections of penicillin in the doses which would now be required to treat infection with penicillin-resistant gonorrhoea.

Once a drug becomes useless, doctors have to switch to using another drug, but unfortunately bacteria that have developed resistance to one antibiotic have a tendency to develop resistance to others as well — for example, some strains of gonorrhoea have become resistant not only to penicillin, but possibly also to tetracycline and to spectinomycin. Ultimately, more expensive, more potent drugs — with more side effects — have to be used.

A fourth reason for avoiding self-diagnosis and treatment is that you may give yourself a false sense of security that your disease has been cured when, in fact, it has subsided, only to reappear at a future time in a more dangerous form.

Prophylactic treatment For similar reasons, you should also avoid the prophylactic use of antibiotics or other drugs in an attempt to prevent infection: the drug you choose may well not be effective against any infection you pick up; it will give you a false sense of security, probably increasing the risk of infection; and its indiscriminate use will encourage the development of drug resistance.

Correct treatment

When prescribed a treatment, the most important thing is to take it in the correct amount for the correct time. Taking a drug for a shorter time than advised may not effect a cure and may encourage drug resistance.

It is usual during treatment to have the symptoms subside after 24 to 48 hours, so it is often tempting to stop the treatment then rather than complete the full course — especially if the medicine you are taking is one that makes you feel lousy.

The recommended treatment schedules of the Centers for Disease Control, USA, are listed in Table 10.2. Space does not permit a listing of all effective and alternative treatment schedules. I have provided these *not* so that you can treat yourself, but rather to enable you to compare them with any treatment you are offered abroad. If you are diagnosed as having an STD and are offered treatment which appears to be substantially different, request an explanation. HIV-infected individuals may require a different treatment schedule and should automatically seek expert medical advice.

Anyone given treatment for an STD should always return to a clinic for a follow-up examination, to confirm that treatment has been successful.

Sexual activity should be avoided during treatment, both to prevent further spread of disease and to avoid confusion: it is rather easier to distinguish recurrence from reinfection if one remains celibate during treatment.

Contacts

In some countries, it is the law that all sexual contacts of individuals who have contracted an STD be named, traced, and treated. This is good practice, as it is the only way to stop the spread of the diseases. Even where it is not the law, mere concern for others should prompt anyone who is being treated for an STD to tell their contacts so that they, in turn, can seek medical advice. Although this may be embarrassing, it is to be highly recommended.

End of journey

I strongly advise travellers with any possibility of exposure to STD to take the precaution of seeking a physical and laboratory examination on their return home — to protect subsequent, unsuspecting sexual partners from unwelcome gifts from abroad.

Travel, sex, and cancer

A British study has shown that wives of frequent travellers are at higher risk of contracting cervical cancer than any other women. For example, wives of airline pilots were four times more likely to develop the disease than wives of civil servants or school teachers. A sexually transmitted virus is believed to be partly responsible, so that having multiple partners is a major risk factor. The study did not show, however, if the high rate was caused by husbands who passed the virus to their wives on return home, or by the wives themselves taking advantage of their husbands' absence to find other partners.

What to do in an emergency

In the unusual situation of a traveller developing symptoms of a sexually transmitted disease in a remote place, where no medical advice can be obtained, no laboratory facilities are available, but there is access to a supply of medicines, I advise the following approach — bearing in mind the warnings given in the text regarding self-treatment.

Penile discharge in males

The most likely causes of this are gonorrhoea and chlamydia. Previously, one drug could have treated both. Antibiotic resistance now makes this impossible.

Some strains of gonorrhoea are resistant to tetracycline. If you can find cefixime you can take 400 mg orally, in a single dose; or ceftriaxone, 125 mg (intramuscular) in a single dose; or ciprofloxacin, 500 mg orally, in a single dose; or ofloxacin, 400 mg orally, in a single dose. To treat chlamydia, you should take doxycycline 100 mg orally twice a day for 7 days or azithromycin orally once in addition to one of these drugs. Where available, a one dose treatment with cefixime 400 mg by mouth and azithromycin 1 mg by mouth would be optimal.

Even if treatment succeeds, I strongly recommend a check-up after your travels. You might have contracted syphilis at the same time, and this treatment may not have eradicated it.

Vaginal discharge in females

I would advise the same treatment as given above for males, for the same reason. If this treatment fails I would then give 2 g metronidazole (Flagyl), orally, in a single dose to treat trichomoniasis. If that failed, I would then give treatment for vaginal thrush — miconazole or clotrimazole, 200 mg inserted into the vagina once daily for three days. If this also fails, then specialist medical advice must be sought, even if this means changing your travel plans. *This treatment schedule is not appropriate for pregnant women.*

Genital ulcers

In addition to penile and vaginal discharge, the other major manifestation of an STD is genital ulceration. There are several diseases that can produce genital ulcers. A good treatment to start with would be tetracycline hydrochloride, 500 mg orally, four times a day for 15 days. This would treat syphilis and lymphogranuloma venereum. If this treatment failed you could take a treatment for chancroid: erythromycin 500 mg, orally, four times a day until the ulcer has healed. These treatment schedules should give you enough time to find medical assistance.

Finally, I would caution you once again to seek medical assistance if at all possible, and not to attempt to diagnose and treat yourself unless there is no alternative. There are side effects to all medicines. These treatments may not be suitable in your particular case, and tetracycline is unsuitable for use in pregnant women.

Sexual assault

The most commonly diagnosed STDs following sexual assault on women are trichomoniasis, chlamydia, gonorrhoea, and bacterial vaginosis.

If possible, a physical examination, gonorrhoea/chlamydia cultures, microscopic examination of vaginal discharge, and serum samples should be obtained. A follow-up examination for STDs should be repeated after two weeks, and serological tests for syphilis and HIV infection should be performed after 12 weeks.

Although not all experts agree, most victims will benefit from prophylaxis because follow-up may be difficult and victims are reassured if given treatment. Prophylactic measures should include:

- Hepatitis B vaccination
- Antibiotics including: ceftriaxone, 125 mg intramuscularly, in a single dose; metronidazole, 2 g orally, in a single dose; and doxycycline, 100 mg orally, two times a day for seven days. This treatment should deal with chlamydia, gonorrhoea, trichomoniasis, and bacterial vaginosis.

Table 10.2 Recommended treatment schedules for various STDs

Disease	Recommended treatment	Dose/route (Tablets/capsules unless stated otherwise)	Alternative
URETHRAL / CERVICAL INFECTION			
Gonococcal infections	Cefixime (Suprax)	400 mg, single dose	Azithromycin 2 g, single dose
	OR		Spectinomycin 2 g, single dose by i.m. injection
	Ciprofloxacin	500 mg, single dose	
	OR		
	Ofloxacin	400 mg, single dose	
	OR		
	Ceftriaxone (Rocephin)	125 mg, single dose by i.m. injection	
Chlamydial infections	Azithromycin (Zithromax)	1 g, single dose	Erythromycin base 500 mg, 4 times daily for 7 days
	OR		Erythromycin ethylsuccinate 800 mg, 4 times daily for 7 days (Erythromycin is 80% effective — may need to be repeated)
	Doxycycline	100 mg, twice daily for 7 days	Ofloxacin 300 mg, 4 times daily for 7 days
Epididymitis	Ceftriaxone (Rocephin)	250 mg, single dose by i.m. injection	Ofloxacin 300 mg, twice daily for 10 days
	+ Doxycycline	100 mg, twice daily for 10 days	
Pelvic inflammatory disease	Ceftriaxone (Rocephin)	250 mg, single dose by i.m. injection	
	+ Doxycycline	100 mg, twice daily for 14 days	
	OR		
	Cefoxitin	2 mg, single dose by i.m. injection	
	+ Probenecid	1 g, single dose	
	+ Doxycycline	100 mg, twice daily for 14 days	
	OR		
	Ofloxacin	400 mg, twice daily for 14 days	
	+ Metronidazole (Flagyl)	500 mg, twice daily for 14 days	

Table 10.2 (continued)

Disease	Recommended treatment	Dose/route (Tablets/capsules unless stated otherwise)	Alternative
INFECTIONS WITH ULCERATION			
Syphilis *Early disease*	Benzathine penicillin G (Bicillin)	2.4 million units, single dose by i.m. injection	Doxycycline 100 mg, twice daily for 14 days
Chancroid	Azithromycin (Zithromax)	1 g, single dose	
	OR		
	Ceftriaxone	250 mg, single dose by i.m. injection	
	OR		
	Ciprofloxacin	500 mg, twice daily for 3 days	
Genital herpes simplex (HSV) *First clinical episode of genital, anal, or oral HSV*	Acyclovir (Zovirax)	400 mg, 3 times daily for 7–10 days	
		OR	
		200 mg, 5 times daily for 5 days	
	OR		
	Famciclovir (Famvir)	250 mg, 3 times daily for 7 days	
	OR		
	Valacyclovir (Valtrex)	1 g, twice daily for 7–10 days	
Episodic recurrent infection	Acyclovir	400 mg, 3 times daily for 5 days	
		OR	
		200 mg, 5 times daily for 5 days	
		OR	
		800 mg, twice daily for 5 days	
	OR		
	Famciclovir	125 mg, twice daily for 5 days	
	OR		
	Valacyclovir	500 mg, twice daily for 5 days	

Table 10.2 (continued)

Disease	Recommended treatment	Dose/route (Tablets/capsules unless stated otherwise)	Alternative
VAGINAL INFECTION			
Trichomoniasis	Metronidazole (Flagyl)	2 g, single dose	Metronidazole 500 mg, twice daily for 7 days
Bacterial vaginosis	Metronidazole (Flagyl)	500 mg, twice daily for 7 days	Metronidazole 250 mg, 3 times daily for 7 days
	OR		
	Clindamycin cream 20%	One 5 g application intravaginally, four times daily for 7 days	Metronidazole 2 g, single dose
	OR		
	Metronidazole gel 0.75%	One 5 g application intravaginally, twice daily for 5 days	Clindamycin 300 mg, twice daily for 7 days
Candidiasis	Fluconazole (Diflucan)	150 mg, single dose	
	OR		
	Butoconazole	2% cream, 5 g intravaginally for 3 days	
	OR		
	Clotrimazole	1% cream, 5 g intravaginally for 7–14 days	
		OR	
		10 0 mg vaginal tablet, daily for 7 days	
	Miconazole (Monistat)	2% cream, 5 g intravaginally for 7 days	
		OR	
		200 mg vaginal suppository, daily for 3 days	
	OR		
	Nystatin	100 mg vaginal suppository, daily for 7 days	
		100 000-unit vaginal tablet, daily for 14 days	

Table 10.2 *(continued)*

Disease	Recommended treatment	Dose/route (Tablets/capsules unless stated otherwise)	Alternative
MISCELANEOUS			
Human papilloma virus (HPV) *External genital warts and perianal warts*	Podophyllin resin 10–25% **OR** Trichloracetic acid (TCA) **OR** Bichloracetic acid 80–90%	Apply small amount, dry. Wash off in 1–4 hrs. Repeat weekly as required.	Intralesional interferon Laser surgery
Pediculosis pubis *Pubic lice*	Permethrin 1% cream rinse **OR** Lindane 1% shampoo **OR** Pyrethrins with piperonyl butoxide	Apply to area, wash off after 10 mins. Apply to area, wash off after 4 mins. Apply to area, wash off after 10 mins.	
Scabies	Permethrin 5% cream (Elimite)	Apply to all areas of body from neck down. Wash off after 8–14 hrs	Lindane 1%, 1 oz of lotion or 30 g of cream. Apply thinly to body from the neck down. Wash off after 8 hrs.

Notes:
Tetracycline, doxycycline, and clindamycin cream should not be used in pregnancy.
Oil-based creams and suppositories may weaken latex condoms and diaphragms.

Risk of acquiring HIV infection following assault

HIV infection has been reported by people whose only known risk factor was sexual assault; however, the risk in most instances is minimal. Although the overall rate of transmission of HIV from an HIV-infected person during a single act of heterosexual intercourse is thought to be low (less than 1 per cent), the risk depends on many factors. The Centers for Disease Control, in the 1998 STD treatment guidelines, states that prophylactic treatment for HIV is effective for healthcare workers who have had percutaneous exposures to HIV. However, all persons should have HIV counselling and testing after the assault. Based on available information, a recommendation for prophylactic HIV treatment after sexual exposure to HIV cannot be made. Healthcare providers need to evaluate the risks versus the benefit (see also p. 475).

Conclusion

Scare tactics have never yet been successful in campaigns to stop any epidemic. The best protection against STDs is education and a commonsense approach to prevention, combined with prompt treatment of both partners if treatable disease occurs.

Risk for STD and HIV infection is determined by what you do, not by who you are or where you go. If you are not monogamous or abstinent, you must use condoms regardless of your sexual orientation. Both male and female travellers who consider sexual contact a possibility on their travels should carry condoms with them and use them every time.

If you have difficulty resisting temptation abroad, you should consider travelling with your usual partner whenever possible.

Acquired immunodeficiency syndrome (AIDS) and its cause: human immunodeficiency virus (HIV)

AIDS has become one of the most widely and intensively researched public health issues in the world, since its recognition in 1981, because it is still relatively new, it is serious, and it mainly affects young adults. AIDS cases have been reported from virtually every nation, and the number of cases reported continues to rise. HIV infection is a world-wide problem and the risks to travellers depend more upon their own behaviour than upon their choice of destination.

Dr D. Peter Drotman has been a medical epidemiologist with the Centers for Disease Control and Prevention, Atlanta, since 1979. He has worked with AIDS public health issues and treated AIDS/HIV patients since 1982.

Acquired immunodeficiency syndrome (AIDS) is the name given to a group of health problems first recognized by epidemiologists at the Centers for Disease Control and Prevention (CDC) in the USA in 1981. By year's end, the World Health Organization (WHO) had received reports of AIDS cases from eight nations. By October 1991, that figure had risen to 162 countries. By 2001, more than 36 million persons were estimated by the WHO to be living with AIDS or HIV infection, and 15 000 new infections are estimated to occur daily around the world, mainly in adults aged 15–49 (see Maps 10.1 and 10.2). AIDS is clearly a global public health problem of immense magnitude.

People with AIDS have developed a specific defect in their natural immune (defence) system, which has left them vulnerable to illnesses that would not otherwise be a threat. These illnesses are referred to as 'opportunistic' diseases. The cause of the defect is an infection with a virus called human immunodeficiency virus (HIV). The many strains of HIV all are transmitted in the same way and cause the same clinical syndrome. HIV preferentially infects certain cells of the immune system (T-helper lymphocytes, often referred to as CD4 cells) and destroys them. When a sufficient number are destroyed, the characteristic immunodeficiency results. There is no cure for AIDS, nor any effective vaccine to prevent HIV infection. Extensive research efforts for both better treatments and effective vaccines are ongoing world-wide.

Who is at risk?

Virtually all reported cases of AIDS occur in people who:

- Have had heterosexual intercourse with an infected man or woman
- Have had sexual intercourse with gay or bisexual men
- Have used injectable or intravenous (IV) drugs and have shared needles, syringes, or injecting paraphernalia
- Have been treated for haemophilia (or certain other severe bleeding disorders) with contaminated clotting factor concentrates
- Have received transfusions of whole blood or its components (in countries where donations are not adequately screened)
- Are children born to or breastfed by mothers infected with HIV.

World-wide, the largest proportion of HIV infections is attributable to heterosexual intercourse. The age of those diagnosed with AIDS ranges primarily from 25 to 44 years, but the age at infection with HIV is much younger. All races and ethnic groups have been affected.

In the industrialized nations, HIV infections are more common in gay men and IV drug users. In non-industrialized nations, infection also occurs in these populations, but tends to be more prevalent in heterosexuals with multiple sex partners, including prostitutes and other men and women employed in the sex industry. In Africa, men and women are affected in about equal numbers, and transmission via heterosexual contact and unscreened blood transfusion seems more common, along with transmission to newborn babies from infected women during pregnancy. The precise magnitude of the AIDS problem in Africa is poorly documented, but available evidence indicates it is certainly substantial.

Although the number of AIDS cases reported from Asia has so far been smaller, the WHO estimates it to be growing rapidly. Sexual and needle-sharing transmission have both been documented. In Thailand, in 1985, 2–3 per cent of IV drug abusers were

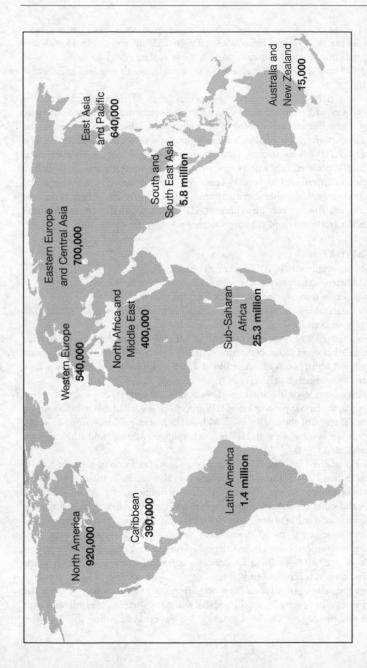

Map 10:1 Adults and children estimated by the WHO to be living with HIV/AIDS at the end of 2000 (reproduced by kind permission of the Joint United Nations Programme on HIV/AIDS (UNAIDS))

Western Europe
540,000

North Africa and
Middle East
400,000

Eastern Europe
and Central Asia
700,000

East Asia
and Pacific
640,000

South and
South East Asia
5.8 million

Australia and
New Zealand
15,000

Sub-Saharan
Africa
25.3 million

North America
920,000

Caribbean
390,000

Latin America
1.4 million

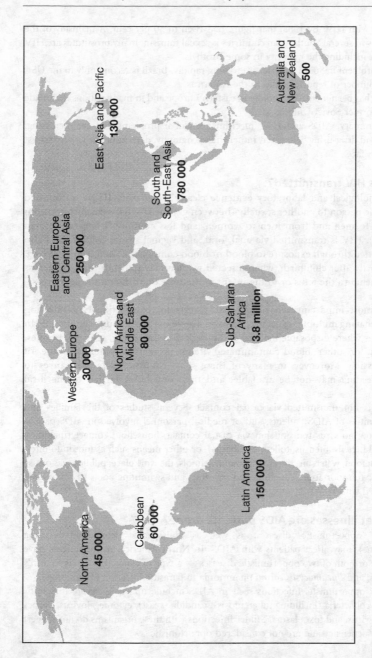

Map 10.2 Number of adults estimated by the WHO to be newly infected with HIV during 2000 (reproduced by kind permission of the Joint United Nations Programme on HIV/AIDS (UNAIDS))

North America
45 000

Caribbean
60 000

Latin America
150 000

Western Europe
30 000

North Africa and
Middle East
80 000

Eastern Europe
and Central Asia
250 000

Sub-Saharan
Africa
3.8 million

East Asia and Pacific
130 000

South and
South-East Asia
780 000

Australia and
New Zealand
500

infected with HIV. By 1988, that figure had risen to 30 per cent. A mainstay of the economy in several South Asian countries is sexual tourism; many prostitutes are HIV infected, including the majority in some brothels.

The problem in South America is growing rapidly. Brazil is second only to the USA in the number of reported cases in the Americas.

AIDS has been increasing rapidly in eastern Europe and in many nations that made up the former Soviet Union.

In summary, AIDS and HIV infection are global problems and are increasing. Sexual and drug-using behaviour, rather than geography, determine the risk that most travellers face.

How is HIV transmitted?

Epidemiological and laboratory evidence clearly show that HIV is transmitted from one person to another sexually (between gay men, heterosexually both from women to men and from men to women, and less commonly between lesbian women). HIV is transmitted via anal, oral, and vaginal sexual contact. It is also transmitted through exposure to blood or blood components; and before, during, and shortly after childbirth, when infected women may transmit the virus across the placenta to the fetus or to the infant at the time of birth and through breast-feeding.

The most important behavioural risk factors for contracting HIV infection include having multiple sexual partners and needle sharing among drug abusers. In countries where disposable medical equipment is not available, re-use of needles, syringes, or other blood-contaminated items presents a potential route of transmission. Moreover, in many of these same countries, safe alternatives to breast-feeding may not be available, and this contributes further to the local problem.

HIV is not transmitted via casual contact. Several studies of the families and communities of AIDS patients, and of medical personnel involved in AIDS patient care, show no virus transmission via casual contact, household contact (including sharing kitchens, utensils, toilets, and baths), or other means such as mosquito bites. Animals, food, water, air, the environment, schools, the workplace, public areas or use of public transportation, coughing and sneezing, and swimming pools have not been associated with HIV transmission.

To what illnesses are AIDS patients prone?

Various 'opportunistic' diseases, as well as non-specific debilitation (wasting syndrome), may affect patients with AIDS. In North America, many patients have had one or both of two opportunistic diseases — a type of cancer known as Kaposi's sarcoma, and *Pneumocystis carinii* pneumonia (a parasitic infection of the lungs).

Other opportunistic infections seen in AIDS include unusually severe infections with mycobacteria (including tuberculosis), candida (yeast), cytomegalovirus, herpes simplex virus, and toxoplasma. Milder infections with these organisms do not suggest immunodeficiency and are not considered opportunistic.

Kaposi's sarcoma

The opportunistic diseases that characterize AIDS are not new. Kaposi's sarcoma was first described over 100 years ago. Before 1980, in Europe and North America, it primarily affected elderly men and was seldom fatal, even five or ten years after diagnosis. It was also seen in children and young adults in some parts of equatorial Africa and in a few other locations where it had a more severe clinical form. Kaposi's sarcoma is caused by a newly discovered virus, human herpes virus-8.

Kaposi's sarcoma usually occurs anywhere on the surface of the skin or in the mouth. In the early stages, it may look like a bruise or blue-violet or brownish spot. The lesions grow larger and may ulcerate. It may arise in other organs, including lymph nodes, causing them to enlarge. Some AIDS patients with Kaposi's sarcoma have responded to treatment with interferon.

Pneumocystis carinii pneumonia (PCP)

PCP affected a few hundred adults and children in the developed nations each year before its increase was noted in the USA in 1978–9, but usually it was seen only in patients with a severe underlying illness (such as leukaemia) or in patients receiving therapy with drugs known to suppress the immune system (such as the drugs used with kidney transplant patients to prevent organ rejection). In fact, an increase in cases of PCP without such underlying predisposing factors was one of the first clues that the epidemic of AIDS was beginning.

PCP has symptoms similar to any other form of severe pneumonia, especially fever, cough, and difficulty in breathing. Specific antibiotic treatments for this pneumonia are available, such as trimethoprim/sulfamethoxazole and pentamidine, but the case-fatality rate is still high and PCP remains the leading cause of death in AIDS patients in many countries. Patients whose T-helper lymphocyte count falls below 200 cells per millilitre of blood should receive chemoprophylaxis with a regimen of trimethoprim 160 mg/sulfamethoxazole 800 mg tablets daily.

Tuberculosis (TB)

TB is the most common major manifestation of AIDS in many nations. HIV-infected immunosuppressed persons are both more susceptible to TB and more likely to transmit it to others once infected (see also p. 93).

How serious is AIDS?

AIDS has a very high fatality rate, and no credible reports have been published of any patient with AIDS who has regained lost immunity. There is no cure for AIDS or HIV infection as yet, but experimental trials are under way with drugs that interrupt the replication of HIV. The first such drug was zidovudine (often called AZT), which was shown to prolong the lives of AIDS patients and forestall the onset of AIDS in HIV-infected persons whose T-helper lymphocyte count had fallen below 500 cells/ml.

Since then treatment for HIV infection has evolved rapidly: at least 17 anti-retroviral drugs were licensed by 2001. These medicines have preserved the health and prolonged the lives of persons living with HIV and AIDS. Their clinical use is complex. Patients must take combinations of medicines (usually three or more drugs) daily and indefinitely. All the drugs are expensive and have toxic side effects, and adhering to the prescribed regimens has been difficult for many. Treatment must be tailored to each individual patient.

Eventually, more such drugs and others, in various combinations and sequences, will be used to extend therapeutic benefits further and to minimize toxicity and development of viral drug resistance.

Furthermore, additional treatments, as well as information on treatments, are developing rapidly. Updated guidelines are posted on the internet at the HIV/AIDS Treatment Information Service (**www.hivatis.org**), which is sponsored by health agencies of the US government.

Symptoms and diagnosis

Infection with HIV typically begins with a 'flu-like illness that resolves spontaneously. The infected person is then symptomless for up to 10 years or more. However, an infected person can transmit HIV to sex partners and needle sharers during this long asymptomatic period.

There are no clear-cut symptoms that indicate the loss of immunity, but many patients who have developed AIDS experienced fever, loss of appetite and weight, extreme fatigue, and enlargement of lymph nodes. These symptoms often occur over a period of months. In some cases, they are severe enough to result in hospitalization or disability. In parts of Africa (mainly East Africa), this condition is sometimes called 'slim disease' because of the characteristic weight loss. When patients develop opportunistic diseases — such as Kaposi's sarcoma, PCP, or cryptococcal meningitis — or have T-helper cell counts that fall below 200 cells/ml, they are then classified as having AIDS.

HIV can infect the central nervous system directly and produce various disorders including dementia, encephalopathy, sensorimotor deficits, and other problems. This also prompts an AIDS diagnosis.

Tests

No single specific test is available for diagnosing AIDS. The basic pathology of AIDS is that the number and function of certain white blood cells decreases and this can be measured (e.g. by CD4+ lymphocyte count). These tests are becoming more widely available, even outside industrialized nations. They are used mainly for monitoring immune function in HIV-infected patients. They can be expensive, and are usually done in larger laboratories or research centres. However, other tests may also help the physician to establish the diagnosis of AIDS and its opportunistic diseases.

A test to detect antibodies to the virus that causes AIDS became available in 1985. This test does not indicate the presence of the virus directly, but a repeatedly reactive and confirmed antibody test does provide evidence of infection. This test is used to screen donors of organs, blood, plasma, and other tissues for transfusion, transplantation, or manufacture of clotting-factor concentrates for people with haemophilia, and for other blood products. It is used to diagnose HIV infection and to assist in prevention-oriented counselling of sexually active men and women at risk of HIV infection, women contemplating pregnancy, IV drug abusers, and others.

Some countries require HIV antibody testing before granting certain classes of visas (usually longer-term immigrant, resident, work, or student visas). The WHO does not endorse or approve of this practice, and travellers should check testing requirements of nations on their itinerary with appropriate consular authorities.

Prevention

Many public health services have adopted the following recommendations for prevention:

- A mutually monogamous sexual relationship with a non-infected person is a safe way to avoid HIV infection.
- Use of condoms is recommended for all other sexual relationships. Condoms reduce, but do not eliminate, risk of HIV transmission.
- Do not have sexual intercourse with people who have or might be suspected of having AIDS or HIV infection.
- Do not use IV drugs or have sexual intercourse with people who abuse them.
- Be aware that having multiple sexual partners increases the chance of contracting AIDS or HIV infection.
- People whose behaviour puts them at risk of HIV infection should not donate blood or plasma or organs for transplantation.
- Blood transfusions (see p. 589) should be given only when medically essential and should be screened.
- Use extreme care when handling hypodermic needles. Do not recap, bend, or clip needles. Dispose of them into impervious containers.

Prevention of HIV infection following possible exposure (post-exposure prophylaxis)

Health care workers exposed to HIV in the course of their work have been able to reduce their risk of becoming infected with HIV via post-exposure prophylaxis (i.e. taking a course of anti-retroviral drugs for several weeks or months, beginning within hours of sustaining a needle-stick injury or other documented exposure to HIV). This has prompted the hypothesis that such post-exposure prophylaxis might also be effective for non-occupational (i.e. sexual or drug-injecting) exposures.

Travellers who wish to avail themselves of post-exposure prophylaxis would almost certainly need to carry the supply of anti-retroviral medicines with them (particularly when travelling to developing nations) and be fully aware of their use and side effects before any medical or other exposure might take place. They should therefore consult a knowledgeable physician well in advance of their anticipated travel.

This is an issue that needs to be considered particularly carefully in relation to medical students travelling overseas for electives, and health care and international aid workers travelling to developing countries.

UK post-exposure prophylaxis guidelines may be found at **www.doh.gov.uk/eaga/pepgu20fin.pdf.**

Summary of advice for travellers

- Travellers are normally at no special risk for HIV infection or AIDS unless they engage in sexual or drug-taking behaviour that puts them in contact with people who might be infected with HIV.

- Gay men and sexually active heterosexual men and women should take particular note of the recommendations listed above. Engaging only in safer sexual practices, in particular using condoms for all sexual intercourse (vaginal, anal, or oral) can reduce the risk of infection with HIV and other sexually transmitted organisms.

- IV drug abusers risk multiple health problems outside the scope of this chapter. Suffice it to note that needle sharing is very dangerous.

- When living or travelling in countries where re-use of medical equipment is common, it is important to make sure that medical staff who look after you are trained in and practise good infection control techniques, such as sterilizing needles, syringes, and surgical equipment before re-use. Blood transfusion abroad is discussed further on p. 589.

- Unless you are certain that new or sterile equipment is being used, skin piercing, such as tattooing, ear piercing, acupuncture, or electrolysis, should always be avoided.

- An epidemic of HIV infection precedes an epidemic of AIDS by several years. HIV infection is usually not clinically obvious; travellers should not assume that AIDS is an insignificant risk in countries that may have so far reported only a small number of cases, and should always take appropriate precautions.

Contraception and travel

Contraception is a neglected aspect of health care for travellers, but can make all the difference between an enjoyable trip and a miserable one. Not all methods of contraception are equally problem-free in travellers, and an appropriate method should be chosen carefully before departure.

Dr Elphis Christopher has been involved in family planning for over thirty years and is a Consultant in Family Planning and Reproductive Care for Haringey NHS Trust. She lectures to medical students and has made numerous radio and TV appearances to discuss sex education, family planning, and related topics.

Glossy brochures use covert promises of sexual adventure to sell travel. Away from everyday stresses and routines, and far from the influence of anyone who might disapprove, vacations and travel bring relaxation of inhibitions, a sense of freedom, and are undoubtedly a time of increased sexual activity both for couples and for men and women travelling on their own.

Too many travellers leave home unprepared. Single people — particularly women, who are most at risk from the consequences — may be unwilling to anticipate a sexual adventure on vacation on the grounds that 'I am not that kind of girl'; they may find it difficult to believe that pregnancy might begin on a vacation, or that contraceptive precautions may be necessary in advance of a romantic attachment. Others, men and women, simply don't bother.

Avoiding an unwanted pregnancy, an unintended souvenir of an otherwise enjoyable vacation, is not merely a question of chance; travelling prepared must not be confused with promiscuity, and it is always better to be safe than sorry.

If you are sexually active and settled on a particular contraceptive method, all you may need to do is visit your own doctor or family planning clinic for a check-up and obtain any contraceptive supplies you will need while away — and also confirm that the method you are using is appropriate for the length and nature of your trip. For prolonged periods abroad it is worth finding out what is available in the country or countries you intend to visit before you leave: the International Planned Parenthood Federation (IPPF)* can provide information on this.

Travelling may reduce the effectiveness of contraceptive precautions which are otherwise perfectly adequate at home, and the specific problems that arise for each method are discussed below. Normally these problems are not serious enough to warrant changing from your established method, but you should be aware of them, and perhaps travel prepared to switch to an alternative method in an emergency.

Once you have decided upon a method, or if you plan to switch to a new method, it is worth getting used to it well in advance of your trip, to enable any side effects or problems to reveal themselves in time to be sorted out. This is a particularly important consideration with the Pill — nausea and tiredness and slight spotting (breakthrough bleeding) are common when taking it for the first time, but usually settle by the third packet — and with the intrauterine device (IUD).

The various methods available are discussed below along with their advantages and disadvantages, although travellers may well need to consult their doctor or family planning clinic in order to make the most suitable choice for their own circumstances.

It may be advisable to travel with *two* methods to ensure against failure of one of them.

The combined oral contraceptive: 'the Pill'

The Pill is a popular method of contraception, familiar and convenient to use; with correct use its reliability is 99–100 per cent. If you are on the Pill be sure to travel with an adequate supply, because further supplies of your particular brand may not necessarily be easy to obtain — especially in remote areas. Make allowances for delays and any unexpected extension of your trip.

If you run out, keep an empty pack so that a doctor or a pharmacist can identify your brand — brand names of the same variety of the Pill usually differ from country to country. Thus a widely prescribed variety like Microgynon 30 occurs under well over 20 other brand names around the world. If exactly the same Pill cannot be obtained and a different one is prescribed, do not leave a seven-day gap between packets, but go straight on to the new Pill regardless of any bleeding. Other contraceptive precautions will not then be necessary.

Stomach problems and diarrhoea affect most travellers at some time or another. *Stomach problems and severe diarrhoea reduce absorption of the Pill, and may leave the traveller without protection.* All travellers on the Pill should be aware of this, and should be prepared to use an alternative method when necessary.

* International Planned Parenthood Federation (IPPF), Regent's College, Inner Circle, Regent's Park, London NW1 4NS, UK. Tel: +44 (0)20 7487 7900 Fax: +44 (0)20 7487 7950 **www.ippf.org**

A barrier method (see below) should be used to protect intercourse over the duration of the stomach problem and for seven days after it has ended. If vomiting occurs within three hours of taking a pill, an additional pill should be taken. If vomiting continues another method of contraception will have to be used.

Using the Pill with antibiotics, anti-malarials, and other medicines
Antibiotics such as tetracycline or ampicillin also reduce the absorption and effectiveness of the Pill, and another method of contraception should be used during a course of antibiotics and for seven days afterwards. *Doxycycline, widely used as an anti-malarial, is a tetracycline and has the same effect.* Anti-fungal medication such as griseofulvin, and anti-epilepsy drugs may also reduce the effectiveness of the Pill. Additional precautions are needed when these are being taken.

In both instances, if the seven days coincide with the seven pill-free days, do not take a break of seven days but carry straight on with another packet of pills. Do not worry if there is no withdrawal bleeding.

Using the Pill across time zones
Time zones cause another potential hazard to travellers on the Pill. When time zones are crossed, make sure that you take a pill every 24 hours, and continue to do so every day at the same time. If that means having to wake up in the middle of the night to take a pill, take it *earlier* before going to sleep rather than later; no more than 24 hours should elapse between doses — particularly with newer varieties of the low-dose Pill — both for protection against pregnancy and to prevent breakthrough bleeding or spotting.

Flight attendants who are continually travelling may find it useful to have two wristwatches, and to keep one of them on 'home time' for this purpose.

Altitude
High altitude, dehydration, and extreme cold stress, are all associated with changes in blood viscosity. Although as yet there is no clear evidence of an increased thrombosis risk among women taking the Pill at high altitude, it would seem wise not to do so (p. 325).

Using the Pill to avoid menstruation
Travel can interfere with periods even when a woman is on the Pill; so a missed period does not necessarily mean that she is pregnant (p. 440) — provided of course that the daily doses have been taken regularly. Women who prefer not to have periods at all while travelling can take the Pill continuously, without a seven-day break in between packets; *but remember to take extra packets to allow for this*. This is not advisable with the biphasic or triphasic Pills because the dose in the first seven pills is too low to prevent possible breakthrough bleeding; triphasic brands are probably best avoided for long journeys that cross time zones, since the margin of error is less with this type and the risk of pregnancy increases if they are not taken regularly.

The progestogen-only Pill (POP)

The progestogen-only Pill, or POP, is sometimes used by women who cannot take the combined Pill, although the same considerations apply. It is *not* 100 per cent effective (about 96–98 per cent) and it *must* be taken at a fixed time each day, one every 24 hours in order to remain effective. If a pill is forgotten, take one as soon as it is remembered, but use an additional method for seven days. *Antibiotics do not affect the progestogen-only Pill.*

The patch

Hormonal contraception is also becoming available in the form of a patch. OrthoEvra was approved in the USA in 2001, and offers many advantages for travel, such as usability by women taking doxycycline for malaria protection and those with travellers' diarrhoea. More information can be found at **www.orthoevra.com**.

The intrauterine device (IUD)

Women who already have an IUD should have it checked before going abroad. If it is a copper-bearing device such as a ParaGard T, make sure that it is not due for a change. All-plastic devices such as the Lippes Loop can remain in the uterus for many years provided that there are no problems.

The IUD is about 97–99 per cent effective. It has the advantage that it is not affected by stomach upsets or time zones. It can, however, be expelled by the uterus, so it is a sensible precaution to check after each period that the threads can still be felt. If a 'hard bit' (part of the IUD itself) can be felt as well as the threads, the IUD may be coming out and will need to be checked by a doctor or nurse. An examination is not necessary once the IUD has come out; obviously protection ceases immediately, and another method must be used.

The IUD is not suitable for women with heavy or prolonged periods — it may make these worse. A newly fitted IUD may also cause irregular and sometimes heavy bleeding in the first couple of months — hardly ideal if you are just off on a beach vacation in a new bikini! Heavy or continuous bleeding may make you feel tired and ruin your vacation. It is therefore a good idea to have the IUD fitted well in advance, so that any problems can be sorted out before you travel. Modern studies show conclusively that where a woman is in a mutually faithful sexual relationship infection is not a problem with IUD use. Although an IUD may exacerbate a sexually transmitted disease (see p. 439), it is not the IUD that increases the risks but the woman or her partner and their sexual practices. The IUD is most suitable for older women who have had children, since side effects such as heavy, painful periods are less common and there is less chance of the IUD being expelled.

Mirena — the levonorgestrel-releasing system (IUS)

This is a NovaT-shaped IUD that releases levonorgestrel, a progestogen hormone, at a rate of 20 μg per 24 hours. It works locally, suppressing the womb's lining, changing the mucus of the neck of the womb, and impairing sperm migration. It is effective for five years, is 99 per cent reliable, and is convenient, with few side effects.

It is different from other IUDs in that it reduces the amount and duration of the periods. Its main side effect is frequent though light bleeding during the first few months of use, so it is is best fitted several months before travelling. Eventually the periods may cease; this is not harmful — fertility returns rapidly after the IUS is removed. It appears to reduce the frequency of clinical pelvic inflammatory disease. Fitting may be slightly more difficult than other types of IUD, and a local anaesthetic may be needed.

Barrier methods

The condom

The condom is about 85–98 per cent effective when used correctly. It provides some protection against sexually transmitted disease including HIV (see p. 458), and is particularly useful for the man or woman travelling alone. It can be put on as part of love play.

It is also valuable for women or couples who want to take along a reliable alternative, in case of problems with the Pill, or in case the IUD is expelled. The condom is a good method for the chance sexual encounter, and travels well.

Female condom This is a condom that is put inside the vagina and the area just outside the vagina. There are two soft plastic rings, an inner one to help put the condom in the vagina, the outer one to help the condom to stay in place outside the vagina. Reliability is probably the same as for the male condom. It protects both partners against sexually transmitted disease including HIV. It is used once only and is sold under the brand name *Reality*.

The diaphragm and cervical cap

The diaphragm, covering the cervix and front wall of the vagina, and the cervical cap, covering the cervix, are useful methods with about the same effectiveness as the condom. They need to be fitted by a doctor or family planning nurse, and the woman must be taught how to use them correctly. A diaphragm or cap lasts for about six months to one year, so on a long trip it may be advisable to take along a spare.

They must be used with a spermicide. These come in the form of creams, gels, foams, vaginal suppositories, or film. Creams may become more messy in hot climates but do not lose their effectiveness. Foams in aerosol containers can be a useful alternative. In addition, vaginal suppositories should be inserted if a second act of intercourse takes place soon after the first. They are designed to melt at body temperature, and this can be an obvious problem in hot countries; brands wrapped individually with silver foil travel best, and should be kept in a cool place.

Foaming tablets also travel well, although if conditions are humid the lid of their container should always be firmly closed: moisture will make the tablets dissolve. The diaphragm and cap provide some protection from sexually transmitted diseases (see p. 459).

Injectable contraceptives

Injectable contraceptives (Depo-Provera and Noristerat) are virtually 100 per cent effective and work in a similar way to the progestogen-only Pill.

Depo-Provera is given by injection into the muscle of the buttock or upper arm and remains effective for three months. It is useful for women going on long trips and crossing time zones frequently. It is not affected by stomach upsets or antibiotics. Side effects often occur, such as irregular and occasionally heavy bleeding, especially with the first injection. With subsequent injections, the periods may stop altogether. This is how the injection *should* work, which makes it an ideal method for the woman who does not want regular periods. If Depo-Provera is chosen, the woman needs to be settled on it before she travels.

A second injectable contraceptive, Noristerat, has similar properties (and side effects) to Depo-Provera and is equally effective. Noristerat is also available in many countries, including some where Depo-Provera is unavailable.

Implanon is a long-acting (up to three years) hormonal method for women. It works rather like the oral contraceptive Pill, preventing ovulation and thickening cervical mucus. A single rod, 40 mm long and 2 mm in diameter, is inserted just under the skin in the upper arm, under local anaesthesia. The procedure takes five minutes. It provides a high level of protection against pregnancy (99–100 per cent). Its main side effect is irregular vaginal bleeding, which is occasionally prolonged.

Using contraception for the first time

The Pill is probably the most sensible method for a couple going on honeymoon, who have not had sex before and who do not want a pregnancy straight away. Although honeymoons are often pictured to be idyllic and carefree, in reality they can be a time of great anxiety and stress, with both partners worrying whether sex will be alright.

Sexual adjustment to each other may take time, and methods that directly interfere with intercourse — such as the condom or diaphragm — may interrupt love play and can make that adjustment more complicated. If you choose the Pill, begin taking it a few months in advance, so that any problems can be dealt with before you leave.

Emergency or postcoital contraception: PCC (the 'morning after' Pill)

This method of birth control may be used in an emergency. It works by preventing implantation of the fertilized egg in the uterus. It is preferable to abortion but should not be used on a regular basis. It is useful on those occasions when a contraceptive method fails (e.g. a condom splitting), or for the woman who has had unprotected intercourse.

One tablet of the progestogen-only pill Levonelle (levonorgestrel 0.75 mg) must be taken within 72 hours of an unprotected act of sexual intercourse, and then one tablet 12 hours later. Nausea and vomiting are rare. The next period may arrive slightly earlier or later than expected but usually within three weeks of prescribing PCC.

Table 10.3 Legal status of abortion

Countries where abortion is illegal or only permitted to save a women's life

Afghanistan	Indonesia	Nigeria
Angola	Iran	Oman
Bangladesh	Ireland	Panama
Benin	Ivory Coast	Papua New Guinea
Brazil	Kenya	Paraguay
Central African Republic	Laos	Philippines
Chad	Lebanon	Senegal
Chile	Lesotho	Somalia
Colombia	Libya	Sri Lanka
Congo	Madagascar	Sudan
Dominican Republic	Mali	Syria
Egypt	Mauritania	Tanzania
El Salvador	Mauritius	Togo
Gabon	Mexico	Uganda
Guatemala	Myanmar	United Arab Emirates
Guinea–Bissau	Nepal	Venezuela
Haiti	Nicaragua	Yemen
Honduras	Niger	

Countries where abortion is illegal but be permitted both to save a mother's life and to protect her physical health

Argentina	Eritrea	Rwanda
Bolivia	Guinea	Saudi Arabia
Burkina Faso	Kuwait	South Korea
Burundi	Malawi	Thailand
Cameroon	Morocco	Uruguay
Costa Rica	Mozambique	Zimbabwe
Ecuador	Pakistan	
Ethiopia	Poland	

Source: the Alan Guttmacher Institute, New York. See web directory, Appendix 8.

Postcoital contraception can be obtained from pharmacies in the UK without a prescription, or from family planning clinics or your own doctor or gynaecologist. Ideally a follow-up visit should be arranged after taking PCC.

Abortion
Travellers who become pregnant abroad and want an abortion may find this difficult to arrange. At the last count 53 out of 128 countries listed by the IPPF (see Table 10.3) prohibit abortion except in extreme circumstances (e.g. rape or life-threatening illness). Skilled medical care may be very expensive, or almost impossible to obtain (see p. 441).

RU 486 (mifepristone, Mifegyne: the 'abortion pill')

RU 486 is a synthetic steroid that counteracts the hormone progesterone. Progesterone is produced naturally in the body and is essential to maintain a pregnancy. By blocking the action of progesterone, RU 486 induces a miscarriage. It is more effective when used with another drug, prostaglandin. RU 486 is given as a single dose (three 200 mg tablets) by mouth, and a suppository of prostaglandin is inserted into the vagina 48 hours later. The abortion or miscarriage happens spontaneously about six hours later. This treatment can be given to women who are up to nine weeks pregnant and is effective in 95 per cent of cases. Side effects include period pains and prolonged bleeding. Less than 10 per cent of women have severe pain lasting about an hour. This responds to a strong painkiller. It has no adverse effects on future fertility. It is licensed for use under medical supervision in France and Britain; it has been approved though not as yet introduced for use in China.

11 Travellers at higher risk

Travel in pregnancy

There is absolutely no way of knowing in advance that a pregnancy will be trouble-free, and for travel, some extra precautions are necessary.

Dr John Naponick is a public health physician with specialist training in gynaecology, obstetrics, and tropical medicine. He has worked in the USA, Canada, Cameroon, Bangladesh, Thailand, Burma, and El Salvador. He currently works in Louisiana.
Professor Herbert A. Brant was formerly Professor of Clinical Obstetrics and Gynaecology at University College Hospital, London.

Increasingly, we take travel for granted, but its implications for women who are pregnant or may become pregnant while travelling are worth a little thought. Large numbers of women do travel in pregnancy, and they sometimes travel long distances; most have no real problems, but an unlucky few regret having ventured forth. The widely varying standard of medical care and its availability in different countries is more important than the direct effects of travel on pregnancy. But at least being aware of the problems may help you to minimize their effects.

Possible problems

Why should pregnant women be more concerned about travel? The likelihood of a problem needing medical attention arising is greater during pregnancy than at other times. On statistical grounds alone, women should hesitate before travelling to any area where medical services will be of doubtful quality or where misunderstandings due to language or cultural problems are going to make communication and therefore diagnosis and treatment more difficult.

No woman can be realistically assured in advance that she will have a trouble-free pregnancy. It is worth remembering that pregnancy is normal only when viewed in retrospect — that is, *after* no problems have occurred.

Antenatal care and routine tests in early pregnancy

Don't miss out on antenatal care and important tests that need to be completed in the first half of pregnancy — postpone your trip, if necessary. Serious blood conditions of the fetus such as thalassaemia (in those of Mediterranean or Asian origin) or sickle cell anaemia (in those of African origin) can be detected early in pregnancy — in time for a pregnancy to be terminated if the fetus is affected. The blood test for spina bifida (AFP) is carried out at 16–18 weeks, and amniocentesis for Down's syndrome in older women at about 16 weeks. (In some situations, the chorion biopsy test can be carried out as an alternative to amniocentesis, between 9 and 11 weeks.) An ultrasound examination is usually carried out at some time in the first 24 weeks (but usually at 18 weeks) to confirm the age of the fetus in case of problems later in pregnancy, and also to detect abnormalities that might have arisen during development of fetal organs.

Folic acid

Between 50 and 70 per cent of neural tube defects (birth defects such as spina bifida and anencephaly) could be prevented by taking sufficient folic acid in the diet — at least 400 micrograms a day — before conception and during early pregnancy. Folic acid is present in green leafy vegetables, beans, and legumes, and also in specially fortified foods such as breakfast cereals, but these can be an unreliable source, especially when travelling. So all women who might conceive while travelling — and arguably all women of childbearing age, anywhere — should take a daily supplement of at least 400 micrograms of folic acid. (There is no known toxic level, and a higher dose should be taken when using proguanil (Paludrine) for malaria prevention — see below.)

Miscarriage

Spontaneous abortion (miscarriage) is the commonest problem of early pregnancy. It usually occurs within the first three months. If it merely threatens, as evidenced by vaginal bleeding, the eventual outcome will *not* be altered because the woman travels.

Miscarriages in the early months are due to the inevitable errors of a biological system — errors in cell division during the early stages of development of the fetus or the placenta, and errors concerned with the attachment of the placenta to the wall of the uterus (womb). Travel won't cause miscarriage other than *indirectly*, through the effect of, say, high fever associated with infection or severe dehydration associated with diarrhoea.

Of more pressing concern are the immediate complications of miscarriage, which include the occasional life-threatening haemorrhage, the occasional serious infection, or the problems of inept medical treatment employed to cope with them.

Miscarriage, although uncommon at a later stage of pregnancy, can occur at any time, though once the fetus is able to survive, it is termed premature labour; the above complications are more common with later miscarriages. Any pregnant woman who has had a previous late miscarriage, or has any condition predisposing to miscarriage, is ill-advised to travel in mid-pregnancy.

Ectopic pregnancy
This may be a problem in the first few months, and affects 1 pregnancy in 200. The fetus grows in the fallopian tube instead of in the uterus, and this can lead to life-threatening haemorrhage. If abdominal pain occurs in pregnancy, always consult a doctor.

Premature labour
If labour starts early but at a time when the resulting baby could live (any time after 24 weeks) then the whole future of the baby can depend on the availability of expert care. Without this, the baby is likely to be seriously mentally or physically handicapped for life — if he or she survives. If expert care is available it can be extremely expensive, especially if prolonged intensive care is necessary. Where good obstetric care is available, treatment can sometimes be given to stop or delay premature labour.

Other complications
In late pregnancy, other possible problems are haemorrhage from a normally situated placenta or from a placenta growing near the cervix (placenta praevia); pregnancy-induced hypertension (previously called toxaemia of pregnancy); and premature rupture of the membranes. Such complications threaten both mother and fetus, and ready availability of expert care reduces the risks.

Many of the complications that occur in pregnancy may result in haemorrhage and the need for a blood transfusion, and some of the risks associated with this are discussed on p. 589.

Before you go
If you are planning to live overseas, you should ensure that you will have access to good-quality antenatal advice and care, and also that you will have all the social and emotional support you may need.

Insurance
Be sure to check that any travel or medical insurance covers medical care for the consequences of pregnancy; many policies specifically exclude this, and additional cover often needs to be arranged separately (p. 569).

If you are British and travelling to an EU country, you should obtain form E111 (p. 572).

Immunization
Vaccinations that involve a live virus or are likely to lead to a high temperature should be avoided during pregnancy. A medical certificate can circumvent the vaccination requirements for travel.

Poliomyelitis (the oral vaccine), measles, rubella, and yellow fever vaccines all involve live viruses. Vaccination against rubella and poliomyelitis should have been carried out *before* pregnancy. Diphtheria and typhoid vaccines may cause increased temperature and should be avoided. BCG (against tuberculosis) can affect the fetus, and is therefore also not given. (see also p. 565.)

Anti-malarial medication

If you are pregnant and are thinking of travelling to an area where there is a risk of contracting malaria, it is vital to be adequately protected (see pp. 143–4) — malaria is far more common and more serious in pregnancy. Chloroquine (Avloclor, Nivaquine) and proguanil (Paludrine) are generally agreed not to cause harm in pregnancy, but resistance to these drugs means that there are many parts of the world where they provide insufficient protection. The combined tablet Savarine, popular in France but unlicensed in the UK and USA, contains a larger dose of chloroquine and may be a little more effective. Folic acid supplementation (5 mg daily — a larger dose than is used for supplementation to prevent spina bifida) is advised when taking proguanil.

Of the other, more effective options, mefloquine (Lariam) can be used in pregnancy but is not usually recommended to UK travellers during the first 12 weeks (though in the USA this restriction does not apply): it is not believed to harm the fetus. Doxycycline is unsuitable for use in pregnancy, and there is insufficient experience with Malarone for this drug to yet be an option.

Expert help in balancing the various risks and benefits may sometimes be needed, and, in general, travel to high-risk malarial regions is best avoided during pregnancy.

Travel

Air

Provided that the cabin is pressurized, reduced pressure on board an airliner (p. 252) should have no adverse effect upon healthy women with a normal pregnancy. If a significant problem with the function of the placenta is suspected, however, air travel should be avoided because the slightly reduced oxygen level may harm the fetus.

Most airlines will not accept you for travel after 32 weeks of pregnancy, but will sometimes stretch this to 36 weeks if you can produce a medical certificate stating that all is well. Policy varies between airlines and also depends on the length of the flight. It is obviously difficult to obtain medical assistance in the air if labour begins unexpectedly! Between 1999 and 2001, three babies were born during flights on British Airways.

Pregnant women and those in the first month after delivery have a small but definitely increased risk of developing a blood clot in the deep veins of the legs (deep-vein thrombosis). These clots occasionally travel to the lungs via the bloodstream and can prove fatal. When travelling by air do not sit in a cramped position for a long period, because pressure from the seat and from the fetus slows the circulation in the legs (see pp. 257–8). Tense up the legs and wriggle the toes from time to time; stand up and walk about at least every hour, and consider wearing compression stockings.

Other forms of travel

Sitting in a cramped position in a car, bus, or train has the same effect of impairing blood circulation in the legs. Stand up and walk about every hour or so; if you are travelling by road, stop the car every hour, get out and take a walk.

During pregnancy, women should drive with more care and more slowly, as pregnancy sometimes affects concentration and reaction time in an emergency.

Pregnant women should wear seat-belts, because in a crash injuries are more serious without them.

Nausea and vomiting
The tendency to nausea and vomiting in early pregnancy is likely to be aggravated by travel. All travel sickness tablets cause some unwanted effects, such as drowsiness, altered reaction time, dry mouth, and blurred vision, and so should be used only when symptoms warrant (and not at all when driving). Drugs based on hyoscine (e.g. Kwells) and anti-histamine preparations such as promethazine (Phenergan, Avomine) are safe for use in pregnancy.

At your destination

Food and drink
Dehydration Try to avoid dehydration during air travel or in a hot climate — this aggravates the tendency to thrombosis and also the problem of constipation, which is common in pregnancy. Drink plenty of fluids, preferably in the form of plain water — bottled or boiled if the local supply isn't safe (p. 71).

Take an extra supply of natural bran and increase your intake of fruit and vegetables to counteract the constipation that often goes with changed daily routines and possibly a more refined diet than you are used to at home.

Avoid alcohol, not only because of its dehydrating properties but also for its possible harmful effects on the fetus. *Severe* dehydration — such as may follow prolonged diarrhoea —increases the risk of miscarriage. Smoking and addictive and recreational drugs also have an extremely detrimental effect during pregnancy (addtional harmful effects are coming to light all the time).

Toxoplasmosis Don't eat undercooked meat; the condition toxoplasmosis may result. It causes only mild illness in adults but occasionally has serious effects on the fetus. You could be checked to see whether you are immune, but it is a difficult test, not generally available.

Listeriosis This infection is acquired from contaminated food, particularly poultry that is either fresh or frozen and then *incompletely* cooked. It also occurs in cows' and goats' milk and is not always eliminated by pasteurization. Soft, ripened cheeses often contain the bacteria in high numbers and pre-prepared salads are not safe, as the bacteria can survive in the refrigerator. All these points should be borne in mind by the pregnant traveller, as the infection has little effect on most healthy adults but can cause serious effects in the fetus. If a 'flu-like illness develops in pregnancy, then it is probably wise to have antibiotic treatment (such as amoxycillin), just in case.

Drug treatment abroad
Prescribing habits vary considerably from country to country, and awareness of potential hazards from drug treatment in pregnancy is far from universal; it is safest to

avoid medicines altogether if you can, other than iron supplements and vitamins. One group of drugs that may possibly be prescribed for you, but which should be avoided in pregnancy, are the tetracycline group of antibiotics. Other drugs to avoid include bismuth subsalicylate (Pepto–Bismol); metronidazole (Flagyl), which should not be taken during the first trimester unless absolutely necessary; and the fluoroquinolone antibiotics (e.g. ciprofloxacin and norfloxacin). Amoxycillin and ampicillin are safe.

Recreational drug use may be extremely dangerous in pregnancy; in particular, 'crack' cocaine causes serious brain abnormalities in the fetus.

Summary of advice for travellers

- You will probably have gathered that we are rather against travelling to remote spots at any time in pregnancy, but if a time for a break has to be selected, between 18 and 24 weeks is probably the best. This is after the risk of nausea and miscarriage — and after the necessary tests should have been completed — but before the problems of premature labour loom. You should be back at base for late pregnancy, just in case!

Radiation and flying

Exposure to cosmic radiation at normal flying altitudes (35 000 feet) is more than 100 times greater than at ground level. There has been increasing concern about the effects of low-dose radiation, and it is certainly possible for frequent fliers to build up a significant radiation exposure. Solar flares — bursts of energy on the surface of the sun — account for periodic increases in such exposure, and occur in unpredictable patterns. The radiation exposure for a return trip between London and New York is roughly equivalent to the exposure from a single chest X-ray (0.1 millisievert); a return flight between London and Los Angeles would clock up 0.16 mSv. Because Concorde flies at higher altitudes, radiation exposure might be expected to be higher; this is balanced by the shorter flying time, and overall exposure is generally reduced.

Calculations on the extent of harm associated with radiation exposure are generally based on the effects of much larger doses — such as at Hiroshima. It is difficult to know how such data extrapolate to lower doses, and it is conceivable that low doses may be relatively more harmful. It is also difficult to document the effects, and to know whether subtle changes such as differences in intelligence or minor defects can be attributed to such exposure rather than nature. For this reason it has been suggested that pregnant women should avoid unnecessary long-distance flights during the early, most vulnerable stages of pregnancy, and most airlines now have a policy of 'grounding' any flight crew who become pregnant.

Children abroad

Problems of travelling with children vary according to where you intend to go, how you will be getting there, and how long you will be away. Whether you are moving abroad to live or are merely off on a short trip, careful preparation will be amply rewarded.

Dr Tony Waterston is a paediatrician who has worked for several years as a doctor and teacher in Zambia and Zimbabwe and has spent shorter periods in several other parts of Africa and Asia. His wife (a doctor too) and three children have also contributed to this chapter.

Parents travelling abroad often anticipate all sorts of problems with their children, some concerned with the journey itself, others with what will happen at the destination. Will the change of environment be good for the children or bad? Will the food be suitable? Will it be safe for them to play outside? What dreadful diseases will they get? How will the baby take the heat?

Fortunately, the reality of travelling with children is usually much better than you might expect and is generally a formative and valuable experience for the whole family. In this chapter, I hope to answer some of the most common questions about children's health abroad and help you prepare for your trip, whether it is a package tour to the Mediterranean or a long-term posting to some faraway destination in a developing country.

I will discuss three aspects of the trip with respect to children. First, what preparations to make, and the journey itself; second, health hazards encountered while living abroad; and third, some points about children's diet, and baby care.

Before you go

The longer you intend to stay away, the more preparation will be needed. Plenty of time spent finding out as much as you can about the country you plan to visit will be amply repaid, and if you are going to live abroad, this includes attending any special courses that may be laid on for you before you leave. Try to find out all you can (from friends or colleagues who have already been, or through your embassy) about the following.

The local health system

Make sure that you have adequate insurance for the whole family, and find out if the cost of return travel home will be paid in case of major illness. What are the facilities available for treating sick children? Wherever you are, a child may get appendicitis, a fracture, or a severe infection and need specialized care. This might be available only at a major centre and could be a factor in deciding where you are to live.

Can medicines be obtained easily? You will quite likely need anti-malarials if visiting a tropical zone and may need antibiotics. A small supply of over-the-counter remedies will come in useful for minor illnesses and should be bought in advance. If you have a baby and are going for more than a few weeks, find out where and how routine immunizations can be carried out (see below for schedule). There should not be any difficulty in obtaining immunization in any country you visit, although there may be a queue.

In many developing countries, the emphasis in the medical system will be on *primary health care*. This means basic care concentrating on common ailments and on prevention, delivered by workers with a short training. Do not therefore be surprised if you do not see a doctor at a clinic — the health worker you see should be trained to recognize and treat the common childhood complaints.

Be sure to avoid all treatment by injection unless it is absolutely essential, and unless you are certain that the needle has been sterilized (see p. 588).

Dental care

Dental care abroad is often expensive or non-existent. The whole family should have a dental check and receive essential treatment before going (see p. 420). Fluoride drops or tablets are recommended for infants and young children (see below).

The main diseases

In Europe, North America, and Australia, the diseases are very similar to those encountered in the UK, whereas the developing countries of Africa, Asia, and South America share a wide spectrum of infectious diseases, which are discussed elsewhere in this book.

Find out what the main problems are in the country you intend to visit (e.g. whether drug-resistant malaria is present) and what specific precautions you should take. Do not feel that it would be unsafe to take children to a country where tropical diseases such as malaria and bilharzia are common: simple precautions will protect against these diseases, and it is often more trivial complaints such as cuts, bites, diarrhoea, and respiratory infections that become important when you are there. These problems are dealt with below, but you would be wise also to take with you one of the many child care books that deal with the management of minor illnesses at home.

Water and food

Find out whether the local water supply is drinkable — if not, you should pay careful attention to the information in this book about water purification (pp. 71–83). Clean water is essential for young children, as stomach upsets are the commonest disorders encountered. It always pays to be careful about water quality when travelling — even bottled carbonated drinks are not necessarily always safe. It may be wise to stick to tea when in doubt.

What are the major local foods? If they are not of a kind you feel up to preparing (such as maize meal, sweet potato, plantain, yam) you will need to depend on imported foods. Is there always a constant supply of these?

Foreign exchange is scarce in many countries, and Weetabix or even wheat may not be at the top of the list of priorities. Can you bake bread? Sacks of flour can sometimes be obtained and will allow you to live through temporary bread or flour shortages. You could arrange to have limited stocks of food sent out, but this will prove expensive and it is sensible to try to 'live off the land'.

Is the milk drinkable and if not, is powdered milk available? This is something you could quite easily take and may need to if you have a formula-fed baby (see notes below under baby care).

Table 11.1 Immunization schedule for children

Vaccine (disease)	Comment	Age
Diphtheria/tetanus/pertussis/ *Haemophilus influenzae* type B (DTP Hib), polio, meningococcal meningitis type C	Primary course (3 doses, a month between each dose)	2 months, 3 months, 4 months
Measles/mumps/rubella (MMR)	First dose	12–15 months (can be given at any age over 12 months)
Diphtheria/tetanus (DT), polio	Booster dose	3–5 years (3 years after completion of primary course)
Measles/mumps/rubella (MMR)	Second dose	3–5 years
Tuberculosis (BCG)		10–14 years, or newborn at high risk
Tetanus/low-dose diphtheria (Td), polio	Booster dose	13–18 years

In most cases it is quite easy to provide a balanced diet for children, but it will pay if you learn something about the nutritional content of the foods you will encounter abroad.

Immunization

Children should have had the normal schedule of immunization set out in Table 11.1, before travelling abroad — and the same schedule should be used for babies living abroad (but see note on p. 588 about injections abroad).

In the UK, tuberculin or 'Heaf' testing is also normally carried out at 12 years and BCG vaccine given to protect against tuberculosis for those who are not already immune (see pp. 96–7). However, this can be carried out at any age from infancy for children going to a country with a high prevalence of tuberculosis. BCG should be given at birth to babies born in countries where tuberculosis is common. It should always be given intradermally in the left upper arm.

Boosters against tetanus (unless immunized within the last 10 years) and polio should be given before departure.

In addition, yellow fever immunization may be mandatory for the country you are to visit. Protection can optionally be obtained against typhoid, hepatitis A and B (see below), and rabies. All these additional vaccines may be safely given to children of six months and over, but not earlier. Malaria prevention is dealt with separately below.

The domestic situation and education abroad

Find out in advance what kind of house you will have and whether you will be put first in a hotel or small flat. If so, and you have several children, it may be better for them to follow once the house has been obtained. How well equipped will the house be? For a family, a refrigerator is essential, and you may need to take this out yourself.

If you do not intend to employ domestic help, then a washing machine should also be considered, and in a developing country it will be much cheaper to take it with you than to buy there.

If you have school-age children, find out something about the schools, whether there is a choice, and whether the teaching is what you are used to. If not, and you intend to return them to their original schools later, seek advice from their teachers on whether books should be taken with you to help bridge the gap. For pre-school children, you should take out plenty of books, toys, and playgroup materials and obtain addresses of web-sites and mail order firms who will send things out.

If both parents are to be working, then care arrangements will be needed for pre-school children. Home helps are generally childminders rather than educators and this should be borne in mind: nursery schools of the quality available at home may not be easy to find. You may find it necessary to organize your own playgroup.

If you have a baby, it may be wise to take several sets of baby clothes to expand into as he or she grows. Cotton clothes are preferable to those made of stretch nylon, and plastic pants should be avoided. A hat or sunshade is a must. Further aspects of baby care are dealt with below.

The journey

Travelling long distances with children can be stressful. Here are some tips on how to reduce the stress:

If you have a baby, breast-feeding on the move is far easier than formula feeding, especially if you are not inhibited about feeding in public. If you are flying, ask for a 'sky cot' well in advance (and check again before travelling), otherwise you will be balancing the baby on your knee all the way. Disposable nappies are a boon for the journey, even if you normally despise them, and often they will be supplied by the flight attendant on the aircraft. If you bottle-feed, prepacked milk is very useful for the journey.

Suitable books and toys or games should be kept handy, as bored children sitting in an enclosed space for a long period will not stay happy. 'Looking at the view' may be fun for parents but not for a two- or even a six-year-old.

A small supply of food and drink should be taken (for example, some sandwiches, biscuits, and a bottle of water), as the meals available *en route* may be neither palatable nor healthy, if you can get them at all. Allow extra for delays.

Travel sickness should be prevented in advance if your children are prone to it. Kwells (containing hyoscine) is a suitable medication. Avoid overdosage, which leads to sleepiness, dry mouth, and irritability.

*A **light sedative*** may help children get through an especially long journey, and may provide some respite for parents, though most medication tends to have side effects. A suitable choice is promethazine (Phenergan), in a dose of 15 mg for one- to five-year-olds, and 10–25 mg for over-fives. It is available as tablets or elixir (prescription not required in the UK).

Health hazards at your destination

Short visits (under one month)
For short periods abroad, you do not need to be too concerned about exotic diseases — the most likely infections to crop up are the everyday ones. Make sure that you are prepared to deal with problems like diarrhoea or respiratory infections (sore throat or ears). The contents of a simple first–aid kit for young children on a beach holiday are shown in the box.

You should *always* be aware of the risk of malaria if you are going to a part of the world where it is endemic: babies and young children must be protected even on a short visit (see below). Check what immunizations are needed, and make sure that children are up to date with tetanus and polio vaccinations if they will be going to a tropical or subtropical country — boosters are required every 10 years once the primary course has been completed.

First-aid kit for short holiday trips

- Rehydration solutions (Dioralyte, Rehidrat)
- Paracetamol tablets or elixir (Calpol, Disprol) — for fever
- Antiseptic solution (TCP, Dettol)
- Elastoplast, band-aids
- Sunscreen
- Calamine lotion — for sunburn
- Mosquito repellent
- Simple eye ointment

Longer visits (over one month)
For longer visits, more careful preparation will be needed, as well as an awareness of the endemic diseases in the country concerned. You will also need to find out about the local health system, and where you will be able to obtain advice after your arrival.

Malaria
Malaria is fully covered in another chapter (see pp. 130–150), and the manifestations, treatment, and the choice of anti-malarial tablets will not be discussed again here, although you should note these points:

- A baby is at risk of malaria from birth, so in a malarial area, protective measures should be taken from then on.
- The main anti-malarial drugs are safe for children, in reduced dosages (not doxycycline).
- In malarial areas, taking the tablets or medicine should become a routine, like brushing your teeth.
- As with adults, children should commence taking anti-malarials one week before departure and continue for at least four weeks after returning (one day before, and seven days afterwards, if using Malarone).
- Keep the tablets or syrups in a safe, secure place — even the most trustworthy toddler may swallow a bottleful.

As well as the use of anti-malarial tablets or syrups, other control measures should also be used to reduce the likelihood of mosquitoes biting (see pp. 207–216). Netting is valuable, though hot to sleep under. You may obtain insecticide impregnated netting which is more effective in protecting against mosquitoes. If the windows are screened, an individual cover will not be necessary — but check for holes in old window netting. Infants should always be covered with a separate net. It may be wise to take nets with you for use when travelling outside urban areas.

Mosquito control consists of ensuring that there is no standing water near the house to act as a breeding ground, and spraying the bedroom at night.

HIV and AIDS

The risk to children is mainly from contaminated injections or blood transfusions. Check needle sterility before allowing your child to receive an injection; if necessary take a small supply of needles and syringes with you when travelling to a high-risk country (see p. 588). It is worth knowing your child's blood group, and your own; if they are compatible, you may be able to act as a donor in an emergency.

Fever

Fever is a much more worrying complaint in children overseas than at home, because of the fear of exotic tropical infections. Although malaria is an ever-present worry

---

Some safety tips

- Children should know how to use child seats and safety belts.
- They should be taught not to go anywhere with a stranger.
- They should know the name of their hotel, and should always know what to do if they get lost. (If necessary, they should carry a written note of their name, address, and other appropriate information.)
- Parents should always carry at least one full-face photograph of all children they are travelling with.
- Never leave children alone to watch luggage or to keep a place in a queue.
- Never leave children alone in a car in the sun.

(even in the child on anti-malarial tablets or syrup), the vast majority of fevers in children have the same causes anywhere — namely, viral nose and throat infections (coughs, colds, tonsillitis, and the like). The symptoms of these will usually include cough and a runny nose, with perhaps a sore throat or earache and general malaise with loss of appetite, and sometimes vomiting due to swallowed phlegm. Warning signs of another cause would be these:

1. A very high fever (40°C, 104°F) with headache (? malaria)
2. A severe headache and vomiting with neck stiffness and possibly a non–blanching rash (? meningitis)
3. The presence of jaundice, with yellow eyes (? hepatitis or malaria)
4. Blood in stools or severe diarrhoea (? dysentery)
5. A feeling of burning on passing urine or needing to visit the toilet frequently (? urinary infection)
6. Refusal to feed in a baby (? blood infection)
7. Severe cough with breathing difficulty (? pneumonia)
8. Persistent abdominal pain (? appendicitis)

If these signs are not present but cold symptoms are, then it is quite reasonable to give the child paracetamol and extra fluids, keep him or her cool, and carry on as normally as possible (an antibiotic does not help most throat and nose infections, which are usually caused by a virus, but may be needed for severe sore throats or earache). If one of the above features is present, if the fever is in a baby under a year, or if it lasts over two days without improvement and fever is the only symptom, then medical help should be sought.

Should a fever in a malarious area be routinely treated with anti-malarial drugs, just in case it is malaria? This is difficult to answer (see pp. 448–451). Certainly a supply of suitable medication (such as Malarone) should be kept in the house and you should know how much to give. If medical aid is not readily available, the child has been exposed to mosquitoes, and the features are not typical of a cold, then a course should be given.

However, a *blood test should, if practicable, always be taken for malaria* before giving the treatment — only a few drops of blood on a slide are needed for this. Otherwise it will be hard to decide later whether it was malaria or not. The local hospital or clinic may show you how to take the test yourself.

Respiratory infections

These seem to be worse in children living in the tropics, perhaps because of more frequent swimming leading to ear infections, or perhaps because of exposure to a new set of infective agents.

The commonest serious infections are *tonsillitis* (throat infection) and *otitis media* (middle-ear infection), both of which may need antibiotic treatment, though it is commonly advised to treat ear infections symptomatically (i.e. with paracetamol) as most are due to viruses. Penicillin, amoxycillin, or cefuroxime are the most effective antibiotics used for these conditions and they are available world-wide. If your child is allergic to penicillin make sure that this is clear to anyone giving treatment.

Diarrhoea

Diarrhoea is extremely common in children when travelling or in another country (see pp. 17–40). 'Gastroenteritis' is simply the technical name for a stomach or intestinal infection leading to diarrhoea and is not necessarily severe or life threatening. The seriousness of diarrhoea depends on how much fluid is lost from the body: because a child's total fluid volume is greater in proportion to body weight than an adult's, the effect is greater the younger the child. A baby can become dehydrated (dried out) within a few hours of the onset of severe diarrhoea.

Diarrhoeal disease is usually contracted by contact with infected food or fluid, but also from hands that have touched infected material. Faeces of an infected person are highly contagious, and therefore very careful hand-washing is essential after using the toilet. These diseases spread more easily in the tropics and also certain causative agents are commoner — the features of some of these are given in Table 11.2.

Suspect one of the causes in Table 11.2 if the diarrhoea is bloody, very profuse and watery, or associated with a high fever. If one of these symptoms is present, or if the diarrhoea goes on for longer than three days (one day in a baby), medical help should be sought. However, in most cases a rotavirus or similar infection will be the cause, and the natural course is only two or three days.

Replacement of fluid loss is the most important part of treatment. Drugs are quite ineffective in the vast majority of cases. A suitable fluid-replacement solution may be made with a finger pinch of salt and a teaspoon of sugar added to 250 ml (about one mugful) of boiled water, with a squeeze of orange juice to provide flavour (and a token amount of potassium). The concentration is very important as the sugar helps aid the absorption of the salt, but too much of either is harmful. Taste the solution before giving it to your child, and if it tastes saltier than tears, discard it and start again (see also p. 31–32).

Special packets of powder (e.g. Dioralyte, Electrolade) for adding to water may be obtained from your doctor or at a pharmacy before you go and are valuable for journeys. Give one cupful of mixture for each loose stool. Seek medical help if the child vomits or appears drowsy, has fast breathing, or is dehydrated (eyes become sunken, tongue is dry, skin loses elasticity). Profuse diarrhoea in a baby is also a reason for seeking assistance early.

Table 11.2 Some causes of children's diarrhoea in the tropics

Cause	Symptoms
Rotavirus (commonest cause)	Mild fever, watery diarrhoea, vomiting
Salmonella (food poisoning)	Diarrhoea and vomiting, abdominal pain, fever, malaise
Shigellosis (bacillary dysentery)	Bloody diarrhoea, high fever
Cholera	Profuse watery diarrhoea, leading rapidly to dehydration
Typhoid	Diarrhoea or constipation, fever, headache, rash, persistent weakness
Giardiasis	Offensive stools, recurrent diarrhoea, malaise, abdominal pains (this is a more chronic or longer-lasting condition)

Whilst awaiting assistance or on the way to a doctor, you should give oral rehydration solution in small amounts frequently. A baby may take fluids better by cup and spoon than from a bottle and there is less likelihood of vomiting.

Diet Feeding should be continued during diarrhoea if the child feels like eating — especially high-calorie, low-residue foods. Bananas, cereals, bread and margarine or butter, biscuits, eggs, and milk are all suitable — concentrate on the foods the child likes most. It is undesirable to starve a child with diarrhoea, though often the child will not be keen to eat.

Drug treatment is necessary only for some of the specific types of diarrhoea mentioned in Table 11.2, such as severe dysentery, typhoid, cholera, and giardiasis — all of which are much less likely than a viral cause. Anti-diarrhoeal agents such as kaolin, codeine, diphenoxylate (Lomotil), and over-the-counter mixtures should be avoided in children under five years. Lomotil in particular has toxic side effects (depression of the respiratory system) and should not be used in young children, nor should preventive drugs such as clioquinol (Entero–Vioform). For the older child (over five years), loperamide (Imodium, Arret) is the most acceptable drug if parents feel that symptomatic treatment is absolutely necessary.

Prevention The likelihood of diarrhoea can be minimized by observing these tips:
• Pay close attention to household hygiene — particularly handwashing before meals and after using the toilet.
• Maintain good hygiene in the kitchen by washing hands before food preparation; keeping stored food in the fridge (especially meat); covering all food left out in the open, even for short periods; cooking meat thoroughly; boiling water if there is any doubt about its purity (then keeping it in the fridge — it will taste better); washing fresh fruit and vegetables thoroughly before eating; and not permitting flies in the kitchen.
• Avoid the use of pre-cooked foods bought in the streets; milk and milk products (especially ice cream) unless you are quite sure they are manufactured hygienically; salads and other uncooked foods, and cold meat eaten in hotels and restaurants.

Viral hepatitis

Hepatitis comes in two main forms — named A and B. Of these, hepatitis A or 'infectious hepatitis' is more common in children; it is usually spread by the faecal–oral route and resembles diarrhoea in its origins. It is not usually a serious disease in children, and indeed may sometimes not be noticed ('subclinical') but is nevertheless best avoided. The features of the illness and how to deal with it are covered in another chapter (pp. 54–62).

Prevention depends mainly on food hygiene and avoiding dubious foods, as discussed under diarrhoea. Hepatitis A vaccines are available in children's formulations and provide long-lasting protection. A vaccine is also available against hepatitis B.

Swimming hazards

Bilharzia is present in most rivers and lakes in Africa, the Middle East, Asia, and some parts of South and Central America. It prohibits swimming with only a few exceptions (see p. 104). Some areas are treated against snails (which infect the water), but be sure you have a reliable local source of information on this. The infective risk of a single, brief exposure is not great and may be reduced by showering in clean water immediately afterwards, but it is better to be safe than sorry.

Before swimming in pools, check that the chlorine supply has not run out — a common problem in developing countries.

Babies may be encouraged to swim from a very early age quite safely as long as the water is safe and you are careful to avoid sunburn. See also p. 370.

Ear infections occur quite frequently in hot countries and swimming should be avoided until well after recovery from an episode.

Drowning is sadly still an important cause of accidental death in children, and parents need to be aware of it as an ever-present risk in young children. The first rule is to teach your children to swim at the earliest opportunity. The second is to fence off any swimming pool to which your (or visitors') children might have access. Thirdly, always to keep a watchful eye on any young child (below five) or a non-swimmer of any age when there is water about, whether in baths, in a pool, at a lake, or at the seaside. Toddlers have been known to drown in quite shallow pools.

Other hazards

Sunburn is an obvious environmental hazard, particularly in high or mountainous countries where the tropical sun burns very quickly (see p. 351). Also, beware of burning even when it is cloudy. The usual advice of big hats and covering the arms and legs should be followed rigorously until all the children are mahogany-coloured. Fair children's hair usually bleaches pale blond, but will darken on returning to cooler climates. Sunscreens, preferably water-resistant, are advisable when at the swimming pool or seaside.

Sunburn should be treated by puncturing blisters and draining the fluid. Clean the burned area and paint with calamine lotion. Protect against contact and further exposure to the sun.

Prickly heat is common in hot climates and particularly in humid countries, and can be very troublesome. It is caused by sweating, with blockage of the sweat ducts leading to itching red spots and tiny blisters, usually on the neck, back, and chest.

Treat by washing the area with an antiseptic soap, then dry and powder with talc. Calamine lotion may also be used.

Prevent prickly heat by avoiding sweating as much as possible, by frequent bathing, by wearing loose clothing (p. 339), and by drying the skin whenever it becomes wet.

Walking barefoot should be avoided even in your garden or land you know well. Snakes are more afraid of people than we of them, but if stood upon will bite defensively (p. 232).

A more common hazard for the barefoot is *hookworm*, acquired from soil contaminated with human faeces (see p. 116). The worm passes through the skin of the feet and circulates through the lymphatics and lungs before eventually settling in the small intestine, where chronic bleeding leads to severe anaemia.

Tumbu fly (also known as 'Putsi' in some areas) is another infestation commonly picked up from soil in which eggs of the fly have been laid (see p. 197). It does not depend on faecal spread and may occur even where sanitation is perfect (e.g. your garden). Larvae may enter the skin directly from the soil or from eggs laid in clothes left hanging in the shade or laid on the ground to dry. Lesions resembling boils develop under the skin and may be very painful. The main preventive measure is to iron all clothes and sheets which have been left out to dry, so as to kill the eggs.

Cuts, sores, and insect bites are common in hot countries but heal more slowly than at home, probably because of greater sweating. Treat them meticulously in the early stages by cleaning, disinfecting, and covering. Gentian violet is a good standby for skin disinfection despite its messiness — the tropical bathroom should preferably be painted purple so that the stains don't show up. Gentian violet is no longer licensed for use in the mouth as it may be an irritant; it should only be used on the skin.

For itchy skin lesions and bites, calamine lotion is effective.

Bike-riding Safety helmets will not be available in most places and should be brought from home (see p. 7 and p. 300).

Roads Road traffic accidents are now becoming as common in tropical countries as they are in Europe. Don't let young children out on the road on their own, and ensure that car seats and seat-belts are always used in cars. If possible, don't travel in cars with defective seat-belts.

Poison prevention Syrup of ipecac to induce vomiting after the ingestion of a poison is a must for families with young children, and may not be available locally. The dosage is:

Infants, 6 months to 1 year:	5 ml
Children, 1–12 years:	15 ml
Over 12 years:	30 ml

The syrup should be followed by one or two glasses of water; repeat the dose if vomiting does not occur within 20 to 30 minutes. Gastric lavage will be necessary if no vomiting occurs within a further 20 minutes.

Pets If you keep a dog, ensure that rabies vaccine is given at the right time and that the dog is dewormed. Also be on the lookout for ticks and remove them immediately (drop into methylated spirits or paraffin). They can cause *tickbite fever* in animals and humans.

Cats (as well as undercooked meat) may be a source of toxoplasmosis which causes a glandular fever-type illness. An infected pregnant woman may transmit the disease to the fetus causing congenital deformities, although this condition is rare (p. 488). Cats and dogs may both spread toxocariasis, another parasitic infection which is a rare cause of blindness in children. Infection may occur through contamination of food by cat and dog faeces, so scrupulous hygiene is necessary when handling food if there is a pet around — and be sure to keep animals away from food dishes and to dispose of their litter effectively.

Remember that if you bring a pet back to the UK, quarantine rules still apply unless you are returning from a country that participates in the Pet Transport Scheme (PETS) and your pet has an official PETS certificate. Details are available from vets. (In the UK, more information is available from the PETS helpline: 0870 241 1710, email: helpline@defra.gsi.gov.uk
www.defra.gov.uk/animalh/quarantine/pets/index.html.

Stray animals should be avoided and children warned carefully of their risks. Animals in the street should never be petted because of the risk of rabies and other diseases.

Children's diet abroad
Children tend to eat less in a hot climate, so it is all the more important to ensure a balanced intake of nutrients. Foods obtainable will generally be healthier (few junk foods and sweets) and vegetables and fruit will be abundant and fresh (but always wash them thoroughly if eaten raw). Remember that too many mangoes/guavas/pawpaws may cause intestinal upsets. Here are some tips:
- **Meat** should be thoroughly cooked, particularly beef which may carry tapeworms.
- **Eggs** are likely to be readily available.
- **Milk and milk products** (particularly cream and ice-cream) should be viewed with caution, and milk boiled unless you are sure it has been hygienically prepared.
- A reasonable **salt** intake is necessary but usually this may be obtained by adding extra to food, without the need for salt tablets.
- **Vitamins** should be readily available from the following sources:
  Vitamin A: carrots, highly coloured or dark green vegetables/fruit (e.g. mango, guava, pawpaw, spinach)
  Vitamin B: nuts, cereals, milk, eggs, meat
  Vitamin C: oranges, lemons, guavas, potatoes
  Vitamin D: margarine, eggs, fish, sunlight
  Folic acid: green leafy vegetables
- **Fluoride** is valuable in preventing dental caries but water supplies overseas are rarely fluoridated. Fluoride supplements are quite safe but best obtained before departure; they are recommended from infancy to 12 years of age *if the local water supply is deficient*. Drops are available for babies. A prescription is not needed in the UK but is necessary in the USA (see also p. 426).

Baby care abroad

In general, the care of babies in hot countries does not differ from anywhere else, but a few tips may be helpful.

Breast-feeding

Breast-feeding should be carried out if possible in preference to bottle-feeding, not just because it is better for the baby, but because of the example the expatriate mother sets to the local community. Bottle-feeding is a major cause of death among babies in poor countries because of the difficulty mothers face in boiling water, keeping bottles clean, and just buying milk powder. One reason why the local mother may turn to bottle-feeding is because it carries 'prestige' — since expatriate mothers do it.

Extra water is not needed routinely by the breast-fed baby, even in hot climates, unless he or she is feverish or suffering from diarrhoea. But the mother must be sure to maintain a high fluid intake herself.

Infant foods

For the same reason, it is preferable to use natural foods rather than commercial tins or jars for weaning the baby — it is also cheaper and probably healthier, as some proprietary foods have a high concentration of salt and other additives. The first food will probably still remain a proprietary cereal but when mixed feeding is commenced, then liquidized vegetables, fruit, meat, cheese, and eggs may all be used quite safely (this will usually be over the age of six months).

Nappies and nappy rash

Disposable nappies may be unobtainable or in short supply, so it is wise to take terry nappies and nappy liners for long-term stays. Use cotton pants, because plastic pants predispose to nappy rash, and leave the baby without a nappy for some of the time. A nappy rash will clear up well if the baby is allowed to play out in the sun without anything on the bottom. Remember to press terry nappies on both sides with a hot iron, in tropical countries, to kill the eggs of the tumbu fly.

Sunshine

Babies have a sensitive skin and burn easily. Always protect them from direct sunlight by using a sunhat or sunshade. Cars left in the sun become very hot inside — never leave children unattended in a parked car, and ensure that there is always sufficient ventilation.

Malaria prevention in babies

Malaria prophylaxis in babies should be started immediately after birth. Even if you are breast-feeding and taking a drug yourself, an insufficient amount will reach the baby to be effective. Use nets carefully to avoid mosquito bites.

Cots

A basket is a better place for a baby to sleep than a carry-cot, as it will be cooler. Often you will find that special baskets can be made locally. If using a straw basket, line the inside with netting to prevent mosquitoes and ticks from getting in. After dark, always put a net over the basket, even in a room with screened windows — mosquitoes are expert hole-finders.

Be sure to take with you items you will need as the baby grows, such as a potty, toilet seat, baby chair, travelling cot, car seat, and toddler toys. Clothes should usually be obtainable locally. For the other items, mail order may be possible, but in some countries there may be long delays at customs.

Children with special problems

If you have a child with diabetes (see p. 509), cystic fibrosis, coeliac disease, or another chronic disorder or a disability, you will need special advice before travelling abroad. Obtain this early from your usual specialist or one of the support organizations, as a lot more advance planning will be required.

Conclusion

- Do not let the above list of exotic diseases and problems overwhelm you with horror. Most can be prevented by simple precautions and, on the positive side, there will be the outdoor life, the absence of junk foods and TV, and the exposure to quite different cultures and traditions. You and your children should come back with a much deeper understanding of people of other races and cultures, and of the nature of the problems facing developing countries. It will be worth it.

Elderly travellers

Retirement is the cue for growing numbers of people to reach for their passports and to start making the most of their new-found leisure. Many older travellers take long and adventurous journeys; the key to doing this safely and successfully is to plan a sensible itinerary, and to be aware of the special health concerns that may arise.

Dr Iain B. McIntosh is a General Practitioner, GP trainer and assessor in Stirling, Scotland. He has been an expedition leader and mountaineer, from the Arctic to Antarctica; he has a special interest in geriatrics, and has written six books on travel health.

A vague dictionary definition of elderly is 'quite old' or 'very old', but age alone does not determine health risk in post-retirement global wanderers. Britain's ageing population retires with a state pension at 60 or 65 years of age, but attracts health screening from only 75, implicit recognition that most older people enjoy at least a full decade of sound health. Many, freed from the burden of work, supporting a growing family, and mortgage commitments, satisfy ambitions to travel the world.

One in five people in the UK, as in many Western societies, are over 65, and most are retired. At any one time, a third of these will have travelled abroad during the previous three years. Over 2.8 million overseas trips are made by British residents aged over 65 annually; 20 per cent embark upon lengthy, often exotic, adventurous journeys. Popular destinations are Borneo, Thailand, China, South Africa, Nepal, and India — places with a variable quality of health care available to visitors if things go wrong.

Most elderly people travel safely, but all of them need to be aware of the effects of ageing, as well as of travel-associated health risks and preventive measures. Planning a sensible itinerary, and suitable precautions both en route and on arrival, can ensure safe, healthy travel, and avoid illness, accidents, and the need for medical aid or emergency repatriation.

Common health problems abroad

Between 20 and 45 per cent of travellers abroad suffer from diarrhoea and vomiting. Elderly people are not only more susceptible, but more vulnerable to complications such as fluid loss and dehydration, particularly in the heat.

Ageing brings some loss of balance, suppleness, and agility. In many destinations, roads, pavements, stairs and lighting may be poorly maintained. Falls with fractures are more likely and potentially much more serious in older people

As one gets older, pre-existing health problems become more likely: people suffering from such conditions as heart and lung problems, diabetes mellitus, arthritis, may be less able to cope with a hostile environment.

It is the combination of all these factors that makes health problems more frequent in elderly travellers. Despite the difficulties and potential pitfalls of a hostile environment, older people should not be unduly deterred from their globetrotting ambitions. They will meet their fellows and contemporaries on cruises to distant waters, on the approach to Everest, in Antarctica, or up the Amazon.

Fitness and planning

Age in years is not the ultimate arbiter of ability to travel and retain good health. Few will be denied foreign ventures on medical grounds. Sound professional advice

---

Age-related impairments to travel

Physical and physiological changes that occur with advancing years and that can restrict travel include:

- Loss in lung function — a 90-year-old has half of the lung capacity of a 30-year-old.

- There is a poorer tolerance of low oxygen pressures, e.g. in air travel or high altitude

- The heart is not as effective a blood pump as in youth

- Kidney function is poorer.

- Water and salt regulation are less effective

- Decreased acid in stomach juices may make intestinal infection more likely.

- Decreased immunity to infection, e.g. influenza

- Acquisition and retention of new information is more difficult, and memory poorer. Older people cope less well with the travel stressors and information overload associated with international relocation.

Travel-related hazards to which the elderly may be more vulnerable

- Motion sickness and jet lag
- High temperatures — causing heat-related illnesses and dehydration
- Low temperatures — leading to hypothermia
- Excessive humidity — which can upset body temperature balance
- Air travel and high altitude — leading to reduced oxygen levels, especially in those with chronic lung problems and anaemia
- Enforced immobility in coaches, trains, and aeroplanes — leading to deep vein thrombosis and pulmonary embolism
- Fatigue and exhaustion — from long journeys and travel delays
- Physical stress — especially in airports, train, and coach stations — from walking longer distances and carrying heavy luggage
- Risk from infections uncommon in the home environment
- High risk and more severe consequences of road traffic accidents and other sources of injury.

---

on health risks, and precautionary counselling, can contribute much to maintaining good health while away. A pre-travel health consultation at a travel clinic or GP surgery is strongly recommended, ideally some weeks before departure.

Issues to consider at an early stage include:

- Appropriate routing and travel arrangements
- Appropriate choice of final destination
- International travel can bring added health risks, from infection, trauma, and the environment. Might illness abroad exacerbate the effects of ageing?
- What are the risks of poor or delayed emergency medical care, in the event of illness or accident?
- Will purchase of adequate travel health insurance be difficult?
- What about evacuation and repatriation — will it be possible or prolonged?
- Sensible preplanning of the trip as a whole.

Travel health insurance considerations

- Foreign emergency health care can be expensive
- GPs, ship's doctors, and hospital services may all be chargeable
- Travel health insurance is a priority for older travellers
- Premiums are loaded for those aged over 65 years
- Exclusions on grounds of pre-existing illness may remove cover for the conditions most likely to occur while abroad
- Cover must be adequate and provide home repatriation

Elderly travellers and risk

It is helpful to consider the following categories of risk:

Low risk: the 'young' old: those journeying to low risk destinations — Western Europe, the USA; those taking short-haul air journeys; and those with no pre-existing illness.

Medium risk: as above, but where travel involves environmental extremes or tropical countries; and medium to long-haul air travel. The frail old and those with pre-existing chronic illness.

High risk: those who are medically unfit or terminally ill. Those with pre-existing illness going to high-risk areas, such as developing and exotic countries; and where there will be prolonged travel under cramped conditions.

A pre-travel health consultation and assessment at a specialist travel health clinic or by a doctor or nurse with appropriate expertise is advisable for travellers in Groups 2 and 3.

Pre-travel consultation

This should include an assessment of risk, according to past and current physical status, current medication, transport mode, destination, travel itinerary, nature of the trip, and environmental hazards en route and at the destination, plus advice on:

- Appropriate vaccinations
- Malaria prevention and personal protection from mosquito bites
- Medication for motion sickness
- Changes to medication that may be needed because of time zone changes with travel
- Hazards of air travel, jet lag, and avoidance of deep vein thrombosis
- Effects of high altitude and prophylaxis
- Coping with travellers' diarrhoea and dehydration
- Chronic illness and functional disability and its effects on travel
- Quality and availability of medical and emergency resources

The elderly are more likely to be suffering from chronic health disorders and be on medication than the young. Problems with medication are common — pitfalls include:

- Omitting to take routine medication on the day of travel
- Failing to carry routine medication/prescriptions in hand luggage
- Failing to take sufficient medication to cover duration of trip
- Forgetting that overseas pharmacies and ship dispensaries may not carry required medicine, and
- Not recognising that pharmacies may be far distant, absent, or closed when required A pre-travel consultation provides a good opportunity to consider and forestall such problems.

The effects of pre-existing health problems

Air travel and pre-existing medical conditions

There are few absolute contraindications to flying — examples include a stroke, coronary, or cerebral infarction within two to three weeks of intended travel; severe anaemia; and angina or breathlessness while at rest, abdominal surgery, stomach or intestinal bleeding within the previous three weeks (see table 7.1, p. 251).

Anyone with pre-existing health problems should complete an airline form (MEDIF) advising the airline of their condition. (see Table 11.3.)

Anyone who is able to walk about 80 metres and climb 10–12 steps without symptoms should be able to fly without medical incident.

Deep vein thrombosis (DVT) and lung effects

Sitting down for a prolonged period in coaches or aircraft can cause leg clots (DVT) and lethal pulmonary embolism (see pp. 257–60). Older age appears to increase risk. A single dose of aspirin (75 mg) or a few cod liver oil capsules may be beneficial and are

Table 11.3 Effects of pre-existing health problems

Problem		Precaution
Heart and circulatory problems	Unaccustomed physical stress and increased activity may cause angina and heart disturbance	• Anticipate physical and mental stress and take anti-anginal medication • Consider the use of compression stockings for long-haul flight or coach journeys • Use (and when possible, pre-book) porters for luggage, wheelchairs, and buggies for transit, at stations and airports
Lung problems	People with breathlessness at rest theoretically should not fly	• Those with considerable breathing difficulties can arrange supplemental oxygen to assist breathing during flights
Arthritic disability	May create problems in cramped airline seating and difficulties in toilets	• Book wider seating near entrance doors and the toilet • Consider travelling in business class
Diabetics	Travel across time zones, long journeys, delays, unfamiliar foods, and disruption of the home routine, can lead to problems with blood sugar control	• Carry adequate insulin and medication on the person • Avoid 'diabetic' meals on aeroplanes but have the ordinary meal and count calories instead. See also pp. 491–92

unlikely to promote adverse effects in those who can tolerate them and have no history of intestinal bleeding — the risk may be worth discussing with your own doctor.

Advice for the fit older traveller

- Ageing skin is more fragile and vulnerable to the effects of strong sunlight
- Dehydration and extreme heat can increase the risk of a stroke
- Extremely cold or hot environments are better avoided
- Enter high altitudes above 4000 m with forethought
- Carefully consider availability and quality of medical resources and evacuation facilities at your destination

Advice for older travellers with pre-existing illness

- Check before departure that alteration in drug dose is not required en route or at destination
- Take medications as usual on the day of departure
- On flights crossing many time zones adhere to home time until arrival at destination for taking medication
- Carry medication in hand luggage and never stow it in hold baggage
- Carry enough medication for duration of trip and allow 10 per cent extra for unexpected delays
- Carry a list of medications routinely taken and a synopsis of past medical history
- Take precautions against DVT (see p. 257–60)

Summary

- Old and very old people travel the world
- Most can do so safely and will return in good health
- Some will be in a higher health risk group, and need to take extra care and precautions
- They should consider seeking skilled pre-travel health advice
- All should plan their itinerary carefully and
- Take sensible precautions to minimize health risks

Further reading

McIntosh I. (1996) Pitstops and Pitfalls — a health guide for older travellers. Salisbury Quay books, Mark Allan Publishers.

Lovegrove, J. (1996). *Travel trends: a report on the 1995 passenger survey.* London, HMSO. The global view. *High Life.* January, 87–8 (2001).

Carmen, B. (1997) The psychology of normal ageing. *Psychiatric Clinics of North America.* **20**: 15–24.

Patterson, J.E. (1992) The pretravel medical evaluation: the traveller with chronic illness and the geriatric traveller. *Yale Journal of Biology and Medicine.* **65,** 317–27.

Help the Aged publish a holiday Factsheet, available at: **www.helptheaged.org.uk** or from: 207–221 Pentonville Road, London N1 9UZ, Tel: 020 7278 1114

The diabetic traveller

Provided that some important, basic guidelines are followed carefully, travel poses few problems to the majority of diabetics.

Dr Peter Watkins is honorary Consultant Physician at King's College Hospital, London, and is an authority on diabetes.

Diabetes mellitus is a very common disorder. In developed countries, 2–3 per cent of the population have diabetes, so that in the UK, for example, approximately one million people are diabetic. Since diabetes is commonest in middle age, there are always a great many diabetic travellers!

Types of diabetes

There are two main types of diabetes — Type 1 (insulin-dependent) diabetes usually begins in youth (especially childhood) but can appear at any point up to about the age of 40; Type 2 (non-insulin-dependent) diabetes usually begins after the age of 40. Common to both forms, and the main cause of symptoms in each, is an above-normal level of glucose in the blood — a condition called 'hyperglycaemia'.

Glucose arrives in the blood from the intestine after absorption from food and is also made in large amounts by the liver. Normally, the hormone insulin then facilitates the use of the glucose as an energy source by various parts of the body. In this way insulin keeps the blood-glucose level under control. Type 1 (insulin-dependent) diabetics are unfortunately unable to make their own insulin, so need daily insulin injections throughout their lives. Without these injections their blood-glucose level would rise uncontrollably, leading to ketoacidosis and eventually to death.

With Type 2 (non-insulin-dependent) diabetes, the cause of the raised blood-glucose level is more complex: insulin deficiency is responsible in some cases, but other factors such as obesity may also play a role by causing insulin resistance. Whatever the cause, the blood-glucose level can be kept in check, usually without resort to insulin injections.

The initial symptoms are the same with both forms of the disorder. In older people they may be vague, and not recognized for months or years, so that diagnosis may come at a routine medical examination. Typically, patients describe thirst or dry mouth, pass large amounts of dilute urine, lose weight, and feel tired. Sometimes itching of the genital organs occurs because of thrush (yeast) infection, and a few people experience blurring of vision.

Treatment is aimed at restoring health by lowering blood glucose to as near normal a level as possible. Dieting is a key part of treatment for both types of diabetes and at the very least, all simple sugars must be eliminated.

Type 1 diabetics must inject insulin under the skin between one and four times each day, and must carefully balance food intake and exercise. Type 2 diabetics may just need a special diet, sometimes supplemented by tablets that help to lower the blood-glucose level. These tablets will not work in Type 1 diabetics requiring insulin injections. Most diabetics monitor their 'control' by performing their own blood-glucose tests after pricking a finger to obtain a small sample of blood. Good diabetic control requires much self-discipline, but reduces the rates of long-term diabetic complications.

Modern insulins include quick-acting (clear or soluble) insulins and longer acting (cloudy) insulins. Individual patients will use different combinations of these. When making changes during travel, it is best to confine these to changes of the soluble insulin. Modern insulin 'pens' that deliver metered doses from a cartridge make this very simple.

Travel

Travelling generally presents few real problems to diabetics provided that they follow the simple guidelines presented below. It is obviously more difficult for those taking insulin, especially when major time changes occur when travelling long distances by air. No country need be off limits, although places very remote from medical services might not be ideal for those lacking confidence. Those who wish to work abroad can generally do so, but diabetics on insulin ought to remain within reach of medical services, and some remote areas may not be appropriate for long spells. Many of the comments that follow apply only to Type 1 diabetics.

Before you go

Immunization and malaria protection

Diabetics should be immunized in exactly the same way as non-diabetics (see pp. 553–67). There are only a few reasons for not undertaking immunization and they apply equally to non-diabetics. Malaria medication is safe in diabetes and does not interact with medication commonly used in diabetes.

Supplies

Ensure that ample supplies of tablets or insulin, syringes, needles, and blood-testing equipment are carried — take twice what you need, and keep supplies in at least two separate items of luggage or with a companion (except through customs) in case of loss. Insulin should not be put in baggage that will travel in the hold of an aircraft, where it may freeze. As a result of the terrorist attacks of 11 September 2001, most airlines no longer permit sharp objects to be carried as hand luggage. It is essential that you carry clear identification as a diabetic (see below).

Storage of insulin is not generally a problem. Refrigeration is not necessary during the journey and in temperate climates insulin will keep for some months at room temperature. Refrigeration (but not deep freezing) is recommended for long-term storage, especially in the tropics. For handling at extreme temperatures, specialist advice should be sought.

Disposal

Some items are better suited to travel than others — Baylet lancets, for example, have caps that cover used points. A special clipper is useful for de-arming syringes and pen needles. Depending on local waste disposal facilities, it may be more appropriate to bring back used items, although on long trips this may not be feasible.

Insurance
Adequate insurance cover is always essential, and travellers to EU countries should always obtain the E111 (see p. 572). It is important to declare any pre-existing conditions so as to avoid loss of cover. If a company asks for an increased premium, there are many other companies to try. Some insurance policies exclude loss of drugs, but even a considerable supply of insulin generally costs less than the average policy excess. In case of loss or theft, the main problem is finding a doctor, pharmacist, and the appropriate products. National and local diabetes associations may be able to offer information on special schemes (see 'Further information', p. 514).

Motion sickness
Diabetics can use the same anti-motion-sickness tablets as non-diabetics (see pp. 275–7). These tablets do not affect diabetic control. Don't forget that many preparations cause drowsiness, and it is best not to drive while under their influence. If vomiting should occur, the method of managing the diabetes is described below.

Identification
Some form of identification is most valuable in case of problems. All diabetics should carry with them at all times a clear statement that they are diabetic with details of their treatment, indicating their usual physician or clinic. *Medic–Alert Foundation International* (see addresses on p. 245) offers a valuable service in this regard, and their bracelet is widely known. Identification will also help if there are any problems with regard to customs officials (syringes and needles may be confused with the paraphernalia of drug addicts) and security. You should not under any circumstances hand in your equipment to any official.

Travelling companions
Type 1 diabetics travelling to remote parts of the world should ideally be accompanied, so that immediate help is available, especially in the event of a low blood-glucose level (hypoglycaemia — see below).

The journey

Time changes during long-distance air travel
This will cause minor temporary upset of diabetic control in insulin-treated diabetics.

Flying west
The time between injections can, with little problem, be lengthened by two to three hours twice daily. Regular tests should be performed and if they are very 'sugary' a little extra soluble insulin (perhaps 4–8 units) can be given. If the time gap between injections is lengthened still further, a small supplementary injection of soluble insulin (4–8 units) is given between the usual injections.

Flying east

The time between injections will need to be shortened by two to three hours each time, which could result in rather low blood-glucose readings. Careful testing should be performed, and if required each dose can be reduced by a small amount (4–8 units on average). Regular meals should be taken as normal. Many airlines will make special provision for diabetics if notified in advance.

Flight delays can happen, so always carry spare food in case of hypoglycaemia (see below). Certain items such as fruit, vegetables, nuts, and meat can be problematic with regards to customs, and on Australian interstate buses and trains, and are best avoided. Cereal bars, biscuits, and sweets or Dextrosol are generally suitable — get into the habit of carrying a few of these with you at all times, wherever you are.

Some airlines have sharps' bins, useful for disposing of needles.

Abroad

Whilst away, the chief problems are:

1. Vomiting, either from motion sickness or stomach upsets.
2. Other illnesses affecting diabetic control e.g. infections.
3. Hypoglycaemia (a low blood-glucose level).
4. Alterations of diabetic control due to major changes in diet or activity.
5. Minor injuries or burning feet on hot sand or stones — so foot protection with sandals or trainers is important, as well as careful attention to minor injuries and insect bites. If infection develops, take medical advice at once.

Vomiting and other illness

The blood-glucose level tends to increase during any illness, even if little food is being taken, and quite often the insulin dose needs to be increased. At the very least, *insulin should never be stopped*, otherwise deterioration of diabetes is inevitable, leading to diabetic ketoacidosis (pre-coma) and hospital admission.

Take the following steps:

1. Monitor blood-glucose levels carefully at least four times daily. If the results are poor (blood-glucose readings greater than 15 mmol/l) then extra insulin is needed. This can be done either at the normal times by increasing the soluble insulin by about 10 per cent (normally 4–8 units) or as additional doses of soluble insulin at noon or bedtime if tests remain poor then.
2. Carbohydrate should be maintained if possible by taking the normal quantity in fluid form. Table 11.3 shows the amounts of various fluids and simple sugar preparations containing 10 grams of sugar.
3. If vomiting persists, or if the general condition deteriorates, it is best not to delay seeing a doctor or attending hospital.

Hypoglycaemia

Low blood glucose develops if too much insulin is taken, too little food is eaten, or if there is a marked increase in physical activity. The symptoms fall into three phases: early warning, when the person may shake or tremble, sweat, and note 'pins and needles' in the lips and tongue, palpitations, or headache; a more advanced phase, with

Table 11.4 Items containing 10 grams carbohydrate

Milk	One third of a pint
Coca-cola	90 ml (six tablespoons)
Sugar	Two teaspoons
Sugar lumps	Three small lumps
Lucozade	60 ml (four tablespoons)
Ribena	15 ml (one tablespoon)
Dextrosol	Three tablets
Hypostop gel	(see text)

double vision, slurring of speech, difficulty of concentration or even confusion and odd behaviour; and eventually, without treatment, the person may become unconscious.

All diabetics taking insulin should be aware of the possibility of hypoglycaemia, and all are supposed to carry with them, at all times, some form of sugar, usually as sugar lumps, candy, or dextrose tablets (see Table 11.4). About 10–20 grams of sugar should be taken at the first warning of hypoglycaemia; if a diabetic becomes confused, his or her companions should compel the person to take two or three glucose tablets (dextrosol) or three sugar lumps. Hypostop gel is also useful in this situation, delivering glucose into the mouth directly from a compressible tube.

To help people who are seriously prone to troublesome hypoglycaemia with unconsciousness, an injection of glucagon (1 mg intramuscularly) can easily be given by a companion. Glucagon causes a rapid increase of the blood glucose. Glucagon is supplied in a small kit; it must be prescribed by a doctor, and those carrying glucagon must learn how to use it before the emergency arises.

Alteration of diabetic control

Lifestyle and routine during travelling are likely to be very different from those at home, and this change may alter diabetic control.

If physical activity is much greater than usual (hiking or swimming, for example), hypoglycaemia is more likely to occur. Food intake needs to be increased, or a small decrease in insulin dose will be required. Most diabetics know that extra carbohydrate is needed *before* considerable physical exertion in order to avoid hypoglycaemia.

If the level of activity on vacation is much less than usual, then blood glucose tends to increase. This needs to be monitored and, if necessary, a little more insulin given. Beers and lagers contain large quantities of sugar and may also cause hyperglycaemia.

Keeping to a diet abroad can be difficult. However, even with foreign foods it should still be possible to keep to the usual amount of carbohydrate. Do your best not to exceed your normal amount.

Type 2 (non-insulin-dependent) diabetes

There are few problems for those not taking insulin but diabetes should not be neglected, and regular tests should be conducted as if at home. Above all, diabetics should not overeat as this will very probably lead to poor control. If any illness occurs, control must be monitored with special care, and attention from a doctor may be necessary. Remember that with this type of diabetes, insulin may occasionally be needed temporarily during an illness, especially if there is an infection.

Large quantities of spirits increase the effect of sulphonylurea drugs sometimes used for treatment; they can provoke serious hypoglycaemia, especially if taken without food.

Summary of advice for diabetic travellers

If careful preparations are made and proper precautions followed, travelling should not present any problems for diabetics.

- Don't give up travelling!

- Carry a doctor's letter, in the local language, explaining the condition and your need to carry syringes.

- Have adequate insurance.

- The major hazard, as at other times, is hypoglycaemia — remember to carry sugar and make sure someone else knows how to help you if hypoglycaemia occurs.

When I was diagnosed with diabetes, at a diving medical, aged 30, I was devastated and thought it meant the end of so much that matters most to me, especially travel and outdoor activities. However, in the intervening years, I've learned much and worked out a few useful strategies for myself.

The most important thing is to encourage those with diabetes to go somewhere, follow their dreams, and not be too discouraged by dire warnings and difficulties placed in their way. Diabetics can obtain advice from patients' organizations like Diabetes UK, and product manufacturers, in addition to medical and nursing staff. However, the best source is often someone with a similar condition and experience of travelling in a similar area and mode.

Some destinations are easier than others — for example, anywhere the traveller speaks the language or can at least recognize food names on menus. Extremes of temperature need special precautions with equipment. A few countries, such as Saudi Arabia and Malaysia, are particularly suspicious of syringe carriers — a letter in the appropriate local language from a doctor may help. Diabetes UK can supply fact sheets for about 60 countries, covering general advice and useful vocabulary and phrases.

It may help to begin with a familiar and easy destination, and work up to more exciting places. Soon after starting insulin, I stayed in a French farmhouse and hitch–hiked with a friend in Belgium. Later, I led a small youth expedition in Costa Rica, travelled independently around the Dominican Republic, hiked alone around Mallorcan mountains, kayaked the Caledonian Canal, hiked and travelled independently with a boyfriend in Ecuador, and sailed around the Inner Hebrides.

Copies of a doctor's letter, in English and translated into the local language, can ease passage through customs and security. The only time I've ever had any hassle was when flying from Luton to Belfast, when a guard insisted on searching what was obviously an insulin pen.

Jean Sinclair

Further information

The following organizations may be able to help with further information and details of travel insurance schemes:

The American Diabetes Association, 1701 North Beauregard Street, Alexandria, VA 22311. Tel. (800) 342 2383; **www.diabetes.org**

The Canadian Diabetes Association, 15 Toronto Street, Suite 800, Toronto, ON M5C 2E3. Tel. (416) 363 3373 or (800) BANTING; **www.diabetes.ca**

Diabetes Australia, 1st Floor, Churchill House, 218 Northbourne Ave, Braddon, ACT 2612. **www.diabetesaustralia.com.au**

Diabetes New Zealand, 4 Coquet Street, PO Box 54, Oamaru, South Island. Tel. (3) 434 8110; Fax (3) 434 5281; **www.diabetes.org.nz**

Diabetes UK, 10 Queen Anne Street, London W1M OBS. Tel. 020 7323 1531; **www. diabetes.org.uk**

Frio, PO Box 10, Haverfordwest, SA62 5YG. Tel. 01437 741700; Fax 01437 741781; E-mail *frio@btinternet.com*; **www.friouk.com**

Other national associations can be located via the International Diabetes Federation **www.idf.org**

Travellers with HIV infection

Infection with human immunodeficiency virus (HIV) poses additional risks during travel, particularly for those who are severely immunocompromised. Travellers should be aware of their HIV status and of their level of immunosuppression and should consult their physician before travel.

Dr Jonathan E. Kaplan has been a medical epidemiologist at the Centers for Disease Control and Prevention (CDC), Atlanta, since 1980. He currently specializes in issues related to the care of persons with HIV infection and acquired immunodeficiency syndrome (AIDS), including prevention of opportunistic infections. He is a Fellow of the Infectious Diseases Society of America and attending physician at the HIV clinic at the Veterans Affairs Medical Center, Atlanta, Georgia.

Dr David L. Swerdlow has been a medical epidemiologist at the CDC since 1989. He specializes in gastrointestinal infections and issues related to the care of persons with HIV infection.

Dr Mary E. Wilson is an infectious diseases physician who specializes in infections associated with travel. She is Associate Professor of Medicine, Harvard Medical School, and Associate Professor of Population and International Health, Harvard School of Public Health. At Mount Auburn Hospital, in Cambridge, Massachusetts, she is Chief of Infectious Diseases and Director, Travel Resource Center.

Dr D. Peter Drotman has been a medical epidemiologist at the CDC since 1979. He worked exclusively with AIDS from 1982 to 1996 and has worked with HIV as well as other emerging infections since then. He is a Fellow of the Infectious Diseases Society of America and attending physician at the HIV clinic at the Veterans Affairs Medical Center, Atlanta, Georgia.

International travel exposes travellers to pathogens that are absent or uncommon in their country of residence, and increases the potential for exposure to familiar pathogens such as those transmitted through food and water. The level of risk depends on the location of travel, types of accommodation, activities pursued, and length of stay. In general, travel within developed countries such as the United States, Canada, western Europe, Australia, and Japan poses few incremental risks for travellers. However, travel to developing countries, particularly those in tropical or subtropical regions, exposes travellers to greater risks.

The risk of severe illness is increased for those who are severely immunocompromised. Therefore, all HIV-infected persons, particularly those who are severely immunocompromised, should consult a physician well in advance of travel to a developing country, or before beginning any long-distance or arduous journey. Additionally, persons who are at risk for HIV infection (see p. 469) should be tested for HIV before travel, if they have never been tested.

HIV-infected travellers and their physicians should be aware that some countries may inquire about HIV status, some may require HIV testing as a condition of travel or long-term residence, and some may even deny entry to HIV-infected persons, although the public health merit of such regulations is low. Information on such regulations and requirements may be obtained from appropriate consular authorities.

Travellers should review whether their medical insurance will cover them during travel and, if not, should consider obtaining special travel insurance before departure.

Vaccinations

Preparation for travel to developing countries often requires specific vaccinations, and HIV infection imposes some restrictions on the types of vaccines that should be received, particularly vaccines that contain living viruses or bacteria (see Table 13.3, p. 565).

In general, vaccines that include live viruses (such as oral polio and yellow fever vaccines) should be avoided because of the possibility that they may cause disease in HIV-infected persons. One exception is the measles vaccine, since measles is prevalent in many developing countries, and infection can be severe and even fatal for immunocompromised persons. However, measles vaccine is not recommended for persons who are already severely immunosuppressed; immunoglobulin should be considered for persons with no immunity to measles (i.e. no history of measles or vaccination against measles) who fall into this category. Another exception is varicella (chickenpox) vaccine, which may be given to asymptomatic, non-immunosuppressed children.

Oral (live) polio vaccine should be avoided. Instead, inactivated (killed) polio vaccine should be used when polio vaccination is indicated.

Yellow fever vaccine should not be given to persons with advanced (symptomatic) HIV infection. Travellers with asymptomatic HIV infection who must travel to a region where yellow fever is being transmitted should be offered the choice of being vaccinated. If travel to an area with yellow fever is necessary and immunization is not performed, the traveller should be advised of the risk, instructed in methods to avoid mosquito bites, and provided with a vaccination waiver letter. Such a letter should also be carried by travellers whose destinations or transit stops include countries requiring yellow fever vaccination

Live bacterial vaccines that should be avoided are the live, attenuated, oral typhoid vaccine and Bacille Calmette–Guerin (BCG) vaccine to prevent tuberculosis (TB).

Persons at risk for exposure to typhoid fever should receive one of the injectable typhoid vaccines. TB is discussed below.

In general, inactivated vaccines such as rabies, Japanese encephalitis, hepatitis A and B, and diphtheria–tetanus toxoids should be used as they would be for non-HIV-infected travellers. It is important to be aware that these vaccines may not result in a normal protective (antibody) response in HIV-infected travellers, and appropriate antibody testing should be considered before travel.

Medications

Travellers should obtain an appropriate supply of their usual medication before travel (such as anti-retrovirals and trimethoprim–sulfamethoxazole to prevent *Pneumocystis carinii* pneumonia (PCP)). They should discuss with their physician possible interactions between their medication and other drugs (such as anti-malarials) they might take during travel. Medication should be appropriately labelled to prevent confiscation at a port of entry. Travellers should discuss with their physician, before departure, where they might seek medical help in case of illness.

Water and food

Perhaps the greatest risk for HIV-infected travellers visiting developing countries — as is the case for all travellers — is that of food- and water-borne diseases. Such diseases can be more severe and even fatal for the immunocompromised traveller. For example, *Salmonella* bacteria, which may be present in unpasteurized dairy products or raw or undercooked eggs, poultry, or meat, usually causes diarrhoeal illness in the healthy traveller, but may cause a life-threatening bloodstream infection (septicaemia) in persons with HIV.

Similarly, infections caused by *Shigella* and *Campylobacter* can be more severe in the immunocompromised traveller. Therefore, HIV-infected travellers should follow the advice in this book and should be extremely careful to avoid consuming raw fruits and vegetables that are not peeled by the traveller, unpasteurized milk and dairy products, raw or undercooked eggs, raw or undercooked meat or seafood, tap water or ice made with tap water, and items purchased from street vendors. Items generally safe for consumption include steaming-hot foods, fruits that are peeled by the traveller, bottled (especially carbonated) beverages, hot coffee or tea, beer, wine, and water brought to a rolling boil for one minute. Treatment of water with iodine or chlorine may not be as effective as boiling but can be used, perhaps in conjunction with filtration, when boiling is not practical.

Water-borne infections may also result from swallowing water during recreational activities. Therefore, HIV-infected travellers should avoid swallowing water during swimming and should not swim in water that may be contaminated with sewage or animal waste.

Whether HIV-infected travellers should take antibiotics to prevent traveller's diarrhoea is controversial. Antibiotics are not routinely recommended because they can cause adverse effects (drug reactions) and may also cause bacteria to become resistant, therefore making it harder to treat infections. However, in some circumstances, such as when the risk of infection is very high and the period of travel is brief, the traveller and physician may decide that antibiotics are advisable. In such cases, fluoroquinolone-class drugs, such as ciprofloxacin, may be used. These drugs require a prescription from a physician and should not be given to pregnant women or to children.

Trimethoprim–sulfamethoxazole may also be effective, and persons taking this drug to prevent PCP may derive some protection against traveller's diarrhoea. However, HIV-infected persons not already taking this drug should be very cautious about using it for this purpose because of the high rate of drug reactions. Regardless of whether antibiotics to prevent travellers' diarrhoea are used, all HIV-infected travellers to developing countries should carry with them a supply of antibiotics to be taken if diarrhoea develops. Again, a fluoroquinolone-class drug is the best choice.

Travellers should consult a physician if any of the following occurs:
• Diarrhoea is severe and does not respond to antibiotics.
• Stools contain blood.
• Fever is accompanied by shaking chills.
• Dehydration develops.

Drugs to slow diarrhoea, such as diphenoxylate or loperamide, may be used, except by patients with high fever or with blood in the stool. These drugs should not be used for more than 48 hours.

Other preventive measures

All travellers, including HIV-infected persons, should take other appropriate measures to prevent infection during travel such as drugs to prevent malaria, protection against insect bites, and treatment with immunoglobulin (if not vaccinated against hepatitis A). All travellers should avoid direct contact of the skin with soil and sand (by wearing shoes and protective clothing and using towels on beaches) in areas where faecal contamination is likely (such as beaches where dogs are present).

Also, in reviewing the itinerary before travel, the traveller should be aware of risks pertinent to specific areas and ways to reduce those risks. Such infections that pose a high risk to HIV-infected travellers include leishmaniasis (a parasitic infection transmitted by the sandfly in tropical and subtropical areas, p. 179) and several fungal infections acquired from the soil or dust, such as histoplasmosis (found in many areas of the world), coccidioidomycosis (in desert areas of the American Southwest, Mexico, and some parts of Central and South America), and *Penicillium marneffei* infection (in Southeast Asia).

Sinus infections are common in HIV-infected persons and may be precipitated by the changes in air pressure that accompany air travel. Travellers who experience frequent bouts of sinusitis should consider using a decongestant during air travel.

Tuberculosis (TB)

TB poses a significant risk to the HIV-infected traveller and such travellers should be aware that this aerosol infection is highly prevalent in many areas of the world. All HIV-infected persons should receive a skin test for TB. Since this test becomes less reliable as immunodeficiency advances, any symptoms suggestive of TB (prolonged cough, fever, weight loss, night sweats) should prompt evaluation by a physician even if the skin test is negative. Travellers should consult with their physician regarding appropriate skin testing or other testing for TB before and after travel. In addition, any known exposure to TB (such as to a patient with TB while in a hospital) should prompt evaluation for preventive treatment even if the skin test is negative.

Preventing transmission of HIV to others

Finally, HIV-infected travellers should take measures to prevent transmission of HIV to others during travel. The excitement inherent in travel may impair otherwise good judgement and may predispose travellers to risky behaviour. The HIV-infected traveller should avoid sexual contact, but if such contact is not avoided, latex condoms should be used to prevent transmission of HIV as well as other sexually transmitted diseases. The use of alcohol and other drugs that might impair judgement should be avoided.

In areas where infection control practices are below the standards of developed nations, HIV-infected travellers should ensure that health care providers take appropriate precautions to prevent contact with blood and mucous membranes. If confidentiality is a concern, revealing one's HIV status should be done carefully.

Summary of advice for HIV-infected travellers

- Review your itinerary with your physician well in advance of travel to developing countries, particularly if you are severely immunocompromised.

- Obtain appropriate vaccinations before travel. Live virus and bacterial vaccines should generally be avoided. However, measles, varicella, and yellow fever vaccines may be used in non-immunosuppressed persons if needed.

- Follow the advice in this book about avoiding food- and water-borne diseases, since some of these diseases can be particularly dangerous for HIV-infected persons.

- Although medicine to prevent traveller's diarrhoea is generally not recommended, there may be some situations in which it is advisable; discuss with your physician.

- Carry a supply of antibiotics to take in the event of diarrhoea, but consult a physician if they don't work or if you develop shaking chills, bloody diarrhoea, or dehydration.

- Be aware of health risks in the specific regions in your itinerary; know how to avoid them.

- Prevent transmission of HIV infection to others by abstaining from sexual intercourse or by using condoms consistently and correctly.

The disabled traveller

Being disabled or experiencing a chronic health condition need be no bar to the change of scene and opportunity for relaxation provided by getting away from it all.

Agnes Fletcher is disabled and has worked with disability organizations for 10 years. She is currently Parliamentary Affairs Manager at the Disability Rights Commission based in London.

These days, taking a holiday is no frivolous luxury. It can make a huge difference to your health, outlook, and how you cope with life during the rest of the year. Increasingly, holiday accommodation in the UK and abroad has accessible features, such as ramps, handrails, and raised toilets, which can make life that bit easier for the disabled traveller. Also increasing is awareness of meeting the needs of people with visual and hearing impairments and health problems.

In fact, there are now few places on earth that have not been visited by disabled travellers. Most have returned to tell the tale! Disabled people and their friends and families are making journeys, for work or pleasure, in increasing numbers and transport and holiday providers are slowly starting to recognize this group as an important sector of their customers. Indeed, disabled people number more than 10 per cent of the population in most countries. If you add their friends and families, who may be travelling with them, you are talking about significant numbers of people.

People often assume that disability equals use of a wheelchair. In fact, most disabled people are not wheelchair users, though many will have mobility difficulties that make walking long distances or carrying heavy items difficult. Some will have visual impairments. Some will be deaf. Others will have health needs that mean particular considerations when it comes to travelling and spending time away from home. For example, people with diabetes, heart conditions, kidney disease, or respiratory ailments might not be visibly 'disabled' but may have particular requirements when travelling or at their destination, such as a special diet or piece of equipment.

While many disabled people are seasoned travellers, experienced in the art of getting from A to B in difficult circumstances and impeded by ignorance or even prejudice, others need the reassurance of knowing exactly what the journey and the destination will bring. For some, comfort — and indeed safety — demand precision planning and support from key staff.

Planning and booking a holiday

Successful travel depends upon careful planning, and planning depends upon correct information. Ask questions that are sufficiently detailed, for instance:

Aeroplanes Is there a ramp or sleeve for boarding? A wheelchair-accessible lavatory? An aisle chair for moving disabled passengers to their seats? Does any leg of the journey involve a small airline that may not be able to accommodate a collapsible wheelchair? What are the oxygen regulations? Is a companion necessary?

Buses Is there a mechanical wheelchair lift? Are employees permitted to lift passengers manually? On group tours, are buses available in which passengers can remain in their wheelchairs, and can these be safely secured to the floor? Do rest stops have accessible lavatories and restaurants?

Ships How wide are the cabin, bathroom, and lift doors? Is there enough turning space to allow a wheelchair user to get into the bathroom? Is there room for a wheelchair user at restaurant tables? Are there ramps over doorsills? If not, are portable ramps available? Is there accessible transport for sightseeing in port?

Trains Are there accessible lavatories? Where are they located? Can food be brought to the passenger? Is there a difference in height between the platform and the train? Do the stations have accessible lavatories? Are porters and ramps available?

Specialist guides and agencies can take the uncertainty out of planning a holiday. In the UK, the Holiday Care Service or Tripscope are good places to start your holiday planning (see 'Contacts' section, p. 525). They offer free information and advice on all aspects of holidays from the perspective of disabled people.

Before you book, be clear about what type of trip you are making. Will you travel on your own, with your family and friends, or as part of an organized group? Do you want to stay somewhere where all the meals are provided or would you feel more comfortable in self-catering accommodation? What part of the country or the world do you fancy? Local general tourist publications should give some information on accommodation and attractions suitable for people with mobility difficulties. It pays to be honest about your level of needs: you are the expert. Some accommodation providers may make assumptions about what you can or cannot manage. Getting things right at this stage will ensure that you have fewer headaches during the holiday itself. Think about what is essential and what is desirable to meet your needs, including whether you need any particular services or equipment. Next, make arrangements for getting to and from your holiday destination and make sure you have adequate insurance cover — particularly for health care if you are going abroad.

If you take medication, make sure you have adequate supplies. You could also take relevant written prescriptions for use in an emergency (see p. 573).

Disabled travellers should follow the same general guidance on health found elsewhere in this book, and should carry the E111 form, which must be completed and stamped by the post office to make use of reciprocal health agreements with a number of other countries, particularly in the European Union (p. 572).

Details of specialist immunization clinics can be found in Appendix 8.

Particular conditions and travel

Blindness
Logistically, blindness presents fewer difficulties than one might suppose. Restaurants are beginning to offer Braille menus and hotels to provide safety instructions in Braille.

If flight attendants do not volunteer the information, they should be asked the number of rows to the nearest exit. Blind passengers should check whether guide dogs are permitted in passenger cabins and what quarantine restrictions apply. Some countries require medical certificates for dogs (see p. 501). Check with the embassy or consulate of the destination country and don't rely on airlines for complete information.

Deafness

The hearing population tends to be unaware of how much information is conveyed through the ear rather than the eye. Announcements of departures and delays, meals and bar service, fire alarms, 'abandon ship' signals, train and bus stops — these are some of the many pieces of basic information that may swirl unheeded around the hearing-impaired traveller.

> A growing number of physically handicapped people are discovering that, in the near-weightless conditions of the underwater environment, they are as capable as any ablebodied diver. Also, everybody is deaf under water. The Handicapped SCUBA Association has a network of more than 1000 instruction centres in 30 countries, specializing in helping handicapped divers. More information can be found at **www.hsascuba.com.**

Transport and hotel staff should be informed and asked to make sure that emergency warnings are delivered visually or in person. Many hotels have installed fire and smoke detectors with flashing lights as well as sirens. Hearing guide dogs, trained to alert their owners to specific situations, are becoming more common. The same precautions apply as for other guide dogs — though officials may need more convincing that these are indeed legitimate guide dogs. In some countries, text telephone (minicom) reservation systems for those with hearing or speech impairments are widely available. In the UK, the Typetalk system provides an operator service 24 hours a day, seven days a week, to allow someone using a text phone to communicate with a standard phone user. Dial 0800 95 95 98 from a text phone to use this interpreter service. Further details are given at **www.rnid-typetalk.org.uk**

Diabetes

Major requirements for people with diabetes are refrigeration facilities for insulin and 24-hour-a-day access to food. It is best to carry small snacks at all times, since meals in transit may be delayed or even skipped. On long journeys, remember to move about at regular intervals.

Diabetes UK offers information to people with diabetes on travel planning including a travel guide leaflet and specific guides for popular holiday destinations; (see the 'Contacts' section for details, p. 525, and see also p. 509).

Heart disease

Heart conditions should not preclude travelling, unless constant medical supervision is necessary, but it is obviously important to take sensible precautions. Avoid high altitudes and extremely cold weather, keep schedules flexible enough to avoid stress, and use luggage with wheels or a collapsible luggage carrier. If you prefer the convenience of an organized tour but want to avoid the often frenetic pace, consider going with a tour specifically for disabled people. This can be an excellent choice for people with heart conditions or anyone who simply requires a slower pace. Cruises, too, provide an especially low-key mode of travel, but be sure that all decks of the ship are accessible by lift.

Kidney disease

With their doctor's approval, people with kidney problems can travel abroad and maintain their dialysis routine at hospitals and renal centres that give treatment to visitors. A doctor's summary and recommendations for treatment will be required. If travel plans are delayed or cancelled, the host unit should be notified immediately because failure to appear could disrupt scheduling and inconvenience regular patients.

The international Directory of the European Dialysis and Transplant Association lists the dialysis facilities available for people who wish to travel and should be available at your local centre. If you would like to use any of them you must arrange this well in advance with your local centre.

Respiratory problems

If you have a respiratory condition and use an oxygen-powered respirator, you must make special arrangements with airlines and shipping companies. Most ships, but not all, permit passengers to bring their own oxygen aboard. Airlines require 24 to 48 hours' notice and must abide by strict safety regulations, so it is best to consult as far in advance of travel as possible. Often, only airline-supplied oxygen may be used, for which there may or may not be an additional charge. Dry-cell battery respirators are permissible on aircraft. If your respirator needs a domestic electrical supply, you must be able to manage without it for the length of your air journey, plus a couple of hours' leeway (in case of delay in take-off or landing).

While the USA and Canada use a 110-volt electrical system, most other countries operate on a 220-volt electric current. A converter is necessary to use a respirator on an incompatible current, plus adapters for differently shaped plugs even with similar current.

Some helpful travel tips

Access when flying

- Phone the airline in advance and ask to be allocated bulkhead seats, which allow more room for manoeuvre.
- Check in early.
- Arrange in advance to take your own wheelchair to the aircraft door or have it in the cabin with you. You will almost certainly need to be insistent, but it is important (for your comfort, to avoid pressure sores, etc.).

- Take advantage of early boarding even if you are not visibly disabled — it is there for your convenience and may mean you don't have to stand for long periods in a queue.
- Business-class lavatories are likely to be bigger and the seats and aisles wider — upgrade if possible.
- If you can walk a short distance, ask for a seat near the entrance doors.
- For details of UK airlines' access rules, visit **www.allgohere.com**
- For details of US airlines' access rules, visit **www.faa.gov/acr/dat.htm**

Travel by car
Many European countries operate national schemes of parking concessions similar to the UK's orange badge scheme. Often these concessions apply to visitors who are orange badge holders. Details are available from the Department of the Environment, Transport, and the Regions (DETR).

Insurance
Be particularly careful about getting good cover. A lot of insurers exclude 'pre-existing conditions', but some don't. Shop around to get adequate coverage — it could be important.

Further information

Holiday and travel guides and resources
The Royal Association for Disability and Rehabilitation (RADAR) produces several guides for older people with mobility difficulties in Britain and elsewhere in the world. Its annual *Holidays in Britain and Ireland: A Guide for Disabled People* includes detailed information on over 1300 places to stay in all parts of the UK and the Republic of Ireland. These include hotels, guest houses, self-catering cottages and flats, holiday parks, activity centres, campsites, and centres where specialist care is provided. Individual listings include the size of entrance doors, ground-floor bedrooms, lifts, whether there are specially designed bathroom facilities and if waterproof or feather-free bedding is available.

Getting There: A Guide to Long Distance Travel for Disabled People helps people plan long-distance travel, especially journeys that involve more than one means of transport. It includes information on air travel and airports in Britain and Europe; sea travel and ferry companies in Britain and abroad; rail travel in London, Europe, and elsewhere; the Eurotunnel; coach travel; and insurance.

Access to Air Travel is a booklet for first-time disabled travellers. If you have recently lost some mobility and fear that travelling by air has become too difficult, this guide should help to reassure you, giving practical advice on planning and booking a flight, medical matters connected with air travel, aids and equipment, insurance, getting to and from the airport, and what to do when you get there and while on the plane.

Also, from RADAR, *Access in Paris* and *Access in London* are guides for older and disabled people. They include maps, information on how to get around, accommodation, places of entertainment, sights, and attractions.

The RNIB provides *Plane Easy*, a tape and leaflet giving information about air travel and assistance at UK airports for people with visual impairments.

If you feel that you may have been discriminated against by a travel operator, you can contact the Disability Rights Commission for advice.

Contacts: UK

Diabetes UK (formerly the British Diabetic Association), 10 Queen Anne Street, London W1M 0BD, UK. Tel: 0207 636 6112. E-mail: *bda@diabetes.org.uk* Web-site: **www.diabetes.org.uk/** Has a number of country guide information sheets for travellers with diabetes.

Holiday Care Service, 2nd Floor, Imperial Buildings, Victoria Road, Horley, Surrey RH6 7PZ, UK. Tel: 01293 774535. Minicom: 01293 776943. This service gives information on suitable accommodation and organizations which provide holidays.

RADAR, 12 City Forum, 250 City Road, London EC1V 8AF, UK. Tel: 020 7250 3222. Fax: 020 7250 0212. Minicom: 020 7250 4119. E-mail: *radar@radar.org.uk* Web-site: **www.radar.org.uk**

RNIB, PO BOX 173, Peterborough PE2 6WS, UK. Tel: 0845 702 3153. Minicom: 0845 58 5691. E-mail: *cService@rnib.org.uk* Web-site: **www.rnib.org.uk**

Tripscope, Alexandra House, 241 High Street, Brentford, Middlesex TW8 0NE, UK. Tel: 08457 585641. Provides travel information for disabled people.

Disability Rights Commision Helpline, Freepost MID 02164, Stratford–upon–Avon CV37 9BR, UK. Tel: 08457 622 633. Minicom: 08457 622 644. E-mail: *ddahelp@stra.sitel.co.uk* Web-site: **www.drc-gb.org**

Contacts: elsewhere

Mobility International, PO Box 10767, Eugene, Oregon 97440, USA. Tel/Text: +1 541 343 1284. E-mail: *miusa@igc.apc.org*

National Information Communication Awareness Network, PO Box 407, Curtain, ACT 2605, Australia. Tel: +06 285 3713. E-mail: *nican@spirit.com.au*

Web-sites

Access-Able Travel Source — **www.access-able.com**

Global Access — **www.geocities.com/Paris/1502**

Expedition health

An expedition is an 'organized journey with a purpose', and health — not just of individual participants, but of the group as a whole, and of local people as well — is a key factor in determining its success or failure.

Jean Sinclair is a registered nurse, a public health specialist, and a marine biologist who has taken part in expeditions in Greenland, Svalbard, Canada, Costa Rica, Indonesia, and Australia, as well as travelling independently throughout the Americas, Asia, and New Zealand. She is a medical trainer for the Voluntary Service Overseas.

Most health considerations on expeditions are variations of those that apply to all overseas travel. Some, however, are unique. Some key characteristics of expeditions are addressed in this chapter.

Expedition aims

These are generally either scientific or physical, often involving exploration of places or participation in activities that may be unfamiliar to many of the expedition team. Some expedition activities are associated with specific risks and hazards, ranging from mountaineering accidents to rabies from handling bats and other animals, or histoplasmosis from working in caves.

Histoplasmosis

Histoplasmosis is caused by inhalation of spores of the fungus *Histoplasma capsulatum*. Symptoms are a 'flu-like illness with fever, headache, and a dry cough; the illness usually lasts 3–7 days, and almost always gets better without treatment, though more serious infections can also occur.

Spores are found in bird and bat droppings, and in the soil, and occurs world-wide. Cases have occured in travellers to Central America and wihtin the USA, and are particulary associated with inhaling dust from bat-infested caves during dry weather, which should be avoilded — cavers and speliologists are at particular risk.

Avoid disturbing accumulations of bird or bat droppings, and minimize exposure to dust in potentially contaminated places — wear a mask or wrap a scarf around your mouth and nose. Before stirring up the soil, spray the area with water if you can.

RD

Expedition members

Expedition teams range in size from three or four members, in the case of a university student expedition, to over a hundred in the case of a major project. In a large expedition, members often operate in smaller subgroups. When such concentrations of people live and work together, issues like water supply, food hygiene, sanitation, and waste disposal, need special consideration to prevent infectious disease spreading to the entire group and affecting the local population.

Expedition members are generally young to middle-aged adults, fit and healthy. Being disabled or having a pre-existing illness need not prevent participation, but types of disabilities that can be accommodated need careful consideration. Uncontrolled epilepsy would be difficult to cope with, for example, and the value of going on a largely scientific expedition might not be as great to a person with a learning disability as to a person without. Many young people with well-controlled diabetes, hearing loss, or mild cerebral palsy have taken a full part in British Schools Exploring Society expeditions, although rough terrain can exclude people dependent on walking aids or wheelchairs.

Though each member is responsible for his or her individual health, it is usual to nominate one or more members to take on overall responsibility for the health of the group.

Expedition organization

An expedition may last from a few weeks to a year or more. This means that diseases with relatively long incubation periods may become apparent while still in the field.

Expeditions often operate in areas that are naturally challenging (in terms of the climate, terrain, altitude, and wildlife) and that are relatively remote from medical aid. They may operate in areas where there are no other people within many miles, or in conjunction with people local to the area or from another part of the country.

If very remote, an expedition needs self-sufficient health provision, as far as is practical. Expedition subgroups may be relatively remote from each other — a day's walk or boat trip is not unusual — and so each of these may also need to be self-sufficient.

In remote places, expeditions depend on local accommodation, tents, bivvies, or vehicles for shelter. Such accommodation may pose intrinsic risks — for example, of fire in tents, of carbon monoxide poisoning from cooking over a stove in any small, enclosed area or from sleeping in a vehicle cab with the engine running, and of Chagas disease in adobe huts in South and Central America (see p. 183).

All methods of travel have specific risks associated with them. Both conventional types (such as motor vehicles, trains, passenger boats, commercial aircraft) and less conventional options (such as micro-light aircraft, sailing yachts, small hovercraft, kayaks, and trekking with pack animals) are used on expeditions.

General preventive measures

As with any type of overseas travel, the most important consideration is to prevent health problems. Key methods in preventing disease on expeditions are:
- Immunization (see p. 533, 553)
- Malaria prophylaxis (see p. 130)
- Avoiding insect bites (see p. 207)
- Food hygiene (see p. 17, p. 531)
- Safe water (see p. 71.)
- Sanitation (see p. 77 and p. 537)
- Waste disposal (see p. 538)
- Environmental considerations — heat and cold (see p. 326) and altitude (see p. 314)
- Safety considerations (see p. 311)
- Foot care (see p. 435)

Ordinary colds, sore throats, and indeed every other routine problem that can occur at home, can and will also occur on expeditions; they need to be planned for.

Perhaps surprisingly, the problems faced by expeditions working under very different conditions, in different climates and environments, are often the same. For example, insect bites can cause severe discomfort and nuisance in arctic and temperate regions just as much as in the tropics.

An extensive study examined the health problems that occurred during expeditions leaving the UK from 1995 to 1997 (Anderson and Johnson, 2000). Among 2381 participants, in 105 countries and 130 000 person days in the field, 835 medical incidents were reported. The most common problems were gastrointestinal (33 per cent), orthopaedic trauma (e.g. broken bones) (12.5 per cent), altitude (7 per cent), insects (5.25 per cent), sun/heat (4.75 per cent), and malaria (2.75 per cent). Of these, 40 incidents were considered serious, of which 25 required temporary or permanent evacuation. Malaria was the single most important cause of serious medical problems.

One of the more unexpected causes of problems are football matches between expedition members and local people. These often result in serious grazes and sprains, particularly when players wear walking boots and play on rough gravel pitches.

Common expedition issues

Alcohol
Alcohol in any form, for fuel or for drinking, can be very dangerous at low temperatures, causing frostbite if poured over skin or drunk. It is important to remember that alcohol remains liquid below 0°C and that as it evaporates, it removes much heat from its surroundings.

Being under the influence of alcohol (or drugs) is a major contributing factor in road traffic accidents and drowning.

Dabbing the skin with alcohol should not be used to cool a person with a fever, as this can cause shivering, which paradoxically increases the body temperature. Instead, tepid water, applied with a wrung-out cloth or sponge, should be used.

Confidentiality
Information about the medical history or status of any member of an expedition should remain confidential unless a situation arises where the safety of the whole group might be compromised.

Non-medical professionals may not consider confidentiality very important, but medical professionals taking part in expeditions should be reassured to note that professional codes of conduct acknowledge the unique situations that can arise on expeditions or on board ship.

Contact lenses
Contact lenses are sometimes discouraged on expeditions, but my own experience is that they can be worn successfully and safely under all conditions. See p. 433 for more information, but additional considerations include:

- Eye hygiene: disposable soft contact lenses, worn for one day only, are the most hygienic, followed by hard gas-permeable, and then extended — wear soft lenses
- Poor hand hygiene can increase the risk of infection. Disposable hand wipes may be useful
- Overwear: expedition members sometimes have to work, travel, or take part in rescues, unable to rest, sleep, or remove lenses; be certain your eyes can cope with such conditions
- Handling in cold conditions: loss of fine feeling in the fingertips means that handling lenses requires more care
- Loss and damage: take spare lenses, plus glasses in a rigid case.

Emergency skills

Ideally everyone on an expedition, and certainly one or two nominated 'medics' (see below), should have undertaken some basic, formal, first-aid training. For remote conditions, it may be worthwhile for one or more of the participants to learn specific skills that are beyond the usual first-aid repertoire. The choice of techniques to learn should take account of the following:

- The risk of an injury/condition occurring that would be helped by the technique
- Its value in saving life, easing pain, or preventing further complications
- The skill/training required to become safely proficient in the technique, and the availability of such training
- The equipment required, its cost or availability to borrow, its weight, bulk, fragility, and any dangers associated with carrying it.

Doctors taking part in expeditions will generally be proficient in most of the skills listed in Table 11.5 — but may need to brush up! Nurses and other health professionals can sometimes learn techniques in appropriate hospital departments (usually accident and emergency or anaesthetics). Other sources of training, and indeed potential sources of people to act as expedition medics, include fell, mountain, and cave rescue teams, the ambulance service, and Territorial Army medical units. There are some excellent manuals (such as *Kurafid* [the British Antarctic Survey Medical Handbook], and Siderfin's chapter in *Expedition Medicine* — see 'Further reading'), but remember that these are not a substitute for practical experience.

Evacuation procedures

A genuine emergency is not the time to begin thinking about how to get medical help for a sick or injured expedition member. Communication methods (radio, telephone or satellite, flares, runner, vehicle, boat, etc.) and transportation (e.g. vehicle, boat, helicopter, aircraft) need to be worked out in the early stages of expedition planning and checked carefully when out in the field. It is useful if the expedition medic (see below) can visit the nearest hospital and/or evacuation services soon after arrival in the area to introduce him/herself.

The 'expedition medic'

Medically qualified personnel are not essential. The requirements are for a person with standard first-aid level skills, commonsense, and a caring attitude. Experience in

Table 11.5 Some useful medical techniques requiring special training

Technique	Purpose
Blood pressure — recorded using an electronic measuring cuff	For monitoring following injury or illness
Broken bones/splinting	First aid following injury; reduces pain, facilitates transportation of casualty
Cardio-pulmonary resuscitation	Maintains ventilation and circulation pending arrival of skilled help; life-saving
Chest drains	Relieves trapped air or fluid from chest cavity; life-saving.
Chest percussion	For loosening secretions in person with severe chest infection
Dental fillings, etc. using emergency kits See also p. 422	Pain relief until reaching a dentist
Ear drops, administering	Typically, for treatment of infection
Endotracheal intubation	Insertion of tracheal tube in person unable to breathe, pending arrival of help; life-saving
Eye drops, administering	Typically, for treatment of infection
Foreign body in ear, removing	
Foreign body in eye, removing.	See also p. 432
Glasgow coma scale	For monitoring people with head injuries
Guedal airway	Insertion of curved tube to facilitate breathing in an unconscious person; life-saving
Intramuscular injections	For giving medication; can be life-saving
Intravenous cannulation	Insertion of intravenous drip for fluids; can be life-saving
Intravenous injection	For giving medication; can be life-saving
Nail trepanning (for sub-ungual haematoma), in which the nail is pierced with a sterile or heated needle or paper clip	Allows trapped blood to escape; pain relief
Nasogastric (stomach) intubation	For drainage of secretions in bowel obstruction, or for giving fluid or medicines in person unable to swallow
Needle cricothyroidotomy	Slightly easier alternative to endotracheal intubation, in dire emergency; life-saving
Pulse oximeter, using a simple	For measuring blood oxygen e.g. at high altitude finger sensor
Pulse, recording	For monitoring ill person.
Recovery position (p. 401)	Life-saving
Subcutaneous injections	For giving medication; can be life-saving
Suturing wounds (stitching)	For closing gaping cuts/wounds
Temperature, recording	For monitoring ill person
Urinary catheterization	For relieving bladder obstruction or emptying bladder; for monitoring unconscious person

health problems outside the hospital/surgery setting is highly desirable. The expedition medic should be responsible for briefing all members and preparing and maintaining medical kits. On a larger expedition, particularly with young people, it may be appropriate to have a medical team of two or three members, preferably of both sexes.

Medical professionals should check with their professional bodies and/or insurance companies about their liability when on expedition.

Female health

Generally, women encounter no more problems than men on expeditions. However, there are a few points to make, all concerning sanitation.

- Women use more toilet paper than men — a fact to consider when planning supplies!
- Any paper-based items, including sanitary products, are particularly susceptible to getting wet. Double-plastic-bagging is the minimum protection required.
- Generally, used sanitary protection can be disposed of in the same way as toilet paper. If it is to be burned, then a hot and well-established fire is required, and a suitable container for holding it until incineration must be available. Special care is required to cover bloodied items where predators such as bears, dogs, and large cats are present.
- Most women find that their menstrual cycle is disturbed on expedition, and for some time afterwards. The most common change is a reduction in the frequency and intensity of bleeding i.e. periods are less troublesome than at home. The contraceptive Pill can be used to control the cycle, but its effectiveness is limited, especially where episodes of diarrhoea are common (e.g. Indian Himalayas, see Cohen *et al.* 1989). My own studies during expeditions in Greenland, Svalbard, Russia, and Canada have shown it is not worth starting the Pill especially to control menstruation on an expedition. For the young women studied (16.5–20 years), the Pill either did not work (i.e. did not prevent bleeding) or they felt that the slight advantage of lighter bleeding was not worth the hassle of taking it for several months.
- For some, dysmenorrhoea (painful periods) and menorrhagia (heavy periods) can both be worse in hot or cold climates, owing to changes in pituitary and hypothalamic function. Weight and/or body fat changes also play a part. Ibuprofen (Brufen or Nurofen) or mefenamic acid (Ponstan) is often helpful.
- If not included in the medical kit, women should take their own post-coital (emergency/'morning after') contraception. Responsibilities for normal contraception remain unchanged on expedition.
- In theory, menstruating women are at higher risk from attack by sharks and estuarine crocodiles (if they swim) and bears, big cats, etc on land (see also p. 440).

Food hygiene

This is the responsibility of everyone involved in buying, packaging, storing, washing, preparing, and cooking food, disposing of waste food, and cleaning utensils. A rigorous system needs to be devised and adhered to, for the sake of the health, morale, and success of the expedition.

Most travellers are dependent on other people to prepare and provide food, but expeditioners are responsible for this themselves. In many ways, this makes it easier to control and prevent many of the problems that occur in less developed countries.

Whenever a group of people lives and eats together, the scope for transmission of food-borne diseases can be high. Normal standards of hygiene, such as hand washing, not sharing utensils, protecting food from flies, and maintaining safe temperatures, become even more important where pathogens in food are more common (see Melville, 1981). A golden rule is that no-one with an intestinal infection goes anywhere near anyone else's food, and that they are responsible for washing their own utensils, unless they are really too sick to do so.

Foot care

On many expeditions, foot troubles are the largest single group of problems — regardless of whether or not the expedition is primarily on foot. Yet many of the problems are easily preventable. This is an area where the experienced expeditioner probably knows more than an expedition-inexperienced but medically qualified person. The main problems are blisters, cuts and abrasions (grazes), and fungal infections (athletes' foot) and these are discussed in detail on pp. 435–9.

General hygiene

Where water is limited or very cold, washing only the 'essentials' may be possible. This means washing hands after using the toilet and before preparing food or eating, and washing feet and the groin area once a day. Nothing else is essential, certainly not hair washing, so some people prefer to have very short hair or to afro-plait long hair.

When there is insufficient water for body washing, washing clothes is also likely to be a problem, and again only the 'essentials' — in this case, socks and underpants — may be washed. Even if they cannot be washed, alternating and airing sets of underwear is at least better than nothing. Silk clothing has the advantage of not absorbing body smells.

Placing water in a black plastic bag and leaving it in the sunshine is a simple way of warming water to make washing in cold climates more pleasant.

Insurance

Insurance is best organized for the expedition as a whole, rather than individuals arranging their own cover. This particularly helps those with pre-existing medical conditions, which must be declared. Expedition cover means a standard level of cover for all members, and should include cover for search and rescue, third party liability, medical treatment, nursing, physiotherapy, repatriation, and compensation for injuries. Insurance against delays, missed connections, and lost or damaged equipment may need to be taken separately.

Local people

An expedition may be operating in an area where other people live, year round or transiently. When planning water use, sanitation, and waste disposal, their needs must be considered along with those of the expedition.

Members of an expedition also need to decide their policy towards local people who come seeking medical aid. To give worthwhile aid, greater medical knowledge is required (e.g. child and maternal health), plus additional supplies of expedition drugs and perhaps a broader range of medicines; knowledge of the local language and customs (perhaps through an interpreter) are also necessary. Inappropriate aid does more harm than good.

It is also important not to undermine confidence in any permanent local source of aid — such as village health workers, traditional birth attendants, nurses, and doctors — that will remain in place, perhaps long after the expedition has gone.

Even placebos, such as vitamin tablets, that seem harmless enough, encourage a dependence on medicines that is often less helpful than promoting preventive measures such as breast-feeding, sanitation, adequate nutrition, and immunization.

The best reference book on looking after local people is David Werner's *Where There is No Doctor*, preferably a local language edition that can be left behind when the expedition departs. See also Bezrucha, 1992.

Immunizations; medical and dental check-ups

All expedition members should be encouraged to visit their dentist for a check-up, at least a few months before departure, to allow time for any necessary course of treatment.

Where immunizations and malaria medication are appropriate, the schedule of injections should ideally be planned several months before departure. Usually, it is possible to plan to avoid injections during revision or exam periods and specific physical training periods.

Participants inevitably compare the vaccines and advice they have received; inconsistencies can lead to unnecessary anxiety. The best option is for an expedition's medical co-ordinator to draw up some general guidelines or a formal policy, seeking specialist advice if this is needed, and then to circulate copies of guidelines to all of its members, to give to the individual clinics or practices that will carry out immunization. Where participants come from different parts of the world, differences in advice are more likely — vaccines and malaria tablets are not licensed at the same time and in the same way in all countries.

A short screening examination with your doctor may also be appropriate, consisting of, for example, a blood pressure check, urinalysis, and chest examination. For women considering using the contraceptive Pill to control their menstrual cycle during the expedition, now is the time to discuss it. For those who have not used it before, it is wise to take it for a few cycles before departure to allow time to change the brand if necessary. Even without taking the Pill, bleeding tends to be less frequent and lighter when travelling in unfamiliar places.

You cannot donate blood for several weeks or months after immunizations and overseas travel, so expedition members should be encouraged to do so beforehand. The promise of obtaining reliable documentary evidence of your blood group, for use when abroad, is usually a good incentive, although it is always advisable that full cross-matching is carried out before any blood transfusion (p. 589). People under 18 years of age are not allowed to donate blood in the UK.

Now is also the time to get spare glasses and/or contact lenses if worn. For post-tropical check-ups on your return, see Appendix 7.

Medical kits

Some general principles (see also p. 573):

- Tablets are more convenient than liquids, and plastic bottles are better than glass. Sachets of liquids (such as antiseptics) are fragile and tend to burst, so should be avoided if possible
- Oral medicines are preferable when possible e.g. fluconazole (Diflucan), 1 x 150 mg capsule for vaginal thrush, instead of days of pessaries
- Pack medicines such as antibiotics in complete courses — wherever possible, using short courses of high doses, with fewer doses per day; and consider using combination antibiotic capsules (e.g. Magnapen, which contains both flucloxacillin and ampicillin) rather than carrying the two drugs separately
- Allow for common allergies — take alternatives to penicillin, for example, and take special note of any allergies reported by expedition participants in pre-departure questionnaires
- Try to settle on one treatment for each problem e.g. just one type of anti-diarrhoeal and just one anti-histamine
- Try to take items that can be used to treat several conditions e.g. codeine for pain, diarrhoea, and coughs; Trimovate ointment for most skin problems
- Mercury thermometers cannot be carried on aircraft. Alternatives are bulky, heavy, and expensive electronic devices or cheap devices with coloured dots (available from TALC). In cold climates, low reading thermometers (below 35.5°) are vital for monitoring hypothermia.

The number, size, and contents of kits depends more on the nature of the expedition and its organization than on the number of members. In general, there should be three types of kit — 'personal', 'group', and 'base camp', and some examples of possible contents are given below (note that many of the items require a doctor's prescription):

In addition to the above items, a head torch and a waterproof watch with second markings have many non-medical and medical uses. In temperate and polar regions, at least one bivvy bag between two people is essential.

Manufacturers of medical supplies are sometimes generous in donating products. If funding is no problem, there are many specialist suppliers of complete kits — these can save a great deal of time and effort.

Packaging Kits must be packed, stored, and handled carefully to protect the contents from mechanical damage, water, and extremes of temperature. Suitable containers are usually made of plastic e.g. cases with drawers such as those used for art supplies or tools, sandwich and ice-cream boxes, old large drug tubs (usually donated free by a local or hospital pharmacy), BDH chemical containers. Courses of drugs can be

---

Personal kit — for each expedition member

- Plasters, dressings, and adhesive flexible tape
- Antiseptic solutions, e.g. iodine
- Mild painkiller/anti-inflammatory (aspirin and/or paracetamol and/or ibuprofen).
- Lip salve (in lipstick form, not a glass pot)
- Sunscreen (high protection factor) – can be decanted from large bottle to plastic 35 mm film pots
- Insect repellent (containing DEET)
- Cough sweets (often any suckable sweet is adequate)
- Personal drugs for any chronic condition (e.g. asthma, diabetes, epilepsy, eczema, hypertension) or intermittent condition (e.g. thrush, haemorrhoids, cold sores)
- Any appropriate additional medication for problems specific to the area e.g. for diarrhoea treatment, malaria prevention, high altitude, hand cream for cold dry areas

---

packed in small, ziplock plastic bags or foil strips of tablets can be used. Labelling and documentation of contents is vital, both for expedition use and when passing through customs. All writing must be in water-resistant ink, on either plastic or on card protected by plastic.

Controlled drugs See p. 576.

Disposal Medical supplies remaining unused at the end of the expedition can be retained by members for future expeditions (provided they will be used before their expiry dates) or passed on to another expedition. They can also be donated to local people, keeping in mind the comment made earlier about appropriate care.

Medical research
Performing unpleasant medical procedures on one's colleagues for any purpose that does not benefit the individual needs to be carefully considered. It is also a sure way to make the researcher extremely unpopular! Approval by an ethics committee should always be sought. No one should be compelled to be a research subject — the right of the individual to withhold informed consent does not vanish in the expedition setting. However, not all research involves unpleasant procedures, and much useful information can be obtained by interviews and questionnaires. As a matter of common courtesy, anyone used as an experimental subject should be given an explanation of results obtained.

Paperwork and records
Any relevant information about members' medical histories needs to be available in the field. Suggested information includes: previous personal or family illnesses, previous injuries or operations, blood group, immunizations, and allergies. Filing

Group kit — needs to be reasonably portable

- Dressings, bandages, and tape
- Wound closure strips e.g. Steristrips or Ciragraf
- Sterile blades
- Antiseptic (iodine solution), for cleaning infected wounds and to purify water
- Oil of cloves, for dental pain
- Ear drops e.g. hydrocortisone, nystatin, and oxytetracycline (Terra-Cortril Nystatin), combines a mild steroid, an anti-fungal, and an antibiotic
- Strong analgesia e.g. morphine 10 mg ampoules and anti-emetic e.g. prochlorperazine (Stemetil) 12.5 mg — both administered by intramuscular injection — and syringes, etc. or buprenorphine (Temgesic) sub-lingual tablets
- Anti-histamine tablets e.g. chlorpheniramine (Piriton), or loratadine (Clarityn). Note: chlorpheniramine can cause drowsiness, but sometimes this is useful, especially as it limits scratching while asleep
- Courses of approximately three antibiotics e.g. co-fluampicil/flucloxacillin and ampicillin (Magnapen) or amoxycillin (Amoxil) — penicillin-based, for a broad spectrum of infections, especially pneumonia and wounds; erythromycin (Erythrocin, Erythomid, Erythroped, Erymax, Ilosone), for people allergic to penicillin; metronidazole (Flagyl, Tiloryth, Metrolyl), for dental, urinary, and vaginal infections, and also for amoebiasis. (Greater quantities of all are required in the tropics)
- Sedative tablets e.g. diazepam (Valium) 5 mg or Zimovane 7.5 mg, for sleeping, and following a severe injury
- Anti-fungal cream e.g. Canesten and/or multi-purpose cream such as Trimovate (which combines a mild steroid, an anti-fungal, and an antibiotic, and so covers most skin problems)
- Silver sulphadiazine (Flamazine) ointment, 50 g tubes, and clear, limb-sized plastic bags and clingfilm, for burns
- Laxative tablets e.g. senna
- Travel sickness tablets e.g. cinnazarine (Stugeron)
- Chloramphenicol eye ointment
- Gentamicin eye drops (don't require refrigeration)
- Anti-diarrhoeal tablets e.g. Imodium
- Oral rehydration salts and/or sugar and salt spoon
- Post-coital (emergency/'morning after') contraception and/or condoms — a decision for the expedition, rather than the medic
- Thermometer
- Any specific medication for local problems e.g. diarrhoeal diseases, high altitude, intestinal parasites

---

Expedition 'base camp' kit

Supplies to be left at a central point or carried by medic(s) depending on expedition organization.

- Further supplies of all items in personal and group kits
- Emergency supply of personal hygiene items e.g. spare soap, toothbrushes, toothpaste, sanitary protection
- Metal nit comb
- Medical equipment — see section on 'Emergency skills' (above)
- This book
- Latest available edition of *British National Formulary*
- Copy of *Where There Is No Doctor* (see text)

---

cards are particularly suitable. Keeping records and books dry is often a major problem — waterproof ink, thick paper, and plastic bags are essential.

Notes can be kept either by the individual member or by the medic, depending on expedition organization, but notes about any injury or illness should accompany the casualty if evacuated.

I recommend carrying a copy of the book *Where There Is No Doctor* and a copy of the most recent edition of the *British National Formulary* (BNF), which is updated every six months and usually available free from a doctor or pharmacist. The *BNF* is helpful for identifying foreign equivalents of familiar drugs, as chemical names do not vary much between languages. However, adrenaline in the UK is called epinephrine in the USA, and paracetamol in the UK is acetaminophen in the USA.

Physical fitness

A good standard of physical fitness is required by all members, and does much to reduce the risk of injury. Usually all members are fit, but for young people taking important exams just before the expedition training can be a problem. It is simply a question of priorities, and expedition preparation must be made a top priority — and usually helps relieve exam stress too.

Sanitation

Toilet pits must be carefully located — away from any water used for drinking or food preparation; above the high-water mark and not cut off by the tide; downwind and downhill from the camp, and preferably 100 m away; and screened or out of site of the main camp. Ideally, there should be a 'loo with a view'! If toilets are overlooked, inaccessible, or unpleasant, people tend to go anywhere they feel like — or get constipated!

They must be deep enough so that a final surface covering of 20-30 cm of substrate is possible. A slit-shaped trench is easiest, as it can be crouched over. If the substrate is loose, some reinforcement of the trench edge (e.g. with wood) may be necessary. Some means of indicating that the toilet is occupied is required — such as raising a flag or removing a shovel from the centre of camp. Toilet paper is usually best kept by the individual, as it tends to blow away or get wet if left at the toilet. If flies are a problem, the pit must have an insect-proof cover (see Warrell and Anderson 1998).

Chemical toilets are not recommended because of the environmental impact, bulk and weight, need for rubber gloves, and the organization involved in emptying them — people always seem to leave this task until they are full to the brim and very difficult to move.

Smoking

Most people are fully aware of the health risks of tobacco smoking, both to the smoker and to the passive recipient of the smoke. On expeditions, the smoker has a few extra problems, not least being the fire risk of smoking inside a tent or sleeping bag or near fuel stores, and the considerable problem of ensuring an adequate supply of dry and uncrushed tobacco. For the non-smoker, sharing a tent with a smoker is extremely unpleasant. There is also the issue of setting a good example for local people.

So, there are additional reasons for not smoking on an expedition, and the complete break with normal life — routine, work, friends — can help if the decision is made to break the smoking habit, too.

Waste disposal

This is another area that requires a system to be devised and then enforced. Both public health and environmental considerations are important.

Usually the following facilities are necessary:

- A wet or grease pit for cooking water, washing-up water, and waste fatty food.
- A compost pile or pit for waste food — but not fatty food (which impedes breakdown and should be placed in the wet pit). Where flies are a problem, this facility must be insect-proof.
- Paper and card disposal — this can usually be burned; the area must be kept dry until incineration. One large, well-managed fire is safer and less environmentally damaging than several small ones.
- Medical 'sharps' (e.g. needles and scalpels) need to be stored in secure plastic or metal containers until they can be incinerated at high temperature. Insulin users have needle-chopping devices for disarming needles/syringes.
- Remaining waste that cannot biodegrade or be burned usually needs to be removed from the field to the nearest waste disposal facility; in some areas it can be buried or sunk at sea. To reduce the bulk of waste items, especially tin cans, a sledge hammer or heavy boots can be useful.

Waste disposal may be controlled by the laws of the area in which the expedition is operating, and these suggestions are not intended to replace such requirements. See also Cohen *et al.* 1989 and Sinclair *et al.* 1996.

Water

Water is used for drinking, cooking, washing-up, cleaning wounds, bathing, keeping cool in very hot conditions, and for washing clothes; and the order for removing water from a water course is roughly as in this list. Therefore, drinking water should be taken from the highest point upstream. However, other users of the waterway must be considered, especially if people upstream release faeces directly into it. Of course, expeditions do not always obtain their water from a river or stream — lakes, ponds, wells, collection of water from roofs, etc. are other possibilities. Flowing water is nearly always safer though. For drinking water, bottled water and certain jungle vines and bamboo can be used.

Where water treatment by filtration, boiling, or chemical means (see p. 71) is necessary, the equipment required needs to be considered carefully. In particular, the number of large containers in which to allow water to stand during chemical treatment is easily underestimated. Some coding system, colour or otherwise, is needed to identify different grades of water.

Water from glacier-fed streams is usually microbiologically clean, but can cause diarrhoea if it has a high silica sediment content. Any cloudy water should be cleared by allowing it to run slowly through a settling pond, usually a diversion from the main stream.

Where water must be obtained by melting snow or ice (preferably snow), the advice is obvious — 'Don't eat the snow where the huskies go' or, even more simply, 'Don't eat yellow snow'.

Where water-borne infections are a particular problem, or if a person is suffering an infection, drinking bottles and vessels must not be shared.

References and Further information (see also Further reading p. 679)

American College of Surgeons. Advanced Trauma Life Support Course Student Manual. 1989. ISBN 0962037052 (available only to course participants)

Anderson, R. and Johnson, J H. (2000). Expedition health and safety: a risk assessment. *Journal of the Royal Society of Medicine*, **93**, 557–62.

Bezrucha, S. (1992). Medical treatment of local people by travellers. (Editorial) *Journal of Wilderness Medicine*, **3**, 1–3.

Cohen J., Morley C., Bass C. (1989), Menstrual disturbances and the pill on an expedition in the Western Himalayas, 1988. *British Journal of Family Planning*, **15**, 44–6.

Dent J. On Thin Ice. Nursing Times, 2 April 34–5.

Roberts, M. (1991) Rabid Dogs and Snake Bites? *Nursing Times*, **87**: 62–4.

Sinclair, J. (1990) Planning an Expedition. *Nursing Times*, **86**: 46–7.

Sinclair, J., Cohen, J. and Hinton, E. (1996). Use of the oral contraceptive pill on treks and expeditions. *British Journal of Family Planning*, **22**: 123–6.

12 Living and working abroad

Becoming an expatriate

Expatriates are in a better position than other travellers to avoid diseases and accidents — they have time on their side and a degree of stability — but psychological and cultural pressures take their toll. A degree of 'culture shock' is inevitable, but good preparation, careful briefing, and an understanding of some of the factors involved in adjusting to a new environment, can contribute much to the success of an overseas posting.

Dr David Snashall is an occupational physician at Guy's and St Thomas' Hospitals and was Chief Medical Adviser to the British Foreign and Commonwealth Office and Department for International Development from 1990 to 1998. He travels extensively in the developing world assessing medical hazards and facilities and has himself been a working expatriate in Canada, France, Peru, and Tanzania. Since 1998 he has been Chief Medical Adviser to the Health & Safety Executive.

Going to a foreign country for a period of time is quite a different matter from being a short-term visitor or tourist. Living in a less developed country will inevitably confront the expatriate with health and safety hazards, but there may also be cross-cultural and psycho-social difficulties. Going in the other direction — to a more sophisticated country — can provoke psychological problems too. This chapter deals with the more common situation, where an individual, with or without spouse and family, leaves home for a year or more to take up residence in a developing country.

For the intending expatriate who has never lived or even been there, the developing world is impossible to envisage, because apart from the difficulties of even defining what it is, countries considered to be part of it present entirely different challenges, frustrations and satisfactions. For example, two adjacent countries with similar climates, geography, and standards of living, but with different alcohol laws and restrictions on women driving, present totally different problems for a man for whom alcohol is a daily necessity or for a woman who needs or wants to drive her car.

Who goes to live abroad?

The number of long-term expatriates in developing countries has diminished considerably since colonial and immediately post-colonial times. Administrators in khaki shorts, bellicose rubber planters, and shipping agents gone to seed in tropical climes are no more. These men, with or without their families, would prepare themselves for many years overseas with no ticket home, and devised for themselves, for better or worse, a particular expatriate lifestyle. The main tenet seemed to be that 'abroad' was different, and somewhat difficult, and that you had to adapt yourself forcefully to it or else it would get the better of you.

That is probably the main difference in approach between those hardy individuals and today's expatriates, who, despite the fact of living abroad in a variety of countries, often regard themselves as essentially home-based: however extensive, their foreign tour almost always falls far short of a lifelong commitment. Today's expatriates are, in the main, diplomats with their families, aid workers, businessmen employed by multinational corporations, construction workers, students, and a diminishing number of teachers and missionaries.

There is inevitably a difference in attitude, and in the resulting experience, between those who go abroad motivated purely by financial reward, those whose work overseas represents an integral part of their career, and those whose aims are actually to live abroad and achieve an understanding of the country and its culture. The desire or necessity to accomplish any of these objectives may not always be shared by the rest of the family, and in health terms — both physically and psychologically — they may be the ones who suffer most.

A shock to the system

What is likely to be different about living abroad? How can it cause ill health and how can this be prevented, or at least coped with, should it occur?

Adjustments

Moving to a new country demands a number of adjustments. The following categorization is based on a study by Craig Storti of problems in Peace Corps Volunteers — mainly young, healthy Americans going abroad for a two-year tour of duty.

1. There has to be an adjustment to the new country. The climate may be very different from that at home. In the tropics, some people find the uniform limitation of daylight to about 12 hours, and the lack of marked seasons, surprisingly unsettling. There is usually a totally different kind of food, a different language, and different people. With the months preceding departure spent hectically preparing to move, no wonder some people start expatriate life in a state of complete exhaustion.
2. There are adjustments to a new working environment — a new job, new skills and responsibilities to be learned, and new colleagues to get used to. Even worse is learning to live without a job — the unenviable position occupied by many spouses or partners of individuals who have gone abroad to work.
3. There are adjustments to be made to the local community, learning to cope with a different transportation system, perhaps an erratic post and telephone system, and a different pattern of shops and services.
4. The most profound adjustments are cultural. Local customs may be very different. I once worked in a community where 268 saints' days were celebrated. Quite a nice custom, you might think, but it led to very few full working weeks. People's behaviour may appear quite alien, even though such behaviour may once have

been the norm in the expatriate's own home country, in days gone by: habits like spitting in public and refusing to form queues. Coming to terms with different sets of values and apparent attitudes can be most difficult. In some countries there would seem on the face of it to be a lesser value placed on human life, as evidenced by crazy driving and a certain lack of urgency in dealing with emergencies or serious injuries. Attitudes to time may be different: to the expatriate for whom time management has been an essential part of an efficient working life, coming to a country where punctuality is a rarity can be seriously destabilizing. If this extends to the full-blown 'mañana' culture, goal-orientated Westerners must adjust — or they will go under.

5. Life in developing countries tends to be more 'raw'. Expatriates may find the experience of being non-aggressively jostled in crowds to be an invasion of their personal space and if they have been brought up to value privacy, the loss of it can be very threatening. Witnessing cruelty to animals, being expected to give bribes, and abet other minor forms of corruption are facts of life which may have to be faced. Curiously, one's own appearance and cultural reputation may rebound in wounding ways. '*We*' are the foreigners and are liable to be judged fairly or unfairly by a population who, because they have seen it on TV, believe that extravagant lifestyles, naked pursuit of money, drug dependence, and loose morals are the norm in '*our*' countries.

The expression 'culture shock' describes the impact which all these simultaneously occurring differences can have, and the attempts to adjust. Whatever the cause of the shock — it may be cultural or a variety of new stimuli, depending on the individual — it can and frequently does cause real psychological problems that range from insomnia and irritability to profound home sickness, depression, drug dependence, and general inability to cope to the extent of packing up and going home.

Prevention in practice

How can you prevent these problems from becoming overwhelming?

1. It is important to recognize that you will almost certainly experience some of them — and that this is normal. Everyone suffers from a degree of culture shock, even the most seasoned of travellers.

2. Limit your expectations. Do not expect to be able to achieve on a daily basis what you do at home. Most developing countries are simply not set up to nurture the achievement ambitions of foreigners. Indeed, some expatriates feel that the thwarting is almost deliberate. This can be the first step towards paranoia.

3. Be satisfied with small tasks, especially at the beginning when five telephone calls and getting a letter posted take all day and leave you feeling as though you have done a week's work.

4. Remember you have successfully survived what once seemed like tough transitions before — from junior to high school, from school to work — and recognize that you really will survive *this* transition.

5. Take care of your physical health in a positive way: as well as taking the advice in the rest of this book, get adequate sleep and take regular exercise.

6. Don't abuse drugs like alcohol; they make things worse and make you look foolish.

7. Find a mentor, someone with experience and commonsense to whom you can tell your troubles and with whom to share your successes.

8. Don't withdraw, even if you feel like it, even if some of the people with whom you have to mix are not entirely to your liking.

9. Keep in touch with home to a reasonable degree by cultivating the disappearing art of letter writing or e-mail and by buying a short-wave radio.

10. Learn the local language, however useless you think it might prove in the future to be able to speak rudimentary Quechua or Vietnamese.

11. Make an effort to reach out beyond your own expatriate community and make friends and acquaintances with other expatriates and local people. It is a great mistake to try to create a little England, a little America, or a little anywhere in the middle of a foreign country. It only serves to reinforce cultural caricatures and ends with the community becoming a laughing stock. Of course it is necessary to keep elements of your national identity, some national foods, and celebrations of national events (I have attended many more and much better Burns' nights in the most remote outposts of the world than I ever did as an expatriate in Scotland). This kind of patriotism is fine and healthy. When it mutates into nationalism and the development of a collective concept by an expatriate community that they represent a superior cadre living in the midst of a backward populace, it becomes very ugly.

12. Most important of all, cultivate a positive attitude. To actively seek out the good things and the interesting people and to deal with the bad things with a measure of humour will help you immeasurably.

Stages of adjustment

However well or badly you cope overseas, the following states are usually experienced. Enthusiasm and excitement which can last from a few hours to a few months — rather like a honeymoon. This is usually succeeded by a negative phase which may be manifested by rejection of the new country and everyone who lives in it, withdrawal into your own little world of expatriate clubs or coffee mornings and even into yourself, with consequent loneliness. This does not look or feel good but it is normal. By familiarizing yourself with a few new places or practices, sometimes helped by a friend, it is succeeded by re-emergence and adjustment to the new country. This gradually paves the way to achievement and a return of enthusiasm.

Throughout the process it helps to try to understand the cultural elements of the new country as different from your own — not necessarily better or worse, but just different for reasons which are interesting and possibly worth studying. Then, look at yourself and your own expatriate group. Go through the same process and try to appreciate the impact *you* have on your host country.

There is no doubt, however, that after some years in the developing world many people can become worn down by the effort that has to be maintained to survive, and they become jaded and unproductive. Then is the time to move on.

Spouses

Someone who goes abroad to work is not likely to find much time to be bored, but this can easily be the fate of their spouse, partner, or family members, and boredom overseas is a significant health hazard. In some countries partners are not allowed to work, but it may often be possible to find voluntary work somewhere. If even that is not possible then perhaps enrolment in an academic course, either locally or by correspondence from home, might be feasible. If there really is much spare time, make use of it to learn about the country, to travel, to learn to play a musical instrument, to cook better — maybe even to think about starting or extending a family!

Physical health

The physical health of expatriates need in general be no worse than it is at home; given a pleasant climate and an interesting life, it should in fact be even better. 'Tropical' diseases, many of which are actually diseases of poverty and under-development, still occur of course, but as an overseas resident you are in an excellent position to protect yourself against them — especially in comparison with tourists and short-term visitors. After all, you have much better control of your immediate environment; you can ensure that your food is hygienically prepared, that your water supply is pure, that your home is protected from mosquitoes and other pests, and that vehicles are properly maintained. No longer do doctors see expatriates who are chronically debilitated by amoebic dysentery, recurrent malaria, or tropical sprue. This is because of better living conditions, better awareness of food hygiene principles, a better understanding of health precautions, vaccinations, and better provision for medical treatment. Diarrhoeal illness is still common, however, (especially if meals are eaten away from home) and immunity takes over a year to develop.

Table 12.1 US Peace Corps experience

	No. of cases per 100 volunteers per year
Non-specific diarrhoea	45.3
Amoebiasis	18.4
Problems requiring counselling	18.2
Dental problems	17.2
Bacterial dermatitis	15.8
Injuries	15.3
Malaria	13.9
In-country hospitalization	9.6

Figures from the Peace Corps Medical Office, Washington

Unfortunately, the quality of available medical care in many developing countries, is still unsatisfactory despite a burgeoning private system in the cities. In tropical Africa it is probably deteriorating. Previously improving general health is being reversed by the AIDS epidemic. Serious illnesses do occur amongst expatriates, but because of their lifestyle and the length of time they are abroad, these are more likely to be the same kind of illnesses they would get at home, such as heart disease, high blood pressure, and diabetes (affluent locals are increasingly suffering the same conditions). The seeds of these kinds of diseases are sown many years before, sometimes in childhood, and the fact of residence in a developing country does not have anything to do with their appearance. What is important, however, is that there should be adequate arrangements for ensuring access to good care should a medical emergency arise, with evacuation to another country if necessary.

Local diseases vary from region to region. Sub-Saharan Africa provides employing organizations with the biggest headaches, followed by south and Southeast Asia, and then by the Far East, South America and the Caribbean, and the Middle East.

US Peace Corps volunteers are the subject of intense medical surveillance, and are probably the best studied expatriate group. A summary of the health problems that have been reported in them is shown in Table 12.1. The experience of German aid workers is summarized in Table 12.2. Certain infectious diseases will increase in incidence with increased length of stay — hepatitis and worm infestations, for example, and malaria if prophylaxis is not maintained.

Expatriates have a higher chance of dying early than if they had stayed at home — mostly due to trauma (70 per cent, US Peace Corps) and then mainly on the road (Dutch development workers).

Table 12.2 German aid workers abroad, 1990

	Of 1550 adults
After 2 years abroad:	
No serious health problems	1063
Serious illness or abnormal findings on return	487 (47 of which were 'tropical')
Repatriations 1987–9	64
Severe accidental injury	19
Internal medical problem	18
Slipped disc	6
Psychological problem	6
Cancer	4
Malaria	3
Gynaecological	3
Amoebiasis	3
Hepatitis	2

Figures from GTZ, Eschborn, Germany

A recent study of British expatriates
(2000 subjects over 1 year)

- New event reported to a doctor: 20 per cent
- Major event needing secondary care: 13 per cent
- New events requiring hospital admission: 19 per cent
- New events requiring evacuation to home country: 10 per cent

Causes

- Injury: 21.9 per cent
- Muscoloskeletal: 16.4 per cent
- Infectious disease: 13.06 per cent
- Psychological: 4.75 per cent
- Trauma (50 per cent sports injury; 32 per cent slip, trip, fall; 11 per cent road traffic accident)

Psychological problems were the most common cause of a terminated posting.

Patel, D (2001)

Risky behaviour

People enjoy taking risks, but in their home environment have a much fuller appreciation of the pitfalls and consequences. Freedom from the constraints and conventions of home can make some of the risks much more tempting.

Drugs

The penalties for buying, selling, or using drugs or even alcohol can be severe, despite the fact that in the same countries they are often easy to get hold of, more widely used, and very much cheaper than at home.

Alcohol can become a major problem, and every expatriate group has its core of abusers. Many become problem drinkers as a result of prolonged consumption of cheap or subsidized alcohol, especially if their job involves selling goods or services and entertaining or being entertained. Yet others, unable to work, drink to relieve boredom or anxiety. Above about 20 drinks per week, the incidence of medical problems including frank alcoholism increases dramatically. The sensible expatriate will try to keep below this number, if necessary by keeping to rules like not drinking until the sun goes down, never drinking spirits, having two days a week off drinking, or switching to low-alcohol or alcohol-free drinks.

Addiction to tobacco constitutes a major health hazard, but giving up in a developing country can be more difficult, particularly for people who smoke because of stress. Cigarette smoking is furthermore increasingly common and well accepted in developing countries, which have become a major target for tobacco companies losing their grip on Western markets. Well-known brands often have a much higher carcinogen content than they do at home, and may also be considerably cheaper.

Sex
People tend to become more sexually promiscuous when they are away from home. One study from the Netherlands showed that 23 per cent admitted to unprotected sex with partners from HIV-endemic areas whilst overseas. Particularly prone were younger males and single men who were lonely and bored. This means that the incidence of sexually transmitted diseases in expatriates is relatively high, (see p. 454, and p. 58). HIV infection and hepatitis B are spread mainly heterosexually in developing countries, and anybody who has sex with more than one partner or with prostitutes without using a condom nowadays is simply crazy. The same applies to homosexual promiscuity.

Naturally, many expatriates find a partner. Mixed-race marriages are increasingly common, and probably more readily accepted, but one still sees problems of adjustment in couples who return together to the expatriate's home country.

Driving
Driving overseas can be a hair-raising experience, and not only on dirt-track roads. Road accidents are all too common, and frequently have a fatal outcome because of poor rescue and medical facilities. Road traffic accidents are the major cause of death in expatriates — particularly in the age group 20–29. Not all countries have seat-belt rules, but not to install and wear front and rear seat-belts, in a dangerous driving environment, is asking for trouble. If you are going to have to drive an off-road vehicle, it is worthwhile getting some practice in your home country first — manufacturers of such vehicles often run training courses.

Swimming
Swimming is another risky activity, especially when under the influence of alcohol. Amongst the many additional hazards of swimming in developing countries, is that the beaches and swimming pools are rarely patrolled. Children should be particularly closely watched.

More people die in Britain from swimming accidents than in any other sport. Amongst US Peace Corps staff 18 per cent of injury deaths were due to drowning — the second most common cause of accidental death. Abroad, seas and rivers may well be polluted with sewage, but many expatriates will have experienced the same thing at home. It may be safer to stick to swimming pools and bilharzia-free lakes.

Home life abroad

Clothing
It should not be necessary to give advice on what to wear, but one still sees expatriates in the tropics with prickly heat and peeling scalps, caused by wearing tight denim jeans

and no hat. Long-term exposure to the sun ages skin and causes cancer. Protect yourself and your children with sunscreens and suitable clothing, or stay in the shade. Pure cotton clothing is still the most comfortable because of its absorbent qualities, and the looser the better.

Servants

For most expatriates, having servants is a new experience. They may themselves constitute a health hazard, and it makes sense to arrange for them to have a medical check-up by a known and trusted medical practitioner before they start work. Transmitted diseases are common (in many developing countries), like open pulmonary tuberculosis and intestinal infections such as amoebiasis. HIV positive servants are not an infection risk but may well become ill and need medical care.

Oddly enough, the hazards are more often psychological, with servant and employer causing annoyance to each other. There is nothing wrong or embarrassing about having servants as long as you employ them properly and honestly. Stick to local laws on employment (for example, you may find yourself responsible for medical care), pay them according to local rates, tell them and show them clearly and repeatedly exactly what you want them to do. If they can't or won't, terminate their service according to the proper process. Never get into the dreadful habit of complaining about your servants to expatriate colleagues.

Violence

Criminal attacks, robberies, and muggings are all too frequent in developing countries, especially in cities. Even where personal crime is uncommon, such as in many Muslim countries, there may be terrorism or violent fanaticism. Rape is also common in some places. Make personal protection and security a part of your everyday life, and follow local safety advice carefully. This may involve dressing inconspicuously, not driving at night, securing the sleeping quarters of your house, or any number of other strategies, depending on the actual security situation. See also p. 304.

Before you go

Not everybody is fit to go overseas for a prolonged period. A medical check may be required before going, and other family members may also need to be examined (see p. 550). This is also a time to review your general health, any existing problems, and also to discuss specific concerns (contraception, for example). Your family doctor is not always the best person to advise, because he or she may be unfamiliar with the country to which you are going; it may also be worth visiting a travel clinic or a specialist department. Attending a first-aid course could be useful.

It may sound obvious, but find out as much as possible about your *exact* destination before you go. 'Latin America' or 'Asia' may sound exotic — in reality you may be living in a city with worse traffic and air pollution problems than the one you left.

If you are being sent by an institution or company, it is very important to find out exactly what your contractual rights are as far as health care is concerned, and what facilities will be provided for medical support, including evacuations and general welfare. Is there a nurse or GP to register with? Where is the recommended hospital?

Many of the problems referred to in this chapter could be avoided if employers took more care in choosing their expatriate staff and provided sensitive, accurate information and good working conditions. Try to meet others who have recently returned from a posting in the same country, and try to attend any briefing courses that may be available.

The return home

For many expatriates, living abroad is a wonderful experience: the problems start when they come home. Much research remains to be done on the phenomenon that the French term 'la réinsertion en metropole des cadres expatriés' — also sometimes called 'reverse culture shock'. The return to horrible weather and life in the fast lane, with no home help, can indeed be quite a shock. Friends often seem depressingly parochial and secretly jealous. Getting back to work, commuting, and the old routine can be almost as difficult as becoming an expatriate in the first place. Employers can do much to help, by arranging educational and other programmes to enable the returning expatriate to settle in with minimal trauma.

Depending on where you have been, it may also be worth a simple medical check on a blood and stool sample to detect any parasites you may have acquired during your sojourn overseas (Appendix 7).

Fitness for working abroad

Choose an overseas assignment with care, and make sure you are fit, mentally and physically, before you go.

Dr Carol Dow has worked for the Foreign and Commonwealth Office since 1989, and has been their Chief Medical Adviser since 1998.

The success or failure of an overseas assignment often depends on the ability of the individual to remain physically and mentally healthy under difficult circumstances. Many people travel, but the transition from simply travelling abroad for pleasure, to living and working overseas, is a considerable one. All too often, the difficulties may be underestimated in the excitement of an attractive job offer. It is important to think about your fitness and suitability for the particular assignment you are contemplating well in advance; the wrong decision has far-reaching consequences for your own career and for your employer.

Why this job? Why now?

Your reasons for going are important. If the assignment will help your personal development, satisfy your desire for new challenges, give you work in an interesting field, and advance your career, the chances of success are high. If, on the other hand, you take the job because you want to escape — from a job failure, a broken marriage, or financial difficulties — or because you have been given no choice by your employer, then problems may well develop.

Psychological factors

The mental attributes for success in those who work overseas include: adaptability, confidence, proven ability in stressful situations, and a capacity to cope with separation (from family, friends, business associates, and security of the home environment). A personal history of success, particularly abroad, and a family history of stability and achievement, bode well.

A high degree of mental toughness and emotional flexibility are needed to cope with the challenges imposed by the move to any new environment, particularly a tropical one. Surroundings are not the whole story, and New Yorkers may find it as difficult in Aberdeen as Abuja. A lack of self-motivation and self-confidence, a rigid outlook, no hobbies, and an unhappy marriage/partnership — particularly one in which communication is poor — are adverse factors. Many families go overseas to better the employment of one partner. As a result, the spouse may have to give up work completely and children will have to move into a new education system. Anger, resentment, jealousy, and homesickness can turn success into failure.

Those who work overseas have to adapt to a variety of psychologically adverse stimuli which may include: heat, humidity, bright light, poor diet, noise, road traffic accidents, boredom, language difficulties, racial tension, and the risk of being physically assaulted and robbed or maimed. If you are considering working abroad and are not sure whether you and your family will cope, don't go.

Before committing yourself, make sure you have all the information there is about the job — the place, any likely problems, the medical facilities, and evacuation arrangements. You need all this before you can make an informed decision. Unfortunately, some organizations still regard developing countries as somewhere to dispose of their misfits, playing down the difficulties and deliberately concealing the pitfalls.

Physical fitness and preparation

Those working overseas should be fit, whether disabled or not. 'Fitness' includes adherence to sensible lifestyle guidelines regarding moderate alcohol intake, physical activity, height to weight ratio, and no addictive drug-taking.

Prepare for your trip by becoming fitter than usual. Whatever you will be doing, whether office-bound or leading treks, you will cope better if you are in good physical condition.

If you have a disability that affects your mobility, you need to find out as much as you can about the likely conditions. Wheelchair access and adequate emergency exits are not internationally recognized requirements. Lifts are unreliable where the electricity supply is intermittent, and even *getting into* your eighth-floor office could pose problems, let alone getting out in a hurry (see pp. 520–5).

A sensible, informed attitude to any pre-existing illness is important, along with knowing what to do (and carrying the medicine/equipment you need) if an emergency arises because of it. Individuals should take direct responsibility for confirming that medical services at their destination will indeed be capable of looking after someone with their condition. Many travel clinics keep information about medical facilities abroad — ask them.

Anyone with a pre-existing medical problem should carry a letter from their doctor giving full details of the condition, including how it is normally treated, medicines, and dosages. A medical alert bracelet or neck pendant can be useful. It may be helpful to have the name, telephone number, and e-mail address of your home-based GP and/ or specialist.

Individuals should also carry information on any known allergies, blood group, and vaccination record.

Those with pre-existing psychological conditions should discuss the suitability of the proposed posting with their regular medical attendant as well as with a medical travel specialist who has information about available services at the destination. There is no doubt that overseas life is not suitable for some individuals, and there is no job opportunity that justifies placing your long-term health and stability at risk.

Consider doing a first-aid course if you are going to a destination with poor medical facilities — and even if you are not. Knowing what to do in an emergency is not only immensely reassuring, it also saves lives.

Pre-posting medical check-up

A thorough medical check-up is advisable before undertaking any long-term overseas assignment. Spouses and children should also be examined. Conditions such as high blood pressure and diabetes may cause no symptoms, but can produce devastating and sudden effects, and medical facilities in many countries may be poor and difficult to access in an emergency.

Often the most beneficial aspect of the check-up is to reveal a lifestyle that may be putting your health at risk. Take such information positively — you need your body to last as long as you do, and abnormal liver function results today, for example, are perhaps a warning of future liver failure if your alcohol intake is not reduced. Your body is not lying to you: it is in trouble!

You will also need vaccination and anti-malarial advice, and a visit to a travel clinic means you will also be given advice on disease prevention for example, hygiene rules, insect bite avoidance, and preventing sexually transmitted diseases.

Finally, don't forget to visit your dentist (p. 420). You should always go abroad with your teeth in good order.

13 Preparations for travel

Immunization

Large numbers of travellers are exposed to the risk of infectious diseases abroad. Although there are now fewer mandatory vaccination certificate requirements for travel, immunization is an effective measure against some important diseases, and there have been significant improvements in the vaccines available. Every traveller should make the most of the available protection, and at the same time get the latest information and advice about malaria prevention and other precautions.

Dr Gil Lea has been advising vast numbers of travellers for over 25 years. She is now Consultant Medical Adviser to the Trailfinders Travel Clinic in Kensington, London, and provides travel health information to medical professionals at the Communicable Disease Surveillance Centre of the Public Health Laboratory Service in Colindale, London.

International travel is increasing, and so are opportunities for more adventurous holidays in ever more exotic places. Relaxation of immunization regulations has made it easier — though no less hazardous — for travellers to visit risk areas without first having to seek specialist medical advice.

Mandatory and non-mandatory immunization

Travellers should understand that there are now very few *mandatory* immunization requirements for travel — vaccination against yellow fever is now the only example, and even then is required only for travel to or through certain parts of Africa and South America. Most vaccines are *non-mandatory*, but one or more such vaccinations are nevertheless still strongly advised for most destinations — the only exceptions being for direct travel to countries in northern Europe, the USA, Canada, Australia, and New Zealand. In terms of personal health protection, these non-mandatory vaccinations are often far more important than mandatory ones.

Unfortunately, many travel agents and embassy officials mention only the mandatory immunization requirements for a particular country (i.e. those for which a certificate is required as a condition of entry), omitting to mention other advisable precautions. So travellers may gain the impression that no vaccinations are necessary for destinations such as India or Thailand simply because there are no mandatory requirements. In fact, several immunizations *should* be considered, and the opportunity should also be taken to seek medical advice about malaria prevention (see p. 130) and other health precautions.

Travel companies cannot reasonably be expected to provide detailed information about optional vaccinations and the specific choice of anti-malarial tablets, and should not try to do so; they should, however, certainly inform travellers of any mandatory requirements and remind them to consult a doctor or a travel clinic to receive personal advice. An outline of the current position is given below and in Appendix 1, but all travellers should check their individual needs several weeks before departure. A full immunization schedule may take two months or more to complete, but if less time is available valuable protection can still be gained.

About vaccines

Strictly, the word 'vaccination' refers only to that given (in the past) against smallpox. However, international regulations refer to other immunizations by the same term, and the words 'vaccination' and 'immunization' have come to be used interchangeably.

Vaccination stimulates the body's defence systems by the introduction of a small amount of the bacteria or virus concerned into the tissues. Some vaccines contain the killed or inactivated germ organism or its toxin; others contain a related live organism known to be safe for inoculation. The vaccine stimulates the production of antibodies, which are then ready to act if the real infection is encountered.

The number of doses required and the spacing between them depends on whether it is a 'live' or 'killed' vaccine and on any previous protection received. Once the initial courses of polio and tetanus vaccines have been completed, single 'booster' doses every few years are all that is required to maintain protection. The period of protection conferred by a vaccine varies from one vaccine to another (see Table 13.1).

It is important to realize that few vaccines provide 100 per cent protection, and other precautions such as care with food, drink, and personal hygiene are still necessary even when you have been vaccinated.

The only travel injection that is not a vaccine is gamma-globulin, previously used to protect against hepatitis A. Instead of stimulating the body's defences, gamma-globulin is ready-made antibody. It does not last long in the body after injection, so it has to be given close to departure, after the other injections. It is no longer readily available.

Not every vaccine is suitable for every person, for reasons such as allergy, pregnancy, age, or because of certain medical conditions; these problems are considered below.

Obtaining immunization

Where?

Travel clinics can provide accurate and up-to-date advice on both mandatory immunization requirements and non-mandatory recommendations and can also give the vaccine themselves. Their staff are specialists, and will usually be able to provide a quick service. Alternatively, your own GP can give the vaccines — although not all give yellow fever. Some GPs do not have much experience with some of the less common vaccines (e.g. Japanese encephalitis, rabies, tick-borne encephalitis) and prefer to refer

Table 13.1 Dose intervals for travel vaccines

| Vaccine | No. of doses | Primary course | | Booster doses |
		Interval between 1st & 2nd dose	Interval between 2nd & 3rd dose	Usual repeat interval after primary course
Yellow fever	1			10 years
Typhoid (injected; Vi)	1			3 years
Typhoid (oral; Ty21a)	3	On alternate days	On alternate days	3 years
Tetanus	3	4 weeks	4 weeks	10 years
Polio	3	At least 4 weeks	At least 4 weeks	10 years
Rabies (pre-exposure)	3	7 days	21 days	2–3 years
Meningitis (meningococcal A+C / ACYW)	1			3 years
Japanese encephalitis	3	1–2 weeks	2–4 weeks	2–4 years
Tick-borne encephalitis (East European)	3	1–3 months	9–12 months	3 years
Hepatitis A	2	6–12 months		Approx. 10 years
Hepatitis B (standard course)	3	1 month	5 months	Approx. 5 years
Hepatitis B (rapid course)	4	7 days	21 days	1 year, then 5 years approx.

Vaccines abroad

Dangers from injections abroad under unhygienic conditions are discussed further on p. 588, but counterfeit or ineffective vaccines can also be a serious problem. Vaccines need careful manufacture, storage, handling, and preparation. There are well-documented cases of people dying from rabies in Pakistan, for example, or acquiring hepatitis A in the countries of the former Soviet Union, despite 'vaccination'. This is a further reason for having all vaccinations before you leave home; or if that's not possible, ensuring that you go only to a reputable clinic, that can satisfy you that all vaccines come from a safe and reliable source.

---

travellers to specialist centres. Such centres usually provide a complete range of travel immunizations plus current advice, and are mostly found in major cities. Some of the main centres are listed in Appendix 8.

When?

A full travel vaccine immunization schedule could take a month or more to complete. This assumes the traveller has had a full course of childhood immunizations including tetanus, diphtheria, and polio. However, anyone born before the second World War may not have had such protection unless they have travelled extensively or been in the armed forces.

As far more retired people travel than ever before, and many on adventurous trips, they should start their travel vaccines at least two months (or preferably three months) prior to departure to allow for the primary courses to be completed. People are often surprised to learn that the oral (sugar lump) polio vaccine was introduced only in 1962. Some younger people may not have received full courses of these routine vaccines and so travel is a good opportunity to check.

Non-booster immunizations usually take 7–10 days to become effective, while booster doses generally take less than this. However, even when there is insufficient time for the ideal course to be followed, some worthwhile protection can often still be gained at short notice.

Common reasons for vaccination requests being delayed to the last minute are unexpected business trips or news of sudden outbreaks of disease. Another reason may be the discovery that 'no vaccinations are necessary for your trip' actually means that there may still be optional immunizations that are advised, at which point there be little time left. People who may need to travel at short notice can avoid most problems by keeping their protection up-to-date by means of booster doses, particularly for the vaccines they are most likely to need. Tetanus, diphtheria, polio, and the new hepatitis A vaccines need boosters only every 10 years, once the initial courses have been completed; typhoid may also be worth keeping up-to-date, though its boosters are needed more frequently (see Table 13.1). Those who may have to travel at short notice to tropical Africa or South America should also ensure that they have an up-to-date yellow fever vaccination certificate. The certificate is not valid until 10 days after injection but then remains valid for 10 years.

The dates for booster injections are not critical to the exact week and can be taken at any convenient time before travel. If there is time for only a single dose of vaccine before your trip, it is usually worth completing the course afterwards, to avoid the likelihood of the same problem occurring again and so that only booster doses will be needed in the future.

Another reason for allowing plenty of time in advance of your trip is that vaccine production and supply problems do occasionally occur. This has happened recently with rabies, yellow fever, and polio, and only the larger specialist centres have consistently maintained stocks.

Immunization schedules

For many package type holidays, a single visit may be all that is necessary.

Where both yellow fever and oral polio are recommended, they should ideally be at least three weeks apart. The next option is to have them on the same day. Where several (other) vaccines are recommended, it may be decided to divide them between two visits, more for the idea of being comfortable than for any proven medical advantage.

For some vaccines the initial course requires three visits: rabies, Japanese encephalitis, and hepatitis B. The three doses can be spaced over at least four weeks, preferably completing the course at least two weeks prior to departure. A third visit is also necessary for tetanus, diphtheria, and polio vaccines for someone who did not have the routine vaccines as a child.

Where many vaccines are required, it is probably easier to go to a travel clinic if there is one in a convenient location. Don't forget to take your previous vaccination certificates and details with you, for every visit.

Some typical examples of immunization schedules are shown in Table 13.2, but schedules generally need to be planned on an individual basis.

The injections

A surprising number of people are frightened by the thought of an injection. Young adults may not have had one since childhood, and the memory may still loom large. However, modern disposable needles are very small and sharp, and anyone who is well practised can give these shots almost painlessly. Smaller doses and purer vaccines are often used, and adverse reactions are now less common.

Most travel vaccines are given into different layers of the skin, or into the muscle, and the outer part of the upper arm is a convenient site. (Preferences vary: the French often give travel injections into the back, just below the shoulder blade.) The only injection given into the buttock is immunoglobulin, which contains more fluid and is more comfortably given into a large muscle. A lot of travellers are relieved to hear that this is now rarely used.

Those attending for injections (and especially anyone who is prone to feeling faint) should eat normally beforehand. In general, there are no special rules regarding alcohol before or after an injection. However, it may be advisable to avoid strenuous exercise or alcohol for several hours, especially if several injections are given on one day. But each individual should be guided by how he or she feels. Anyone who feels

Table 13.2 Examples of immunization schedules (which should be planned individually for each traveller)

A. **Overland trip through Africa, with about 4 weeks before departure:**

First attendance:	Yellow fever
	Typhoid: injection *or* 3 doses of oral vaccine commenced immediately with 2 further doses on alternate days
	Diphtheria/tetanus (booster)
	Hepatitis A
	Hepatitis B: first dose
	Rabies: first dose
Second attendance:	Meningitis
(1 week later)	Rabies: second dose
	Hepatitis B: second dose
Third attendance:	Polio (booster)
(4 weeks after first visit)	Rabies: third dose
	Hepatitis B: third dose

B. **Rushed schedule, with only one attendance possible**:

For Africa:	Meningitis
	Typhoid
	Diphtheria/tetanus (booster)
	Polio (booster)
	Hepatitis A vaccine
	Yellow fever
For Asia: (Indian subcontinent or Southeast Asia)	Meningitis (some areas)
	Typhoid
	Diphtheria/tetanus (booster)
	Polio (booster)
	Hepatitis A vaccine
For South America:	Typhoid
	Tetanus (booster)
	Hepatitis A vaccine
	Yellow fever

These schedules assume that the UK schedule of immunizations have been given including BCG and primary courses of diphtheria/tetanus and polio, and MMR in those born after 1988 faint after the injections should immediately lie down with his or her legs raised. Anyone with a tendency to faint should ask to have the shots lying down, and should lie down or stay sitting for at least 15 minutes afterwards.

The doctor or nurse who gives the injections should advise about malaria protection without being asked, but it is sensible for travellers to check on this if it is not mentioned. Similarly, this is a good time to ask about other travel medical problems like travellers' diarrhoea or what medication to include in a medical kit.

Individual vaccinations

Yellow fever (see p. 160)

The only remaining international vaccination certificate requirements relate to yellow fever vaccination. The vaccine provides virtually 100 per cent protection against a serious disease, and for at least the 10 years that the certificate lasts, so it is understandable that many countries maintain their yellow fever regulations, although a traveller visiting only a capital city at high altitude, e.g. Nairobi or Addis Ababa, of a country within the endemic zone may not be at risk.

Yellow fever exists only in two endemic zones, one across tropical Africa and the other in the northern part of South America (see Map 5.3, p. 162). Not all these countries report disease all the time, but when planning to travel through these areas, it is considered sensible to be immunized, since epidemics may flare up after decades without a single case. Some countries require a certificate from all travellers; the rest may not require a certificate from those on direct flights from North America or Europe, but may do so for travel from one country to another within the zone. In addition, it may be worth taking the vaccine for personal protection even if a certificate is not required (Appendix 1).

There are many misconceptions about the yellow fever regulations, and travellers often ask for yellow fever vaccination when they do not need it. Conversely, some do not realize that it may be mandatory for travellers leaving yellow fever zones and going to other countries.

As yellow fever does not exist in Asia, yellow fever vaccination is unnecessary for travel to Asian countries, provided travel is by the usual direct routes. However, for travel via Kenya to India, for example, a certificate would be required, as India wishes to avoid the introduction of the disease from Africa. There are many 'yellow fever receptive' areas outside the zones in which yellow fever infections occur. These are countries that have similar climates (and mosquitoes) to the countries where yellow fever is endemic, and naturally wish to prevent introduction of the disease.

Staff at embassies have on many occasions appeared to know the regulations only for direct travel to their countries; it is therefore important to find out about yellow fever vaccination from a reliable source, and to be sure to mention all the countries you will visit, in the correct sequence. Yellow fever centres should have access to the current regulations and if in doubt, the staff of the centre can check with the World Health Organization regulations for the current year.

All of the vaccines mentioned below are optional, except that meningitis vaccination is required for the pilgrimage to Mecca.

Tetanus and diphtheria

As tetanus can follow an injury (p. 100), everyone should be protected whether travelling or not. Certain kinds of travel — hiking, outdoor activities, and camping trips, for example — carry an increased risk of injury and good medical facilities may not always be readily available.

Recently, a combination of diphtheria with tetanus vaccine has become available for adults. It is particularly useful for those who will be in close contact with children in developing areas, for example, nurses and teachers (p. 103). These, and other long-term travellers, should take a booster if they have not done so in the last 10 years. The epidemic of diphtheria in the states of the former USSR during the mid-Nineties is an illustration of how diseases can flare up following poor availability of routine immunizations. In the UK, the combination diphtheria/tetanus vaccine is increasingly used routinely for adults as well as children.

Polio (see p. 52)

Oral (Sabin) polio vaccine, taken on a sugar lump or as drops on the tongue or in water, is also included with the childhood vaccines, usually starting at two months of age. Any child who has not completed the course should do so prior to travel, and unprotected adults of any age should take the basic course of vaccine. Boosters are given after 10 years (since the last dose) for travel to everywhere outside Europe, the American continent, Australia, and New Zealand. Persons who have previously had polio disease should still receive the immunization: they may have immunity to only one type of polio virus.

There are three types of polio virus and three doses in the initial course of vaccine. Each dose contains all three viruses and one of them has an opportunity to 'take' each time. This provides a high level of protection, although sometimes not all types have taken, so booster doses may be recommended after 10 years for travel.

An injected (killed) polio vaccine is also available. This is an up-to-date version of the Salk vaccine used before the oral (live) vaccine was developed. The modern injected vaccine is used by choice in a few countries, and is given especially to those for whom the live vaccine is unsuitable.

Measles

All children going overseas who have not completed their routine childhood immunization course, including measles vaccine, should do so (see pp. 492).

Hepatitis A (see p. 55)

Hepatitis A is the most frequent vaccine-preventable infection in travellers, although not the most serious. Protection against hepatitis A is particularly important for overlanders and for travellers to rural areas, but an increasing number of travellers prefer to be immunized even for short trips, rather than risk a possible period of protracted illness after return home.

Hepatitis A vaccine is a good choice for long-term or frequent travellers (since the second dose, given 6–12 months after the first, lasts about 10 years). The initial dose should be taken two to four weeks prior to departure for best protection. The course does *not* need to be started from scratch if the first dose is delayed.

There is a combined hepatitis A and typhoid vaccine available, and also a combined hepatitis A and B vaccine.

The original gamma-globulin injection gave immediate protection lasting only for two to six months (depending on the dose). It is a blood product, and is now seldom used.

An attack of hepatitis A gives lifelong immunity to the disease; a blood test is available to confirm immunity. The likelihood of previous infection increases with age and in people who have lived in the tropics during childhood. A positive result would mean that no further immunization was necessary.

Although a high level of protection can be obtained against hepatitis A, there are other forms of hepatitis transmitted similarly by food and water, so careful hygiene precautions are advised even for people who are immunized. The same precautions are recommended for those who take typhoid vaccine.

Typhoid (see p. 27 and p. 29)

As typhoid is a food- and water-borne disease, the risk is bound to be greater where hygiene conditions are poor, and the vaccine is certainly justified for rural travel through developing countries. The risk is less for those on short visits who will eat only in good hotels.

There are two routes of administering the vaccine: injected or oral (swallowed). The old typhoid and paratyphoid vaccine (once combined with cholera) was infamously associated with uncomfortable vaccine reactions. Those reactions are less common now, and the new single-shot vaccine usually causes only a slightly sore arm. The oral vaccine sounds attractive because of the absence of a needle, but as the modern vaccines, skilfully injected, are hardly felt, this is not such an important issue. The oral vaccine is also 'live', which means that it has more contraindications and possible problems when taken with other tablets and vaccines.

Vaccines against typhoid do not provide complete protection; like travellers' diarrhoea and some hepatitis strains, typhoid is transmitted by infected food and water, so care with hygiene is still important even if vaccine is taken.

Cholera

There are now no official international cholera certificate requirements. The last territory to abandon this requirement was Pitcairn, in June 1991, so any request for a cholera certificate may now be immediately identified as unofficial. Backpackers crossing remote land borders in South America and Africa, especially where there have been recent cholera outbreaks, may rarely be asked for a certificate. Anyone who is concerned about this can request a *certificate of exemption* when receiving their other immunizations.

The reason that cholera vaccination is no longer required or given is that the traditional vaccines are not very effective. Prevention is by food and water hygiene.

New vaccines are in development, and some are already available in Switzerland and Scandinavia (see p. 42). These could be useful for aid workers and the few travellers at particular risk from the disease. One of these vaccines may be combined with a new vaccine against the commonest form of travellers' diarrhoea.

Hepatitis B

The hepatitis B vaccine tends to be given mostly to travellers going on longer or repeated trips, and is fairly expensive. The full course of vaccine takes several months to complete and does not always produce protection; accelerated courses (with more doses over a shorter period) are sometimes more practicable for travellers.

Hepatitis B is transmitted by the same routes as HIV — such as sexual contact, blood, serum, non-sterile needles and medical instruments, acupuncture, or tattooing. Ideally, anyone who might need medical or dental treatment in a developing country should be protected, as should health care professionals going to work in those areas, and anyone who might have sexual contact with new partners while travelling. This is discussed in greater detail on p. 57. Such travellers should also take full precautions against HIV.

Rabies (p. 217)

Until relatively recently the only rabies vaccine available was so unpleasant that it was not used until *after* a bite, when the victim was faced with an imminent threat of rabies. Modern vaccines are effective and safe, though fairly expensive; they produce very few reactions (a small per centage of people seem to be allergic and should not continue the course). These vaccines make immunization *prior* to possible exposure to rabies feasible for the first time.

Pre-travel immunization does not preclude the need for treatment after a bite but will reduce the amount necessary (usually fewer doses of vaccine and no serum injection) and is likely to be effective even if there is a short delay before the treatment booster doses of vaccine are obtained. A growing world shortage of anti-serum makes this increasingly worthwhile.

Vaccine is recommended for longer stays in rabies areas and for those travelling off the beaten track, more than a day's journey from good medical care. It is important to avoid any delay in starting treatment after a bite or a scratch, especially in people who have had no vaccine in advance.

Meningococcal meningitis

Vaccines are available against the A and C meningococcal strains, and against A/C/Y/W-135. The group A strain has caused outbreaks in countries of the endemic zone that stretches across Africa — especially in the meningitis belt stretching from Senegal to Sudan and Ethiopia (see p. 112). From 1989 onwards, some disease was also reported from Kenya, Uganda, Tanzania, Rwanda, Burundi, and other countries south of the usual belt. Brazil has had outbreaks in several strains in the last few decades. India and Nepal reported some group A meningitis from 1984 onwards, as did Mongolia in the early 1990s.

In view of the increase in reports of meningitis in the home countries of Muslim pilgrims travelling to Mecca, and the fact that there had been a number of cases in the

Middle East the previous year, the health authorities in Saudi Arabia took the unprecedented step of making vaccination against meningococcal meningitis and a vaccination certificate mandatory for those joining the Hajj pilgrimage in 1988. Meningitis is not a disease for which an international certificate of vaccination is required under World Health Organization regulations, and this example illustrates how countries may, from time to time, impose their own restrictions on visas, making them conditional upon additional health certificates and requirements. Since the Hajj of 2001, pilgrims from the UK are advised to take A/C/Y/W-135 vaccine as cases of the W meningitis developed in some pilgrims the previous year.

Travellers from the UK rarely contract the disease overseas, and in general the vaccine is advised only for those going to areas with outbreaks in progress, or staying in endemic zones during the dry season, particularly if there is likely to be close contact with the local population. (See the note on p. 114 regarding protection of travellers who have had their spleens removed.)

In the UK, there has been a highly successful vaccination campaign against meningitis C in children and young adults. However, people who have had this vaccine should still receive the A+C vaccine (or ACYW) if they need protection for travel.

'Flu

'Flu (influenza) occurs seasonally around the world, and outbreaks may occur from time to time. There have been outbreaks of 'flu on board cruise ships, and outbreaks have also been documented in relation to air travel. Those for whom influenza vaccine is normally recommended should also take it prior to travel in the seasons when the vaccine is available. The same applies to *pneumococcal* vaccine.

Japanese encephalitis (see p. 164)

This disease is endemic across Asia, affecting many countries from India to Japan. It is seasonal in the temperate zones affected, but may be all-year-round in the tropics.

The virus is transmitted to humans by mosquitoes that have bitten farm animals or birds, so that prolonged travel through agricultural regions constitutes the highest risk. The disease can be serious or fatal, but it has fortunately been reported only in a tiny number of Western travellers. As the vaccine has to be imported from Japan or Korea in small amounts, the course tends to be rather expensive.

Travellers intending to visit rural parts of Asia for any length of time should enquire about the likely risk before they travel. The vaccine is not licensed in the UK, but can be ordered specifically by GPs or taken at a specialist travel clinic. It is available at some clinics in Canada, Australia, and many Asian countries. The Japanese version of the vaccine is now licensed in the USA.

Tuberculosis

BCG vaccination (against tuberculosis — see p. 98) is usually given in the UK at 11–13 years but can be given from birth in those going to live in higher-risk areas. Adults going to work or stay in similar areas and who may be unprotected can be tested and vaccinated if necessary. (The public health approach to TB in the US is different, and American travellers are not generally encouraged to have BCG vaccinations.)

Plague (p. 181)

Plague still exists in Africa (particularly Madagascar) and other developing areas. A 'plague' scare in India in 1995 caused widespread panic as far away as Europe and the USA, which was totally unjustified. No visitors were affected and it was never proved to be plague.

The disease is passed by rodent fleas, so only those whose work makes it difficult to avoid rats are likely to be at risk, apart from the medical carers of acutely ill patients. There is no vaccine available for general use.

Tick-borne encephalitis

Tick-borne encephalitis (TBE) is an arbovirus infection that occurs especially in summer in the forests of central (mainly Austria, Germany, and Switzerland) and Eastern Europe , including parts of the states of the former USSR and Scandinavia. It is a risk to walkers, campers, hikers, and foresters, using paths not only in the wooded areas but also through shrubbery on forest fringes, where undergrowth can brush against their legs or arms, allowing the ticks to attach themselves (see p. 165). The virus can also be transmitted by drinking unpasteurized milk.

The vaccine is not licensed in the UK, but can be obtained specifically by a GP or a specialist travel clinic for those going to walk or camp in risk areas. For people travelling at short notice, an injection of TBE gamma-globulin is occasionally used to give rapid protection. This is also an unlicensed product.

Smallpox

Smallpox was eradicated world-wide in 1978. There is now no reason for any traveller to have smallpox vaccination under any circumstances, and the vaccine is no longer available.

In the aftermath of the anthrax attacks in the USA in 2001, the position is being re-evaluated. The American government has ordered 210 million doses of smallpox vaccine from the British biotechnology company, Acambis, to be held in reserve.

When not to be vaccinated

Each case should be considered individually, but there are some general guidelines.

Vaccines are not generally administered during an acute infection.

Vaccines to which the recipient has a known allergy are not normally given, and vaccines should not be given during acute illness or some serious chronic diseases. Otherwise, there are no particular circumstances when *killed* vaccines (see Table 13.3) should be avoided — with the exception of the injected polio vaccine and rabies vaccine, which contain trace quantities of rare antibiotics. *Live* vaccines are generally contraindicated in disorders of immunity or pregnancy (see below).

Gastrointestinal infections at the time of vaccination may inhibit the oral typhoid and polio vaccines from 'taking'. Antibiotics and mefloquine (anti-malarial tablets) may also inhibit oral typhoid vaccine,

Other specific cautions are allergy to eggs for yellow fever, tick-borne encephalitis, 'flu, and measles vaccines, and to several rare antibiotics for yellow fever and polio.

Table 13.3 Live and inactivated vaccines

Live vaccines	Inactivated vaccines
Yellow fever	Injected typhoid
Oral polio	Injected polio
BCG (TB)	Tetanus ⎫
Measles ⎫	Diphtheria ⎬ Toxoid
Mumps ⎬ MMR	Meningitis
Rubella ⎭	Rabies
Oral typhoid	Hepatitis A
	Hepatitis B
	Japanese encephalitis
	Whooping cough
	Influenza
	Pneumococcal vaccine

Immune disorders

People with an impaired immune system, whether due to serious disease, steroid medication, or cancer chemotherapy or radiotherapy, should not usually take live vaccines (see Table 13.3). HIV-positive people are a special category who should avoid BCG and other live travel vaccines where possible; but those requiring yellow fever or polio protection should discuss with their physician the risk/benefit ratio that applies in their individual situation. HIV-positive children travelling should usually have measles protection. (See also pp. 515–19)

Pregnancy

Live and inactivated vaccines are listed in Table 13.3. During pregnancy (see p. 486) live vaccines are generally avoided, but in some circumstances they may still be advisable. There is no evidence that yellow fever vaccine during pregnancy has ever caused harm to the fetus (the vaccine does not cross the placenta), and where there is a *real* threat from the disease (not just a certificate requirement), it may be considered. Where urgent polio protection is vital, experts recommend using the oral vaccine; where there is time, the killed one is used. Oral typhoid vaccine is not used in pregnancy.

Tetanus vaccine has been used for many years without any known ill effect. Experience with the newer typhoid and hepatitis A injections is limited, although there is no expectation that they would cause harm. Japanese encephalitis and rabies are usually avoided unless there is a definite risk, such as already having been bitten by a potentially rabid dog.

Small children

Routine childhood vaccinations are very important. Injected typhoid vaccine is not usually given below 18 months of age and oral typhoid under 6 years. Yellow fever is not usually given below 9 months to a year, depending on the risk of disease. The issue of hepatitis A protection is debatable, since the disease usually causes few symptoms in small children, although theoretically they could return and infect others. Children going to live overseas can be vaccinated against TB (BCG), hepatitis B, rabies, and Japanese encephalitis if the areas to be visited are considered sufficiently risky. In the UK, the latter two are usually delayed until after one year of age.

Exemption

Where a certificate would normally be required, a letter or medical certificate of exemption signed by a doctor is usually acceptable to the authorities. People who cannot be vaccinated on medical grounds have to consider the risks of travel without protection.

Reaction to vaccines — what to expect

Yellow fever and oral polio vaccine usually produce virtually no reaction. Occassionally 'flu-like aches are reported several days after yellow fever vaccination. The other injected vaccines tend to produce a slightly sore area at the injection site on the arm, but the arm does not usually become stiff and difficult to use. When gamma-globulin is given, the discomfort is at the top of the buttock, and this can be walked off quite quickly. It is more comfortable not to tense the muscle while an injection is being given.

These days, people are much less likely to feel unwell after travel vaccines, although the injected typhoid and occasionally other vaccines have this effect for a few hours. The oral typhoid can produce nausea and other gastric upset. BCG (TB vaccine) can produce an open ulcer which can take several weeks to heal and leaves a scar. Other vaccines cause only red marks which disappear quickly or fade slowly, but virtually never produce permanent scars.

Side effects

Isolated cases of more serious side effects have been recorded following several vaccines *but are extremely rare.* Oral polio vaccine has been known to produce polio-like symptoms in some recipients or their close contacts on very, very few occasions (about 3 per 5 million doses). It is recommended that unprotected parents take the vaccine at the same time as their babies.

Polio vaccine is excreted in the faeces for several weeks and careful personal hygiene is important to protect anyone in the household with a poor immune system (e.g. from HIV or cancer treatment).

Many millions of doses of yellow fever vaccine have been given safely world-wide. There are a handful of reports of yellow fever-like symptoms developing with fatal consequences.

> **Summary of advice for travellers**
>
> - If you are travelling through Africa or South America, check whether you need an international certificate of vaccination against yellow fever.
> - All other immunizations are optional (apart for meningitis for the pilgrimage to Mecca).
> - Obtain medical advice on planning a course to provide the best protection for your individual trip.
> - Immunizations are only *part* of your health protection, so don't forget to find out about the other measures you can take to protect yourself, such as food and water precautions, malaria protection, and precautions against insect bites.

Health insurance for international travel

Costs of health care abroad can be very high, and so can the cost of air ambulance rescue, should you be unlucky enough to need it. It is vital to make sure that all your requirements are adequately covered before you travel.

Dr Richard Fairhurst is a Consultant in Accident and Emergency Medicine; Medical DIrector of Lancashire Ambulance Service and NHS Direct North West Coast. He was former Chief Medical Officer of Green Flag Travellers' Medical Service and Europ Assistance, London.

Health insurance is an important part of health care for travellers. It is becoming an increasingly complex field, so travellers need to think about and specify exactly what they require. Remember that health insurance provides money after the event, *not* medical care itself.

It is very important that the amount of money provided by the policy is adequate for any likely need. There has been a growing tendency to increase the amount of medical cover provided — indeed, some policies now provide unlimited medical cover — but, in my experience, $500 000 is perfectly adequate even in the USA, provided repatriation expenses are covered separately in another section of the policy.

Medical assistance for travellers

Traditionally, health-care insurance benefits are paid out against a completed claim form, filled in after an episode of illness is over and the patient is back at home.

This begs a number of questions. Will the amount of money insured be adequate to reimburse the costs of treatment abroad? How easy will it be to obtain money in an emergency to pay for treatment? Not all hospital authorities and doctors abroad necessarily accept travel insurance documents as evidence that they will eventually be paid, although when prolonged treatment abroad is necessary it is often possible to make arrangements for insurance companies to pay the costs directly.

UK and European Community nationals are entitled to free or reduced cost medical treatment in certain countries (see p. 572), but additional insurance is still necessary to cover the costs of repatriation and any other expenses.

However much money is available, will adequate facilities for treatment exist at the site of the incident?

These problems resulted in the development of combined health insurance and assistance services, which endeavour to provide on-the-spot help, together with repatriation for further treatment if necessary. In practical terms, this demands expertise in obtaining air ambulance facilities at short notice, medical and logistic support, and the ability to judge which circumstances justify evacuation — and to where. *Remember that it is not necessarily appropriate to repatriate every single case of illness abroad by air ambulance, and in many countries poor communications and lack of airport facilities may make this impossible anyway.*

The concept of assistance originated in France and was to provide practical help to travellers. Sadly, over the years in the UK, the insurance industry has emasculated assistance to an emergency claims handling service. As a result, complex medical decision are taken, in some instances, by lay insurance managers advised only by trainee junior doctors supplied by locum agencies, without even the qualifications to act as independent practitioners in the National Health Service. The complexity of insurance intermediaries means that before you buy any cover you should insist on reading the policy conditions and finding out exactly who will be making the decisions if you become ill or are injured.

However, neither insurance nor assistance can *prevent* accidents, only you can do that. Equally, insurance cannot protect you from the actual or perceived risks at the destination. If you are not prepared to be treated by Spanish doctors if you become ill in Spain, you should not go to that country. If you are worried about the risks of contracting AIDS should you be injured in some African country, you should be aware that insurance has nothing to offer: if you are injured and unconscious, you will be taken by the emergency service to the local facilities. Even if your so-called 'AIDS kit' had sufficient medical supplies to treat you, which is improbable, it would be more likely to be in your hotel room than in your hip pocket!

The risks

So what are the risks to the international traveller? We know from insurance company records that 1 in 500 travellers will call their assistance service whilst abroad with a medical problem, 1 in 10 000 will require repatriation by air ambulance for medical reasons, and 8 in 100 000 will die abroad. Table 13.4 shows the type and number of medical problems requiring help or advice.

Pre-existing illness

The basis of all insurance is that a contract is taken against a risk, before that risk occurs. This is summed up neatly by the saying that it is impossible to insure a house that is already on fire. When this principle is applied to medical risks, certain problems become clear.

Many policies exclude cover for pre-existing illness, or 'risks which could be reasonably foreseen by the client', or 'travelling against the advice of a medical practitioner'. Disputes about pre-existing conditions are among the leading causes of

Table 13.4 Causes of medical problems abroad (Travellers' Medical Service survey)

Problem	per cent
Trauma	30.9
Gastrointestinal problems	17.1
Respiratory problems	14.1
Heart and circulatory problems	10.3
Skin problems	5.9
Genitourinary problems	4.5
Nervous system	3.8
Generalized infections	3.7
Musculoskeletal problems	3.2
Mental problems	1.5
Cancers	0.7
Miscellaneous	4.3

all complaints about travel insurance. If anyone has any type of pre-existing medical condition, it is important that they should notify the company with which they are proposing to insure, and obtain confirmation in writing that the problem *will* be covered in the event of a claim. Any medical certificate that accompanies this should state that the person is unlikely to need medical treatment during the trip, not that the person is fit to fly.

There is of course a moral issue here. Is it reasonable for insurance companies or doctors to encourage people who have a pre-existing illness to travel abroad on holiday? Often a person who is ill perceives the holiday as being a valuable part of convalescence and looks forward to the benefits it will bring.

No less often, however, neither the patient nor his doctor gives adequate consideration to what will happen if the patient becomes ill again outside his home environment. Even in countries with good medical facilities, being ill in a hospital where the doctors do not speak your own language and cannot refer to your previous records can be a dangerous and unpleasant experience. In countries where medical facilities are poor, what was conceived as a period of convalescence and relaxation can be transformed all too readily into a nightmare.

People with a pre-existing illness (and their doctors) should therefore satisfy themselves that adequate facilities for treatment really will be available if the condition recurs or deteriorates, and should think carefully about whether or not the risks are justified.

The young, the old, and the pregnant

These special groups are worthy of particular comment. In general, children and young people are accepted on the same terms and the same premium as adults. A small number of companies offer a discount for children. The elderly obviously have an increased chance of making a claim under a health insurance policy and are more likely to have pre-existing medical conditions which should, as mentioned before, be notified specifically to the insurance company. Disabled people in general are no more likely to become ill than anyone else, though disabilities can cause problems with repatriation from time to time, and it is therefore prudent for disabled people to notify insurance companies of their disability in advance.

Pregnancy poses a great problem. Some companies completely exclude cover in pregnancy. Others say that pregnancy is not a medical illness and therefore include only abnormalities of pregnancy. In any event it is very difficult to arrange insurance cover for the result of a pregnancy — the newborn child (see p. 486). Remember that if a pregnancy ends unexpectedly early and produces a premature baby, the baby's medical care in a neonatal intensive care unit could be very expensive. Many insurers take the view that a child who does not exist at the time the contract is taken can never be covered by a contract, though others would be prepared to write special (and very expensive) contracts to cover this possibility.

Check that you are covered

Other problems occur with insurance contracts, which should be foreseen before difficulties arise. Contracts for holiday insurance almost always exclude manual labour and work, and anyone who is going abroad to do any sort of manual work should check carefully that they are covered.

Similarly many policies do not cover mountaineering, scuba diving, parascending, or motorcycle riding. All these activities are becoming increasingly common, particularly with holidaymakers. If you intend to indulge in any of these activities it is vital to make sure that the risks are covered. Some policies also do not cover driving or driving rented cars. It may be necessary to 'shop around' to find an insurance company that will cover you for the particular sport you are interested in.

Medical insurance policies often also cover baggage, cancellation, and curtailment of the trip, and indeed almost half the claims under such policies are in these sections. Make sure the sums insured under each section are appropriate for your needs, remembering that personal belongings may already be covered under other policies that you may have. Most policies include some sort of death benefit following an accident: note that this is not life cover and covers only *accidental* death; it should not be confused with life assurance.

Check your policy carefully

The Financial Ombudsman Service — The UK insurance industry watchdog — says complaints about travel insurance rose by 25 per cent in 2001, and make up one in eight of the problems it deals with. Check the wording of your policy carefully: for example, many policies restrict cover for 'valuables' or stipulate that 'valuables' — such as spectacles — are covered only whilst in your possession.

Recently, government regulation has changed the way in which travel insurance is sold in the UK. The tying of discounts to travel agents' own brand insurance has been made illegal, and at the same time travel insurance bought through a travel agent incurs a higher rate of VAT than that sold by an insurance company or broker.

Annual insurance

Traditionally, health insurance has been bought on a trip basis, — in other words, you purchase fixed-term insurance to cover the duration of a single trip. More recently there has been a trend towards providing annual policies, albeit with a limit to the duration of any one trip. These annual policies are particularly attractive to frequent travellers, especially because they do not require prior notification of trips and are always in force.

Expatriates

Expatriates need a form of permanent health insurance that will provide for their normal health care needs wherever they are living. This usually includes some form of repatriation cover, which may be limited to repatriation to the nearest place of medical excellence rather than all the way to their home country. The policies are usually taken out by their employer, rather than on an individual basis. Employees are best advised to demand such policies as a condition of employment.

Summary of advice for travellers

- In conclusion, a wide range of health insurance contracts is available. Each individual traveller should define his or her needs and then study the full insurance proposal or contract in order to make sure it meets these needs exactly. If there are any queries, these should be raised in writing with the insurer before going abroad.

- Carry the telephone and fax number and e-mail address of your own physician at home. Communicating directly with your own GP, or putting a local doctor in touch with him or her, is a quick way to resolve conflicting advice and put your mind at ease.

- Take a generous supply, and always keep it with you, of ANY essential medication you might need. The same drug may be impossible to obtain locally.

- Carry sufficient cash to cover emergency expenses. Medical care abroad is expensive: take the best advice you can, and don't attempt to save money if you need emergency care, by shopping around for a cheaper option.

- Be flexible and adaptable, stay calm, and follow medical advice: immediate evacuation may not always be in your best interests, however much you might want to get home if you are injured or unwell.

- Think carefully about safety and accident prevention.

Reciprocal healthcare arrangements

Eligible nationals and residents of the UK and EU countries are entitled to emergency medical treatment either free or at reduced cost, when visiting other Community countries.

- Travellers from the UK will need form E111, available from any main Post Office, in order to obtain treatment in the countries listed below. When completed, take it to a Post Office, where the form will be stamped and signed and returned to you. The E111 is free and remains valid indefinitely so long as you remain ordinarily resident in the UK.

Austria*	Gibraltar	Luxembourg
Belgium	Greece	Netherlands
Denmark	Iceland	Norway
Finland	Irish Republic*	Portugal
France	Italy	Spain
Germany	Liechtenstein	Sweden

*Proof of entitlement, such as a passport, is all that is necessary

A more detailed description of what is covered can be found at **www.doh.gov.uk/traveladvice/eeachecklist.htm**

- There are also reciprocal arrangements between the UK and the following countries for free or reduced-cost emergency medical care, and a more detailed description of what is covered can be found at **www.doh.gov.uk/traveladvice/hcagreements.htm**

Anguilla	New Zealand
Australia	Poland
Barbados	Romania
British Virgin Islands	Russia (and other former Soviet
Bulgaria	Republics except Latvia, Lithuania, and Estonia)
Channel Islands	
Czech Republic	Slovak Republic
Falkland Islands	St Helena
Hungary	Turks & Caicos Islands
Isle of Man	Yugoslavia (i.e. Serbia & Montenegro &
Malta	successor states Croatia, Bosnia,
Montserrat	Slovenia, Macedonia)

Medicines and medical kits

What should a medical kit contain? This is a much more personal question than most people realize: individual needs vary widely, and also depend upon precise travel plans — the destination, nature, and duration of a trip — and whether skilled medical care, medicines, and medical supplies will be available locally.

Dr Richard Dawood devised this project and is the Editor of this book. He has travelled in over 80 countries around the world, and his work at the Fleet Street Travel Clinic includes providing medical supplies and training for journalists and business travellers working in hostile environments all over the world.

Dr Larry Goodyer is the superintendent pharmacist at the Nomad Travel Pharmacy, London, which specializes in preparing personalized medical kits for travellers of all kinds, and is a Senior Lecturer in Clinical Pharmacy in the Department of Pharmacy, King's College London.

Creating the perfect travel medical kit is a matter of striking the right balance between size, weight, cost, and practicality, and thinking clearly about the medicines and supplies you are most likely to need. So the purpose of this chapter is to review some of the commonest medical problems travellers are likely to come across, and the kinds of remedies that might be worth taking along for them. A concise checklist of these items is given in Appendix 6.

Some general points about medicines

Safety

All drugs known to have any useful effect may also be potentially harmful, especially if taken inappropriately or in excess. No drug is suitable for everyone: if at all possible, you should begin by seeking advice from your own doctor about any medication you intend to use abroad. Read manufacturers' instructions carefully, and take notice of them; ask your pharmacist for a copy of the manufacturer's data sheet.

Don't forget to keep all drugs and medicines out of reach of children.

Do check the 'expiry date' of any medicines you purchase abroad, as well as any medication left over from previous trips that you propose to take with you again. 'Out-of-date' medicines can be harmful or ineffective, especially if they have not been stored correctly.

A further problem can be that of a language barrier when describing medical problems to a pharmacist or doctor. It is particularly important that they appreciate any serious drug allergies and it may be worthwhile to carry a written translation of the problem if this is of particular concern. It is also vital to ensure that you fully understand any instructions you are given.

Dosage

- Keep strictly to recommended doses — twice as much is not necessarily twice as effective!
- Always complete a full course of treatment if you are taking antibiotics (usually five to seven days), but discontinue any drug you suspect of causing adverse effects.

Counterfeit drugs

Counterfeit drugs and medicines are a major problem in developing countries; some products cause harm because they are ineffective, while others may actually be toxic. There have been many reports of cases involving well-known brand names, particularly in Africa and the Far East, where drug counterfeiting occurs on a large scale. The first known case of counterfeit drugs penetrating the British market occurred in 1989, when a large quantity of fake Zantac tablets (the anti-ulcer treatment) was found to have been illegally imported, probably from Greece. There have been several subsequent cases. In an incident in Nigeria, industrial solvent in paracetamol syrup killed 109 children and maimed 600. In Burma, scores of villagers are believed to have died after fake anti-malarials flooded the market. In another recent example, one brand of the bilharzia treatment drug praziquantel, on sale in the Sudan, and purportedly made in Canada, was found to contain no trace of the active drug. According to the Russian Health Ministry as many as 3.6 per cent of all drugs on sale there are fakes.

In some countries manufacturing standards of pharmaceutical preparations are poorly controlled, leading to the production of substandard medicines. A well-known example of this occurred in Venezuela when a large number of patients with vivax malaria failed to respond to treatment with primaquine tablets. On analysis, the tablets, which had been obtained from the Venezuelan Health Ministry, were found to be dangerously substandard with some containing as low as 19 per cent of the correct amount of drug. Fake anti-malarials, are also known to be a major problem in Cambodia (one third of samples tested contained no active drug). A recent analysis of medicines purchased in Lagos and Abuja found that almost half of the 581 samples studied contained the wrong dose of drug; too much, too little, or none. And, according to the Pharmaceutical Society of Nigeria, 70 per cent of the drugs on sale in Nigeria are fakes.

It can be very tempting to buy medicines locally in parts of the world such as India and Thailand, where there may be a thriving pharmaceutical industry, and where 'copies' of well-known international brands are produced quite legally at a fraction of the cost (there are more than 20 000 pharmaceutical companies in India alone). However, it is always much safer to take along anything you know you will need, particularly anti-malarials and antibiotics, rather than to rely on being able to buy supplies locally. Inspect all packaging carefully — although fakes have certainly been concealed in authentic packaging. And bear this problem in mind, if locally purchased medication fails to produce the desired effect.

Counterfeit vaccines are discussed on p. 556.

Drug names

Most drugs have two names — a *generic*, or scientific name, which is usually the same or similar in most countries, and a *trade* or *brand* name which may vary from one country to another (some drugs are sold under several different brand names even in the same country). For example, in the UK there is a popular motion sickness remedy called Kwells; a British traveller asking for this brand name at an American pharmacy might easily be given a bottle or two of Kwell, a lotion for killing lice, and American travellers reading this book will probably be surprised to see it listed as a motion sickness remedy. (Kwell is called Quellada in the UK.)

To complicate matters still further, tablets containing combinations of more than one drug have been given *special* generic names. For instance, the combination of

Never allow yourself to be separated from any medical supplies when you travel

In 1997 a 75–year-old American woman was forced to check in a bag that contained her lifesaving asthma medication; the bag was lost, and she died following an asthma attack. There was no suggestion that the bag was too bulky or overweight. This tragic case received much publicity when her family successfully sued the airlines responsible and may at least serve to make airlines more aware of the possible consequences of separating passengers from medicines that they need.

The rule of thumb, when travelling with any essential medicines, is to take more than you need, to ensure that they are clearly labelled, and to divide your supply carefully between hand luggage and checked baggage or between yourself and your travelling companion. Bear in mind that you may not be able to recover the cost of replacement medication from your travel insurance if your baggage is delayed rather than actually lost; and if you need a prescription to get a fresh supply while you are abroad, you will have the added hassle and cost of trying to find a doctor.

paracetamol with codeine tablets is now called co-codamol, and the antibiotic amoxycillin/clavulanic acid is called co-amoxiclav. Make sure that you get what you *want* at a pharmacy abroad, not just what you have asked for.

Current and existing medical problems

Travellers with any pre-existing medical condition requiring drug treatment, should not only take along an adequate supply of their usual medication, but should also carry a separate prescription or written record of their medication giving its *generic* name, in case further supplies are needed in an emergency. It is also sensible to take an adequate supply of medication to cover any condition that might recur, even if this has not recently been a problem — for instance, women who experience cystitis with some regularity or asthmatics who may have recently been symptom-free. In the case of hay fever (p. 358) and asthma in particular, unusual environments may readily precipitate a severe attack. If you need to take psychoactive drugs, see p. 403.

It is also a good idea to tell the pharmacist about any medication you are currently taking, whenever buying medicines from a pharmacy. The same advice applies when seeking treatment abroad from any source.

In the UK, only three months' supply of medicines intended for use abroad can officially be obtained through the National Health Service.

Prescriptions

In this chapter, medicines marked * are available in the UK only on a doctor's prescription. Some doctors — especially those unused to dealing with travellers — may be unwilling to prescribe 'prescription only' items, especially antibiotics and stronger painkillers, to be carried on a 'just in case' basis. Such items should be used, wherever possible, under medical supervision, and are carried only because of the potential unreliable nature or lack of availability of such medicines in certain destinations.

In many countries, you may find that you can buy 'prescription only' medicines at any pharmacy or dispensary without restriction; you should treat all such medicines with respect and note the points made earlier regarding potential problems.

Herbal remedies

Don't try herbal cures and medicines when you travel, however harmless they may seem — just because a medicine is herbal or 'natural' does not mean that it is without dangerous side effects. There have been cases where such products have been found to contain quite toxic adulterants, such as lead, or occasionally to be 'spiked' with conventional medicines such as powerful steroids.

A Korean man died recently after drinking herbal tea made with hai ge fen — powdered clam shell. It was heavily contaminated with lead. Hard-shell clams, barnacles, oysters, mussels, and sea urchins are all able to accumulate toxic levels of lead, copper, chromium and arsenic — which are frequently found in marine paints and preservatives. There is seldom any control on the way these creatures are harvested or prepared, and sea urchins are a particularly 'perilous comestible substance' according to a recent report in the *Journal of the American Medical Association*. A list of possible side effects and interactions between herbal remedies and other medicines can be found at **www.asahq.org/publiceducation/list2.htm**.

When travelling with medicines, the risk of customs difficulties can be reduced by making sure that they are all clearly labelled and in their original containers, and that a prescription or letter from the prescribing doctor is carried whenever possible. Unidentified pills carried loose in a bag invite interest from customs officials, not to mention errors with instructions regarding dosage and usage.

Packaging for travel

It is often more convenient to carry tablets in blister packs rather than loose in a bottle. After a few months rattling around in a backpack, loose tablets can be reduced to powder. The strip packs can be kept in small sealable plastic bags, together with the manufacturers' instructions. A sealable plastic container (e.g. Tupperware) can be used to store medicines and first-aid equipment, although backpackers may find a plastic zip wallet or waterproof pouch less bulky.

Jars of creams readily become contaminated with bacteria that grow rapidly in a hot climate and might introduce infection into open wounds. Tubes of creams are less likely to become contaminated than jars, and are easier to carry, though care should still be taken to keep the cap of the tube clean and away from direct contact with the skin surface.

Controlled drugs

'Controlled drugs' include strong painkillers, particularly those related to morphine. In the UK, anyone intending to carry these into or out of the country may require a licence. For further details, contact the Home Office, tel. 020 7273 3806. Applications take 10 days to process.

These import/export licences facilitate passage only through UK Customs and Excise control. For clearance in the country to be visited, it would be necessary to apply to the consulate of the country concerned.

It is good practice to keep a careful record of all use of controlled drugs while abroad, including their safe return and disposal.

Pessaries and suppositories need to be protected from extreme heat — they are designed to melt at body temperature.

Treating local people

It can be an act of kindness to help local people in cases of emergency, but travellers need to be extremely cautious about giving medicines and indeed any form of medical treatment to local people. They may cause harm and, in particular, it is easy by doing so to undermine confidence in the local health system, which can be even more damaging in the long term. Travellers, and even travelling doctors and nurses, may not be in a position to understand locally prevalent diseases and problems such as drug resistance. If you have any medical supplies left over, find a local doctor or nurse or health worker to give them to, don't distribute them to people who may not know how to use them. See also p. 533.

Athletes abroad

Athletes packing a travel kit should know that some of the medicines listed here may be banned from use in competitive sport, and should be especially wary of any remedies purchased abroad: banned ingredients may not be obvious from the packaging. There may be important differences in formulation between the same brand of product sold in different countries: a British skier in the 2002 Winter Olympics was stripped of a bronze medal after using a US version of Vicks Sinex nasal inhaler. Unlike the UK product, the US formulation contains amphetamine derivatives, banned from sports. In the UK, futher information can be obtained from the Anti-Doping Directorate, UK Sports, 40 Bernard St, London WC1N 1ST (020 7841 9500); they operate a special Drug Enquiry line (020 7841 9531), and also a website (**www.uksport.gov.uk**) with links to other international bodies. British athletes travelling abroad are also advised to contact the British Olympic Association Medical Centre (020 8864 0609). Elsewhere, athletes should contact appropriate national sporting bodies.

Diarrhoea

The advantages and disadvantages of the use of anti-diarrhoeal agents for symptomatic treatment of diarrhoea are discussed in detail on p. 35. One of the following should suffice

- Loperamide hydrochloride (e.g. Arret, Imodium)
- Codeine phosphate*
- Diphenoxylate with atropine (Lomotil)*

Of these, loperamide is generally preferable, since it is the fastest acting and has fewest side effects. It acts locally on the intestine, without entering the general circulation. It is suitable for use by athletes, since it does not influence the results of drug tests. In the recommended dosage, Lomotil often causes a dry mouth and headache; it is unpleasant to take, and is now seldom used.

The theoretical place of anti-diarrhoeal drugs continues to be the subject of debate, but most doctors seem to use them when they themselves have troublesome symptoms, particularly when symptoms threaten to disrupt travel plans. They should *not* be used in children.

Pepto-Bismol is a popular remedy in the USA, but is of only moderate effectiveness; it too should not be used on children.

Hidrasec (racecadotril) is a new drug that dramatically reduces secretion of fluid into the gut; it appears to be safe and highly effective. It is available in France and many other countries, though not in the UK. Other, similar drugs are under development.

See below for antibiotic treatment/prevention, and treatment of dehydration.

Intestinal infections

Treatment
Treatment of diarrhoea with antibiotics is discussed at length on p. 32. Useful antibiotics to consider carrying if you might need to treat yourself are:

- Ciprofloxacin (Ciproxin)*
- Azithromycin (Zithromax)*
- Metronidazole(e.g. Flagyl, Zadstat)*
- Tinidazole (e.g. Fasigyn)*

A single dose of ciprofloxacin is sufficient to treat 80 per cent of cases of travellers' diarrhoea — if symptoms persist, a three to five day course should be completed. Ciprofloxacin should not be used in pregnancy or in children.

Azithromycin is a possible alternative to ciprofloxacin. It is a macrolide antibiotic — belonging to the same family as erythromycin, but with less likelihood of gastro-intestinal side effects; it is a suitable choice for travellers to parts of Southeast Asia where there may be a high rate of resistance to ciprofloxacin; it has the added advantage of being suitable for use in children.

A relatively large quantity of metronidazole would be needed to treat a bout of amoebic dysentery, so tinidazole might be a more practical alternative — just four tablets a day for two or three days would be required for the complete course of treatment. The tablets are film-coated, and are therefore a good way of avoiding the unpleasant taste of metronidazole.

All of them may be used safely in people who are allergic to penicillin.

Mebendazole (Vermox)* can be used for the treatment of some of the worm infestations mentioned on pp. 48–9. For the treatment of threadworm a single tablet of mebendazole 100 mg (e.g. Ovex) can be purchased in the UK without a prescription.

Prevention
Prevention of travellers' diarrhoea with antibiotics is discussed on pp. 36–7.

Dehydration

Severe diarrhoea causes rapid loss of fluid and salts, which can be particularly dangerous in small children, but can also cause symptoms in adults. Glucose promotes intestinal absorption of salts and water, and an understanding of this mechanism led to the formulation of special oral rehydration solutions. These solutions are easy to prepare, and instructions for making one's own are given on pp. 31–2. They are an effective remedy. A double-ended plastic spoon for measuring the correct amounts of sugar and salt can be obtained free from TALC, PO Box 49, St Albans, Herts, UK (send a stamped, addressed envelope and, if possible, a donation to support their excellent health educational work in developing countries).

Oral rehydration powders such as Electrolade and Dioralyte provide all the necessary ingredients in convenient sachets, which can simply be added to water, and should be carried in high-risk zones, especially when travelling with children. Similiar products are generally readily available worldwide. In the UK, Dioralyte is also available as effervescent tablets.

Salt losses increase through sweating if undertaking a lot of physical activity under tropical conditions and salt replacement may be necessary. Depending on the nature of your trip, it may be worth travelling with a small supply of ordinary table salt in a small, waterproof container. Salt *tablets* should not be used.

Constipation

Of those in the UK who have a problem with constipation, 10 per cent are 'regular' sufferers. Travel can often tip the balance, even for people who normally have no problem. Dehydration, long journeys, readjustment of bowel habits after crossing time zones, dietary changes (including low-residue airline food), and initial reluctance to use dirty toilets may each contribute to the problem. A high fluid intake and a high-fibre diet are preferable to medication; it may be worth travelling with a small supply of natural bran (also available in tablet form). Senokot tablets are a safe and effective laxative if this is required.

Heartburn and indigestion

This is a common complaint at home and abroad, and can be exacerbated by unfamiliar foods and over-indulgence in alcohol. There is little to choose between the various antacid preparations; select one that is to your taste and not too bulky to carry (e.g. Bisodol).

Gastric acid has a slight protective effect against several intestinal infections, so antacids should not be used unless symptoms warrant — nor should drugs that reduce acid secretion, like cimetidine (Tagamet) and ranitidine (Zantac). 'Proton pump inhibitors' (PPIs) are a new class of drugs that stop acid secretion almost completely — the effect is so powerful as to justify preventive antibiotic use in some circumstances. (The most popular brands include Losec, Zoton, Pariet, and Protium.)*

Vomiting

Specific treatment of vomiting in food poisoning is not generally advised or considered necessary unless symptoms are sufficiently severe as to require skilled medical treatment.

Once vomiting has begun, treatment with tablets is unlikely to afford relief and prochlorperazine suppositories 25 mg (Stemetil, Compazine)* would be an alternative to injections, although they could melt in very hot climates. There is also a preparation of prochlorperazine (Buccastem)* that can be placed between the upper lip and gum, and so is absorbed through the lining of the mouth. The dosage is one or two 3 mg tablets twice daily.

Metoclopramide tablets (Maxolon, Primperan, Reglan)* 10 mg are occasionally useful to treat nausea unrelated to motion sickness.

Motion sickness

Motion sickness is, by definition, almost exclusively a complaint of travellers, although individuals vary considerably in their susceptibility. It is discussed in greater detail on p. 271.

Since different anti-motion-sickness drugs appear to suit different people, susceptible individuals may need to try several different pills on successive occasions until they find an effective remedy or regimen — and then keep to it. Both hyoscine-containing pills such as Kwells and anti-histamine-containing remedies such as promethazine (Avomine, Phenergan) can have unwanted side effects; in particular, do not drive after taking them, as they may cause drowsiness (see also pp. 275–6). Cinnarizine (Stugeron) is also very effective and will take effect more quickly if the tablet is sucked.

Hyoscine is called scopolamine in the USA. It is also available in the form of an adhesive patch (Scopoderm TTS)* that allows absorption of the drug through the skin, which remains effective for up to three days (see p. 276). These should not be used in children or the elderly, and may also cause drowsiness.

Some preparations of hyoscine (e.g. Kwells) contain instructions to dissolve the tablets in the mouth, for rapid absorption. Otherwise, remember that anti-motion-sickness pills are of little use once vomiting has started — and make a point of taking the pills some hours before your journey begins.

Urinary tract infections

Symptoms of 'cystitis' are common in women and troublesome when they occur during a trip. Sufferers from cystitis should discuss the problem with their own doctor before leaving home.

Trimethoprim* in a dose of 200 mg, twice daily for 3–5 days, is likely to be effective for most urinary tract infections, but will not treat gonorrhoea, which is a possible cause of urinary symptoms in travellers. Dr Naponick's comments about this on pp. 442–3 are worth noting. Other options include ampicillin* (two doses of 3 g, or 500 mg eight-hourly), co-amoxiclav (Augmentin)* 250–500 mg 8-hourly, and ciprofloxacin (Cipro) 250–500 mg twice daily. Three days' treatment is usually sufficient.

Vaginal infections (candidiasis, thrush, yeast)

Like cystitis, a vaginal infection can be a particularly annoying problem when it occurs abroad. Treatment is discussed on p. 442, and it is well worth travelling with a suitable remedy, especially if you are prone to such an infection. An effective single-dose oral treatment, fluconazole (Diflucan 150), is available. If a pessary (vaginal suppository) is to be used, one clotrimazole 500 mg pessary (Canesten 1, Mycelex) will clear up an infection. See also p. 464.

Other infections

Causes of fever in travellers are discussed on p. 449. Do not rely upon antibiotics to treat a fever without seeking medical advice unless the cause of the fever is obvious. It is sometimes worth travelling with a course of antibiotics in case of throat, chest, or middle ear infections. Amoxycillin (Amoxil)* is probably a good choice with erythromycin (Erythrocin)* as an alternative for those allergic to penicillin, although the latter tends to cause a high incidence of nausea and vomiting. The other type of infections which may cause problems in travellers are those of skin and wounds; again erythromycin could be used but co-amoxyclav (Augmentin)* would be a better choice, although more expensive. Antibiotics for use in a fever are discussed further on p. 431.

Generally the first sign of allergy is a rash and any antibiotic should be discontinued if this develops.

Pain

Headache, toothache, sunburn, minor injuries, and other causes of mild to moderate pain respond well to aspirin, paracetamol, or ibuprofen. If you have a history of more severe pain (e.g. from backache or arthritis), if you will be away for a long time, or if you will be involved in activities that might put you at higher risk of injury, it might be worthwhile taking along a more powerful, prescription painkiller, if your doctor is willing to prescribe one. Here are some of the options:

Aspirin Water-soluble preparations reduce the chance of gastric symptoms, and are absorbed more rapidly. Aspirin reduces temperature in a fever. It should be avoided by sufferers from stomach ulceration, and should not be given to children. The dosage for pain relief is 300–900 mg (usually 1–3 tablets) 4–6 hourly whereas the dosage to achieve a blood–thinning effect (such as for DVT prevention) is 75–150 mg daily.

Paracetamol (Panadol, Tylenol) has a comparable pain relieving effect to aspirin, and causes no gastric symptoms. It also reduces temperature in fever, though less effectively than aspirin. (It is called acetaminophen in the USA). Available for children as Calpol, in bottles or sachets.

Codeine phosphate is often used by travellers to relieve diarrhoea, as a constipating agent; in a dose of 30–60 mg, four-hourly, it is also a valuable remedy for moderate pain, and codeine in smaller doses can be purchased without a prescription in the UK when combined with paracetamol (e.g. Panadeine) or aspirin (e.g. Codis).

Ibuprofen (e.g. Nurofen) has anti-inflammatory properties that make it particularly useful for treating muscle and joint aches and pains. Like aspirin, sufferers from stomach ulcers must avoid it.

Diclofenac (Voltarol)* belongs to the same category of drugs, but is more suitable for moderate to severe pain. It is available in a variety of preparations, including soluble and suppositories, but the most suitable form for travel is probably the long-lasting 75 mg tablet — the dose is one tablet 12–24 hourly. This should also be avoided by those with a history of stomach ulcers.

Buprenorphine (Temgesic)* has often been recommended to travellers in case of moderate to severe pain, because although it is a powerful drug, at one time it could be prescribed without the kind of restrictions that apply to drugs like morphine, and therefore was unlikely to cause problems with customs officials. It has now been reclassified as a controlled drug within the UK, although up to 10 tablets can be carried without a licence. *Tramadol* (Zydol, Ultram)* is a new painkiller, which while probably not quite as potent as buprenorphine, is not yet classified as a controlled drug.

Dihydrocodeine An alternative, although not as useful in controlling very severe pain, would be dihydrocodeine tablets (DF118)*, taken at a dose of 30 mg every eight hours. Dihydrocodeine is also effective as a combined preparation with paracetamol, called co-dydramol (Paramol)*, which is also available in a non-prescription formulation that contains less dihydrocodeine. Hydrocodone is similar to dihydrocodeine and more widely available in the USA, also combined with paracetamol (e.g. Lortab).

Codeine, dihydrocodeine, and hydrocodone are all quite closely related to morphine, and regulations regarding their use can vary in different countries. As well as carrying a copy of the original prescription it is perhaps advisable to have a letter from the prescribing doctor explaining why they are necessary. This would not normally apply to the small amount of codeine in the compound preparations. However, in 1987 there was a single report regarding a nurse who was arrested and fined for carrying 10 tablets of Panadeine into Greece. The Greek government has since explained that this incident was a result of a misunderstanding and that there is no problem with carrying small quantities of such tablets for personal use, but it is conceivable that similar problems might occur elsewhere.

Children

Anyone travelling with small children should also take along a suitable children's analgesic such as Calpol (available in sachets) or ibuprofen syrup (e.g. Junifen).

Jet lag

Melatonin is discussed on p. 264. In the US and certain other countries, this is classed as a food supplement and so is widely available. In the UK, however, it is considered a medicine. It remains unlicensed and is virtually unobtainable. A short-acting sedative/hypnotic such as zaleplon or zopiclone (see below) may be helpful during readjustment of sleep patterns. (See also p. 268)

Sleep

Sleeping tablets can be helpful on especially long and tiring journeys — particularly across time zones, or overnight journeys in noisy surroundings. However, there has

> The world's worst urban nightmare, or Africa's most vibrant city? The constant roar of traffic, blare of car horns, and wail of loudspeakers competing to summon the Faithful to prayer from several thousand minarets, have forced 62 per cent of Cairo residents to resort to sleeping pills in order to get to sleep, according to a report in *The Times*. The favoured remedy is Valimil, the local brand of Valium, and earplugs are also at a premium.

been increasing concern about the relationship between immobility and the risk of deep vein thrombosis; falling deeply asleep in a cramped, seated position, would seem to increase the risk. Sleeping medication should therefore be used in the lowest possible dosage, if at all, and ideally should be reserved for situations in which it is possible to stretch out fully in a horizontal position.

Following a westward journey, sleep is often interrupted in the small hours of the morning, with difficulty falling asleep again; following eastward journeys, the problem is difficulty falling asleep in the first place. Sleeping medication does not speed up adjustment to a new time zone, but used carefully for the first two or three nights after arrival, it can help cope with readjustment of sleep patterns.

Adults
Zopiclone (Zimovane)* (3.75–7.5 mg) is a suitable option — try starting with the lower dose. It has a metallic taste, which some people don't like but which is quite useful because you can tell when it has been absorbed and when it is out of your system. It provides 6–8 hours of sleep. A similar preparation is zolpidem (Stilnoct, Ambien)*, which is also available in the US.

Zaleplon (Sonata)* (10 mg) is shorter-acting. It can be used at bedtime, or during the night if you awake and cannot get back to sleep (see p. 270).

To prevent early morning waking, such as after westbound travel, a longer acting drug may be appropriate. Temazepam* 10 mg is suitable, but is now a controlled drug in the UK following problems with abuse. Alternatives might be nitrazepam* 5 mg or flurazepam* 15 mg.

Children
Promethazine (Phenergan) in a dose of 5–10 mg for children aged six to twelve months; 15–20 mg for children aged one to five years; and 20–25 mg for children aged six to ten years, may be useful occasionally. (See p. 493.)

Malaria prophylaxis and treatment
A detailed discussion of the choice and dosage of anti-malarial drugs can be found on p. 145. For those who object to the bitter taste of chloroquine, it is worth knowing that the Nivaquine brand of chloroquine sulphate comes as film-coated tablets.

Side effects

As chloroquine-resistant malaria has become more common, large numbers of travellers have had to resort to alternative drugs such as mefloquine* and doxycycline*. There is much debate concerning the true scale of potential problems associated with mefloquine and whether the benefits outweigh any potential risks (pp. 147–8). An important problem limiting the use of doxycycline is a relatively high incidence of photosensitivity reactions, where even high SPF sunscreens are unable to provide adequate protection. Malarone* is a more recent addition to the armoury, with fewer side effects but at greater cost. It is important to seek confirmation that any proposed regimen is both appropriate and safe before travel by contacting one of the sources listed in Appendix 8.

Insect bites

Treatment

Crotamiton (Eurax) cream or lotion is often sufficient to relieve local irritation, and is probably more effective than calamine lotion. An alternative that many people find effective is tea tree oil; the Chinese remedy, White flower lotion, can also be helpful.

Anti-histamines may be required if bites are widespread, with persistent, itchy wheals. Anti-histamine creams and ointments should be avoided — sensitivity to them can occur. Chlorpheniramine maleate (Piriton, Chlor-Trimeton) tablets in a dose of 4–16 mg daily are often helpful, but tend to cause drowsiness. Loratadine (Clarityn) 10 mg once daily is an effective anti-histamine that does not do this.

Steroid creams such as betamethasone (e.g. Betnovate, Diprosone)* are advised for those who develop severe reactions to bites — provided there is no evidence of infection and the skin is unbroken. Hydrocortisone cream (HC45, Lanacort) is a mild steroid cream that may be purchased without a prescription.

Antibiotic treatment is occasionally necessary when bites are scratched and become infected. The antibiotics described for skin infections in the previous section would be suitable. Such bites also need careful local treatment, to prevent formation of a skin ulcer that may take many weeks to heal.

Prevention

Insect repellents are a most sensible precaution, and are an essential part of any medical kit for travel to a hot country — see p. 208.

DEET is the most widely-tested insect repellent, which has been in both civilian and military use since the 1950s. If travelling to malaria endemic areas it is probably the repellent of choice and can be found in a variety of products both on the UK and US market. Its principal drawback is that most products need to be reapplied frequently to the skin; a more concentrated product tends to last longer. A repellent containing between 30–50 per cent DEET would be optimal for skin application, although many are formulated with alcohol, which rapidly evaporates on application leaving behind 100 per cent DEET on the skin surface.

Any worries about the safety of DEET are largely overstated. There have been remarkably few reports of problems after normal use, considering that over a third of the population in the US and UK apply these products at least once a year. Its use in children is sometimes questioned on the grounds of a tiny number of reports of seizures that have emerged over the years. Even in these cases it is difficult to confirm a definite link to the use of DEET.

There are a number of other products available based on various plant extracts, but there is little evidence that they are any safer than DEET or effective enough to give worthwhile protection.

Allergies

Treatment of bee-sting allergy is discussed on p. 245. Travellers who have had a serious allergic reaction of any kind in the past are strongly advised to travel with all they may need in an emergency. If necessary, this includes adrenaline in preloaded syringes (EpiPen, Ana-Guard, Ana-Kit)*.

Chlorpheniramine tablets (Piriton) in a dose of 4–16 mg daily or loratadine (Clarityn) 10 mg daily are often useful to treat allergic skin reactions, and steroid creams may also be useful (see 'insect bites' above). Syrup is available for children.

If you suffer from hay fever, remember to take along any medication you may need. Hay fever seasons vary considerably between different countries (see p. 358).

Sunburn

Prevention is the most sensible strategy. Sunscreens (see also p. 335) should be applied liberally. Water-resistant sunscreens are widely available and are especially recommended for children. Stated protection factors usually refer to protection from UVB; check that any product you propose to use also protects against UVA. It is also a good idea to discard a product after a year, as they tend to lose their potency if not stored in a cool place.

Ibuprofen may also be of value if used soon after exposure to strong sunlight; it can be taken as tablets, or possibly also used as mousse or gel. Calamine lotion may be helpful for treatment of mild cases; calamine-containing creams (Lacto calamine) are less drying on the skin. Aspirin or paracetamol are also useful for pain relief (see 'painkillers' above).

Conjunctivitis

Eye irritation following excessive exposure to sun and dust, and minor eye infections, are common in traveller (p. 430).

Chloramphenicol eye ointment* is worth taking if medical supplies are not likely to be available *en route*, especially if you wear contact lenses. Chloramphenicol drops need to be stored in a fridge so an alternative preparation such as gentamicin (Genticin)* eye drops should be carried if necessary. Gentamicin is preferred to chloramphenicol in the USA. Propamidine eye drops and ointment (Brolene) are probably not quite as effective as the antibiotic preparations but can be purchased without a prescription in the UK.

On long-haul flights, comfort drops (artificial tears) should be used, especially if you wear contact lenses (pp. 433–5).

Colds/sinusitis

Air travellers liable to colds or sinusitis should travel with a decongestant spray (e.g. Sinex, Otrivine) to avoid discomfort from pressure changes during flight. Oral decongestant tablets containing pseudoephedrine (Sudafed) would also be useful.

A nasal saline spray (e.g. Sterimar) may also be helpful to maintain comfort and possibly to reduce the risk of airborne infection.

Cold sores, herpes blisters

Strong sunlight, cold, and wind can trigger cold sores (p. 426). Anyone who is prone to cold sores should use a high protection factor sunscreen on the lips. Applying acyclovir cream (Zovirax) at an early stage can help reduce the duration and severity of attacks. A lip salve (e.g. Chapstick) may also be helpful for chapped and sore lips.

Ear problems

External ear infection can be a problem for swimmers and divers. The problem is just as likely to be due to fungal infection as bacterial, and advice on suitable drops to take is given on p. 379.

First-aid — cuts, grazes, and animal bites

Prompt cleansing of any wound — with running water, or better still, with an antiseptic solution — is the most important step in treatment. Subsequently, keeping a wound clean and dry under arduous travelling and living conditions in a tropical environment can be difficult, but is of great importance.

Treatment

Local people sometimes ask travellers to remote areas to treat minor wounds, and it is worth carrying extra supplies of an antiseptic.

Iodine is a valuable antiseptic agent, and povidone iodine tincture (Betadine paint) comes with a small brush which is very convenient for travellers, although it does tend to sting. A dry powder povidone iodine spray is now available in a small container (Savlon Dry, Betadine Aerosol Spray) which does not sting, and removes the need to touch damaged skin.

Cetrimide and chlorhexidine cream (e.g. Savlon) is also a useful antiseptic for minor grazes. Savlon antiseptic solution can be used for cleaning wounds; it can be conveniently carried in sachets (Savlodil) or plastic steripods rather than a bottle, which might become contaminated with bacteria. In the USA the equivalent preparation contains chlorhexidine alone (Hibiclens).

Steristrips and similar adhesive tapes are useful for holding together the edges of a clean, gaping wound if medical care cannot be obtained.

Wound dressings Band-aids or other sticking plasters are essential for minor wounds and cuts. It is also worthwhile carrying non-adherent dressings (e.g. Melolin) which may be difficult to obtain abroad, together with tape (e.g. Micropore or zinc oxide) with which to attach them. For those engaged in more hazardous activities, a standard wound dressing (BPC No. 14) would be useful in an emergency. Keep wounds clean and dry; if they are weeping, change dressings frequently.

A crepe (ace) bandage may provide relief following a joint injury, but anything less than 7.5 cm would be of little use on a knee joint, for example. Other bandages, dressings, and slings can usually be improvised, and are probably not worth taking. Larger expeditions may need to consider more extensive first-aid supplies, including inflatable or malleable aluminium (SAM) splints.

Antibiotic treatment may occasionally be necessary if infection is more than trivial. Animal bites carry a high risk of infection and warrant antibiotic treatment preventively (see p. 228). Suitable choices include amoxycillin, tetracycline, cefuroxime axetil and co–amoxiclav.

Fungal skin infections
Anti-fungal cream and dusting powder is useful for treatment of athlete's foot and other fungal skin infections. See also pp. 410 and p. 437.

Some other things to take
1. *Water purification supplies* are discussed in detail on pp. 73–83. I usually take along a small plastic dropping bottle of 2 per cent tincture of iodine — one drop will purify a cup of water — which doubles as a useful antiseptic for minor cuts.
2. *Contact lens solutions* Take ample supplies, and do not rely upon being able to obtain your preferred brand abroad. Bottles of sterile intravenous saline can usually be obtained cheaply from pharmacies in most countries, and are useful in an emergency if other supplies run out. Keep solutions with you on long flights.
3. *Contraceptive needs* are discussed on pp. 476–83.
4. *Feminine hygiene* Take all your likely needs with you, unless you know that acceptable supplies will be available locally (p. 440).
5. Male travellers over the age of 65, or who have a history of prostatic symptoms (such as hesitancy or difficulty passing urine, or a poor urinary stream) should talk to their doctor about the possibility of travelling with a sterile urinary catheter that could be used by a local doctor in an emergency. In remote places, and in many developing countries, such items may not be easily available.
6. *Thermometer* If required, a thermometer should be carried in a protective container, and kept away from excessive heat. An ordinary clinical thermometer is

not suitable for detecting or monitoring hypothermia (see p. 343); a special, low-reading thermometer should also be taken if likely to be needed. Disposable liquid crystal thermometers are cheap, lightweight, and accurate.

7. *Toilet paper* In many parts of the world, toilet paper is not used or is not readily available, the preference being for washing or, sometimes, using sand. Away from the beaten track, it is generally advisable to take your own supply; otherwise you risk discovering, in the words of one frequent business traveller to China, 'what socks are for'.

8. *Antiseptic wipes* — wipes soaked in chlorhexidine or alcohol — are also useful for cleaning minor wounds, and at a pinch can be used on suspicious-looking plates and cutlery. Wet wipes are useful for cleaning hands before touching food.

9. *Lancets* These are small sterile needles covered with a twist-off plastic cap. They are normally used for pricking the thumb to obtain a small droplet of blood for testing. They are ideal for use by travellers to remove splinters or burst a blister.

10. *Rubs* If there is much walking to be done, a rub for muscle aches or sprains can provide relief. There are many preparations on the market, from the new anti-inflammatory preparations such as ibuprofen cream, gel, or mousse, which are widely available in the UK, to traditional remedies like Tiger Balm.

11. *Malaria diagnosis* Travellers to remote malarial areas who develop a fever may have to treat themselves presumptively for malaria. If a blood film is made prior to treatment, this can be extremely helpful in confirming the diagnosis at a later stage. The technique is simple to learn, and travel clinic staff may be willing to show you how to prepare your own film. Blood-testing kits are a possible alternative — only a small finger prick of blood is needed for an instant result. They are currently available for the diagnosis of malaria (Malapack, Malaquick) (see also p. 138, p. 449); others, for diseases like dengue (p. 161), will be available soon. The main drawbacks are their relatively high cost and their limited shelf-life plus the fact that careful instruction is necessary for successful use.

12. *Tick tweezers* For safe removal of ticks. Available from pet shops and veterinary suppliers.

13. *Blood group record* (see p. 592)

14. *Toiletries* If you have sensitive skin, consider travelling with your usual brands rather than relying on hotel supplies — these are a common source of skin reactions.

Injections abroad: needle kits

According to the World Health Organization, about 12 billion injections are given each year — 5 per cent are immunizations, and the rest are for medication. World-wide, non-sterile injections cause between 8 and 16 million cases of hepatitis B every year, 2 to 4 million cases of hepatitis A, and 75 000 to 150 000 cases of HIV/AIDS. The situation is worst in India and Taiwan, where more than 60 per cent of hepatitis B infections are attributed to unsafe injections. World-wide, unsafe injections cause an estimated 1.3 million deaths. Further information can be found at **www. injectionsafety.org**

In China 60 per cent of the population is hepatitis B positive — largely as a result of unsafe injections. A UNICEF study in 2000 found that up to 65 per cent of children in rural areas had received injections as a treatment for their most recent cold; many children receive more than six injections a year (other than immunizations) and in one rural county, 88 per cent of the injections given were found to be unsafe. Many patients are culturally attuned to expecting an injection, just as many poorly trained doctors and medical people may be culturally and perhaps financially attuned to providing them.

Hepatitis B has occurred in numerous travellers who have received injections with contaminated needles and syringes, and the HIV risk from this route of infection is also considerable. In the countries where unsafe injections are most common, more than half of all medical consultations result in injections being given, yet most such injections are completely unnecessary: satisfy yourself that there is a genuine need for an injection before agreeing to receive one.

Disposable pre-sterilized needles and syringes are not widely available in many poor countries. If you are going abroad to live in one, or expect that you will need any medication by injection (including dental anaesthesia) while you are away, you should either satisfy yourself that any needle or syringe used has been adequately sterilized (i.e. boiled for at least 10 minutes) or you should take your own supply. Remember that if you have an accident when driving abroad, a blood test for alcohol may be compulsory — in Turkey, for example. (See also p. 402 and p. 425)

In the UK, needles and syringes are available without prescription at the discretion of a pharmacist. They are also available in kits that include other medical items, from travel clinics and the suppliers listed in Appendix 8. In the USA and most other countries, a prescription is necessary, and a prescription should always be carried when travelling. Many airlines prohibit needles and other sharp objects from being carried in hand luggage.

Blood transfusion and the traveller

In the event of injury or illness abroad, blood transfusion may be life-saving, but may bring dangers of its own. It is important to be aware of the risks, and to consider whether 'blood cover' through an organization such as the Blood Care Foundation may be appropriate for your needs.

Colonel (retired) Michael J.G. Thomas is the Clinical Director of the Blood Care Foundation. Previously he served for 34 years in the Royal Army Medical Corps, for the last eight of which he was the Director of the Army Blood Transfusion Service. He was responsible for the transfusion cover for the Falklands campaign, the Gulf War, and the British troops in Bosnia. He is the founder chairman of the Autologous Transfusion Group of the British Blood Transfusion Society.

If you are travelling overseas on business, or are taking a well-earned holiday, and you are involved in an accident and need a blood transfusion, would you know whether the blood provided in that particular country met the standards of your national transfusion service?

Problems

The problems with having a transfusion overseas fall into three groups: availability, transfusion-transmitted diseases, and testing of blood donations.

Availability

In developing countries there is a constant, severe shortage of blood — far worse than anything we ever have to face in Westernized countries. Some countries solve this problem by requiring relatives to donate blood. It is unlikely, however, that sufficient members of your family with the correct blood group (Fig 13.1) will be accompanying you, to cover your needs. In addition, when there are such acute shortages, there is also the ethical problem of whether it is right for a relatively affluent traveller, who has other means of obtaining blood, to use up a local resource, thereby depriving a local resident whose need may be greater.

Transfusion-transmitted diseases

In many parts of the world, the incidence of the common transfusion-transmitted diseases, such as HIV and hepatitis, is as much as 10 000 times higher than in the UK. This means that a donated unit of blood is much more likely to be infected. As the incidence is higher, the chances that an individual is in the early stage of a particular disease are increased. In such a situation the donor is in what is commonly known as the 'window period' — although the screening test has yet to become positive, the unit of blood is infected and would transmit the disease to a recipient. A recent study in Kenya found 6.4 per cent of blood donors to be HIV positive.

In addition, in some parts of the world diseases are prevalent that do not occur in Europe, but that can be transmitted by blood transfusion. Examples of such diseases are malaria, leishmaniasis, Chagas disease (p. 186), and filariasis.

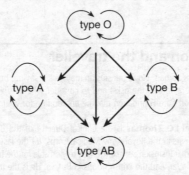

Fig 13.1 ABO blood groups: donors and recipients. For each blood group, the arrows indicate who can be a donor, and who can be a recipient. In addition, people who are 'Rhesus negative' must only receive Rhesus negative blood. People with 'O negative' blood are therefore described as 'universal donors' — in an emergency, they can usually donate blood to anyone: people who are 'AB positive' are described as 'universal recipients' — they can receive blood from anyone.

Ironically, as a result of the BSE outbreak in the UK, with human cases of new variant CJD (Creutzfeld Jakob disease) the USA has imposed restrictions on accepting blood from British and French donors.

Testing
In many countries, the health budget is insufficient to allow units of donated blood to be fully tested. If they are tested, frequently the test kits used are of a lesser quality.

Basic points

Avoidance
There is much truth in the old saying that 'the best blood transfusion is no blood transfusion' — so travellers should always be on their guard, and should do everything possible to avoid needing one.

Medical
Don't travel to countries where the transfusion facilities may be inadequate if:
- You suffer from a coagulation disorder, such as haemophilia or Von Willebrand's disease, or you are not properly stabilized on anticoagulant medication
- You have a medical condition which commonly requires transfusion, such as chronic peptic ulceration or oesophageal varices
- You are pregnant.

Behaviour
Being involved in an accident is the commonest reason for a traveller to require a blood transfusion. Avoiding accidents is, therefore, the most effective way of avoiding a transfusion.
- **Driving on the road** If you are driving in a foreign country take extra precautions, always remembering that you may have to drive on the opposite side of the road from that in your own country (p. 300). Always wear seat-belts; don't drive in the dark; don't drive too fast; and never drink and drive no matter how great the temptation, when you are on holiday and having a good time. In many countries, holiday-makers are encouraged to hire mopeds. If you do, always wear a crash helmet and protective clothing. Peace Corps volunteers have recently been banned from driving mopeds or motorcycles, and there has been a dramatic reduction in their injury rate (see also p. 294, p. 300)
- **Exploring on foot** One of the commonest causes of road accidents amongst travellers is looking the wrong way when crossing the road. If the traffic drives on the opposite side of the road to that to which you are accustomed, take great care, as your natural instinct is to look in the wrong direction and then step off in front of oncoming traffic. As you will be unfamiliar with the surrounding area, keep to well-lit streets where there are plenty of other people. Do not venture into areas where you are likely to be attacked
- **Hazardous sports** Avoid hazardous sports, especially if you are not being properly supervised. Take care when going off on mountain walks or hill climbing

- **Disease** Ensure that you avoid catching any disease that might require a blood transfusion as part of the treatment. The most common such disease is malaria; so when you are in an area where malaria is endemic, take adequate malarial prophylaxis (p. 144), wear long-sleeved shirts or blouses and long trousers after dark, and always sleep under a properly impregnated mosquito net (p. 208).

Be prepared
Before leaving home, there are a number of things that you can do to minimize any risks whilst you are abroad.
- **Blood group** Have your blood grouped before departure and make sure you take a copy of the laboratory report with you. **Knowing your blood group in advance will make it easier to find a blood donor in an emergency**
- **Sterile needles and syringes** Take a supply with you, as these may not be readily available in the countries to which you are going. Most travel clinics can provide packs especially designed for travellers
- **Intravenous fluids** It is possible to take plasma substitutes and/or crystalloid solutions for use in an emergency, though such products require skill to use, and an adequate supply is bulky and heavy. In an emergency, supplies can sometimes be obtained from embassies. Sterile transfusion equipment (giving sets and cannulae) may be difficult to obtain. Large expeditions with trained medical officers may find it valuable to travel with such resources, but these are impractical for the majority of travellers. If you do take such supplies with you, do not attempt to insert an intravenous line unless you are skilled in transfusion techniques. Failed attempts may ruin the only good venous access available and make it much more difficult for a doctor to eventually set up a transfusion
- **Medical assistance** It is vital that you take out adequate health insurance, which includes telephone support as well as emergency evacuation by air ambulance if indicated (p. 567)
- **Blood cover** It is also advisable to obtain cover from an institution that can provide screened blood (see below).

Solutions
One solution that used to be favoured by expatriates living in a small community was to set up and maintain a so-called 'walking blood bank', comprising a group of people who would be prepared to donate blood to meet a particular emergency. However, there are numerous problems associated with such a venture including:
- The number of people involved is so small that there is always a significant chance that sufficient blood of the required group will not be available
- As the members of the blood bank live locally, they will be liable to carry the diseases endemic to that area
- As all the members probably know each other, it is much more difficult for someone to opt out of donation if their social behaviour has put them at risk of transmitting infection

- Adequate quality control of such a small venture is very difficult, and the problems of product liability now make such blood banks non-viable.

For the above reasons, walking blood banks are now no longer clinically acceptable within the international medical community (Walker 1993). Blood, whenever practically possible, should be provided from a major licensed blood bank, to ensure high quality and to increase the likelihood that the requested number of units of suitable blood will be available rapidly. This is especially important for patients with rare blood groups or complicated antibody profiles.

In response to the difficulties in locating reliable sources of blood, and with the active encouragement of the expatriate medical and residential communities in Nigeria, a blood bank was established in Lagos in 1989 as a pilot exercise. The experience gained in setting up and operating, on an international basis, effective procedures for the handling, transportation, importation, and storage of blood, resuscitation fluids, and sterile equipment led, in 1991, to the establishment of the Blood Care Foundation.

The Blood Care Foundation

The Blood Care Foundation is a charitable organization, registered in England, that provides, in emergencies, screened blood (obtained from internationally recognized sources in western Europe), resuscitation fluids, and sterile transfusion equipment to its members in countries where these are not readily available.

Today, the Foundation operates a global network of blood banks, enabling it to provide whole blood, by courier service, to almost any location in the world within 12 hours (subject to the availability of scheduled air services).

It is now well recognized that your heart works most efficiently when your haemoglobin concentration is around 100 g/L. Most people in the UK have a level of between 140 g/L and 160 g/L. Because we all have this spare capacity, people rarely die from the anaemia caused by losing blood. People die from the lack of fluid volume, which is medically termed 'shock'. In emergencies, therefore, resuscitation fluids are normally required and will support the patient until blood can be provided. To ensure these are readily available, the Foundation has set up an integrated network of over 200 Regional Supply Points (RSP) throughout the world, which hold stocks of resuscitation fluids, including plasma expanders, and the sterile equipment needed for transfusion purposes.

Response

Should an emergency occur, one of the Foundation's alarm centres is contacted. The Duty Medical Officer (DMO) in the alarm centre will contact the doctor in charge of the case to identify the transfusion requirements. If required, the DMO will arrange for the provision of resuscitation fluids from an RSP and for a courier to take blood to the patient. The couriers are doctors or paramedics, trained in cardio-pulmonary resuscitation, and capable of putting up a transfusion, even in the shocked patient.

Options for the future

Intensive research into blood substitutes is continuing. One such product, Hemopure, is at an advanced stage of development and has been licensed in South Africa. It consists of a purified solution of haemoglobin, and has a shelf life without refrigeration of two years. More information is available at **www.biopure.com**.

Details of the services provided by the Blood Care Foundation can be found on **www.bloodcare.org.uk**, by telephoning +44(0)1403 262652 or writing to the Blood Care Foundation, Fieldfare, North Heath Close, Horsham, West Sussex, RH12 5PH, UK.

References

Walker, R. H. (1993). Neonatal and obstetric practice. In *Technical Manual*, 11th edu, p. 448. American Association of Blood Banks, Maryland.

14 Postscript: Challenges for the future

Disease eradication and the future

Success with smallpox eradication fuelled optimism that other diseases would follow in its wake. But while eradication of polio and the Guinea worm are also near, formidable challenges remain. Progress is too slow to allow travellers to think about lowering their guard, and there are lingering concerns over the security of laboratory stocks of smallpox virus.

Dr Richard Dawood is the Editor of this book, and first met several of those involved in smallpox eradication in West Africa during the 1970s. Their enthusiams for fighting disease proved contagious, and this book is a direct result!

The global eradication of smallpox was one of the landmark achievements of twentieth century medicine. Not the kind of medicine that I studied as an undergraduate medical student in central London during the 1970s, I hasten to add. While I was learning about the afflictions of industrialized, Western societies, epidemiologists from the World Health Organization and from the Centers for Disease Control (CDC) were tackling smallpox in the front line. Village by village, they immunized entire populations and conducted a tireless hunt for each and every known case of infection, devising ever more ingenious schemes to keep track of their own progress. In the final days of the campaign, telling the authorities about a case attracted a substantial reward, the value rising every week. By the end, more Indians knew the latest bounty on a case of smallpox than knew that Indira Ghandi was Prime Minister of the day.

Targeting smallpox

Smallpox had been responsible for an estimated billion deaths through the ages and its dissemination had always been closely linked to travel: its elimination was the result of an international effort co-ordinated by the WHO, lasting just 10 years. In 1980, just over two years after the last recorded case of smallpox, and following a period of careful surveillance, a Global Commission certified that the disease had indeed been eradicated. The total cost of the eradication programme amounted to just over $300 million — considerably less than the annual global cost of smallpox vaccination and other measures for its prevention and control.

For many reasons, smallpox had been an almost ideal target for eradication: its fearsome reputation made it easy to mobilize the necessary popular and political will;

the existence of a cheap, safe, and effective vaccine made prevention a straightforward matter; and the inability of the virus to persist in the environment meant that cases could only be spread directly from person to person: eliminate the cases, and you have eliminated the disease. Desirable attributes for eradicable diseases have been carefully studied, and some of these are listed in Table 14.1.

Table 14.1 What makes a disease eradicable?

Scientific and technical attributes

- Epidemiological vulnerability (e.g. presence or absence of a non-human reservoir of infection, ease of spread, natural cyclical decline in prevalence, naturally induced immunity, ease of diagnosis, duration of any relapse potential).

- Availabilty of effective options for prevention/intervention (e.g. vaccine, curative treatment, vectoricide. Ideally, these must be effective, safe, inexpensive, long-lasting, and easily deployed).

- Demonstrable feasibility of elimination (e.g. documented elimination from island, or other successful pilot operation).

Targeting other diseases

For a variety of reasons, other attempts at eradication had not been quite so successful: notable failures included malaria, cholera, yaws, and yellow fever.

Successful eradication of smallpox changed everything. The practical economic benefits were obvious to everyone (not least to travellers all over the world who could now tear up their vaccination certificates). Valuable scientific, medical, practical, and political experience had been gained; and veterans of the smallpox campaign were itching for further action: the logical next step was to focus the available experience and expertise on other diseases that might perhaps be eradicable.

In 1988, the International Task Force for Disease Eradication (ITFDE) was formed to systematically evaluate disease candidates for their global eradication potential (Table 14.2).

The ITFDE investigated 21 candidate diseases, and judged two of them — Guinea worm infection and poliomyelitis — to be eradicable; three of them — mumps, rubella, and taeniasis/cysticercosis (tapeworms) to be potentially eradicable; another three (onchocerciasis, yaws and endemic syphilis, and rabies) to be candidates for elimination of transmission or of clinical symptoms; and the remainder not presently eradicable.

Both Guinea worm infection and poliomyelitis are now the subject of active global eradication campaigns, and there has been substantial progress towards their elimination. Guinea worm is still endemic in 14 countries in Africa. Poliomyelitis is endemic in most developing countries outside the western hemisphere (where it has already been eliminated — no cases of polio due to indigenous wild virus have been reported in the Americas since August 1991).

Table 14.2 Communicable, diseases and their potential for eradication

Disease	Current annual toll world-wide	Chief obstacles to eradication	Conclusion
Guinea worm	75 000 cases recorded in 2000	Lack of public and political awareness; inadequate funding	Eradicable
Poliomyelities	2 800 cases in 2000	No insurmountable technical obstacles; increased national/international commitment needed	Eradicable
Onchocerciasis	18 million cases; 340 000 blind	High cost of vector control; no therapy to kill adult worms; restriction	Could eliminate associated blindness
Yaws and endemic syphilis	2.5 million cases	Political and finanical inertia	Could interrupt transmission
Rabies	2 million deaths	No effective way to deliver vaccine to wild animal disease carriers	Could eliminate urban rabies
Measles	2 million deaths, mostly children	Lack of suitably effective vaccine for young infants; cost; public misconception of seriousness	Not now eradicable
Tuberculosis	8–10 million new cases; 2–3 million deaths	Need for improved diagnostic tests, chemotherapy, and vaccine; wider application of current therapy	Not now eradicable
Leprosy	11–12 million cases	Need for improved diagnostic tests and chemotherapy; social stigma; potential reservoir in armadillos	Not now eradicable
Mumps	Unknown	Lack of data on impact in developing countries; difficult diagnosis	Potentially eradicable

Table 14.2 (continued)

Disease	Current annual toll world-wide	Chief obstacles to eradication	Conclusion
Rubella	Unknown	Lack of data on impact in developing countries; difficult diagnosis	Potentially eradicable
Hepatitis B	250 000 deaths	Carrier state, *in utero* infections not preventable; need routine infant vaccination	Not now eradicable
Neonatal tetanus	770 000 deaths	Inexhaustible environmental reservoir	Not now eradicable
Diptheria	Unknown	Difficult diagnosis; multiple dose vaccine; carrier state	Not now eradicable
Pertussis	60 million cases; 700 000 deaths	High infectiousness; early infections; multiple dose vaccine	Not now eradicable
Yellow fever	10 000 deaths	Sylvatic reservoir; heat-labile vaccine	Not now eradicable
Taeniasis/ Cysticercosis	50 million cases, 50 000 deaths	Need simpler diagnostics for humans and pigs	Potentially eradicable
Cholera	Unknown	Environmental reservoirs; strain differences	Not now eradicable
Chagas disease	200 million infected; 20 000 deaths	Difficult diagnosis and treatment; animal reservoirs	Not eradicable
Schistosomiasis	200 million infected;	Reservoir hosts; increased snail-breeding sites	Not now eradicable
Hookworm disease	1.3 billion infected; 65 000 deaths	Widespread	Not now eradicable

Guinea worm eradication

The guinea worm: infection

The medical name for this ancient infection is 'dracunculiasis', after the Latin name for the worm, *Dracunculus*, which means 'fiery serpent'. It is an infection of poor people in rural areas who drink water from infected pools or step wells. Because infection does not confer immunity against re-infection many people suffer from the disease year after year and much time is lost from growing food or schooling.

The female worm is 60–100 cm long and 2 mm in diameter. It travels under the skin and usually appears in the legs. The male worm is much smaller and dies after accomplishing his life"s work — impregnating the female!

The female worm reaches maturity about one year after initial infection, and secretes chemicals that cause ulceration of the overlying skin in the region of the creature"s head. The worm"s uterus protrudes through the resulting ulcer, and millions of living larvae are discharged in a milky fluid each time the ulcer is exposed to water. After about three weeks, birth of the larvae is complete and the worm dies. It is reabsorbed, emerges from the ulcer, or is extracted. This may be the end of the infestation, but unfortunately secondary bacterial infection of the ulcerated skin is common and may lead to serious sepsis in adjacent tissues, infection of neighbouring joints, or even tetanus.

Many villagers are incapacitated for weeks at a time by guinea worms. After the worm has discharged her larvae the old method of attaching the worm to a stick and winding it out of the ulcer slowly day by day is still useful; but the ulcer must be kept clean, well covered, and away from water sources used for drinking. Several drugs are available to facilitate extraction of the worm and antibiotics may be needed for bacterial infection.

Larvae that escape from the worm through the skin ulcer and reach fresh water may be swallowed by tiny shrimp-like creatures called cyclops. Within cyclops the larvae develop and grow, and become infective to humans about four weeks later. Once swallowed in contaminated water the cyclops are digested, freeing the larvae, which then burrow through the intestinal wall; they find their way to the subcutaneous tissues and become adult in about a year.

Contamination of water supplies occurs when people with guinea worm ulceration stand in drinking water or bathe their ulcers there. The larvae can then reach and infect cyclops, which are later swallowed. Transmission is especially common during the dry season when water supplies in ponds and wells dry up or become small in volume.

Travellers are at risk if they drink untreated water from primitive water supplies in areas where guinea worm infection still exists, but this is an unusual infection in travellers unless they are living rough or travelling in poor rural areas in the tropics, and this risk is declining fast, thanks to the eradication programme. Boiling, filtration, or chemical treatment of drinking water removes all risk.

India was the first country to undertake an organized programme to eliminate Guinea worm disease in 1980. In 1986, the WHO officially launched the global eradication programme, and in 1991 it adopted an eradication target of 1995.

Pakistan and India were certified as achieving interruption of transmission in 1997 and 2000 respectively. In Africa, Ghana and Nigeria commenced their own efforts at eradication in 1987 and 1988, successfully reducing their combined total of cases from 850 000 in 1989 to 15 000 in 2000. Most other endemic countries now have active, well-organized programmes.

Protecting drinking water from contamination with *Dracunculus* larvae is the key to interrupting transmission. The ideal approach, provision of safe water sources (usually tube wells) is expensive and slow, and was not sufficient on its own to enable the 1995 target date for eradication to be met. Other approaches include filtering all drinking water through finely-meshed cloth, health education to prevent contamination of drinking water sources in the first place, or applying a chemical, temephos (Abate), to water sources at four-week intervals to kill the tiny water fleas (cyclops) that carry the larvae.

The eradication campaign also involves searching for cases of disease, village-by-village, case reporting and surveillance, coupled with cash rewards as cases become increasingly scarce. Any cases that are found need to be carefully followed up and investigated, and the surveillance system that has been established in the countries concerned will be a valuable legacy to the polio eradication campaign.

The number of offiically recorded Guinea worm cases world-wide fell from 1 million cases in 1989 to 75 000 in 2000, in just 14 African countries. But with 50 000 of these cases coming from Sudan, it is very clear that by far the biggest obstacle to successful eradication is the continuing unrest there. Thousands of villages are still affected, and the challenge now is whether or not the necessary efforts can be sustained.

Polio eradication

By 2000, the number of officially reported cases of polio had fallen to 2800 world-wide (see also p. 52). The true extent of the disease remains hidden, however, because for every paralytic case there are 100 persons who carry the virus and can infect others, but have no symptoms themselves.

The effort to eradicate polio began in 1985, when the Pan American Health Organization (PAHO) declared a goal of eliminating polio from the Americas by 1990. Its progress prompted the WHO, in 1998, to declare a goal of global eradication by the year 2000.

In the Western hemisphere, measures like national vaccination days using OPV (oral polio vaccine) and intensive surveillance for cases, resulted in a fall in the number of reported cases from about 1000 in 1986 to just 9 in 1991. No cases have been detected there since. Success in the Americas demonstrated that eradication is feasible, and the current global strategy draws heavily on this experience: it includes maintaining high OPV coverage levels, improving case surveillance, and maintaining a global laboratory network.

The Western Pacific Region of WHO, which includes the People's Republic of China, was certified formally as polio-free in October 2000. The WHO's European Region has been polio-free since November 1997. Although a number of countries in the African, Eastern Mediterranean, and Southeast Asian regions still report endemic poliomyelitis, regional and national elimination plans have been developed and are being implemented. Major challenges facing the global initiative include funding, maintaining the necessary political and public support, and improving surveillance so as to detect the remaining foci of transmission.

The current target date for eradication is 2005, and more information about the campaign's progress can be found at **www.polioeradication.org**.

The future of disease eradication

Eradication programmes have a unique ability to mobilize resources that would not otherwise be forthcoming. With polio in particular, as with smallpox, the benefits to industrialized countries of being able to abandon mass vaccination have a special appeal. Despite delays in achieving their targets, demonstrable progress towards the eradication of polio and Guinea worm continues to focus attention upon the broader concept of disease eradication.

So too does progress with other diseases: for example, measles transmission has fallen to a very low level in the USA and Caribbean, and the WHO's Expanded Programme on Immunization has resulted in a fall in the number of cases world-wide from almost 4.5 million in 1980. Among the other candidate diseases now waiting in the wings are mumps, rubella, and *Taenia solium* (pork tapeworm) cysticercosis (see p. 49–50). Onchocerciasis (African river blindness) is a disease that had previously been targeted only for 'control'. Improved technology plus successful use of the anti-parasitic drug ivermectin (made available at no cost by its manufacturer) is beginning to make eradication a realistic option here too — especially if the guinea worm eradication programme succeeds in creating a precedent for eradicating a parasitic disease. In January 1998, the WHO launched a programme to eliminate lymphatic filariasis by 2020.

The International Task Force for Disease Eradication set out a rationale for eradication campaigns as a public health strategy that remains valid today:

- Control of a disease required unrelenting effort and investment; eradication is permanent
- Limited campaign duration, and campaign target dates, make concentrated efforts possible
- World-wide eradication targets create a powerful case for co-operation between neighbouring countries
- Eradication campaigns set a standard of success that is unambiguous.

Sequential eradication of diseases would multiply the benefits. The same health workers could be used in successive campaigns, with some of the savings achieved by elimination of one disease being devoted to an attack on the next.

Emerging infections and the international traveller

Far from diminishing, many disease hazards are on the increase: more than 30 previously unknown infectious agents have emerged as a problem in recent years, and others that once seemed to be under control have re-emerged as a threat. For now and for the foreseeable future, travellers need to inform themselves carefully about the likely risks, and take appropriate steps to control them.

Dr David L. Heymann is Executive Director of infectious disease programmes at the World Health Organization. Before joining WHO in 1989, Dr Heymann was a staff member of the US Centers for Disease Control and Prevention. He spent two years working with the Indian government in the smallpox eradication programme, and 13 years in sub-Saharan African ministries of health, strengthening the control of endemic childhood infections such as measles and diarrhoeal diseases, malaria and AIDS; and investigating disease outbreaks, including the first and second outbreaks of Ebola haemorrhagic fever.

The problem

During the past 20 years, well over 30 new infection-causing organisms have been identified ranging from new strains of influenza and hepatitis to haemorrhagic fevers. Many, if not most of these emerging infectious agents are thought to be transmitted to humans by animals, as in the case of bovine spongiform encephalopathy (BSE) in the UK. This disease was first identified during the 1980s and is caused by an infectious agent in cattle that has now been shown capable of infecting humans. Other agents which infect animals enter the food chain either at the time of food production or during its preparation. Emerging infections are a risk to the traveller either from contact with infected humans or animals, or as a result of eating contaminated food.

While new infections are emerging in human populations, known infections such as tuberculosis, cholera, and dengue fever have re-emerged, sometimes with a vengeance, also threatening the international traveller. Outbreaks of tuberculosis and legionnaires' disease have now been linked with travel, and the development of drug resistance to tuberculosis, gonorrhoea, and other common infections has further added to the problem, leading to the conclusion that an infectious disease in one country is the concern of all.

Each year there are countless travellers who cross international borders by land, air, and sea. They travel in small groups for pleasure, business, humanitarian work, or personal reasons such as religious pilgrimage; or they travel in larger groups for reasons of security, to seek safety from wars or natural disasters. With increases in travel, and a decrease in the time required to arrive at the final destination, humans, have become vectors of infection, carrying new and old infectious diseases from place to place within and between countries and continents. Seriously ill travellers who were medically evacuated to hospitals in Switzerland and South Africa were later found to have Ebola infection, and in South Africa fatal infection was spread to a health worker.

In 2000 a sports event in the jungle and rivers of Malaysia (Eco Challenge) — in which athletes from 29 states of the United States and 26 other countries participated — led to the importation of leptospirosis on four continents. (See also Map 14.1 and p. 371.)

In 1997, an outbreak of influenza among passengers and crew on a cruise ship travelling from New York to Montreal clearly demonstrated the ease with which infectious diseases can be transferred across international borders. In this outbreak, 3 per cent of passengers and many crew presented with acute febrile respiratory illness caused by a variant of a common influenza virus, and introduced this variant into both Canada and the USA.

Each year over 10 000 cases of malaria are reported among travellers returning to countries of the European Union. Such cases are misdiagnosed by health care staff, with potentially fatal consequences, if no information is provided about recent travel to a risk area for the disease.

The solution

The role of travel in the spread of infectious diseases has been known for centuries, and their control has long been a concern. Countries have attempted to limit their spread since at least the fourteenth century when the city-state of Venice introduced quarantine legislation aimed at keeping shipboard rats from introducing plague.

Infected humans travelling prior to the advent of air travel often developed illness and then either recovered or died before they arrived at their destination. With air travel today, when a traveller can be in a European or Latin American capital one day, and the next be in the centre of Africa or Asia, an infectious disease can remain in the incubation period and not appear until several days or weeks after travel has been completed.

International co-operation to control infectious diseases among travellers has been documented since 1851, with the first International Sanitary Conference in Paris. Many different treaties followed between countries, but they were often contradictory and remained non-standardized until 1951, when the World Health Organization (WHO) adopted the International Sanitary Regulations. These regulations were amended and renamed the International Health Regulations (IHR) in 1969. The IHR have as their objective to provide maximum protection against the spread of infectious disease with minimum interference with world travel and trade.

Though regulations such as the IHR provide an important structure for dialogue about infectious diseases among countries, and set out standards and norms for preventing and controlling infectious diseases, they are not a replacement for vigilance and response through strong national disease detection and control systems. And none of these are a replacement for the international traveller's personal responsibility and protection. There have been several recent cases of travellers returning to the USA, Switzerland, and Germany who had contracted yellow fever infection while on safari travel in jungle areas in Latin America and Africa. They had not been vaccinated prior to travel, and they returned home endangering not only their lives (they later died), but those of their communities where mosquitoes could have been present and transmitted the disease to others. Had these travellers been vaccinated prior to travel, the risk of a yellow fever infection would have been minimal.

Personal responsibility requires that knowledge obtained in guides such as this, and available from other sources in hard copy or on the world-wide web, be read, assimilated, and applied. National health services and international organizations such as the WHO are good sources of additional information. The responsible traveller should become informed and take the necessary preventive precautions prior to and

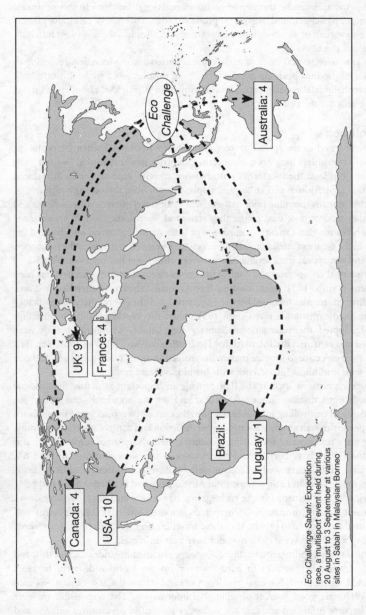

Map 14.1 Outbreak of leptospirosis (confirmed and suspected cases) among 312 participants, Eco Challenge 2000, Malaysia. (Source: World Health Organization).

Eco Challenge Sabah: Expedition race, a multisport event held during 20 August to 3 September at various sites in Sabah in Malaysian Borneo

Eco Challenge

Australia: 4

UK: 9

France: 4

Canada: 4

USA: 10

Brazil: 1

Uruguay: 1

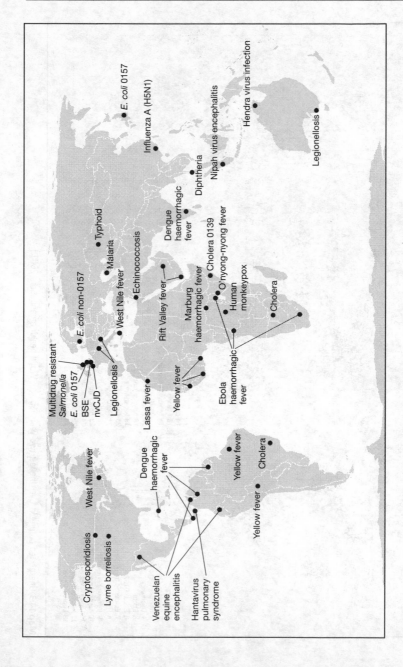

Map 14.2 Emerging and re-emerging infectious diseases, 1996-2001. (Source: World Health Organization, 2001)

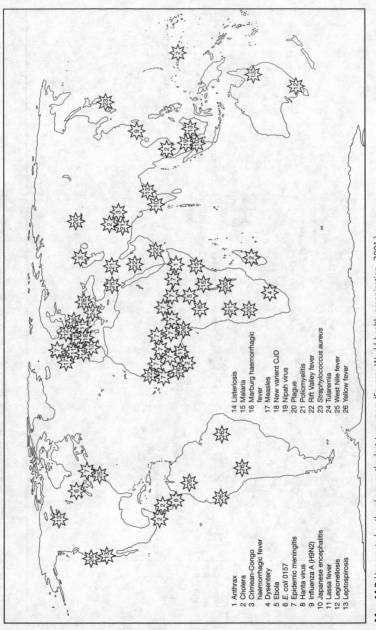

Map 14.3 Unexpected outbreaks over the last two years (Source: World health organization, 2001.)

1 Anthrax
2 Cholera
3 Crimean-Congo haemorrhagic fever
4 Dysentery
5 Ebola
6 *E. coli* 0157
7 Epidemic meningitis
8 Hanta virus
9 Influenza A (H9N2)
10 Japanese encephalitis
11 Lassa fever
12 Legionellosis
13 Leptospirosis
14 Listeriosis
15 Malaria
16 Marburg haemorrhagic fever
17 Measles
18 New variant CJD
19 Nipah virus
20 Plague
21 Poliomyelitis
22 Rift Valley fever
23 *Staphylococcus aureus*
24 Tularemia
25 West Nile fever
26 Yellow fever

during travel, and remain aware of the possibility of travel-related infection after return.

Further information

The WHO issues an annually updated publication containing recommendations for travellers, *International Travel and Health*, which can also be consulted at **www.who. int/ith**

WHO information about outbreaks and disease surveillance can be found at **www. who.int/disease-outbreak-news** and other sources listed in Appendix 8.

Conclusion

The eradication of polio will be the next major public health achievement, but only if adequate resources remain available to sustain the global effort to its conclusion. There are only limited prospects for eradicating the other major travel-related diseases, and for many years to come responsibility for staying healthy abroad will rest firmly with individual travellers themselves.

Eradication is an absolute: until now, it has been defined as the achievement of a status whereby no further cases of a disease occur anywhere, so that continued control measures are unnecessary. Both the United States and the former Soviet Union retained laboratory stocks of smallpox virus, however, and the fate of the former Soviet stock following the break-up of the Soviet Union is not fully known. The anthrax attacks in the USA in 2001 inevitably fuelled anxieties that smallpox virus might already have fallen into the hands of bioterrorists.

Perhaps we can no longer afford to believe that any disease has truly been eradicated while samples lurk unsecured in the deep freeze of an unknown laboratory, available one day for sale to the highest bidder. The U.S. government is re-stocking with smallpox vaccine, and a new drug, HDP-cidofovir, shows much promise as an oral treatment for smallpox. It would nonetheless be an unforgiveable act of betrayal if this terrible human scourge was ever permitted to reappear. Those entrusted with its security may yet have much to answer for.

Further reading

Fenner, F. et al. *Smallpox and its eradication* available at **www.who.int/enc/diseases/ smallpox/smallpoxeradication.html**

I am indebted to Andrew N. Agle, Dr Donald R. Hopkins, Dr William H. Foege, and Dr M. Karam for their contributions to this chapter.

Appendices

Appendix 1:
Vaccination requirements and recommendations

I: Requirements

The only formal international vaccination certificate requirements relate to yellow fever vaccination.

A. The following countries require a yellow fever vaccination certificate from ALL arriving travellers:

Benin	Côte d'Ivoire	Mauritania*
Burkina Faso	French Guiana	Niger
Cameroon	Gabon	Rwanda
Central African Republic	Ghana	Sao Tome & Principe
Congo	Liberia	Togo
Congo Democratic Republic (Zaire)	Mali	

B. The following countries require a yellow fever vaccination certificate **only** from travellers arriving from African or South American countries in the yellow fever endemic zone (Map A1, p. 612). These requirements do not apply to direct travel from the UK, USA, or Australasia.

Afghanistan	Cambodia	Grenada
Albania	Cape Verde	Guadeloupe
Algeria	Chad (R)	Guatemala
American Samoa	China	Guinea (R)
Angola (R)	Colombia (NC, R some areas)	Guinea–Bissau (R)
Antigua & Barbuda	Djibouti	Guyana (R some areas)
Australia	Dominica	Haiti
Bahamas	Ecuador (R some areas)	Honduras
Bangladesh	Egypt	India
Barbados	El Salvador	Indonesia
Belize	Equatorial Guinea (R)	Iran
Bhutan	Eritea	Iraq
Bolivia (R some areas)	Ethiopia	Jamaica
Brazil (R some areas)	Fiji	Jordan
Brunei	French Polynesia	Kenya (R)
Burma	Gambia	Kazakhstan
Burundi (R)	Greece	Kiribati

continued

Laos	Niue	Syria
Lebanon	Oman	Taiwan
Lesotho	Pakistan	Tanzania (R)
Libya	Panama (NC, R)	Thailand
Madagascar	Papua New Guinea	Tonga
Malawi	Paraguay	Trinidad & Tobago
Malaysia	Peru (R some areas)	Tunisia
Maldives	Phillipines	Uganda (R)
Malta	Pitcairn	Venezuela (NC, R some areas)
Mauritius	Portugal (Azores and Madeira only)	Vietnam
Mexico	Reunion	Yemen
Mozambique	Samoa	Zambia (NC, R)
Myanmar	Saudi Arabia	Sri Lanka
Namibia	Senegal (R)	St Kitts & Nevis
Nauru	Seychelles	St Lucia
Nepal	Sierra Leone (R)	St Vincent & the Grenadines
Netherlands	Singapore	Sudan (R some areas)
New Caledonia	Solomon Islands	Suriname (R)
Nicaragua	Somalia (R)	Swaziland
Nigeria (R)	South Africa	Zimbabwe

Key:

R = vaccination recommended even if not mandatory

NC, R = no certificate mandatory, only recommended for some areas

* = except for visits shorter than two weeks, with direct travel from UK, USA, or Australasia

T = required even from travellers who have been in transit through infected areas

Infants: in most, but not all cases, infants under one year are exempt from producing a certificate; however, the vaccine may sometimes nonetheless be recommended for their protection.

These guidelines are based on WHO sources (2002), but are subject to change. Check the exact regulations that apply at the time of travel, and make sure that you have no medical contraindications to the vaccine (see pp. 559, 565–6).

II: Recommended vaccines

Recommendations vary from source to source; for example, WHO and national health departments in different countries often give slightly differing recommendations. Your own special risk factors and circumstances will also need to be taken into account.

Travellers are therefore strongly advised to seek advice from an up-to-date source at least four weeks prior to departure — an ample choice of suitable sources is listed in Appendix 8. The summary below is intended merely as a general guide to current recommendations.

Region 1: North America, western and southern Europe, Australia, New Zealand, Japan

Everyone should be protected against tetanus, and it is good practice for protection against diphtheria to also be maintained. No additional travel vaccinations are likely to be recommended. In some parts of Europe, tick-borne encephalitis can be a risk for people taking part in outdoor activities (see p. 165).

Region 2: Eastern (Asian) Mediterranean and North Africa

Tetanus and diphtheria, polio, hepatitis A, and also typhoid protection are recommended.

Region 3: Tropical Africa

Tetanus and diphtheria, polio, hepatitis A, and typhoid; in addition, yellow fever is recommended for travel to many parts of Central, West, and East Africa. Travellers on prolonged visits should be vaccinated against hepatitis B and rabies. In some areas protection against meningococcal disease may be advisable for long-stay travellers, as well as for short-stay visitors during an outbreak.

Region 4: Middle East

Tetanus, polio, hepatitis A, and typhoid; in addition, travellers on prolonged visits should be vaccinated against hepatitis B and possibly rabies. Meningitis vaccine is required for the pilgrimage to Mecca and is recommended if there are any current outbreaks in the region.

Region 5: Asia

Tetanus and diphtheria, polio, hepatitis A, and typhoid; those staying for prolonged visits should be vaccinated against hepatitis B. In addition, rabies and Japanese encephalitis (see p. 162) may be advisable. Meningitis vaccine is sometimes recommended for parts of India and Nepal.

Region 6: Mexico, Central and South America

Tetanus and diphtheria, hepatitis A, and typhoid; in addition, travellers staying for prolonged visits should be vaccinated against hepatitis B and rabies. Yellow fever vaccination is advised for travel to Panama and the Amazon basin area. Polio has been eradicated from the region.

Region 7: Caribbean and Pacific Islands

Tetanus and diphtheria; in addition, travellers to places other than the usual tourist destinations should be immunized against typhoid and hepatitis A, and this is especially important for travel to Haiti and the Dominican Republic; those staying for prolonged visits should be vaccinated against hepatitis B, and for certain Caribbean islands, rabies. Polio has been eradicated from the region, though a vaccine-related outbreak occurred recently in the Dominican Republic.

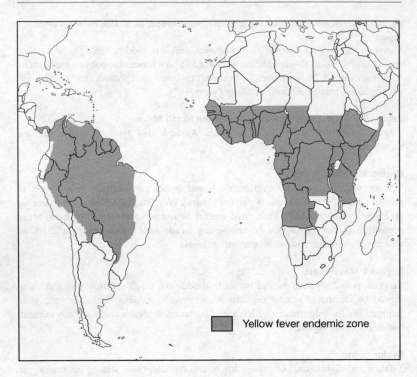

Yellow fever endemic zone

Map A1 Yellow fever (Source: WHO)

Appendix 2:
Malaria: risk areas for disease and drug resistance

1. Countries where malaria occurs

Abu Dhabi*	Ecuador
Afghanistan	Egypt*
Algeria	El Salvador
Angola	Equatorial Guinea
Argentina	Eritrea
Armenia*	Ethiopia
Azerbaijan	French Guiana
Bangladesh	Gabon
Belize	Gambia
Benin	Ghana
Bhutan	Guatemala
Bolivia	Guinea
Botswana	Guinea Bissau
Brazil	Guyana
Burkina Faso	Haiti
Burundi	Honduras
Cambodia	Hong Kong*
Cameroon	India
Cape Verde Islands	Indonesia
Central African Republic	Iran
Chad	Iraq
China	Kenya
Colombia	Korea (South)*
Comoros	Laos
Congo	Liberia
Congo Democratic Republic (Zaire)	Madagascar
Costa Rica	Malawi
Cote d'Ivoire	Malaysia
Djibouti	Mali
Dominican Republic	Mauritania

1. Countries where malaria occurs (continued)

Mauritius*	Sierra Leone
Mayotte	Solomon Islands
Mexico	Somalia
Morocco*	South Africa
Mozambique	Sri Lanka
Myanmar (Burma)	Sudan
Namibia	Surinam
Nepal	Swaziland
Nicaragua	Syria
Niger	Tajikistan
Nigeria	Tanzania
Oman	Thailand
Pakistan	Togo
Panama	Turkey
Papua New Guinea	Turkmenistan*
Paraguay	Uganda
Peru	United Arab Emirates*
Philippines	Vanuatu
Russian Federation*	Venezuela
Rwanda	Vietnam
Sao Tome	Yemen
Saudi Arabia*	Zambia
Senegal	Zimbabwe

2. Countries with a risk of chloroquine-resistant malaria

Afghanistan	Central African Republic
Angola	Chad
Bangladesh	China
Benin	Colombia
Bhutan	Comores
Bolivia	Congo
Botswana	Congo Democratic Republic (Zaire)
Brazil	Côte d'Ivoire (Ivory Coast)
Burkina Faso	Djibouti
Burundi	Ecuador
Cambodia	Equatorial Guinea
Cameroon	Ethiopia
Cape Verde Islands	French Guiana

2. Countries with a risk of chloroquine-resistant malaria *(continued)*

Gabon	Panama
Gambia	Papua New Guinea
Ghana	Peru
Guinea	Philippines
Guinea Bissau	Rwanda
Guyana	Sao Tome
Hong Kong	Saudi Arabia
India	Senegal
Indonesia	Sierra Leone
Iran	Solomon Islands
Kenya	Somalia
Laos	South Africa
Liberia	Sri Lanka
Madagascar	Sudan
Malawi	Surinam
Malaysia	Swaziland
Mali	Tajikistan
Mauritania	Tanzania
Mayotte	Thailand
Mozambique	Togo
Myanmar (Burma)	Uganda
Namibia	Vanuatu
Nepal	Venezuela
Niger	Vietnam
Nigeria	Yemen
Oman	Zambia
Pakistan	Zimbabwe

3. Countries where malaria is chloroquine-sensitive

Abu Dhabi*	El Salvador
Algeria	Eritrea
Argentina	Guatemala
Armenia*	Haiti
Azerbaijan	Honduras
Belize	Iraq
Costa Rica	Korea (South)*
Dominican Republic	Mauritius*
Egypt*	Mexico

3. Countries where malaria is chloroquine-sensitive (continued)

Morocco*	Syria
Nicaragua	Turkey
Paraguay	Turkmenistan*
Russian Federation*	United Arab Emirates*

Notes:

1. In countries marked * malaria is localized and transmission is currently very low: drug protection is not usually necessary for visitors, though precautions against insect bites should never be omitted.
2. Malaria distribution may vary considerably within a country, and from time to time; for up-to-date information, consult a knowledgeable source, such as one of the centres listed in Appendix 8, or check the WHO web site (**www.who.ch/ith**).
3. Malaria transmission does not normally occur above an altitude of 2000 metres.
4. See Chapter 5, pp. 130–50 for further information.

Appendix 3:
Geographic distribution of infectious diseases:

What diseases occur where? This seems a simple enough question for a book like this, but in fact the answers are not straightforward.

In one sense, the answer should not really matter. Travellers who want to stay healthy should adopt healthy habits and precautions wherever they go. Whether there is filariasis on the menu, or dengue fever, the precautions are just the same.

Statistics on disease patterns that filter back to organizations like the World Health Organization in Geneva depend upon:

- An accurate medical diagnosis in the first place, which in turn usually needs doctors and perhaps laboratory facilities for confirmation;
- A public health bureaucratic infrastructure, with sufficient resources and enthusiasm at every level to gather statistics and pass them on;
- Governments' and authorities' willingness to allow frank public disclosure of information that might be seen as a deterrent to tourism or as harmful to their image.

Reliable information about the distribution of disease is therefore most lacking from the countries of greatest interest to readers of this book: countries with plenty of disease but scarce medical resources; and where official statistics do exist, they almost always underestimate the true scale.

The tables that follow are a compromise that takes account of the fact that travellers still need access to this kind of information. They are based on WHO figures and a combination of other sources, with modifications when these are unconvincing or inadequate. Estimates have been sought from doctors working in the countries concerned or with specialist knowledge of particular diseases. (Countries with rabies are listed separately in Table 6.1, p. 223–7)

The figures given here do not correspond directly with the risk to individual travellers: they give a **rough indication** of the occurrence of particular diseases in the local population. There is often considerable variation in the distribution of disease **within** any one country, and all of the figures listed here are based on generalizations that cannot take account of this, or of differences in disease patterns between rural and urban areas. It is hard to make meaningful generalizations, about non-uniform land masses the size of the former Soviet republics, China, India, Brazil, and the Sudan.

The tables are far from flawless, and should be used with caution. In particular, they should **not** be used as a basis for important decisions regarding treatment. If you find any errors, please tell us! — by email to feedback@travellers-health.info.

Key

S: Similiar or smaller number of cases per million population to those occurring in the UK, France, or West Germany (Western Europe); or no cases at all.

L: 3–10 times number of cases relative to Western Europe.
Or
Less than 10 cases per million population (where disease does not occur in Western Europe).

M: 11–100 times number of cases relative to Western Europe.
Or
11–100 cases per million (where disease does not occur in Western Europe).

H: Greater than 100 times number of cases relative to Western Europe.
Or
More than 100 cases per million population (where disease does not occur in Western Europe).

AFRICA (NORTH)

	Cholera	Typhoid	Shigellosis	Amoebiasis	TB	Plague	Brucellosis	Diphtheria	Meningococcal infection	Polio	Yellow fever	Dengue or other arboviruses	Viral hepatitis (A + B)	Typhus	Leishmaniasis	Trypanosomiasis	Syphilis	Gonorrhoea	Schistosomiasis	Liver flukes	Hydatid disease	Tapeworms	Filariasis	Hookworm	Other intestinal worms
Algeria	S	H	L	M	L	S	M	L	S	L	S	S	H	S	M	S	S	S	L	S	H	L	S	L	L
Egypt	S	H	L	L	L	S	L	M	S	M	S	L	H	L	M	S	L	L	H	L	H	L	L	L	L
Libya	S	H	M	L	L	L	L	M	S	L	S	S	H	L	L	S	S	S	M	L	M	L	L	S	L
Mauritania	H	H	L	M	M	S	L	M	S	L	S	S	H	L	L	S	L	S	L	S	L	L	M	S	L
Morocco	S	H	M	M	M	S	L	M	S	L	S	S	H	L	L	S	L	L	H	S	M	L	S	S	L
Tunisia	S	H	L	M	L	S	L	L	S	L	S	S	H	L	M	S	S	L	L	L	M	L	S	L	L

AFRICA (WEST)

	Cholera	Typhoid	Shigellosis	Amoebiasis	TB	Plague	Brucellosis	Diphtheria	Meningococcal infection	Polio	Yellow fever	Dengue or other arboviruses	Viral hepatitis (A + B)	Typhus	Leishmaniasis	Trypanosomiasis	Syphilis	Gonorrhoea	Schistosomiasis	Liver flukes	Hydatid disease	Tapeworms	Filariasis	Hookworm	Other intestinal worms
Benin	H	H	H	H	L	S	M	L	M	L	H	S	H	L	S	M	S	L	H	L	L	M	L	M	M
Burkina Faso	H	H	M	H	L	S	M	M	M	L	H	S	H	L	L	M	L	H	L	S	L	L	L	L	M
Cameroon	H	H	L	M	M	S	M	M	M	L	H	S	H	L	S	S	L	H	M	L	M	L	M	M	M
Cape Verde	H	H	L	M	L	S	L	L	H	L	S	S	H	H	S	M	H	H	S	L	M	M	L	M	H
Chad	S	H	M	H	M	S	M	L	M	L	S	M	H	M	S	L	H	S	H	L	M	M	M	L	L
Gambia	S	H	M	M	M	S	L	S	H	L	H	M	H	L	S	L	S	H	H	L	L	M	L	M	L
Ghana	H	H	M	H	M	S	M	M	M	L	H	M	H	S	S	L	S	H	H	S	L	L	M	H	H
Guinea	H	H	M	M	M	S	S	M	L	L	H	L	H	L	S	M	S	M	M	L	L	L	M	M	M
Guinea-Bissau	H	H	M	M	M	S	S	M	M	L	H	L	H	L	S	S	S	S	M	L	L	M	M	S	L
Côte d'Ivoire	H	H	M	M	M	S	L	M	M	L	H	S	H	L	S	S	S	M	H	S	L	L	L	M	M
Liberia	H	H	L	M	M	S	L	M	L	L	S	M	H	L	S	L	M	M	H	L	L	L	M	L	L
Mali	H	H	L	L	L	S	M	M	M	L	S	S	H	L	S	M	M	M	S	L	M	L	H	L	M
Niger	H	H	L	M	L	S	M	L	M	L	H	L	H	L	S	S	M	M	H	L	S	L	H	L	L
Nigeria	H	H	H	H	L	S	L	L	S	L	S	S	H	L	S	L	S	S	H	L	L	L	H	L	M
São Tomé & Príncipe	M	H	L	H	M	S	M	H	L	M	H	L	H	L	S	L	M	M	L	L	M	L	H	L	L
Senegal	H	H	M	M	M	S	M	S	M	M	H	S	H	L	S	L	M	S	S	S	S	L	L	M	M
Sierra Leone	H	H	H	M	M	S	M	L	M	M	H	L	H	L	S	M	S	H	H	L	M	L	H	M	M
Togo	H	H	L	H	L	S	L	L	M	M	S	S	H	L	L	L	S	S	H	L	S	L	H	M	M

AFRICA (CENTRAL AND EAST)

	Cholera	Typhoid	Shigellosis	Amoebiasis	TB	Plague	Brucellosis	Diphtheria	Meningococcal infection	Polio	Yellow fever	Dengue or other arboviruses	Viral hepatitis (A + B)	Typhus	Leishmaniasis	Trypanosomiasis	Syphilis	Gonorrhoea	Schistosomiasis	Liver flukes	Hydatid disease	Tapeworms	Filariasis	Hookworm	Other intestinal worms
Burundi	H	H	M	H	M	S	M	L	L	L	M	M	H	H	S	M	S	S	L	L	L	L	L	S	L
Central African Republic	H	H	M	H	M	S	L	M	M	L	S	M	H	L	L	M	S	L	L	L	L	M	L	S	L
Congo	H	H	M	M	M	S	L	M	L	L	M	M	H	M	S	H	L	L	M	L	L	L	M	M	L
Congo Democratic Republic	H	H	M	M	L	L	M	M	L	L	H	M	H	M	S	M	S	L	M	L	L	L	M	M	L
Djibouti	H	H	H	H	H	S	M	M	L	L	S	L	H	L	L	S	S	S	L	L	L	L	L	M	L
Equatorial Guinea	S	H	M	H	M	S	S	M	L	L	S	M	H	L	S	M	L	S	L	S	L	L	L	L	L
Eritrea	S	H	M	H	M	L	S	M	L	L	S	L	H	M	S	M	S	S	L	S	H	L	L	L	L
Ethiopia	S	H	M	H	M	S	M	M	L	L	S	L	H	M	M	M	S	L	L	L	H	H	L	L	L
Gabon	S	H	M	M	M	S	L	L	L	L	S	S	H	L	S	M	S	S	L	L	L	L	M	L	L
Kenya	H	H	M	L	M	S	M	M	M	L	H	S	H	M	M	M	M	S	H	L	L	H	M	L	M
Malawi	H	H	M	L	L	L	L	L	L	L	S	S	H	L	S	M	M	L	M	L	L	L	M	H	M
Rwanda	H	H	H	L	M	S	L	M	M	L	S	H	H	L	L	S	S	L	S	S	L	L	M	L	M
Seychelles	S	H	S	L	L	L	S	L	L	S	S	S	H	L	S	S	M	L	L	S	L	L	M	L	L
Somalia	H	H	M	H	M	S	S	M	L	H	S	H	H	L	H	M	M	L	H	L	M	L	M	M	M
Sudan	S	H	M	L	M	S	L	H	M	M	H	L	H	L	L	S	S	S	M	L	M	M	M	M	M
Tanzania	H	H	L	M	M	L	L	M	L	M	S	M	H	L	L	M	S	S	M	L	L	M	L	L	H
Uganda	H	H	M	M	M	L	L	M	M	M	S	L	H	L	L	M	S	S	H	L	L	M	M	H	H

AFRICA (SOUTHERN)

	Cholera	Typhoid	Shigellosis	Amoebiasis	TB	Plague	Brucellosis	Diphtheria	Meningococcal infection	Polio	Yellow fever	Dengue or other arboviruses	Viral hepatitis (A + B)	Typhus	Leishmaniasis	Trypanosomiasis	Syphilis	Gonorrhoea	Schistosomiasis	Liver flukes	Hydatid disease	Tapeworms	Filariasis	Hookworm	Other intestinal worms
Angola	H	H	M	M	M	L	M	L	S	L	H	L	H	L	S	M	S	L	H	L	L	L	H	H	L
Botswana	S	S	L	M	M	L	L	L	L	L	S	S	H	L	S	M	L	S	L	L	M	H	M	L	H
Lesotho	S	H	L	S	M	L	S	L	L	L	S	L	H	L	L	S	M	M	S	S	S	H	S	S	H
Madagascar	H	H	M	L	M	L	S	M	S	L	S	L	H	L	S	S	S	S	L	L	L	H	L	H	H
Mozambique	H	H	L	M	M	L	M	L	S	L	S	M	H	L	S	M	S	S	M	L	L	M	M	H	H
Namibia	S	H	M	L	M	L	L	L	L	L	S	L	H	L	S	M	S	S	L	L	L	M	M	H	H
Reunion	S	H	L	H	S	S	L	M	S	L	S	L	H	L	S	S	M	S	S	L	L	M	L	S	L
South Africa	H	M	L	M	M	L	M	M	L	L	S	M	H	L	S	S	M	M	L	S	S	H	S	M	H
Swaziland	H	H	M	M	M	S	M	L	L	L	S	M	H	S	S	S	M	M	H	S	S	H	S	M	H
Zambia	H	H	M	M	M	S	L	M	L	M	S	S	H	L	L	L	M	L	M	L	L	M	M	M	H
Zimbabwe	H	M	L	L	M	L	L	L	L	L	S	S	H	L	S	L	M	M	H	L	S	M	L	M	H

ASIA: NEAR AND MIDDLE EAST

	Cholera	Typhoid	Shigellosis	Amoebiasis	TB	Plague	Brucellosis	Diphtheria	Meningococcal infection	Polio	Yellow fever	Dengue or other arboviruses	Viral hepatitis (A + B)	Typhus	Leishmaniasis	Trypanosomiasis	Syphilis	Gonorrhoea	Schistosomiasis	Liver flukes	Hydatid disease	Tapeworms	Filariasis	Hookworm	Other intestinal worms
Afghanistan	H	H	M	M	M	L	H	M	S	L	S	S	H	M	H	S	S	S	S	S	M	L	L	H	H
Bahrain	S	S	M	H	M	L	H	L	S	L	S	S	M	M	M	S	S	S	L	S	L	L	L	H	M
Iran	H	H	H	M	L	S	H	L	S	M	S	S	M	S	M	S	S	S	M	S	M	M	S	M	H
Iraq	H	H	H	S	M	S	L	H	S	M	S	S	M	M	H	S	S	S	M	S	M	L	L	L	M
Israel	S	S	H	S	S	S	S	L	S	L	S	S	L	M	H	S	S	S	S	S	S	L	S	S	S
Jordan	S	L	M	M	S	S	M	L	S	L	S	S	M	S	L	S	S	S	L	S	M	M	S	M	M
Kuwait	S	H	M	M	L	S	L	L	M	L	S	S	H	L	M	S	S	L	S	L	M	L	S	S	L
Lebanon	S	M	L	L	S	S	S	L	L	L	S	S	M	M	L	S	S	S	M	L	L	S	S	S	L
Oman	S	M	S	L	S	S	S	H	S	L	S	S	H	M	M	S	S	S	S	S	L	M	S	L	L
Qatar	S	M	S	M	L	S	S	M	S	L	S	S	M	L	S	S	L	L	M	S	L	L	L	L	L
Saudi Arabia	S	M	L	M	L	S	H	M	S	M	S	S	M	M	M	S	S	S	M	S	M	M	L	L	M
Syrian Arab Republic	S	M	M	M	L	S	L	H	H	L	S	S	M	M	M	S	S	S	M	S	H	M	L	S	H
Turkey	S	H	H	H	L	S	L	H	L	M	S	S	H	M	L	S	S	S	S	L	H	M	L	L	
United Arab Emirates	S	M	S	M	L	S	M	S	S	L	S	S	M	M	M	S	S	S	H	S	M	L	L	M	M
Yemen	S	M	H	M	M	L	M	H	M	M	S	S	M	M	M	S	S	S	H	S	M	L	M	S	H
Yemen (South)	S	M	H	M	M	L	M	H	M	M	S	S	M	M	M	S	S	S	M	S	L	L	L	L	L

ASIA: CENTRAL AND SOUTHEAST

	Cholera	Typhoid	Shigellosis	Amoebiasis	TB	Plague	Brucellosis	Diphtheria	Meningococcal infection	Polio	Yellow fever	Dengue or other arboviruses	Viral hepatitis (A + B)	Typhus	Leishmaniasis	Trypanosomiasis	Syphilis	Gonorrhoea	Schistosomiasis	Liver flukes	Hydatid disease	Tapeworms	Filariasis	Hookworm	Other intestinal worms
Bangladesh	L	H	H	H	M	S	S	M	M	M	S	M	H	M	L	S	S	L	S	S	L	L	M	M	H
Brunei	S	H	L	L	L	S	S	S	S	S	S	L	M	M	S	S	S	S	L	S	S	L	L	M	M
Myanmar (Burma)	H	H	M	M	L	S	M	L	S	L	S	M	H	L	S	S	S	S	S	S	M	L	M	M	H
India	H	H	H	M	M	L	H	M	H	M	S	L	M	M	H	S	S	S	S	M	M	M	M	H	H
Indonesia	M	H	M	L	L	L	L	M	L	M	S	H	M	M	M	S	L	L	L	S	S	M	M	H	H
Malaysia	H	H	M	L	M	L	M	L	S	L	S	M	M	L	L	S	S	S	L	L	S	L	M	H	H
Maldives	S	L	L	L	S	S	L	M	S	S	S	L	M	L	L	S	S	S	S	S	S	S	L	S	L
Mongolia	S	H	S	S	M	L	M	M	L	S	S	L	L	L	L	S	S	S	L	L	L	L	L	L	L
Nepal	H	H	L	M	M	S	S	H	H	S	S	M	M	M	L	S	S	L	S	L	M	M	M	H	H
Pakistan	M	H	M	H	M	S	H	L	L	L	S	M	H	L	M	S	S	H	S	S	S	M	L	H	H
Singapore	H	M	L	L	L	S	S	M	S	L	S	M	M	L	S	S	H	M	S	S	S	S	M	H	L
Sri Lanka	H	H	M	M	M	S	M	H	L	M	S	M	M	L	M	S	S	S	S	M	M	S	L	H	H
Thailand	H	H	H	M	L	S	M	H	S	S	S	M	M	L	M	S	S	S	S	M	M	M	M	H	H
Bhutan	H	H	L	M	L	S	L	S	M	S	S	L	H	L	L	S	S	S	L	L	S	L	L	H	H

ASIA: FAR EAST

	Cholera	Typhoid	Shigellosis	Amoebiasis	TB	Plague	Brucellosis	Diphtheria	Meningococcal infection	Polio	Yellow fever	Dengue or other arboviruses	Viral hepatitis (A + B)	Typhus	Leishmaniasis	Trypanosomiasis	Syphilis	Gonorrhoea	Schistosomiasis	Liver flukes	Hydatid disease	Tapeworms	Filariasis	Hookworm	Other intestinal worms
China	H	M	M	L	H	L	L	M	L	L	S	L	M	L	L	S	S	S	M	L	L	L	M	M	M
Hong Kong	S	L	M	L	M	L	L	L	L	L	S	L	H	L	S	S	L	M	L	M	L	L	L	L	M
Japan	S	S	L	L	L	S	L	L	S	S	S	L	L	L	S	S	S	S	L	L	L	L	L	L	L
Cambodia	H	H	M	M	M	S	M	H	S	L	S	M	M	M	L	S	S	S	L	L	M	M	L	M	M
Korea (North, Dem. Rep. of)	S	L	S	L	L	L	M	M	L	L	S	L	M	M	S	S	S	S	S	M	M	L	L	L	L
Korea (South, Republic of)	S	L	S	L	L	S	M	M	L	L	S	M	M	L	S	S	S	S	S	L	L	L	M	L	L
Laos	H	M	S	M	M	S	M	H	L	L	S	L	M	L	S	S	L	L	M	M	M	M	L	M	H
Philippines	H	H	H	H	M	S	M	H	L	L	S	L	M	S	S	S	S	L	M	L	M	M	L	M	L
Taiwan	S	L	M	M	M	L	L	H	L	L	S	L	M	L	L	S	S	L	L	M	M	M	L	M	L
Vietnam	H	M	M	H	M	H	M	H	S	M	S	H	M	L	M	S	L	L	L	M	M	M	M	L	M

AMERICA (NORTH AND CENTRAL)

	Cholera	Typhoid	Shigellosis	Amoebiasis	TB	Plague	Brucellosis	Diphtheria	Meningococcal infection	Polio	Yellow fever	Dengue or other arboviruses	Viral hepatitis (A + B)	Typhus	Leishmaniasis	Trypanosomiasis	Syphilis	Gonorrhoea	Schistosomiasis	Liver flukes	Hydatid disease	Tapeworms	Filariasis	Hookworm	Other intestinal worms
Belize	S	L	L	M	L	S	L	M	S	S	S	M	H	L	M	L	S	L	L	L	L	L	M	M	M
Canada	S	S	L	S	L	S	L	S	S	S	S	L	S	L	S	S	S	S	S	S	S	S	S	S	L
Costa Rica	H	L	S	H	L	S	L	M	S	S	S	L	H	L	H	L	L	M	L	L	M	M	M	M	H
El Salvador	H	L	M	H	L	S	L	M	S	S	S	L	H	L	L	L	L	L	L	L	L	L	L	M	M
Guatemala	H	H	M	M	M	S	L	M	S	S	S	L	H	L	M	M	L	S	L	L	L	L	M	M	M
Honduras	H	M	M	H	S	S	S	L	S	S	S	H	H	L	M	L	L	L	L	L	M	M	L	M	H
Mexico	M	M	M	M	L	S	S	L	S	S	S	M	H	L	H	L	S	S	L	S	M	M	L	M	H
Nicaragua	H	L	M	H	L	S	S	S	S	S	S	S	H	L	H	M	L	L	L	L	L	L	L	M	H
Panama	H	M	M	H	S	S	S	M	S	S	S	M	H	L	S	M	M	M	L	L	L	L	M	M	H
USA	S	S	M	L	S	L	S	L	S	S	S	L	S	L	S	S	S	M	S	S	L	L	S	L	L

AMERICAS: CARIBBEAN

	Cholera	Typhoid	Shigellosis	Amoebiasis	TB	Plague	Brucellosis	Diphtheria	Meningococcal infection	Polio	Yellow fever	Dengue or other arboviruses	Viral hepatitis (A + B)	Typhus	Leishmaniasis	Trypanosomiasis	Syphilis	Gonorrhoea	Schistosomiasis	Liver flukes	Hydatid disease	Tapeworms	Filariasis	Hookworm	Other intestinal worms
Antigua and Barbuda	S	S	L	L	S	S	S	S	S	S	S	M	L	S	S	S	L	L	M	L	L	L	L	M	M
Bahamas	S	S	M	L	S	S	S	S	S	S	S	M	L	S	S	S	M	M	S	S	L	L	L	L	M
Barbados	S	S	M	L	S	S	S	S	S	S	S	H	L	S	S	S	L	L	S	S	S	S	S	L	L
Bermuda	S	L	M	L	S	S	S	S	S	S	S	M	L	S	S	S	L	H	S	S	S	L	L	L	M
British Virgin Islands	S	L	S	M	S	S	S	S	S	S	S	M	L	S	S	S	L	H	L	L	S	L	L	L	L
Cuba	S	M	M	H	S	S	L	M	S	S	S	L	M	S	S	S	L	L	L	M	S	L	L	M	M
Dominica	S	S	M	L	S	S	S	S	S	S	S	M	M	S	S	S	L	L	S	L	S	L	L	M	M
Dominican Rep	S	H	L	H	L	S	L	H	S	L	S	L	M	S	S	S	M	M	S	L	S	L	L	M	M
Grenada	S	L	L	L	S	S	S	S	S	S	S	L	M	S	S	S	L	L	S	L	S	L	L	M	M
Guadeloupe	S	S	L	H	S	S	S	L	S	S	S	L	L	S	S	S	L	M	S	L	S	L	L	M	M
Haiti	S	H	M	M	M	S	L	M	S	S	S	M	M	S	S	S	L	M	M	L	L	L	L	M	M
Jamaica	S	S	S	M	S	S	L	L	S	S	S	M	L	S	S	S	L	M	S	L	L	L	L	M	M
Martinique	S	S	L	L	S	S	S	L	S	S	S	L	L	S	S	S	L	L	S	L	S	L	L	M	M
Montserrat	S	S	M	M	S	S	S	S	S	S	S	M	M	S	S	S	L	H	M	L	S	L	L	M	M
Puerto Rico	S	S	S	L	S	S	S	S	S	S	S	H	L	S	S	S	H	L	S	L	S	L	L	L	M
St Kitts and Nevis	S	S	S	L	S	S	S	S	S	S	S	M	L	S	S	S	L	M	S	L	L	L	L	M	M
St Lucia	S	S	L	L	S	S	S	S	S	S	S	L	L	S	S	S	M	M	S	L	S	L	L	M	M
St Vincent	S	S	L	L	S	S	S	S	S	S	S	M	L	S	S	S	L	L	S	L	S	L	L	M	M
Trinidad and Tobago	S	S	L	L	S	S	S	S	S	S	S	M	L	S	S	S	L	M	S	L	L	L	L	M	M

AMERICA (SOUTH)

	Cholera	Typhoid	Shigellosis	Amoebiasis	TB	Plague	Brucellosis	Diphtheria	Meningococcal infection	Polio	Yellow fever	Dengue or other arboviruses	Viral hepatitis (A + B)	Typhus	Leishmaniasis	Trypanosomiasis	Syphilis	Gonorrhoea	Schistosomiasis	Liver flukes	Hydatid disease	Tapeworms	Filariasis	Hookworm	Other intestinal worms
Argentina	S	L	S	M	L	S	L	M	L	S	S	S	M	L	L	M	L	L	L	L	M	L	L	H	M
Bolivia	H	H	L	M	M	L	L	S	S	S	M	S	M	L	H	M	S	S	L	L	M	L	L	L	M
Brazil	M	H	L	H	M	L	L	M	L	S	L	M	H	S	H	M	S	M	H	L	L	M	L	H	H
Chile	H	H	L	L	L	S	L	M	S	S	S	S	L	S	L	L	S	M	S	L	M	M	S	M	M
Colombia	H	H	H	H	M	S	S	M	S	S	H	H	M	L	M	M	L	L	S	L	S	M	M	H	H
Ecuador	H	H	L	H	L	L	S	M	S	S	L	L	L	L	M	L	S	S	M	L	M	M	M	M	M
Falkland Islands	S	S	S	S	L	S	S	S	S	S	L	S	S	L	S	S	M	M	S	L	H	S	S	L	L
French Guiana	L	M	S	M	S	S	S	S	S	S	S	M	S	S	H	L	M	H	S	L	S	L	L	H	H
Guyana	S	L	M	L	L	S	S	S	S	S	S	S	M	L	L	M	S	S	M	L	L	L	M	H	H
Paraguay	S	L	M	M	M	L	S	M	L	S	S	L	L	L	M	L	L	S	L	L	M	M	L	H	M
Peru	H	H	H	M	L	S	S	M	S	S	S	M	M	L	H	L	S	S	H	M	M	M	L	S	H
Surinam	H	M	M	M	M	L	L	L	L	S	S	S	L	L	M	M	L	L	L	L	L	L	M	H	H
Uruguay	S	L	L	M	L	S	L	M	S	S	S	L	M	L	L	M	M	L	M	L	M	M	L	H	M
Venezuela	H	L	L	L	L	S	L	M	L	S	L	L	M	L	M	M	M	H	M	L	S	L	M	H	M

OCEANIA

	Cholera	Typhoid	Shigellosis	Amoebiasis	TB	Plague	Brucellosis	Diphtheria	Meningococcal infection	Polio	Yellow fever	Dengue or other arboviruses	Viral hepatitis (A + B)	Typhus	Leishmaniasis	Trypanosomiasis	Syphilis	Gonorrhoea	Schistosomiasis	Liver flukes	Hydatid disease	Tapeworms	Filariasis	Hookworm	Other intestinal worms
American Samoa	S	S	H	H	S	S	L	L	S	S	S	S	M	S	S	S	L	L	S	S	S	S	L	M	L
Australia	S	S	M	L	S	S	S	S	S	S	S	L	S	S	S	S	S	S	S	L	L	S	S	L	S
Cook Islands	S	S	S	S	L	S	L	S	M	S	S	L	L	S	S	S	S	M	S	S	S	S	S	L	L
Fiji	S	S	M	M	L	S	S	S	D	S	S	H	L	S	S	S	L	L	S	S	L	S	M	L	L
French Polynesia	S	M	M	M	M	S	S	S	L	S	S	H	M	S	S	S	M	L	S	S	S	S	M	L	H
Guam	S	S	M	M	L	S	S	S	L	L	S	M	M	S	S	S	L	M	S	S	S	S	S	M	M
Kiribati	S	L	L	M	M	S	S	L	L	L	S	L	M	S	S	S	L	L	S	S	S	S	M	M	M
New Caledonia	S	S	M	H	M	S	S	S	S	S	S	L	M	S	S	S	M	M	S	S	S	S	M	M	M
New Zealand	S	S	M	L	S	S	S	S	S	S	S	L	S	S	L	S	S	S	S	S	S	S	M	S	S
Papua New Guinea	S	H	M	H	M	S	S	S	S	L	S	H	M	S	S	S	L	L	S	S	S	S	S	H	H
Samoa	S	M	L	L	L	S	S	L	L	L	S	H	M	S	S	S	S	S	S	S	S	S	H	H	M
Solomon Islands	S	H	L	L	M	S	S	S	L	S	S	M	M	S	S	S	S	S	S	S	S	S	M	H	M
Tonga	S	H	M	M	H	S	S	L	L	S	S	H	M	S	L	S	S	S	S	S	S	S	M	H	M
Vanuatu	S	L	L	H	M	S	S	S	L	S	S	M	M	S	L	S	S	S	S	S	S	S	M	M	M
Wallis and Futuna Islands	S	L	L	H	M	S	S	S	S	S	S	H	M	S	L	S	S	S	S	S	S	S	H	H	H

EUROPE (SELECTED COUNTRIES)

	Cholera	Typhoid	Shigellosis	Amoebiasis	TB	Plague	Brucellosis	Diphtheria	Meningococcal infection	Polio	Yellow fever	Dengue or other arboviruses	Viral hepatitis (A + B)	Typhus	Leishmaniasis	Trypanosomiasis	Syphilis	Gonorrhoea	Schistosomiasis	Liver flukes	Hydatid disease	Tapeworms	Filariasis	Hookworm	Other intestinal worms
Albania	S	S	L	L	L	S	L	S	S	L	S	S	L	L	L	S	L	L	S	S	S		S	S	
Bulgaria	S	S	H	L	L	S	L	S	S	L	S	S	M	S	S	S	H	S	S	S	L	S	S	S	S
Cyprus	L	L	S	S	S	S	M	S	L	S	S	S	S	M	S	S	L	L	S	S	L	S	S	S	L
Czech Republic	S	S	H	L	S	S	S	L	S	S	S	L	M	S	S	S	S	S	S	S	S	S	S	S	M
Denmark	S	S	M	M	S	S	S	S	S	S	S	L	S	S	S	S	S	L	S	S	M	L	S	S	S
Finland	S	M	S	M	S	S	M	S	S	S	S	L	S	S	S	S	S	S	S	S	H	L	S	S	S
Greece	S	S	L	L	L	S	M	S	S	S	S	L	L	L	M	S	S	S	S	L	L	S	L	S	S
Hungary	M	S	H	L	L	S	S	S	S	S	S	L	L	S	S	S	S	S	S	S	L	S	S	S	S
Iceland	S	S	S	S	S	S	S	S	S	S	S	S	S	S	S	S	S	S	S	L	L	S	L	S	S
Norway	S	S	S	S	L	S	L	S	M	S	S	L	S	S	S	S	S	S	S	S	L	S	L	S	S
Portugal	S	M	S	S	S	S	L	M	S	S	S	L	L	L	S	S	S	L	S	S	S	S	S	S	S
Romania	S	S	H	S	M	S	S	H	S	S	S	L	M	S	S	S	H	S	S	S	L	S	S	S	S
Russia	S	L	M	L	L	S	L	H	S	S	S	L	S	L	S	S	H	L	S	S	S	L	S	S	L
Spain	S	M	M	S	S	S	M	S	S	S	S	S	M	S	S	S	S	S	S	S	S	S	S	S	S
Sweden	S	S	L	S	S	S	L	L	S	S	S	L	S	S	S	S	L	L	S	S	L	M	S	S	S
Yugoslavia	S	L	H	S	M	S	L	L	S	S	S	L	M	S	S	S	L	S	S	L	S	S	S	S	S
Slovakia	S	S	H	L	L	S	S	L	S	S	S	L	M	S	S	S	S	S	S	S	S	S	S	S	M
Armenia	L	S	M	L	L	S	S	L	S	S	S	L	M	S	S	S	S	S	S	S	S	L	S	L	L
Azerbaijan	S	L	M	L	L	S	S	L	S	S	S	L	M	S	S	S	H	S	S	S	L	L	S	L	L
Belarus	S	S	M	L	L	S	S	L	S	S	S	L	M	S	S	S	H	S	S	S	L	M	S	L	L
Estonia	S	S	M	L	L	S	L	L	S	S	S	L	M	S	S	S	H	L	S	S	L	M	S	L	L
Georgia	S	L	M	L	L	L	L	L	S	S	S	L	M	S	S	S	H	L	S	S	L	L	S	L	L
Kazakhstan	S	L	M	M	M	L	L	L	S	S	S	L	M	S	S	S	H	S	S	S	L	L	S	L	L
Kyrgistan	S	M	M	L	M	S	L	L	S	S	S	L	M	S	S	S	H	S	S	S	L	L	S	L	L

EUROPE (SELECTED COUNTRIES)

	Cholera	Typhoid	Shigellosis	Amoebiasis	TB	Plague	Brucellosis	Diphtheria	Meningococcal infection	Polio	Yellow fever	Dengue or other arboviruses	Viral hepatitis (A + B)	Typhus	Leishmaniasis	Trypanosomiasis	Syphilis	Gonorrhoea	Schistosomiasis	Liver flukes	Hydatid disease	Tapeworms	Filariasis	Hookworm	Other intestinal worms
Latvia	S	S	L	L	L	S	L	L	S	S	S	L	M	S	S	S	H	S	S	S	L	L	S	L	L
Lithuania	L	S	M	L	L	S	L	L	S	S	S	L	M	S	S	S	H	L	S	S	L	L	S	L	L
Moldova	L	S	M	L	L	S	L	L	S	S	S	L	M	S	S	S	H	S	S	S	L	L	S	L	L
Tajikistan	S	M	M	L	L	S	L	L	S	S	S	L	M	L	S	S	H	S	S	L	L	L	S	L	L
Turkmenistan	S	L	M	L	L	S	L	L	S	S	S	L	M	S	L	S	H	S	S	S	L	L	S	L	L
Ukraine	S	L	L	L	L	S	L	L	S	S	S	L	M	S	S	S	H	S	S	S	L	L	S	L	L
Uzbekistan	S	L	M	L	L	S	L	L	S	S	S	L	M	S	S	S	H	S	S	S	L	L	S	L	L

Appendix 4:
Can you drink the water?

This remains one of the questions that travellers most often ask. Unfortunately, little reliable information is available, and even in countries where water is safe at source, man and nature commonly conspire to contaminate it before it reaches your mouth. The bottom line is to always be sceptical of claims about water purity. If there is any doubt at all, choose water from a reliable bottled source, boil it or purify it — see p. 71 for more information.

The following tables are based on a survey of what long-term British, American, and Australian expatriates actually advise visitors and each other to do in each of the countries listed, plus information from medical and nursing staff at embassies of English-speaking countries.

If you disagree, or have anything to add, let us know! Send any updates to feedback@travellers-health.info.

AFRICA

	Water is safe in:					Unsafe/unreliable			
	Capital?	Main cities?	Hotels & resorts?	Rural areas?	Everywhere?	Everywhere?	Bottled widely available?	Comments
Algeria	No	No	No	No	No	Yes	No	Regarded as unreliable even where chlorinated
Angola	No	No	No	No	No	Yes	Major cities only	Infrastructure in tatters. Choose imported bottled brands
Benin	No	No	No	No	No	Yes	Cities & towns	
Botswana	Yes	Yes	Yes	No	No	No	Yes	
Burkina Faso	Yes	No	No	No	No	No	Yes	
Burundi	No	No	No	No	No	Yes	Yes	
Cameroon	No	No	No	No	No	Yes	Yes	
Cape Verde Islands	Yes	Yes	Yes	Yes	Yes	No	Yes	
Central African Republic	No	No	No	No	No	Yes	Very expensive	Some deep wells are safe
Chad	No	No	No	No	No	Yes	No	
Comores								
Congo	No	No	No	No	No	Yes	Yes	Local bottled water is good quality and safe
Congo Democratic Republic (Zaire)	No	No	None	No	No	Yes	Only Kinshasa	
Cote d'Ivoire	No	No	No	No	No	No	Limited availability	
Djibouti	Yes	No	Yes	No	No	Yes	Yes	
Egypt	No	No	No	No	No	Yes	Yes	Don't trust hotel supplies
Equatorial Guinea								
Eritrea	No	No	No	No	No	Yes	Yes	
Ethiopia	No	No	No	No	No	Yes	Yes	Poor delivery system even when treated
Gabon	Yes	No	No	No	No	No	Yes	
Gambia	No	No	No	No	No	Yes	Yes	Bottled water advised
Ghana	No	No	No	No	No	Yes	Yes	Reliable bottled water available

AFRICA

	Water is safe in:					Unsafe/unreliable		
	Capital?	Main cities?	Hotels & resorts?	Rural areas?	Everywhere?	Everywhere?	Bottled widely available?	Comments
Guinea	No	No	No	No	No	Yes	Yes	Local bottled water is good
Guinea Bissau	No	No	No	No	No	Yes	Capital only	
Kenya	Yes	No	No	No	No	No	Yes	
Lesotho	Yes	No	No	No	No	Possibly	Yes	Bottled water advised
Liberia	No	No	No	No	No	No	Limited availability	
Libya								
Madagascar	No	No	No	No	No	Yes	Except in rural areas	
Malawi								
Mali	No	No	No	No	No	Yes	Major cities / tourist areas only	Unsafe distributor system even where treated
Mauritania	No	No	No	No	No	Yes	Capital only	
Mauritius	Yes	Yes	Yes	No	No	No	Yes	
Morocco	Yes	Yes	Yes	No	No	No	Yes	Good local bottled water
Mozambique	No	No	No	No	No	Yes	Major cities only	Check seals on all bottled water
Namibia	Yes	No	No	No	No	No	Yes	Safe bottled brands widely available
Niger	No	No	No	No	No	Yes	Limited availability	
Nigeria	No	No	None	No	No	Yes	Yes	Choose imported brands
Rwanda	No	No	No	No	No	Yes	Yes	Some locally bottled water available
Senegal	Yes	No	No	No	No	No	Yes	
Seychelles	Yes	Yes	Yes	Yes	Yes	No	Yes	
Sierra Leone	No	No	No	No	No	Yes	Yes	Infrastructure very poor
South Africa	Yes	Yes	Yes	No	No	No	Yes	
Somalia	No	No	No	No	No	Yes	Capital only	

AFRICA

	Water is safe in:					Unsafe/unreliable			
	Capital?	Main cities?	Hotels & resorts?	Rural areas?	Everywhere?	Everywhere?	Bottled widely available?	Comments
Sudan	No	No	No	No	No	Yes	Most cities, but not elsewhere	
Swaziland	Yes	Yes	Yes	No	No	No	Yes	
Tanzania	No	No	No	No	No	Yes	Yes	
Togo	Yes	No	No	No	No	No	Yes	
Tunisia	Yes	Yes	Yes	Yes	Yes	No	Yes	
Uganda	No	No	No	No	No	Yes	Yes	
Zambia	No	No	No	No	No	Yes	Yes	
Zimbabwe	Yes	Yes	Yes	No	No	No	Yes	Infrastructure is currently fragile; caution advised

AMERICAS/CARIBBEAN

	Water is safe in:					Unsafe/unreliable		
	Capital?	Main cities?	Hotels & resorts?	Rural areas?	Everywhere?	Everywhere?	Bottled widely available?	Comments
Anguilla	Bottled water advised							
Antigua & Barbuda	No	No	No	No	No	Yes	Yes	
Argentina	No	No	No	No	No	Yes	Yes	
Bahamas	No	No	No	No	No	Yes	Yes	
Barbados	Yes	Yes	Yes	Yes	Yes	No	Yes	
Belize	No	No	No	No	No	Yes	Yes	
Bermuda	Yes	Yes	Yes	Yes	Yes	No	Yes	
Bolivia	No	No	No	No	No	Yes	No	
Brazil	No	No	No	No	No	Yes	Yes	
Canada	Yes	Yes	Yes	Yes	Yes	No	Yes	
Cayman Islands	Yes	Yes	Yes	Yes	Yes	No	Yes	
Chile	Yes	Yes	Yes	No	No	No	Most places	
Colombia	Yes	Yes	Yes	No	No	No	Yes	Not safe on San Andres island
Costa Rica	Yes	most	No	No	No	No	Yes	
Cuba	Bottled water advised							
Dominica	Bottled water advised							
Dominican Republic	No	No	No	No	No	Yes	Yes	
Ecuador	No	No	No	No	No	Yes	Yes	
El Salvador	Yes	Yes	Yes	No	No	Yes	Yes	
Falkland Islands	Yes	Yes	Yes	Yes	Yes	No	Yes	
French Guiana	No	No	No	No	No	Yes	Yes	
Grenada	Yes	Yes	Yes	Yes	Yes	No	Yes	
Guadeloupe	Bottled water advised							
Guatemala	No	No	No	No	No	Yes	No	

AMERICAS/CARIBBEAN

	Water is safe in:					Unsafe/unreliable			
	Capital?	Main cities?	Hotels & resorts?	Rural areas?	Everywhere?	Everywhere?	Bottled widely available?	Comments
Guyana	No	No	No	No	No	Yes	Yes	
Haiti	No	No	No	No	No	Yes	Yes	
Honduras	No	No	No	No	No	Yes	Yes	
Jamaica	Yes	Yes	Yes	No	No	No	Yes	Avoid tap water during drought periods
Martinique	Yes	Yes	Yes	Yes	Yes	No	Yes	
Mexico	No	No	No	No	No	Yes	Yes	
Montserrat	Yes	Yes	Yes	Yes	Yes	No	Yes	
Neth Antilles	Yes	Yes	Yes	Yes	Yes	No	Yes	
Nicaragua	No	No	No	No	No	Yes	Yes	
Panama	Yes	Yes	Yes	No	No	No	Yes	
Paraguay	Yes	Yes	Yes	No	No	No	Yes	
Peru	No	No	No	No	No	Yes	Yes	
Puerto Rico	Yes	Yes	Yes	Yes	Yes	No	Yes	
St Kitts/ Nevis	Bottled water advised							
St Lucia	Yes	Yes	Yes	Yes	Yes	No	Yes	
St Vincent	Yes	Yes	Yes	Yes	Yes	No	Yes	
Surinam	Yes	Yes	Yes	No	No	No	Yes	
Trinidad	Yes	Yes	Yes	Yes	Yes	No	Yes	
Uruguay	Yes	Yes	Yes	Yes	Yes	No	Yes	
USA	Yes	Yes	Yes	Yes	Yes	No	Yes	
Venezuela	No	No	No	No	No	Yes	Yes	

ASIA

	Water is safe in:					Unsafe/unreliable			
	Capital?	Main cities?	Hotels & resorts?	Rural areas?	Everywhere?	Everywhere?	Bottled widely available?	Comments
Afghanistan	No	No	No	No	No	Yes	No	Complete absence of infrastructure
Armenia								
Azerbaijan	No	Some	Most	Some	No	No	Yes	
Bali	No	No	Some	No	No	No	Yes	
Bangladesh	No	No	No	No	No	Yes	Yes	Heavy arsenic content in some deep well water is a serious problem
Belarus	Yes	Yes	Hotels	No	No	No	Yes	
Bhutan	No	No	No	No	No	No		
Brunei	No	No	No	No	No	Yes	Yes	
Cambodia	No	No	No	No	No	Yes	Yes	
China	Yes	No	No	No	No	No	Yes	
East Timor (Indonesia)	No	No	No	No	No	Yes	Yes	
Georgia	No	No	No	No	No	Yes	Yes	
Hong Kong	Yes		Yes		Yes	No	Yes	
India	No	No	No	No	No	Yes	Yes	
Indonesia	No	No	No	No	No	Yes	Yes	
Iran	Yes	Yes	Yes	Mostly	Mostly	No	No	
Irian Jaya (Indonesia)	No	No	No	No	No	Yes	Yes	
Japan	Yes	Yes	Yes	Yes	Yes	No	Yes	
Kazakhstan	No	No	No	No	No	Yes	Yes	
Korea (North)	No	No	No	No	No	Yes	Cities	
Korea (South)	No	No	No	No	No	Yes	Cities	
Kyrgystan (Kyrgyz Republic)	Yes	No	Yes	No	No	No	Yes	
Laos	No	No	No	No	No	Yes	Yes	
Malaysia	Yes	Yes	Yes	No	No	No	Yes	

ASIA

	Water is safe in:					Unsafe/unreliable		
	Capital?	Main cities?	Hotels & resorts?	Rural areas?	Everywhere?	Everywhere?	Bottled widely available?	Comments
Maldives	No		Some		No	No	Yes	
Mongolia	Yes	No	No	No	No	No	Yes	
Myanmar (Burma)	No	No	No	No	No	Yes	No	
Nepal	No	No	No	No	No	Yes	Yes	
Pakistan	No	No	No	No	No	Yes	Yes	
Philippines	No	No	No	No	No	Yes	Cities	
Singapore	Yes	-	-	-	-	-	Yes	
Sri Lanka	No	No	No	No	No	Yes	Yes	
Taiwan	No	No	No	No	No	Yes	Yes	
Thailand	Yes	Yes	Yes	No	No	No	Yes	
Turkey	Yes	Some	No	No	No	No	Yes	
Turkmenistan	No	No	No	No	No	Yes	Capital only	
Uzbekistan	No	No	No	No	No	Yes	Yes	
Vietnam	No	No	No	No	No	Yes	Capital & main cities	
Yemen	No	No	No	No	No	Yes		

AUSTRALASIA/PACIFIC

	Water is safe in:					Unsafe/unreliable			
	Capital?	Main cities?	Hotels & resorts?	Rural areas?	Everywhere?	Everywhere?	Bottled widely available?	Comments
Solomon Islands	No	No	No	No	No	Yes	Major towns & resorts
Australia	Yes	Yes	Yes	Yes	Yes	No	Yes
Fiji	Yes	Yes	Yes	Yes	Yes	No	Yes
Hawaii	Yes	Yes	Yes	Yes	Yes	No	Yes
New Zealand	Yes	Yes	Yes	Yes	Yes	No	Yes
Papua New Guinea	Yes	Yes	Yes	No	No	No	Urban areas only
Samoa	No	No	No	No	No	Yes	No
Tonga	No	No	No	No	No	Yes	Yes
Vanuatu	Yes	Yes	Yes	Yes	Yes	No	Yes

EUROPE

	Water is safe in:					Unsafe/unreliable			
	Capital?	Main cities?	Hotels & resorts?	Rural areas?	Everywhere?	Everywhere?	Bottled widely available?	Comments
Albania								
Andorra	Yes	Yes	Yes	Yes	Yes	No	Yes	
Austria	Yes	Yes	Yes	Yes	Yes	No	Yes	
Azores								
Belgium	Yes	Yes	Yes	Yes	Yes	No	Yes	
Bosnia	Yes	Yes	Yes	Yes	Yes	No	Yes	
Bulgaria	No	No	No	No	No	Yes	Yes	
Canary Is	Yes	Yes	Yes	Yes	Yes	No	Yes	
Croatia	Yes	Yes	Yes	Yes	Yes	No	Yes	
Cyprus	Yes	Yes	Yes	Yes	Yes	No	Yes	
Czech Republic	Yes	Yes	Yes	Yes	Yes	No	Yes	
Denmark	Yes	Yes	Yes	Yes	Yes	No	Yes	No fluoride in water
Estonia	Yes	Yes	Yes	Yes	Yes	No	Yes	
Finland	Yes	Yes	Yes	Yes	Yes	No	Yes	
France	Yes	Yes	Yes	Variable		No	Yes	
Germany	Yes	Yes	Yes	Yes	Yes	No	Yes	
Gibraltar	Yes				Yes	No	Yes	
Greece	Yes	Yes	Yes	Most	No	No	Yes	
Greenland	Yes	Yes	Yes	Yes	Yes	No	Yes	
Hungary	Yes	Yes	Yes	Yes	Yes	No	Yes	
Iceland	Yes	Yes	Yes	Yes	Yes	No	No	

EUROPE

	Water is safe in:				Unsafe/unreliable			
	Capital?	Main cities?	Hotels & resorts?	Rural areas?	Everywhere?	Everywhere?	Bottled widely available?	Comments
Ireland	Yes	Yes	Yes	Yes	Yes	No	Yes	
Italy	Yes	Yes	Yes	variable		No	Yes	
Latvia	No	No	No	No	No	Yes	Yes	
Luxembourg	Yes	Yes	Yes	Yes	Yes	No	Yes	
Lithuania	No	No	No	No	No	Yes	Yes	
Macedonia	Yes	Yes	Yes	Yes	Yes	No	Yes	
Malta	Yes	Yes	Yes	Yes	Yes	No	Yes	
Moldova	Yes	Yes	Yes	No	No	No	Yes	
Monaco	Yes				Yes	No	Yes	
Netherlands	Yes	Yes	Yes	Yes	Yes	No	Yes	
Norway	Yes	Yes	Yes	Yes	Yes	No	Yes	
Poland	Yes	Yes	Yes	Yes	Yes	No	Yes	
Portugal	Yes	Yes	Yes	Yes	Yes	No	Yes	
Romania	Yes	Yes	Yes	No	No	No	Yes	
Russian Federation	No	No	No	No	No	Yes	Yes	
Slovakia	Yes	Yes	Yes	Yes	Yes	No	Yes	
Slovenia	Yes	Yes	Yes	Yes	Yes	No	Yes	
Spain	Yes	Yes	Yes	No	No	No	Yes	
Sweden	Yes	Yes	Yes	Yes	Yes	No	Yes	No fluoride in water
Switzerland	Yes	Yes	Yes	Yes	Yes	No	Yes	Low fluoride
Ukraine	No	No	No	No	No	Yes	Yes	

MIDDLE EAST

| | Water is safe in: | | | | Unsafe/unreliable | | | |
	Capital?	Main cities?	Hotels & resorts?	Rural areas?	Everywhere?	Everywhere?	Bottled widely available?	Comments
Abu Dhabi	Yes	Yes	Yes		Yes	No	Yes	
Bahrain	No	No	No	No	No	Yes	Yes	
Iraq	No	No	No	No	No	Yes	No	
Israel	Yes	Yes	Yes	Yes	Yes	No	Yes	
Jordan	No	No	No	No	No	Yes	Yes	
Kuwait	Yes	No	Yes	Yes	Yes	No	Yes	
Lebanon	No	No	No	No	No	Yes	Yes	
Oman	Yes	Yes	No	Yes	Yes	No	Yes	
Qatar	Yes	Yes	Yes		Yes	No	Yes	
Saudi Arabia	No	No	No	No	No	Yes	Yes	
Syria	No	No	No	No	No	Yes	Yes	
United Arab Emirates	Yes	Yes	Yes	No	No	No		

Appendix 5:
Some hints on eating abroad under extreme conditions of bad hygiene

1. Choice of food

Diarrhoea is preventable, not inevitable, but precautions often run counter to instinct. At home, we are conditioned to thinking of an attractive salad as being healthier than a plate of chips, and fresh fruit juice as healthier than sugary soda; in hot, poor countries, they are not. At home, we use 'appetite appeal', not safety, to choose from a menu; they don't always go together. When travelling, it is hard to accept that we can't always eat what we want or what we have already paid for, especially when we feel tired and hungry. Cultivate the art of defensive eating — especially if gastronomy is not the major purpose of your trip!

Here are some general principles to follow when you know or suspect that hygiene conditions are very poor:

- When possible, choose food that *must* have been freshly cooked e.g. omelette, chips, items that are not on the menu or on display and so have to be cooked to order
- Freshly boiled food, served piping hot, is always safe e.g. rice, sweetcorn
- Eat fruit or vegetables that are easily peeled or sliced open without contamination e.g. bananas, citrus fruits, melon, papaya, avocado
- Eat food from sealed packs or cans (take emergency supplies!)
- Look for freshly baked bread (find the bakery)
- Choose acceptably prepared local dishes rather than incompetently prepared imitation western-style food
- Regard all cooked food as only safe when *freshly* prepared and served hot (not stored and then reheated)
- Be prepared to send food back and to complain when appropriate.

Whenever possible, prepare your food yourself, or watch it being cooked.

2. Don't eat

- Salads
- Food that you do not *know* to have been freshly cooked, including hotel buffet food left out in warm temperatures
- Food on which flies have settled or may have settled
- Shellfish, crab, prawns, etc. (which need 8 minutes' vigorous boiling as an absolute minimum)
- Intricate dishes that have required much handling in preparation
- Unwashed (in *clean* water) or unpeelable fruit or vegetables
- Ice cream and ices

- Dairy products made from unpasteurized milk. In some countries, not all 'pasteurized' milk has really been pasteurized
- Rare meat, steak tartare, raw fish
- Unpeelable fruit (berries, grapes) or fruit peeled by others (fruit buffets)
- Fruit, butter, or other foods chilled by adding ice
- Food handled with dirty fingers; avoid foods that necessarily require much handling, such as canapés
- Spicy sauces, salsa, relishes, mayonnaise left out on the table; (hot sauces, however spicy, are not self-sterilizing!).

On a two-week trip, you will probably be eating 42 meals prepared by others: the only way to protect yourself is to be selective about what you eat.

Beware of hospitality: if the food is not safe, refuse it, and plead an upset stomach — local people will usually understand. Where there is no alternative to unsafe food, smaller quantities on an empty stomach are safer. Consider missing a meal; many Western travellers can afford to lose a little weight, and it is safer to do so by choice than from illness.

3. Plates and cutlery

These need to be washed with detergent, rinsed with clean water, and protected from flies. When this has not or cannot be done, and you suspect that they are contaminated, the risk can be reduced by rinsing with hot weak tea, a small amount of whisky or other duty free spirit, or by cleaning with an alcohol swab or wet wipes. Use wipes on cutlery, or flame them with a candle or a cigarette lighter.

Otherwise, don't eat the bottom layer of food on the plate — easy when food is served on a bed of rice. Alternatively, use paper plates and your own cutlery. (Plastic airline cutlery is good for emergency use; in Asia, packs of disposable chopsticks are cheap and widely available.)

4. Hands and fingers

Should be washed at every opportunity; if possible, keep a supply of wet wipes. Only eat food that you have handled if your hands are scrupulously clean; otherwise, use a clean tissue, the inside of a clean plastic bag, or a piece of bread to handle food; or use your fingers, but discard any part of the food that you have handled.

5. Drinks

Drinking water should be sterilized with iodine or boiled. Hot tea is often easily available. Bottled drinks should be opened in your presence — safest if carbonated. In the tropics, also try baby coconuts (they contain a pint of sweet water — bring your own straws). Don't drink fruit juices from street vendors. Get into the habit of never using ice. Don't use tap water — even for brushing teeth; if you really must, water from the hot tap is likely to be safer.

6. Cups and glasses

Those that may be contaminated can be swilled out with hot tea or boiling water before use. Flies often settle on rims — pour away a little tea to rinse the rim of a teacup. Otherwise, use your own cup or water bottle, or drink bottled drinks directly from their bottle.

Eating is supposed to be part of the travel experience. In Korea, local delicacies include dried fish heads, roasted locusts, sea slugs, toasted silkworms, snake, and dog meat. In West Africa, you might be offered stir-fried termites; and in New Guinea, roasted palm grubs (they taste of caramel) — in fact, insects are widely eaten in many parts of the tropics*. In French Guiana, endangered species like black cayman ('caiman á l'orange'), red ibises, and anacondas are casually served in tourist hotels. In China, bear paw, deep-fried crunchy scorpion, and rat kebab are further possibilities, and so are bull's genitalia in Vietnam. Meat from monkeys, other primates and game animals – 'bush meat' – is firmly on the menu in many African countries and is often traded illegally. It has been implicated in the spread of foot-and-mouth disease to livestock, and recent reports indicate that one in six monkeys eaten in Cameroon are infected with the simian form of HIV.

Some travellers regard dietary advice as an attempt to rob them of opportunities to try new foods. This is not my intention, though strict health grounds are not always the only reason for foregoing the pleasure. But no matter what food you are offered, and whether or not you are tempted to accept, the same fundamental principles of food hygiene always apply.

---

*Some of global cuisine's most disgusting offerings can be found, beautifully photographed, in *Man Eating Bugs: The Art and Science of Eating Insects* Menzel P, D'Aluisio F, Ten Speed Press 1998, 15800 80510.

Appendix 6:
Medical kit check-list

Here is a checklist of the main things to consider when putting together a medical kit for travel. It is unlikely that all of these would be needed — the exact choice will depend on where you are going, how long you will be away, and what you will be doing. Read the chapter on medical kits p. 573 and the other relevant sections of this book before drawing up your own final list.

The check-list is divided into three parts — items to include in a basic medical kit, additional things to consider for frequent or extended travel to developing countries, and finally, some things to consider for long-haul flights.

1. Basic medical kit
- **Sterile supplies**
  A small selection of syringes and needles (assorted sizes) to reduce the risk of transmission of HIV or hepatitis B in the event of medical treatment.

- **Wound dressings**
  — assorted plasters
  — bandages
  — micropore tape

- **Antiseptic**
  — cream (e.g. Savlon or Germolene) and/or
  — spray (e.g. Betadine) and/or
  — solution (e.g. Chlorhexidine) and/or
  — antiseptic wipes
  — tea tree oil/spotstick

- **Medication**
  — pain relief (e.g. paracetamol or ibuprofen)
  — anti-histamine (e.g. Piriton or Clarityn)
  — anti-diarrhoeal (e.g. Imodium)
  — rehydration sachets (e.g. Electrolade or Dioralyte)
  — malaria medication (if appropriate)

- **Other useful products**
  — scissors
  — tweezers
  — non-sterile gloves
  — anti-insect supplies (insect repellent, etc.)
  — water purification tablets/iodine drops

2. Additional supplies for frequent, extended, or high-risk travel

- **Sterile supplies**
  — sterile gloves
  — disposable sutures
  — local anaesthetic*
  — steristrips (for wound closure)
  — lancets (for popping blisters)
  — sterile non-adherent dressing (melolin)
  — gauze pads
  — dental repair kit

- **More extensive first-aid supplies as appropriate**
  — dressings, paraffin gauze
  — splints
  — cool packs, spray

- **Creams and lotions**
  For itching and insect bites
  — Eurax cream
  — calamine lotion
  — hydrocortisone cream

  For fungal infections
  — miconazole cream or
  — clotrimazole cream (e.g. Canesten)

  For pain and stiffness
  — ibuprofen gel
  — tiger balm

  For lips and cold sores
  — acyclovir
  — lipsalve with UV protection

  For vaginal infections
  — Canesten pessary
  — miconazole cream

- **Additional medication**

  Pain relief
  — diclofenac* (e.g. Voltarol) (stronger painkiller with anti-inflammatory properties)

  Antibiotics
  — ciprofloxacin*
  — co-amoxiclav*
  — metronidazole*/ Tinidazole*
  — doxycycline*
  — amoxycillin*

  Motion sickness/nausea
  — promethazine/cyclizine/dimenhydrinate/ buclizine
  — scopolamine patches*
  — Stugeron
  — metaclopramide*

- **Eye drops**
  — gentamicin drops*

- **Additional items to consider**
  — sleeping tablets (e.g. zimovane*, zaleplon*)
  — vitamins
  — antacids
  — laxatives
  — cold/sinus medicines
  — anti-worm medication (mebendazole)
  — anti-insect supplies (insect repellent, net, clothing treatment, mosquito killer etc.)
  — water purification tablets/iodine
  — thermometer strips

3. In-flight kit

— saline nasal spray or drops
— eye drops (comfort drops) and contact lens supplies
— anti-embolism stockings (for prevention of deep-vein thrombosis)
— dispersible low-dose aspirin (for prevention of deep-vein thrombosis)

Key: * prescription required

Appendix 7:
Post-tropical screening

The need for and format of a medical examination on returning from the tropics depends largely upon where you have been and what you have been doing whilst abroad: some people find it reassuring, and it may occasionally reveal an unsuspected problem.

Dr Carol Dow has worked for the Foreign and Commonwealth office since 1989, and has been their Chief Medical adviser since 1998.

If you have no symptoms or signs of illness

Opinions vary on the value of a check-up in people without symptoms or signs of illness. It is certainly not necessary following short trips, unless there has been a particular risk or problem. It may be worth considering for people who have been ill while away, or who have been living or working in a developing country.

Expert advice may be needed to match a travel itinerary/activity list to the most likely potential infections (e.g. where schistosomiasis is present and transmission likely, or the risk of HIV and hepatitis B), but it should be possible for a GP to carry out all appropriate tests in individuals who are well.

For those with symptoms

If you actually have symptoms, you do not need post-tropical screening, you need examination, investigation, and treatment! Your doctor may well need to seek advice from a tropical disease unit, which will probably offer a gentle reminder that any delay in looking for malaria can be extremely dangerous. It is not good enough simply to send a blood sample off to the local laboratory, expecting the result back after a weekend: you can die from malaria within 24 hours of the first symptom. To think that you and your doctor thought it might be only 'flu!

- **Fever** generally indicates infection and needs investigation.
- **Diarrhoea** may be due to infection and may need investigation if it lasts longer than 48 hours.
- **Jaundice** may be due to infection with a hepatitis virus or malaria and always warrants investigation.
- **Respiratory symptoms** such as sore throat or productive cough are common in travellers and need investigation.

- **Malaria** is a killer, the symptoms often vague and non-specific. Fever, chills, and headache are the cardinal symptoms, but others include diarrhoea, vomiting, cough, abdominal pain, and jaundice.
- **Other infections** such as viral hepatitis can cause vague symptoms initially, including tiredness and loss of appetite.

Examination

A tropical specialist may be able to identify the cause of a rash caused by a tropical infection, and should be more familiar with the detection of an enlarged spleen (following malaria) than a UK-based GP.

Quite often, the abnormalities detected by examination turn out to be due to diseases of temperate zones such as high blood pressure, obesity, and diabetes (on dipstick urine testing), rather than exotic or tropical diseases.

Tests

The most helpful tests are a full blood count with white cell differential to detect a rise in eosinophils — a general indicator of infection with certain parasites — and a stool sample for cysts, ova, and parasites. A dipstick urine test will detect sugar, blood, or protein in the urine — all of which warrant further investigation.

For anyone exposed to fresh water in schistosomal areas, a blood test for schistosomiasis should be performed — at least six weeks after the last possible exposure, so as to avoid false negatives.

High-risk sexual exposure (or exposure to non-sterile needles or medical treatment) might warrant screening for antibodies to HIV, hepatitis B, or possibly syphilis.

And finally

Travel-related symptoms can sometimes take a very long time to appear — remember to tell the doctor about your travels for at least a year after your return. Any visit to a doctor on returning home should be used as a reminder to carry on taking malaria medication for the appropriate period, usually four weeks.

Appendix 8:
Directory: Specialist centres, information sources, and web directory

Although the information provided in the first part of this Appendix is classified by region, many of the resources listed here can readily be accessed from any part of the world via the Internet.

United Kingdom

GPs are able to provide many travel-related vaccines; many are also licensed to give the yellow fever vaccine, though many of these stopped providing it during an extended vaccine shortage in 2000 and 2001, and have not resumed. (A complete list of yellow fever centres in England can be found on the **Department of Health web-site** at **www.tap.ccta.gov.uk/doh/yellcode.nsf/pages/Home?open.** In Scotland, further information is available at **www.show.scot.nhs.uk** or by calling the NHS Helpline on 0800 224488. See also sources below.

For students travelling abroad, the most suitable source of advice will almost always be their university health centre.

Malaria medication and most travel vaccines are not normally available on the NHS.

Dedicated travel clinics tend to have the full range of vaccines in stock and immediately available and, no less importantly, specialist staff who are well informed about the necessary precautions. Time your appointment so that the staff will not be frantically busy and will have time to answer any specific questions you may have.

London's main travel clinics

Hospital for Tropical Diseases, Mortimer Market, Capper St, London WC1E 6JA Tel: 020 7388 9600; **www.thehtd.org**; Premium rate advice line: 09061 33 77 33

Fleet Street Travel Clinic, 29 Fleet Street, London EC4Y 1AA; also custom medical kits and supplies; Tel: 020 7353 5678; **www.fleetstreetclinic.com**

Trailfinders Ltd, 194 Kensington High Street, London W8 7RG; Tel: 020 7938 3999; **www.trailfinders.co.uk**

British Airways Travel Clinics, 101 Cheapside, London EC2V 6DT; Tel: 020 7606 2977; 115 Buckingham Palace Road, SW1W 9SJ, Tel: 020 7233 6661; 156 Regent Street, W1B 5LB. **www.britishairways.co.uk**

Royal Free Travel Health Centre, Pond Street, Hampstead, London NW3 2QG; Tel: 020 7830 2885; **www.travel-health.co.uk**

Outside London

Liverpool School of Tropical Medicine, Pembroke Place, Liverpool, Merseyside L3 5QA; Tel: 0151 708 9393; **www.liv.ac.uk/lstm/clin/clin3.htm**; Premium rate advice line: 0906 708 8807

SCIEH Immunization Clinic, Clifton House, Clifton Place, Glasgow G3 7LN Tel: 0141 300 1100 and Gartnavel General Hospital, 1053 Gt. Western Road, Glasgow G12 0YN Tel: 1410 211 3000 **www.show.scot.ns/scieh**

Travel Clinic, Regional Infections Diseases Unit, Western General Hospital, Crewe Rd, Edinburgh EH4 2RU Tel: 0131 537 1000

MASTA operate several clinics around the UK (they also provide many health-related supplies and services) — for more information see **www.masta.org**

Information from the Department of Health

If you are planning to travel abroad you should obtain a copy of the Department of Health Leaflet T6, '*Health Advice for Travellers*,' updated annually and available from main post offices, and also by freephone from the **Health Literature Line**, 0800 555 777. This gives information on health precautions, reciprocal health agreements, and vaccinations. It also contains Form E111, which entitles you to free, or reduced cost emergency medical treatment in many EC countries.

Health advice for travellers is available at **www.doh.gov.uk/traveladvice/index.htm** and **www.fitfortravel.scot.nhs**

Advice is also available from **NHS Direct** at **www.nhsdirect.nhs.uk**; and from NHS Direct Wales **www.nhsdirect.wales.nhs.uk**; and by telephone on 0845 4647.

For further information, contact one of the following **UK Government Health Departments**:

- The Department of Health, Richmond House, 79 Whitehall, London SW1A 2NS; Tel: 020 7210 4850 Minicom: 0207 210 5025. E-mail: dhmail@doh.gsi.gov.uk **www.doh.gov.uk**
- Scottish Executive Health Department, St Andrew's House, Regent Road, Edinburgh EH1 3DG Tel: 0131 556 8400 **www.show.scot.nhs.uk/**
- Welsh Office, Cathays Park, Cardiff CF1 3NQ, Tel: 0222 825111 Ext. 3395 **www.wales.nhs.uk**
- DHSSPS, Castle Buildings, Stormont, Belfast BT4 3SJ Tel: : (028) 90520500 Fax: (028) 90520572 **www.n-i.nhs.uk**

Major UK centres specializing in tropical diseases

The Hospital for Tropical Diseases, Mortimer Market, Capper Street, Tottenham Court Road, London WC1E 6AU; Tel: 020 7387 9300 or 020 7387 4411; **www.thehtd.org**

Liverpool School of Tropical Medicine, Pembroke Place, Liverpool L3 5QA; Tel: 0151 708 9393; **www.liv.ac.uk/lstm/clin/clin3.htm**

The Centre for Tropical Medicine, Nuffield Department of Clinical Medicine, John Radcliffe Hospital, Oxford OX3 9DU; Tel: 01865 222316; **www.jr2.ox.ac.uk/ndm/Tropical_Medicine/pages/home.htm**

Department of Communicable and Tropical Diseases, Birmingham Heartland Hospital, Bordesley Green Road, Birmingham B9 5ST; Tel: 0121 766 6611

SCIEH, (Scottish Centre for Infection and Environmental Health), Clifton House, Clifton Place, Glasgow G3 7LN; Tel: 0141 300 1130

PHLS Communicable Disease Surveillance Unit, 61 Colindale Avenue, London NW9 5EQ; Tel: 020 8200 6868; **www.phls.co.uk**

Other key resources

The PHLS Malaria Reference Laboratory, at the London School of Hygiene & Tropical Medicine, Keppel St, London WC1E 7BR; **www.malaria-reference.co.uk/** provides specialist advice about anti-malarial precautions for individual countries, on a special premium rate helpline: Tel: 09065 508908. For health-care professionals only, who need to discuss particular problem cases, the laboratory can be contacted on 020 7636 3924.

Official UK guidelines on malaria prevention are published in the British National Formulary (BNF) (**www.bnf.org**) — see Further Reading — and on the Malaria Reference Laboratory web-site (above) and are updated from time to time.

The Foreign & Commonwealth Office, King Charles Street, London SW1; Tel: 020 7270 3000, provides information about political risks abroad, and should be consulted if you intend to visit a part of the world where there is currently unrest or instability. Web-site: **www.knowbeforeyougo.co.uk** The web-site can be 'personalized' to provide e-mail notification and to keep you up to date with news of important developments.

Other useful addresses

Nomad Travellers Store & Medical Centre, 40 Bernard St, London WC1N 1LE, Tel: 020 7833 4114 and 3 Turnpike Lane, London N8 OPX. Tel: 020 8889 7014. Travel pharmacy plus vaccines, medical kits, and supplies. **www.nomadtravel.co.uk**

Expedition Advisory Centre, Royal Geographical Society, 1 Kensington Gore, London SW7 2AR; Tel: 020 7589 5466. Huge variety of resources for travellers and expeditioners of all kinds. Organizes frequent lectures and seminars. **www.rgs.org**

Teaching Aids at Low Cost, (TALC), PO Box 49, St. Albans, Herts AL1 4AX, UK. Tel: 01727 853869; fax: 01727846852; e-mail: talc@talcuk.org; website: **www.talcuk.org**. TALC sells books, instruction slides, Zeal clinical thermometers and sugar and salt measuring spoons.

Ireland

The free booklet '*General health information for people travelling abroad*' is published by the **Health Promotion Unit of the Department of Health and Children**, Hawkins House, Dublin 2, Ireland, Tel: 01–6354000, Fax: 01–635 4001, E-mail: queries@health.irlgov.ie.

The main specialist travel clinics / tropical medicine centres are:

Tropical Medical Bureau, Dun Laoghaire Medical Centre, 5 Northumberland Avenue, Dun Laoghaire, Co Dublin. Tel: 01–280 4996, Fax: 01–280 5603, E-mail dlmc@tmb.ie.

Grafton Street Medical Centre, Grafton Buildings, 34 Grafton Street, Dublin 2, Tel: 01–671 9200 Fax: 01–671 9211 **www.tmb.ie**

Royal College of Surgeons in Ireland Travel Health Clinic, Mercers Health Centre, Lower Stephens Street, Dublin 2, Ireland, Tel: 01–497 6379

Infectious disease monitoring and surveillance

National Disease Surveillance Centre, Sir Patrick Dun's Hospital, Lower Grand Canal, Street, Dublin 2, Ireland. Tel: +353 (0)1 6617346, Fax: +353 (0)1 6617347, E-mail: info@ndsc.ie **www.ndsc.ie**

The **Department of Foreign Affairs** web-site is **www.gov.ie/iveagh/**

United States of America

In the USA, it is historically the responsibility of city, county, and state departments of health to provide information for the public about immunization. Many still do this and they should also be consulted for information about the nearest immunization clinic; health department clinics generally carry a good stock of travel vaccines, including yellow fever. Information can also be obtained from local offices of the **US Public Health Service.**

However, the major source of health information for international travel is now the federally funded **Centers for Disease Control and Prevention (CDC)**, 1600 Clifton Road, Atlanta, GA 30333. A vast range of information is available, and the simplest way to access this is through the internet (**www.cdc.gov/**). Public inquiries: (404) 639–3534 and (800) 311–3435. See Further Reading for official publications.

Directories of travel clinics across the USA (and elsewhere) as well as centres specializing in tropical medicine can be found on the web-sites of the **American Society of Tropical Medicine & Hygiene** (**www.astmh.org**) and the **International Society of Travel Medicine** (**www.istm.org**)

The **State Department** web-site (**travel.state.gov/**) carries the latest information on US government travel warnings, consular information sheets, and public alerts and announcements, and provides access to a host of other important information services.

The **US State Department Citizens Emergency Center**, Tel: (202) 647 5225 (24 hours), provides information about political and other risks abroad, and should be consulted if you intend to visit a part of the world where there is currently unrest or instability; it also provides advice for travellers and their families in distress. Using a touch-tone phone, you can select pre-recorded advisory information for any country, or you can speak directly with a State Department employee.

Canada

Health Canada's Travel Medicine Program provides current information on international disease outbreaks, immunization, general health advice for travellers, and disease-specific treatment and prevention guidelines. Information is accessible via the FAXlink service (613–941–3900) or the Internet (**www.travelhealth.gc.ca**). This web-site also contains a directory of travel clinics throughout Canada, plus links to other key resources such as a PDF version of the *Canadian Immunization Guide*.

Information about safety and security is provided by the **Department of Foreign Affairs and International Travel voyage.dfait-macci.gc.ca/destinations/menu_e.htm**. Government publications on subjects ranging from safety advice for women to adventure travel, business travel, and imprisonment abroad can be accessed at

www.voyage.gc.ca/Consular-e/publications_menu-e.htm. Travellers with specific problems should contact the DFAIT Operations Centre at Tel: (613) 996–8885 Fax: (613) 943–1054 E-mail: sos@dfait-maeci.gc.ca

Main travel and tropical disease clinics in Canada

Quebec: McGill Centre for Tropical Diseases Montreal General Hospital 1650 Cedar Ave., #D7-153 Montreal, quebec H3G 1A4 Tel: 1-514-933-7045 Fax: 1-514-933-9385 E-mail: MD10@musica.mcgill.ca Web: **www.medcor.mcgill.ca/~tropmed/td/txt** (Pre- and Post-Travel)

Travel Medisys Health Group Inc. 500 Sherbrooke Street West, Suite 1100 Montreal. Quebec H3A 3C6 Tel: 1-514-499-2773 Fax: 1-514-845-484 E-mail: tesd:@medisys.ca (Pre- and Post-Travel)

Ontario: Centre for Travel & Tropical Medicine Toronto General Hospital, University Health Network Eaton North, g-208 200 Elizabath Street Toronto, Ontario. M5G 2C4 Tel: 1-416-340-3000 Fax: 1-416-340-3260 E-mail: traveclinic@un.on.ca. Web: **www.tghtravel.ca** (Pre and Post-Travel)

Riverside Travel Medicine Clinic 1919 Riverside Drive, Suite 411 Ottawa, Ontario. K1H 1A2 Tel: 1-613-733-5553 Fax: 1-613-733-2689 E-mail: post@travelclinic.org Web: **www.travelclinic.org** (Pre-Travel)

Alberta: Capital Health Authority Travellers's Health Services 10320-100 St. Edmonton, Alberta T5J 0R3 Tel: 1-780-413-5745 Fax: 1-780-420-0483 E-mail: hbirk@cha.ab.ca Web: **www.ca.ab.ca/travellers** (Pre-Travel)

British Columbia: Travel Clinic Vancouver/Richmond Health Board L-5 601 West Broadway Vancouver, BC V52 4C2 Tel: 1-604-736-9244 Fax: 1-604-736-3917 E-mail: suniboraston@vrhb.bc.ca Web: **travelclinic.vancouver.bc.ca** (Pre-Travel)

Key Canadian travel health information sites for health care professionals:

Committee to Advise on Tropical Medicine and Travel (CATMAT) **www.c-sc.gc.ca/pb/lcdc/osh/reccom_e.tml#catmat**

Canadian Immunization Guide, 5th ed., 1998 **www.hc-sc.gc.ca/pb/lcec/publicat/immguide/index.html**

Canada Communicable Disease Report (CCDR) **www.c-sc.gc.ca/pb/lcdc/publicat/ccdr/01vol27/index.html**

Public Health Information **www.hc.sc.gc./hpb/lcdc/phi_e.html**

Australia

Information about immunization recommendations and requirements is available from GPs and university health centres. Information can also be obtained from regional offices of the **Australian Department of Health and Aged Care**. Complete contact information for these can be found at **www.health.gov.au/contacts.htm**.

Information about approved yellow fever vaccination centres can be obtained from the following **State and Territory departments**, and health department advice on yellow fever can be found at **www.health.gov.au/pubhlth/strateg/communic/factsheets/yellow.htm**

Australian Capital Territory: Communicable Disease Control Unit, Department of Health and Community Care, Tel: (02) 6205 2300

Northern Territory Disease Control Program: Territory Health Services, Tel: (08) 8922 8044

South Australia: Communicable Disease Control Branch, Department of Human Services, Tel: (08) 8226 7192

Victoria: Disease Control Section, Department of Human Services, Tel: (03) 9637 4130

New South Wales: AIDS/Infectious Diseases Branch, NSW Health Department, Tel: (02) 9391 9196

Queensland: Communicable Diseases Unit, Queensland Department of Health, Tel: (07) 3234 1062

Tasmania: Public Health Branch, Department of Health and Human Services, Tel: (03) 6233 3775

Western Australia: Communicable Disease Control, Health Department of Western Australia, Tel: (08) 9388 4863

The **Travel Doctor Group/TMVC** runs a national network of specialist private vaccination centres, as well as a service for returning travellers: Head office: TMVC House 27–29 Gilbert Place, Adelaide SA 5000, Tel: 1300 658 844 **www.traveldoctor.com.au**

Another private group is **Travel Clinics Australia**, Tel: (61 3) 9528 1222 **www.travelclinic.com.au/**

The **Australian Department of Foreign Affairs & Trade** (Tel: 61 2 6261 1111 Fax: 61 2 6261 3111) provides advice on safety and political risks via its web-site at **www.dfat.gov.au/consular/advice/index.html** and in a booklet entitled *Hints for Australian Travellers*. This booklet is updated twice a year and provided free with each new Australian passport; it contains contact details of all Australian overseas posts that provide consular services to Australian travellers, plus useful travel information and advice. Details of reciprocal health arrangements with other countries, health information and safety tips can be found at **www.dfat.gov.au/travel/travelwell.html#8** and **www.dfat.gov.au/travel/index.html**

There is a specialist infectious diseases unit at:

Commonwealth Institute of Health A27, University of Sydney, NSW 2006, Tel: 660 9292

New Zealand

Up-to-date advice on requirements and recommendations, and information about yellow fever vaccination centres are available from general practitioners and Area Health Boards, addresses below. The **Department of Health** also publishes a booklet entitled *Passport to Healthy Travel*, available from Government Print Offices or on application to the Department of Health, 133 Molesworth St, PO Box 5013, Wellington, Tel: 04 496 2000, or by E-mail request to pubs@moh.govt.nz , or from the HealthEd web-site: **www.healthed.govt.nz**. Health information is also available from the **Department of Health Healthline** Tel: 0800 611 166

District Health Boards: addresses and phone numbers:
Auckland: Private Bag 92–024, Auckland 1003, Tel: (09) 638 9908
Bay of Plenty: Private Bag 12 024, Tauranga, Tel: (07) 579 8010
Canterbury: PO Box 1600, Christchurch, Tel: (03) 364 0460
Capital and Coast: Private Bag 7902, Wellington South, Tel: (04) 385 5999
Counties Manukau: Private Bag 94 052, South Auckland Mail Centre, Auckland, Tel: (09) 262 9503
Hawke's Bay: Private Bag 6023, Napier, Tel: (06) 878 8109
Hutt:Private Bag 31 907, Lower Hutt, Tel: (04) 570 9488
Lakes: Private Bag 3023, Rotorua, Tel: (07) 349 7982
MidCentral: PO Box 2056, Palmerston North, Tel: (06) 350 8061
Nelson Marlborough: Private Bag 18, Nelson , Tel: (03) 546 1800
Northland: PO Box 742, Whangarei, Tel: (09) 430 4100
Otago: Private Bag 1921, Dunedin, Tel: (03) 474 0999
South Canterbury: Private Bag 911, Timaru, Tel: (03) 684 1556
Southland: PO Box 828, Invercargill, Tel: (03) 218 1949
Tairawhiti: Private Bag 7001, Gisborne , Tel: (06) 869 0500
Taranaki: — Corporate Services, Private Bag 2016, New Plymouth
Waikato: PO Box 934, Hamilton, Tel: (09) 839 4679
Wairarapa: PO Box 96, Masterton, Tel: (06) 946 9800
Waitemata: Private Bag 93 503, Takapuna, Auckland, Tel: (09) 486 1491
West Coast: PO Box 387, Greymouth, Tel: (03) 768 0499
Whanganui: Private Bag 3003, Wanganui, Tel: (06) 348 1234
TMVC have a network of specialist, private travel clinics. **www.tmvc.co.nz**
There is an infectious disease unit at Auckland Hospital, Tel: 09 379 7440
Additional information:
New Zealand Communicable Disease Centre, Kenepuru Drive, Porirua, Wellington, Tel: 04 370 149
The **New Zealand Ministry of Foreign Affairs & Trade** provides advice on travel security and safety. Web-site: **www.mft.govt.nz** Information by phone, Tel: 64–4 494–8500

South Africa
Up-to-date advice on requirements and recommendations, and information about yellow fever vaccination centres are available from GPs. There is a high degree of awareness generally on travel and tropical health issues.
Specialist travel clinics affiliated with the **TMVC group** can be located via **www.tmvc.com.au.**
South African Airways (SAA Netcare) clinics can be found at **www.travelclinic.co.za.**
The Department of Health web-site is at **www.health.gov.za**.
Travel advice from the Department of Foreign Affairs can be found at **www.dfa.gov.za/travelling/index.html.**

Web directory

Here is a list of some of the main Internet-based resources in travel medicine. Some of these are intended only for travellers, while others are primarily for health professionals.

- **This book also has a web-site — www.travellershealth.info,** on which you will find details of information that has changed since this book went to press, plus an online version of this section with updated links to these sites.

- Please send suggestions, corrections, and additions to webmaster@travellershealth.info

Web-site	Address	Notes
GOVERNMENT AND WHO SOURCES		
CDC (Centers for Disease Control) home page	**www.cdc.gov**	The big daddy of all disease information web-sites, a truly global resource
CDC links	**www.cdc.gov/ncidod/id/links.htm**	CDC links to other resources
CDC Travel Information home page	**www.cdc.gov/travel/index.htm**	Includes link to PDF version of CDC Yellow Book
Health Canada Travel Medicine	**www.hc-sc.gc.ca/hpb/lcdc/osh/tmp.e.html**	Canadian Government advice & resources
NHS Scotland travel health web-site (SCIEH)	**www.fitfortravel.scot.nhs.uk/**	NHS country-by-country guides, with malaria maps
NHS Travax web-site	**www.travax.scot.nhs.uk/**	Information & resources for health professionals. Registered user only
UK 'Yellow Book'	**www.the-stationery-office.co.uk/doh/hinfo/index.htm**	Official advice & information for health professionals
WHO (World Health Organization) home page	**www.who.org**	Links to massive network of WHO site and disease information
CDC Blue sheet	**www.cdc.gov/travel/blusheet.htm**	CDC listing of countries infected with yellow fever & other quarantinable diseases
WHO Travel health advice	**www.who.int/ith/**	Includes link to online version of WHO's *International Travel & Health*
Pan American Health Organization (PAHO)	**www.paho.org/**	Health in the Americas
World Tourism Organization	**www.world-tourism.org/**	Global tourism and travel statistics
Link to health departments world-wide	**www.moh.govt.nz/moh.nsf/wpgIndex/Links -Overseas+Health+Contents**	From the New Zealand Health Department

Web-site	Address	Notes
PROFESSIONAL ASSOCIATIONS		
International Society of Travel Medicine	**www.istm.org**	International organization for health professionals. Links to key resources
Aerospace Medical Association	**www.asma.org/**	Information about aviation medicine & health issues
American Public Health Association	**www.apha.org**	Infectious disease resources
American Society of Tropical Medicine & Hygiene	**www.astmh.org/**	Tropical medicine resources
ASHRAE (American Society of Heating, Refrigerating and Air-Conditioning Engineers)	**www.ashrae.org**	Aircraft cabin air quality issues
British Travel Health Associatio/n	**www.btha.org**	UK organization for health professions
Canadian Society of International Health	**www.csih.org/**	Supports global health & development, links to key sites
Royal Geographical Society	**www.rgs.org**	Country information, maps, key resource for expeditioners
Royal Society of Tropical Medicine and Hygiene (RSTMH)	**www.rstmh.org/**	Tropical medicine resources
Undersea and Hyperbaric Medicine Society	**www.uhms.org/**	Diving medicine resources
Wilderness Medical Society	**www.wms.org/**	Wilderness and outdoors
TRAVEL CLINIC DIRECTORIES		
ISTM Directory of Travel Clinics	**www.istm.org/disclinics.html**	Clinics run by members of the American Society of Tropical Medicine & Hygiene
ASTMH Directory of Travel Clinics	**www.astmh.org/clinics/clinindex.html**	Clinics run by members of the International Society of Travel Medicine
GENERAL TRAVEL HEALTH INFORMATION		
Fit For Travel (Germany)	**www.fit-for-travel.de/en/**	What the Germans do. Advice from University of Munich Tropical Institute
Fleet Street Travel Clinic, London	**www.fleetstreetclinic.com**	Private clinic web-site (my own!) with news and links

Appendix 8**661**

Web-site	Address	Notes
GENERAL TRAVEL HEALTH INFORMATION		
Lonely Planet Health	www.lonelyplanet.com/health/health.htm	Country information, travellers forum, health information
MASTA	www.masta.org	Health information plus travel health products
Medicine Planet	www.medicineplanet.com	Broad-ranging travel health info
SafeTravel Switzerland (French/German)	www.safetravel.ch/	What the Swiss do: Universites of Zurich / Basel
Shoreland Travel Health On-line	www.tripprep.com	Broad-ranging travel health info
TravelMed Web	www.travelmedicineweb.org	Educational site for health professionals
TMVC Australia	www.traveldoctor.com.au/info.html	Private clinic network, locations in Australia, NZ, South Africa and beyond
DISEASE SURVEILLANCE		
Canada Communicable Disease Report	www.hc-sc.gc.ca/hpb/lcdc/publicat/ccdr/index.html	Infectious disease news, statistics, and local outbreak reports
CDR Weekly Report	www.phls.co.uk/publications/cdrw.htm	Infectious disease news, statistics, and local outbreak reports
Communicable Disease Report Weekly	www.phls.co.uk/publications/cdrw.htm	Infectious disease news, statistics, and local outbreak reports
Communicable Diseases Australia	www.health.gov.au/pubhlth/cdi/cdihtml.htm	Infectious disease news, statistics, and local outbreak reports
EuroSurveillance	www.eurosurv.org/update/	Infectious disease news, statistics, and local outbreak reports
Hong Kong Bulletin	www.info.gov.hk/dh/diseases/content.htm	Infectious disease news, statistics, and local outbreak reports
Morbidity & Mortality Weekly Report (MMWR) — US	www2.cdc.gov/mmwr/	Key weekly resource for health professionals, from the CDC
Public Health Laboratory Service, UK	www.phls.co.uk	Infectious disease news, statistics, and local outbreak reports
SCIEH Weekly Report (Scotland)	www.show.scot.nhs.uk/scieh/report.htm	Infectious disease news, statistics, and local outbreak reports
SCIEH Home Page	www.show.scot.nhs.uk/scieh	Communicable disease surveillance — Scotland
US Military — Global Emerging Infections	www.geis.ha.osd.mil/	Surveillance site with links

Web-site	Address	Notes
DISEASE SURVEILLANCE		
WHO Weekly Epidemiological Record	**www.who.int/wer/**	WHO weekly report
EMERGING DISEASES / OUTBREAKS		
Department of Health, UK	**www.doh.gov.uk/cmo/idstrategy/index.htm**	*Getting Ahead of the Curve.* National strategy for combating infectious diseases
Emerging infectious diseases	**www.cdc.gov/ncidod/eid/index.htm**	Online journal
ProMed	**www.promedmail.org**	Unofficial first reports of outbreaks
WHO Surveillance and Response Outbreak	**www.who.int/emc/outbreak.news/index.html**	WHO outbreak news, usually of confirmed outbreaks
DISEASE INFORMATION		
CDC Health Topics A to Z	**www.cdc.gov/health/diseases.htm**	
Cholera statistics	**www.who.int/emc/diseases/cholera/choltbl2000.html**	
Cholera vaccine	**www.bernaproducts.com/Berna.nsf/htmlmedia/wchophymutacolberna.html**	
FluNet—WHO	**oms2.b3e.jussieu.fr/flunet/**	
HIV Post-Exposure Prophylaxis	**www.doh.gov.uk/eaga/pepgu20fin.pdf**	Guidance from the UK Chief Medical Officers' Expert Advisory Group on AIDS
Joint United Nations Programme on HIV/AIDS	**www.unaids.org/**	
Leishmaniasis	**www.who.int/emc/diseases/leish/leisgeo1.html**	
Leishmaniasis	**www.who.int/health-topics/leishmaniasis.htm**	
Leprosy	**www.who.int/lep**	
Lice	**www.nits.net**	
Lyme disease	**www.cdc.gov/ncidod/dvbid/lymeinfo.htm**	Information from CDC

Web-site	Address	Notes
DISEASE INFORMATION		
Lyme disease Foundation	**www.lyme.org**	
Lyme disease Network	**www.LymeNet.org/**	
Malaria Foundation	**www.malaria.org/**	
Meningitis	**www.who.int/emc-documents/surveillance/docs/whocdscsrisr2001.html/Meningitis/Meningitis.htm**	
PAAT (Programme Against African Trypanosomiasis) Information System	**www.fao.org/paat/html/home.htm**	
Pictures of insects	**www.ent.iastate.edu/imagegallery/**	
Rabies information	**oms2.b3e.jussieu.fr/rabnet/**	
Smallpox	**www.who.int/emc/diseases/smallpox/smallpoxeradication.html**	Classic WHO text on eradication
Trypanosomiasis	**www.who.int/health-topics/afrtryps.htm**	
WHO Fact Sheets	**www.who.int/inf-fs/en/index.html**	
WHO Infectious Disease Health Topics	**www.who.int/health-topics/idindex.htm**	
CHARITIES, AID, GLOBAL HEALTH ISSUES		
African Medical Relief (AMREF)	**www.amref.org/**	African Health Charity, air rescue for travellers, African health information.
International Committee of the Red Cross	**www.icrc.org/eng**	Landmines, security & safety, international aid & health issues
Médecins Sans Frontières	**www.msf.org/**	International aid, plus mines information
Mines Advisory Group	**www.mag.org.uk/**	Mines information

Web-site	Address	Notes
CHARITIES, AID, GLOBAL HEALTH ISSUES		
TALC (Teaching Aids at Low Cost)	www.talcuk.org	Low cost books, ORS measuring spoons, thermometers
United Nations Childrens' Fund	www.unicef.org	International aid & health issues
United Nations Development Programme	www.undp.org/	International aid & health issues
United Nations Fund Population Activities	www.unfpa.org	International aid & health issues
World Bank	www.worldbank.org	International aid & health issues
Transplanted organs, organ theft	sunsite.berkeley.edu/biotech/organswatch/	Yes, it can happen
Links to all US Government health initiatives	www.globalhealth.gov	
Norwegian Peoples Aid	www.angola.npaid.org/	Mines information — Angola
GENERAL HEALTH		
American Cancer Society	www.cancer.org	Cancer and prevention
Dr Koop	www.drkoop.com	Beyond travel medicine: useful resource whilst travelling
Netdoctor	www.netdoctor.co.uk/	Beyond travel medicine: useful resource whilst travelling
National Electronic Library for Health (UK)	www.nelh.nhs.uk	A digital medical library
NHS Direct	www.nhsdirect.nhs.uk/	Beyond travel medicine: useful resource whilst travelling
Virtual Naval Hospital — US Naval Medical Department	www.vnh.org	Beyond travel medicine: useful resource whilst travelling
BNF (British National Formulary)	www.bnf.org	Information about medicines; UK guidelines on malaria prevention
Merck	www.merck.com	Search the Merck Manual, and the "Health Infopark"
AVIATION HEALTH & SAFETY		
Air Transport Users Council	www.auc.org.uk	Complaints, UK passenger rights

Web-site	Address	Notes
AVIATION HEALTH & SAFETY		
UK Department of Health	**www.doh.gov.uk/dvt**	Official UK advice on travel
US Department of Transport	**ostpxweb.dot.gov/policy/safety/disin.htm**	Policy on insecticide use in aircraft for different countries, plus airline contacts
Aviation Safety from the FAA	**www.asy.faa.gov/safety.data/**	Main FAA safety page
Flight International	**www.flightinternational.com**	Publication covering safety and other aviation issues
Flight Safety Foundation	**www.flightsafety.org**	Publishes Flight Safety Digest
House of Lords Inquiry / Air travel & Health	**www.parliament.the-stationery-office.co.uk/pa/ld199900/ldselect/ldsctech/121/12101.htm**	Full text online
International Air Transport Association (IATA)	**www.iata.org/**	IATA home page
International Civil Aviation Organization	**www.icao.int**	Safety and other issues
Safety data by airline	**www.waasinfo.net/**	Safety information
Emirates	**www.emirates.com/pr/ek.pr34.1.asp**	News about DVT prevention
British Airways	**www.britishairways.com/health/**	Airline health web-site with section on in-flight health/DVT
Qantas	**www.qantas.com.au/flights/essentials/healthinflight.html**	Airline health web-site with section on in-flight health/DVT
Virgin Atlantic	**www.virgin-atlantic.com/main.asp?page=4,5,5**	Airline health web-site with section on in-flight health/DVT
DIVING & MARINE		
Australian Institute of Marine Science	**www.aims.gov.au/pages/research/project-net/dma/pages/dma-01.html**	Dangerous marine animals of North Australia
Divers Alert Network (DAN)	**www.diversalertnetwork.org/**	Promotes scuba diving safety. Emergency 24/7 helpline: +1 919 684 8111

Web-site	Address	Notes
DIVING & MARINE		
Diving Medicine Online	www.gulftel.com/~scubadoc	Electronic newsletter and information about diving medicine
Electronic Shark repellents	sharkpod.co.za/	Shark attack prevention
Florida Museum of Natural History	www.flmnh.ufl.edu/fish/Sharks/ISAF/ISAF.htm	Statistics on shark bite
Mediterranean Shark site	www.zoo.co.uk/~z9015043/	Shark information
British Sub-Aqua Club	www.bsac.com/	Dive training and resources
PADI	www.padi.com/	Dive training and resources
Royal Navy (UK)	www.royal-navy.mod.uk/content/1204.html	Undersea Medicine Division — emergency advice
HIGH ALTITUDE MEDICINE		
British Mountaineering Council	www.thebmc.co.uk/world/mm/mm0.htm	Key altitude medicine resource for climbers; offers expert advice
CIWEC Clinic, Nepal	www.ciwec-clinic.com/	Also covers other health issues in Nepal
High Altitude	www.high-altitude-medicine.com	High altitude medicine information
SPORTS / ATHLETES		
Sports Council	www.uksport.gov.uk	Information for travelling athletes
SAFETY / ACCIDENT PREVENTION		
General safety issues	www.rospa.co.uk/	General accident prevention
Child safety	www.capt.org.uk	Child safety
International road safety	www.asirt.org/	International road safety statistics and pressure group

Web-site	Address	Notes
SAFETY / ACCIDENT PREVENTION		
Links to injury prevention web-sites	www.euro-risc.net/eurorisc.htm	Injury prevention
National Lightning Safety Institute	www.lightningsafety.com	Lightning safety awareness
Spinal injury awareness	www.spinal.co.uk	Injury prevention
Transport Safety / OECD	www.oecd.org/dsti/sti/transpor/road/index.htm	Transport safety statistics
MEDICAL ASSISTANCE		
E-Med	www.e-med.co.uk/	Information, plus consultations by e-mail
IAMAT	www.iamat.org	Directory of English-speaking doctors world-wide
Association of British Insurers	www.ABI.org.uk	Check before you go — factsheet and information about insurance
International SOS	www.intsos.com/index.htm	Medical assistance and rescue
State Department Medevac Resources List	travel.state.gov/medical.html	Information about medical evacuation (US) and assistance companies
UK reciprocal health agreements	www.doh.gov.uk/traveladvice/hcagreements.htm	UK reciprocal health arrangements
BLOOD TRANSFUSION / INJECTION SAFETY		
Blood Care Foundation	www.bloodcare.org.uk/	Provides safe blood for members, in emergency situations
Hemopure	www.biopure.com	Future developments in blood substitutes
WHO Injection Safety Site	www.injectionsafety.org	Information about injection safety
DISABLED / SELF-HELP		
Access-able Page	www.access-able.com/	Resources for elderly and disabled
Diabetes UK	www.diabetes.org.uk	Resources for diabetics

Web-site	Address	Notes
DISABLED / SELF-HELP		
American Diabetes Association	**www.diabetes.org/**	Resources for diabetics
Canadian Diabetes Association	**www.diabetes.ca**	Resources for diabetics
Dialysis abroad	**www.globaldialysis.com**	Dialysis world-wide
Dialysis abroad	**www.kidneypatientguide.org.uk**	Resources for renal patients
Handicapped Scuba Association	**www.hsascuba.com**	Scuba diving for the disabled
Medic-Alert Foundation — UK site	**www.medicalert.co.uk**	Identification tags for people with allergies & medical conditions
Medic-Alert Foundation International	**www.medicalert.org**	Identification tags for people with allergies & medical conditions
Mobility International USA	**www.miusa.org**	US organization for the disabled
RADAR (Royal Association for Disability & Rehabilitation)	**www.radar.org.uk**	UK organization for the disabled
Diabetes Australia	**www.diabetesaustralia.com.au**	Resources for diabetics
Diabetes New Zealand	**www.diabetes.org.nz**	Resources for diabetics
International Diabetes Federation	**www.idf.org**	Links to international diabetes sites
Royal National Institute for the Deaf	**www.rnid-typetalk.org.uk**	Help with Minicom communication
British Epilepsy Association	**www.epilepsy.org.uk**	Epilepsy resources
Epilepsy Foundation of America	**www.efa.org**	Epilepsy resources
Epilepsy Canada	**www.epilepsy.ca**	Epilepsy resources
AIDS Education Global Information System (AEGIS)	**www.aegis.com/topics/travel.html**	Resources for travellers with HIV
Council on th Ageing, Australia	**www.cota.org.au**	Resources for the older traveller

Web-site	Address	Notes
DISABLED / SELF-HELP		
Help the Aged UK	**www.helptheaged.org.uk**	Resources for the older traveller
American Association of Retired Persons	**www.aarp.org**	Resources for the older traveller
Jim Lubin	**www.makoa.org/travel.htm**	Self-help site with extensive links
CONTRACEPTION & SEXUAL HEALTH		
Family Planning Association	**www.fpa.org.uk**	
Museum of Menstruation	**www.mum.org**	Menstruation & women's health
Toxic shock syndrome	**www.tamponalert.org.uk**	
HAY FEVER / ALLERGY		
Hay fever in the USA	**www.pollen.com/**	Pollen forecasts for all areas of the United States
Pollen	**cat.at/pollen/**	Pollen forecasts for Europe, plus maps
UK National Pollen Network	**www.pollenforecast.org**	Provides regional pollen forecast, UK May–August
The National Institute of Allergy and Infectious Diseases	**www.niaid.nih.gov/publications/eid.htm**	
GOVERNMENT TRAVEL WARNINGS & CONSULAR ADVICE		
Australian Department of Foreign Affairs	**www.dfat.gov.au/consular/advice/advices.mnu.html**	
Canadian Department of Foreign Affairs	**www.dfait-maeci.gc.ca/travelreport/menu.e.htm**	
Foreign & Commonwealth Office	**www.knowbeforeyougo.co.uk**	
UK Consular Information	**www.fco.gov.uk/travel/**	
US State Department Advisories	**travel.state.gov/travel.warnings.html**	
COUNTRY INFORMATION		
Central Intelligence Agency Factbook	**www.odci.gov/cia/publications/factbook**	Updated country-by-country political snapshots

Web-site	Address	Notes
COUNTRY INFORMATION		
State Department Background Notes	**www.state.gov/www/background.notes/index.html**	Background country information
SECURITY		
AKE	**www.akegroup.com**	Security & hostile environment training (ex-SAS run)
Control Risks Group	**www.crg.com/**	Private security information & consultancy
Kroll Associates	**www.krollworldwide.com/home.cfm**	Private security information & consultancy
Pinkerton Global Intelligence Service	**pgis.pinkertons.com**	Commercial security intelligence service
The National Security Institute	**nsi.org**	Commercial security intelligence service
US State Department OSAC	**www.ds-osac.org/**	Overseas Advisory Security Council — free security database
Suzy Lamplugh Trust	**www.suzylamplugh.org**	UK charity for personal safety & safety awareness
LEGAL HELP		
Fair Trials Abroad	**www.f-t-a.freeserve.co.uk/**	Legal assistance resources and pressure group
Prisoners Abroad	**www.prisonersabroad.org.uk/**	Support and pressure group
MISCELLANEOUS		
Conversion tools	**www.onlineconversion.com**	Atmospheres, psi, millibars, kilopascals and more
Conversion tools	**www.digitaldutch.com/unitconverter/**	Atmospheres, psi, millibars, kilopascals and more
Conversion tools	**www.omega.com/techref/techdata.html**	Atmospheres, psi, millibars, kilopascals and more
Online Medical Dictionary	**cancerweb.ncl.ac.uk/omd**	Help with medical technical terms
WOMEN		
Journeywoman online travel magazine	**www.journeywoman.com/**	Resources and links for women travellers
Budget Travel portal	**www.budgettravel.com/women.htm**	Resources and links for women travellers

Appendix 9:
Software tools and databases

In a travel clinic setting, databases and software tools can be a valuable aid to providing travellers with up-to-date advice, appropriate to their destination. They can also be a helpful guide to diagnosis in returning travellers. The following are a selection of the best-known products available:

TRAVAX — UK

An on-line service, provided by the SCIEH, (Scottish Centre for Infection and Environmental Health), Clifton House, Clifton Place, Glasgow G3 7LN. Tel:. 0141 300 1130. Service is free to Scottish GPs, BTHA members, and certain non-commercial organizations, otherwise attracting a fee of £50–£350. **www.travax.scot.nhs.uk** travax@scieh.csa.scot.nhs.uk

MASTA

Medical Advisory Services for Travellers Abroad (MASTA). A well-established UK-based database able to generate health briefs for individual travellers and to support and run travel clinic activities. Dial-up and internet access. (Health briefs are available on the internet at **www.masta.org**)

GIDEON

Global Infectious Disease and Epidemiology Network. Sophisticated, stand-alone PC-based software with frequent updates. Has stood the test of time, and is an excellent aid to diagnosis of travel-related infections, as well as a mine of useful information about the epidemiology of tropical and infectious diseases. $395 per year, with quarterly updates. More information: **www.gideononline.com** C Y Informatics, 34 Keren Hayesod St, Ramat Hasharon, Israel 47248 +972 354901120

EDISAN

Database also includes information about local hospitals and doctors, medical evacuation, climate, environment, etc. PC, Mac & Linux versions. Also available as a 'lite' version — Meditravel. CD updates every 6 weeks (€800 p.a. plus VAT). Information: CD Conseil, 18 Rue Le Sueur, 75016 Paris. **www.edisan.fr** Tel: (33) 0 140 67 78 72, Fax: (33) 0 140 67 78 79, E-mail: conseil@calva.net. French only, at present.

TRAVAX — US (unrelated to TRAVAX — UK)

PC-based system used widely in North America (cost $675-$995 per year). Country-by-country and disease-based information. Online version (TRAVAX EnCompass)

also available ($995-$7200 per year). Available from Shoreland Inc, PO Box 13795, Milwaukee, WI , 53213–0795 USA Tel: 800 433 5256, 414 290 1900, Fax: 414 290 1907 **www.shoreland.com**

EXODUS

A range of PC-based software tools, from travel health information to clinic management; also produce a customizable tool for developing a travel clinic web-site. Exodus Software Ltd, 5 Northumberland Road, Dun Laoghaire, County Dublin, Ireland, Tel: +353 1 280 2535, E-mail: office@exodus.ie **www.exodus.ie**

ADVICE FOR TRAVELLERS

US version of TROPIMED (German) software. Detailed country and disease information, customizable reports for travellers. $125 per year, includes 6-monthly update. Details: **www.medletter.com** The Medical Letter, Inc. 1000 Main Street, New Rochelle, NY 10801 +800 211 2769

Appendix 10
Hay fever seasons world-wide

Professor Jean Emberlin

Europe

Austria

Seasons vary between the mountains and the plain.

Mountains
- Peak grass pollen season is June–August, otherwise counts are low.
- Main tree pollen season is March–May (hazel and alder in March, then birch in April and May — note, these cross-react and can cause a long period of symptoms), otherwise counts are mainly low.
- Weed pollen counts can be high May–September, otherwise generally low.

Lowlands
- The grass pollen season is May–September, otherwise counts are low.
- Tree pollen counts are low generally, apart from February–July.
- Weed pollen counts are low generally, apart from May–September. (Note: ragweed blows into Austria if the wind is from Hungary, where ragweed is prolific. It causes problems for sensitive people. Concentrations peak at night and are lower in the daytime.)

France

Corsica
- Counts low near coasts.
- Generally good after the end of June.
- Weed pollen season over by end of October.

West coast
- Pollen counts are generally low near west coasts, but can be high inland.
- Tree pollen season is over at the end of June.
- Grass pollen season is usually over by August.
- Weed pollen season lasts until the end of October.

North-west
- Counts low on Brittany and Normandy coasts, but can be high inland in rural areas.
- Grass season over by end of July.
- Tree pollen season over by end of June.
- Weed pollen season goes on until September.

South coast
- The mild climate allows plants to flower all year; vegetation is diverse and some grass pollen may be in the air all year, but the peak time is April–July.
- High counts of tree pollen can occur January–July (abundant cypress trees planted in some areas as wind breaks can produce very high concentrations).
- The peak weed pollen season is March–October.

Paris basin
- Grass pollen counts are low apart from in the peak season (May–August).
- Peak season for tree pollen is February through to July, when chestnut pollen is abundant in Paris.
- Weed pollen is abundant May–September.

Greece
- Drought in late summer (from July onwards) tends to reduce grass pollen counts to low in all areas, but some weeds e.g. *Pareitaria* (pellitory) may be prolific locally.
- Counts are lowest on the islands, especially the smaller ones.
- Grass season over by the end of June.
- Tree pollen season over by the end of June.
- Weed pollen season over by the end of September.

Italy
A lot of regional differences because of the geography of the country.

Po Valley including Milan
- Grass season is April–August; very high count in May and June.
- Tree pollen season is February–June.
- Weed pollen season is May–October.

North-west / Tuscany / Pisa
- Grass season is March–June.
- Tree pollen season is February–June.
- Weed pollen season is April–October.

Adriatic
- Grass season is April–August. (N.B. coastal resorts do not always have low counts because land/sea breezes carry pollen and spores out to sea and back again.)
- Tree pollen season is February–June.
- Weed polllen season is May–September.

Central areas, Florence, and Rome
- Grass season is April–July.
- Tree pollen season is January–June.
- Weed pollen season is March–September.

Portugal

Algarve
- Pollen counts are low near coasts, especially from June onwards.
- Grass season is usually over by end of June.

- Tree pollen season is over by end of May.
- Weed pollen season is over by end of September.

Madeira
- Counts generally low.
- Grass season is usually over by end of June.
- Tree pollen season is over by end of May.
- Weed pollen season is over by end of August.

Spain

Northern areas
- Places near coasts have low pollen counts, but counts may be high inland.
- Grass pollen may continue into early August.
- Tree pollen season over by end of June.
- Weeds may flower until November.

Costa del Sol, Costa Almeria, Costa Dorada
- Moderate counts for grass, May and June; low grass pollen counts after June.
- Trees flower January–June and October and November.
- Weed pollen season is over by end of September.

Balearic Islands
- Counts are generally low.
- Very low grass counts after June.
- Tree counts are low, especially after July.
- Weed pollen season over by end of September.

Canary Islands
- Generally low counts, even during pollen seasons.
- Grass season is over by the end of June.
- Tree pollen season is over by the end of May.
- Weed pollen season is over by the end of June.

Central areas including Andalucia
- Olive pollen counts can be very high in May and June, especially near Cordoba.
- Grass season is April–July.
- Tree pollen season is February–June.
- Weed pollen season is April–September.

Switzerland

Mountain areas
- Grass season is May–August.
- Tree pollen season is March–August.
- Weed pollen season is May–September.

Lowlands
- Grass season is April–August.
- Tree pollen season is February–August.
- Weed pollen season is May–September.

Turkey

Coastal areas in West:

- Grass season is May–September.
- Tree pollen seasons are February–June and September and October.
- Weed pollen season is June–September.

North America

Ragweeds are present throughout the whole USA and southern Canada, but are most prolific in central and eastern USA. These flower mostly in July–September causing great problems to sensitive people. In the USA, estimates suggest that over half of the cases of hay fever are caused by ragweeds.

USA

(I have included here some of the most popular destinations, noting the low seasons, rather than pointing out low-pollen venues, many of which are not typical holiday destinations.)

Florida

Lowest counts on coasts; some pollen is in the air all year round.

- Low season for grass pollen is November–April; for tree pollen, June–December; and for weed pollen, December–April.

California

Lowest counts near coasts, but there will be some pollen in the air all year in the south; long seasons elsewhere.

- Grass pollen low season, November–April.
- Tree pollen low season, June–January.
- Weed pollen low season, January–April.

North-east seaboard (e.g. New York, Washington DC)

Low counts on coasts.

- Grass low season, August–April.
- Tree pollen low season, June–January.
- Weed pollen low season, October–April.

South Central (e.g. Mississippi, Alabama)

- Grass low season, December–April.
- Trees flower all year, but lowest pollen times are June–August and October–March.
- Weed pollen low season, November–June.

Hawaii

Some differences between islands and locations.

- Lowest counts are on coasts with onshore winds.
- Grass pollen all year, but lowest December and January.
- Tree pollen low season, May–December.
- Weed pollen low season, December–mid-May.

Canada

British Columbia
- Grass pollen seasons tend to be mild, especially near coasts.
- Grass low season, September–May.
- Tree pollen low season, June–March.
- Weed pollen low season, October–June.

Great Lakes area
Counts are high during season, so avoid main flowering times for allergenic plants.
- Grass low season, August–May.
- Tree pollen low season, July–March.
- Weed pollen low season, October–June.

Prairies
Again, counts are high during the main flowering times.
- Grass low season, September–May.
- Tree pollen low season, July–March.
- Weed pollen low season, October–July.

Caribbean

The tropical climate allows plants to flower all year, but there are peak times. Pollen counts are lowest on coasts with onshore winds. Local topography and climates differ greatly over short distances. Avoid main pollen seasons which are:
- Grass, October–March, June and July.
- Trees, February–May and June–October.
- Weeds, December–August.

Africa

Egypt
- Grass pollen season, February–November.
- Tree pollen season, all year.
- Weed pollen season, March–November.

South Africa
- Grass pollen season, November–January.
- Tree pollen season, September–December.
- Weed pollen season, November–February.

Gambia
- Grass pollen season, all year.
- Tree pollen season, all year.
- Weed pollen season, all year.

Kenya
- Grass pollen seasons, September and October, December and January.
- Tree pollen season, July–December.
- Weed pollen season, June–January.

Zimbabwe
- Grass pollen seasons, July and August, October and November.
- Tree pollen seasons, July and October.
- Weed pollen seasons, July and August, October and November.

Australasia

Australia

South coast of southern Australia
- Grass pollen season, July–March.
- Tree pollen seasons, August–November and March–July.
- Weed pollen season, August–April.

South-west of western Australia
- Grass pollen season, September–March.
- Tree pollen season, July–November.
- Weed pollen season, July–February.

Southeast Australia
- Grass pollen season, August–May.
- Tree pollen season, June–December.
- Weed pollen season, August–March.

New Zealand
Seasons start earlier in the north e.g. in most years there is about one month difference in the grass seasons between the north and the south.
- Grass pollen season, October–February.
- Tree pollen season, August–October.
- Weed pollen season, January–March.

Asia

India
- Grass pollen season, September–January.
- Tree pollen season, October–January.
- Weed pollen season, September–February.

Northern Thailand
- Grass pollen seasons, June and July, October and November.
- Tree pollen season, March–December.
- Weed pollen season, May–July.

Southern Thailand and western Malaysia
- Grass pollen season, all year.
- Tree pollen season, all year.
- Weed pollen season, all year.

Further Reading

Air travel, jet lag

Anderson, N. *The Backseat Flyer: Plane sense about flying as a passenger*, Safe Goods, 1998, ISBN: 1884820352.

*Arendt J., *Melatonin & the Mammalian Pineal Gland*, Chapman & Hall, 1995, ISBN: 041253600.

Barish, R. *The invisible passenger: radiation risks for people who fly*, Advanced Medical Publishing, 1996, ISBN: 188352606X

Bor, R., Josse, J., Palmer, S. *Stress-Free Flying*, Quay Books, 2000, ISBN: 1856421678.

Celentino, T. *Combating Air Rage*, 1st Books Library, 2001, ISBN: 1587212145.

Dowdell N. et al, *British Airways Manual of Inflight Medical Care*, Dorling Kindersley, 2001, ISBN: 0751344354.

*DeHart, R.L. *Fundamentals of Aerospace Medicine*, Lippincott Williams and Wilkins, 1996, ISBN: 0683023969.

Ehret, C., Scanlon, L. *Overcoming Jet Lag*, Berkley Publishing Group, 1988, ISBN: 0425099369, The jetlag diet: now a classic, but does it work?

*Harding, R.M. and Mills, F. *Aviation Medicine*, British Medical Association, 1993, ISBN: 0727908146.

Select Committee on Science & Technology, *Air Travel and Health*, Stationery Office Books, 2000, ISBN: 010 444200X and ISBN: 0104441003.

Yaffe, M. *Taking the fear out of flying*, Constable Robinson, 1998, ISBN: 1854878646.

Children

Gore-Lyons, S. *Are we nearly there? The complete guide to traveling with babies, toddlers and children*,Virgin Books, 2000, ISBN: 0753503999.

Hilton, T., Messenger M., Graham P. *Great Ormond Street New Baby and Child Care Book*, Vermilion, 1997, ISBN: 0091852994.

Morley, D. *The care of young children and babies in the tropics*, National Association for Maternal and Child Welfare (1 South Audley Street, London WIY 6JS). Available from TALC, see p. 630.

Truszkowski, H. *Take the Kids Travelling*, Cadogan, 2000, ISBN: 1860119913.

Weeler M., *Travel with Children*, Lonely Planet, 1995, ISBN: 0864422997

Wilson-Howarth, J., Ellis, M. *Your Child's Health Abroad*, Bradt, 1998, ISBN: 1898323631

Diabetes / Disabled / Elderly / Higher risk.

American Diabetes Association. *Travel Tips for Diabetics*, Available from the American Diabetes Association, 600 Fifth Avenue, NY 10020.

Guide for the disabled traveller, Automobile Association, UK, free for members, otherwise £3.50. ISBN: 08702401456.

Kruger, D.F. *The Diabetes Travel Guide: how to travel with diabetes anywhere in the world*, McGraw Hill, 2000, ISBN: 1580400418.

*McIntosh, I *Health, Hazard & the Higher Risk Traveller*, Quay Books, 1993, ISBN: 1856420817.

RADAR, *Access to Air Travel, Holiday Fact Packs, Mobility Fact Packs, Motoring and Mobility for Disabled People (6th Edn)*, Available from RADAR,12 City Forum, 250 City Road, London EC1V 8AF Tel: 020 7250 3222, Fax: 020 7250 0212, Minicom: 020 7250 4119, E-mail: radar@radar.org.uk.

Ronald, R. *Air Travel Guide for Seniors and Disabled Passengers*, Independent Publishers Group, 2001, ISBN: 096807832X.

Weiss, L. *Access to the World*, Henry Holt, New York, 1986, ISBN: 0871967863. Access guide for the disabled.

Walsh, A. *Able to Travel: true stories by and for people with disabilities*, Rough Guides, 1994, ISBN: 1858281105.

Diving and marine hazards

*Bennett, P.B. and Elliot, D.H. *The physiology and medicine of diving*, WB Saunders, 1993, ISBN: 070201589X.

*Bove, A.A. and Davis, J.C. *Diving Medicine (3rd edn)*, W.B. Saunders, 1997, ISBN: 0721660568.

*Edmonds, C. *Dangerous marine animals of the Indo-Pacific region*, Wedneil Publications, Newport, Australia, 1978, Classic guide to identification and treatment. Out of print.

Wilks, J. Knight J., Lippman, J. *Scuba Safety in Australia*, J L Publications, 1993, ISBN: 0959030670, Sound advice for diving anywhere else in the world too.

Williamson, J., Fenner, P., Burnett, J., Rifkin, J. *Venomous and poisonous marine animals*, Blackwell Science UK, 1997, ISBN: 0868402796.

Drugs and medicines

British National Formulary, Published jointly by the British Medical Association and the Royal Pharmaceutical Society, and updated frequently. Useful technical reference on medicines or drugs. More information: **www.bnf.org**.

Henry, J. *British Medical Association Guide to Medicines and Drugs*, 5th Edn, Dorling Kindersley, 2000, ISBN: 0751327379.

Expeditions (see also Outdoors)

Warrell, A. and Anderson, S. *Expedition medicine*, Profile Books, 2002. Available from the Expedition Advisory Centre, Royal Geographical Society, London (see p. 654).

General first aid

British Red Cross, *New Practical First Aid*, Dorling Kindersley, 1999, ISBN: 0751319635.

British Red Cross Society, *First Aid*, Dorling Kindersley, 1999, ISBN: 0751307092. Compact guide.

Handal, K. *American Red Cross First Aid and Safety Handbook*, Little Brown & Co, 1992, ISBN: 0316736465.

General travel medicine

*DuPont, H., and Steffen, R. *Textbook of Travel Medicine and Health*, BC Decker Inc, 2001, ISBN: 1550090379.

Fry, G., and Kenny V. *Travel in Health*, Newleaf, 2000, ISBN: 0717129888.

*Jong, E.C., and McMullen, R. *Travel and Tropical Medicine Manual*, W. B. Saunders, 2002, ISBN: 0721676782.

*Keystone, J. *et al.*, *Travel Medicine*, Harcourt Publishers Ltd, 2002, In Press.

*Lockie, C., Walker, E., Calvert, L., Cossar, J., Knill-Jones, R., Raeside, F. *Travel medicine & Migrant Health*, Churchill Livingstone, 2000, ISBN: 0443062420.

Steffen, R., and DuPont H. *Manual of Travel Medicine & Health*, BC Decker Inc, 1999, ISBN: 155009078X.

*Townend, M., and Howell, K. *Travel Health for the Primary Care Team*, Mark Allen Publishing, 1999, ISBN: 1856421716.

Travel medicine advisor, American Health Consultants Inc., 3525 Piedmont Rd, Building 6, Suite 400, Atlanta, GA 30305 USA (**www.ahcpub.com**). Looseleaf manual with periodic updates and bimonthly newsletter.

*Walker, E., Williams, G., Raeside, F., Calvert, L. *ABC of Healthy Travel*, British Medical Association, 1997, ISBN: 0727911384.

Wilson-Howarth, J. *Bugs Bites & Bowels*, Cadogan Guides, 1999, ISBN: 186011914X.

Wilson-Howarth, J. *Shitting Pretty: how to stay clean and healthy while travelling*, Travelers' Tales, San Francisco, USA, 2000, ISBN: 1885211473.

*Zuckerman, J. and Zuckerman, A. *Principles and Practice of Travel Medicine*, Wiley, 2001, ISBN: 0471490792.

Government and WHO publications and advice

*Centers for Disease Control, Atlanta, Ga, USA., *Health information for international travel*, Available from the Superintendent of Documents, US Govt. Printing Office, Washington DC 20402, and from **bookstore.phf.org**, 2001, ISBN: 188320576X, Updated every 1-2 years.The official US publication for doctors. PDF version available online (see Appendix 8).

*Department of Health (UK). *Leaflet T6, Health Advice for Travellers*, HMSO, London, 2001, Available from main post offices, and includes the E111 form; and also by freephone from the Health Literature Line, ISBN: 0800 555 777.

*Department of Health (UK). *Health Information for Overseas Travel*, The Stationery Office Books, 2002, ISBN: 0113223293. Also known as the DoH's Yellow Book

National Health & Medical Research Council (Australia). *The Australian Immunisation Handbook — 7th Edition, 2000*. Available online at: **www.health.gov.au/ pubhlth/immunise/handbook 7.pdf**.

US Dept. of State, Bureau of Consular Affairs. Publications for travellers are now all available online at **travel.state.gov**.

*World Health Organization, Geneva. *International Travel and Health*, The Stationery Office Books, 2002, ISBN: 9241580267, Official WHO listing of requirements and recommendations for travel. Also available online (see Appendix 8. WHO also produces many other useful publications, including: *World health statistical quarterly; WHO Weekly epidemiological record; Atlas of the global distribution of schistosomiasis (1987); Yellow fever vaccinating centres for international travel; International medical guide for ships; The rational use of drugs in the management of acute diarrhea in children; Prevention of sexual transmission of HIV; Plague manual.*

World Health Organization, Geneva, *Publications on vaccines can be found at* **www.who.int/vaccines-documents**.

High altitude

*Heath, D. and Williams, D.R. *High altitude medicine and pathology, 4th Edn*, Oxford University Press, 1995, ISBN: 0192625047.

*Ward, M.P., Milledge, J.S., and West, J.B. High altitude medicine and physiology, Arnold, 2000, ISBN: 0340759801.

Immunization

*Department of Health (UK), *Immunization against infectious disease*, HMSO, London, 1995, ISBN: 011321815X. A practical guide for doctors.

*Kassianos, G. C. *Immunization — childhood and travel health, 4th Edn*, Blackwell Science UK, 2001, ISBN: 0632055812.

Living abroad

Kohls, L.R. *Survival Kit for Overseas Living, 4th Edn*, Nicholas Brealey Publishing, 2001, ISBN: 185788292X.

Pascoe, R. *Living and working abroad — a Parent's guide*, Kuperard, 1995, ISBN: 1857330722.

Pascoe, R. *Living and working abroad — a Wife's guide*, Kuperard, 1997, ISBN: 1857331966.

Piet-Pelon, N. and Hornby, B., *Women's Guide to Overseas Living*, Intercultural Press, 1992, ISBN: 1877864056.

Motion sickness

*Benson, A.J. Motion sickness. In: *Vertigo*, (ed. M.R. Dix and J.D. Hood), pp. 391–426. Chichester, J. Wiley & Sons, 1984, ISBN: 0835734692.

*Crampton, G.H. *Motion and space sickness*, CRC Press, 1990, ISBN: 0849347033.

*Ernsting, J. Nicholson, A.N., Rainford, D.. Motion sickness. In: *Aviation Medicine (2nd edn)*, Arnold, 1999, ISBN: 0750632526.

*Health and Safety Executive. *Medications for the Treatment of Motion Sickness during Evacuation, Escape and Rescue Offshore*, HSE, 1996, ISBN: 0717611116.

*Motion sickness: significance in aerospace operations, and prophylaxis, AGARD Lecture Series 175. Neuilly-sur-Seine: AGARD/NATO: NASA, Washington DC. Also available from **www.ntis.gov**, 1991.

*Reason, J.T. and Brand, J.J. *Motion sickness*, Academic Press, London, 1975, ISBN: 0125840500. Out of print.

Outdoors, survival.

Alloway, D. *Desert Survival Skills*, University of Texas Press, 2000, ISBN: 0292704925.

Auerbach, P.S. *Field Guide to Wilderness Medicine*, Mosby-Year Book, 1999, ISBN: 0815109261.

Auerbach, P.S. *Medicine for the Outdoors*, The Lyons Press, 1999, ISBN: 1558217231.

*Auerbach, P.S. *Wilderness Medicine, 4th edn*, Mosby International, 2001, ISBN: 0323009506. Five-star study of everything from plant and wildlife hazards to lightning, forest fires, and drowning.

Bezruchka, S. *Trekking in Nepal, 7th edn*, Cordee, 1997. ISBN: 0898860032. How to do it safely.

Bezruchka, S. *The Pocket Doctor, 3rd edn*, Mountaineers Books, 1999, ISBN: 0898866146

Bollen. *First Aid on Mountains*, British Mountaineering Council, 1989, ISBN: 0903908719.

Forgey, W. *Wilderness Medicine, Beyond First Aid, 5th edn*, Globe Pequot Press, 1999, ISBN: 076270490X.

Forgey, W. B*asic Essentials — Hypothermia*, Globe Pequot Press, 1999, ISBN: 0762704918.

Kamler, K. *Doctor on Everest : Emergency Medicine at the Top of the World*, Lyons Press, 2000, ISBN: 1558219293.

Lehman, C.A. *Desert Survival Handbook, 2nd edn*, Primer Publishers, 1998, ISBN: 093581065X.

Melville, K.E.M. *Stay alive in the desert*, Roger Lascelles, London, 1984. Survival classic, out of print.

Meyer, K. *How to Shit in the Woods: An environmentally sound approach to a lost art*, Ten Speed Press, USA, 1994, ISBN: 0898156270.

Steele, P. *Doctor on Everest*, Hodder & Stoughton, 1972. A mountaineering classic, but out of print.

Thompson, L. *Hypothermia: The silent killer*, Detselig Enterprises, Calgary, Canada, 1989, out of print.

Tilton, B. *How to die in the outdoors: 100 interesting ways*, ICS Books, 1997, ISBN: 1570340196.

Tilton, B. *Backcountry First Aid and Extended Care. 3rd edn*, Globe Pequot Press, 1998, ISBN: 0762704136.

Weiss, E. *Wilderness 911 — A step-by-step guide for medical emergencies and improvised care in the backcountry*, Mountaineers Books, 1997, ISBN: 0898865972.

Wilkerson, J.A. *Medicine for Mountaineering and Other Wilderness Activities*, Mountaineers Books, 1993, ISBN: 0898863317.

Wilkerson, J.A., Bangs, C. *Hypothermia, Frostbite and Other Cold Injuries*, Mountaineers Books, 1986, ISBN: 0898860245.

Sea travel and sailing

Berry, C. and Justins, D. *First Aid At Sea*, Adlard Coles Nautical, 1999, ISBN: 0713649224.

Day, G. *Safety at sea — a sailors complete guide to safe seamanship*, Cadogan Guides, 1999, ISBN: 0399135715.

Maritime and Coastguard Agency, *The Ship Captain's Medical Guide*, The Stationery Office Books, 1999, ISBN: 0115516581.

World Health Organization, Geneva. *International Medical Aid for Ships: including the ship's medicine chest. 2nd edn,* The Stationery Office Books. In the USA, available from the Superintendent of Documents, US Govt. Printing Office, Washington DC 20402, 1984, ISBN: 9241542314.

Security and safety

Andrew Kain Enterprises. *The SAS Security Handbook*, Heinemann, 1996, ISBN: 0434003069.

Bolz, F. *The Counter-Terrorism Handbook*, CRC Press, 1996, ISBN: 0849395011.

Scotti, A.J. *Executive safety and international terrorism: a guide for travelers*, Prentice-Hall, 1996, ISBN: 0132943808.

Wilkinson, P. and Jenkins, B. *Aviation Terrorism and Security.* Frank Cass Publishers, 1999, ISBN: 0714644633.

Wiseman, J. *The SAS Survival Handbook*, Harper Collins, 1999, ISBN: 0006531407.

Self-help

British Medical Association Complete Family Health Encyclopaedia, Dorling Kindersley, 1990, ISBN: 0751336351, Excellent, comprehensive home medical encyclopedia.

Dickson, M. *Where There Is No Dentist*, Hesperian Foundation, Palo Alto, Ca, USA, 1989, ISBN: 0 942364 058.

Halestrap, D.J. *Simple Dental Care for Rural Hospitals. 4th edn*, The Medical Missionary Association, 1981, ISBN: 0950610011.

IAMAT, *IAMAT directory*, Available from IAMAT, 736 Center Street, Lewiston, NY 14092. (**www.iamat.org**), Names and addresses of English-speaking doctors all over the world.

*McLatchie, G.R. Leaper, D.J. *Oxford Handbook of Operative Surgery*, Oxford University Press, 1996, ISBN: 0192620975.

Milne, A.H. and Siderfin C.D. *Kurafid: The British Antarctic Survey Medical Handbook*, British Antarctic Survey, 1995, ISBN: 0856651664.

Werner, D. *et al. Where There Is No Doctor: a village health care handbook.* Macmillan Press, 1993, ISBN: 0333516516, (Available also from TALC, 30 Guilford Street, London WC1N 1EH, and the Hesperian Foundation, PO Box 1692, Palo Alto, Ca 94302, USA).

Werner, D. *Where There Is No Doctor: a village health care handbook for Africa*, Macmillan Press, 1994, ISBN: 0333516524 (Available also as above).

Sex and contraception

Guillebaud, J. *Contraception: Your questions answered*, Churchill Livingstone, 1999, ISBN: 044306153X.

Szarewski, A., Guillebaud, J. *Contraception: a user's guide*, Oxford University Press, 2000, ISBN: 0192632566.

Skiing and sports

*Bloomfield, J., Fricker, P., Fitch, K. *Science and Medicine in Sport*, Blackwell Science, 1995, ISBN: 0867933216.

Thorne, P. *The World Ski and Snowboarding Guide*, Columbus Travel Guides, 1996, ISBN: 0946393702.

Snake bite

*Chippaux, J.P. and Goyfon, M. *Producers of antivenomous sera, Toxicon*, 6 739–52, 1983.

Nicol, J. *Bites and stings: the world of venomous animals*, David & Charles, London, 1989. Includes listing of anti-venom suppliers, world-wide. Out of print.

*Sutherland, S.K. and Tibballs, J. *Australian animal toxins: the creatures, their toxins, and care of the poisoned patient*, Oxford University Press, Melbourne, 2001, ISBN: 019550643X.

*Warrell, D.A. Venomous and poisonous animals. In: *Tropical and geographical medicine* (ed. K.S. Warren and A.A.F. Mahmoud), McGraw-Hill, New York, 1990, ISBN: 007068328X.

Sunlight

Altmeyer, P., Hoffman K. *Skin Cancer and UV Radiation*, Springer Verlag, 1997, ISBN: 3540627235.

Hawk, J., McGregor, J. *British Medical Association Family Doctor Series: Skin and Sunlight*, Dorling Kindersley, 2000, ISBN: 0751308145.

Howard, W. *Attitudes to sunbathing and the risks of skin cancer*, Health Development Agency, 1997, ISBN: 0752107844.

Travel tips

Collis, R. *The Survivor's Guide to Business Travel*, Kogan Page, 2001, ISBN: 0749430745.

Hatt, J. *The Tropical Traveller*, Penguin, 1993, Travel tips classic. Out of print.

Swedo, S. *Adventure travel tips: advice for the adventure of a life time*, Falcon Books, 2001, ISBN: 1560449829.

Tropical and infectious diseases, international health

*Bell, D.R., Gilks, C., Molyneux, M., Smith., D., Wyatt, G. *Lecture notes on tropical medicine, 4th edn*, Blackwell Science, 1995, ISBN: 063203839X. An excellent introduction to the subject. Highly recommended.

*Chin, J. *Control of Communicable Diseases Manual (17th edn)*, American Public Health Association, 2001, ISBN: 087553242X. Also available on CD-Rom.

*Chiodini, P., Moody A., Manser D. *Atlas of Medical Helmillthology and Protozoology*, Churchill Livingstone, 2001, ISBN: 0443062684.

*Cook, G. *Manson's tropical diseases, 20th Edn*, WB Saunders, 1995, ISBN: 0702017647.

*Eddlestone, M., Pierini, S. *Oxford Handbook of Tropical Medicine*, Oxford University Press, 1999, ISBN: 0192627724.

*Hawker, J *et al. Communicable Disease Control Handbook*, Blackwell Science, 2001, ISBN: 0632056495.

*Lucas, A. O. and Gilles, H.M., *A short textbook of preventative medicine for the tropics*, Hodder & Stoughton, 1984. Out of print.

McCormick, J. B. and Fisher-Hoch, S. *The Virus Hunters: Dispatches from the frontline*, Bloomsbury, 1996, ISBN: 0747530300.

*Peters, W. and Gilles, H.M. *Colour Atlas of Tropical Medicine & Parasitology*, Mosby Wolfe, 1999, ISBN: 0723420696, The ultimate picture guide.

*Schlagenhauf, P. *Travellers' Malaria*, BC Decker Inc, 2001, ISBN: 1550091573.

Schull, C.R. *Common medical problems in the tropics*, Macmillan, London, 1999, ISBN: 0333679997. Guide for health workers in developing countries.

*Service, M. *Encyclopedia of arthropod-transmitted infections*, CABI Publishing, 2001, ISBN: 0851994733.

Spielman, A. and D'Antonio, M., *Mosquito: The story of man's deadliest foe*. Faber and Faber, 2001, ISBN: 0571209807

Taipale, I. *et al. War or Health?*, Zed Books, 2001, ISBN: 185649951.

Vanderhoof-Forschner, K, Lieberman, J., Burgdorfer ,W. *Everything you need to know about Lyme disease and other Tick-borne disorders*, John Wiley and Sons, 1997, ISBN: 047116061X.

Wallace, R. B. *Public Health and Preventative Medicine*, Mcgraw-Hill, 1998, ISBN: 0838561845.

*Warrell, D. and Gilles, H.M. *Essential Malariology, 4th edn*, Arnold, 2001, ISBN: 0340740647. A fascinating account of one of the world's most important diseases.

*Wilson, M.E. *A world guide to infections*, Oxford University Press, 1991, ISBN: 0195043855.

Women

Moss, M. & G., *Handbook for Women Travellers*, Piatkus, London, UK, 1987, ISBN: 086188 6151, Out of print.

Mustoe, A. *Lone Traveller — One woman, two wheels and the world*, Virgin Publishing, 2000, ISBN: 075350426X.

Magazines and journals

The following regularly publish articles relevant to travel medicine & health.

Condé Nast Traveler, Condé Nast Publications, New York **www.concierge.com/cntraveler**, Carries travel health news items, and a good read for anyone interested in travel; Tel. (303) 665 1583 or (800) 777 0700 to subscribe.

Holiday Which? and *Which?*, Consumers' Association, 2 Marylebone Road, London NW1 4DX Tel. 020 7486 5544. **www.which.net**, Covers consumer issues relating to travel.

Flight International, Reed Business Press, U.K. **www.flightinternational.com**, Air transport industry information, statistics and news.

Aviation, Space and Environmental Medicine, Journal of the Aerospace Medical Association. **www.asma.org.**

*British Medical Journal, British Medical Association, London. **www.bmj.com**.

*Emerging Infectious Diseases, Online journal from the CDC **www.cdc.gov/ncidod/eid**.

Geographical, Royal Geographical Society, News, features, geographical and environmental issues. **www.geographical.co.uk.**

*Journal of Travel Medicine, BC Decker Inc, Bimonthly journal of the International Society of Travel Medicine (**www.istm.org**).

*Medical Letter, Medical Letter Inc, New Rochelle, NY. **www.medicalletter.com**.

New Scientist, Reed Business Information, UK. **www.newscientists.com**

*The Lancet, the Lancet, London. **www.thelancet.com**.

*Tropical Doctor, Royal Society of Medicine Press. Aimed at doctors working in the tropics. **www.rsmpress.co.uk/pub/td.htm**.

*Tropical Medicine and International Health, Blackwell Scientific Publications. **www. blacksci.co.uk/uk/journals.htm**.

*Wilderness and Environmental Medicine, Allen Press, Journal of the Wilderness Medical Society (**www.wms.org**).

World AIDS, Panos Institute, 8 Alfred Place, London WC1E 7EB, UK. 1409 King Street, Alexandria, VA 22314 USA. **www.oneworld.org/panos**, World-wide news about AIDS.

Glossary

We've done our best to avoid unnecessary technical medical terminology, but it is not possible to avoid it altogether. Here is a brief explanation of some of the terms in the main text.

Acute: An acute illness is one that is sudden in onset, regardless of severity.

Anaphylaxis: Severe, generalized allergic state.

Aneurysm: A sac formed by the dilatation of the wall of an artery, a vein, or the heart.

Antibody: A protein made by the body in response to anything that it recognizes as 'foreign' — such as components of bacteria and viruses called antigens. Antibodies bind to antigens and inactivate them, and are 'tailor-made' for each antigen. The principle of 'active' immunization is based on the fact that exposure to a small amount of harmless antigen — present in a vaccine — stimulates the production of antibodies that remain ready for action when infection threatens. (Vaccines fool the immune system that they are 'the real thing'.) (See also immunoglobulin.)

Antigen: Any substance capable of triggering an immune response. They include components of bacteria, viruses, toxins, and vaccines. Hepatitis B surface antigen (HBsAg) is an antigen present in the blood of people who have had hepatitis B, and can be detected by laboratory tests.

Arrhythmia: Disorder of cardiac rhythm, irregular heartbeat. Potentially dangerous.

Ascites: Fluid in the abdomen.

Attenuated: Live bacteria or viruses, that have been modified to render them harmless.

Bacillus: 'Rod-shaped' bacteria. Anthrax, leprosy, and tuberculosis are examples of diseases caused by bacilli.

Bacteria: Tiny organisms that consist of a single cell and have a cell wall but no nucleus. There are a great many types, not all of which cause disease.

Chemoprophylaxis: The use of drugs to *prevent* disease.

Chronic: A chronic disease process is one that develops gradually or lasts a long time.

Contra-indication: Any disease or condition that renders a proposed form of treatment or course of action undesirable.

Culture: Growth of micro-organisms in the laboratory for testing and identification.

Cutaneous: Of the skin.

Diuretic: A drug that increases urine production.

Dysentery: Severe diarrhoea with blood, mucus, and abdominal cramps.

ELISA test: Enzyme-linked immunoabsorbent assay — a general test for detecting antibodies.

Embolism: The sudden blockage of an artery, usually by a blood clot that has travelled in the bloodstream from elsewhere in the body. A clot (or 'thrombus') sometimes forms in the veins of the legs; 'pulmonary embolism' occurs when it travels to, and blocks, the arteries of the lungs. Gas entering the bloodstream can have a similar effect — 'gas embolism'.

Endemic: A disease that is constantly present in the human population, to a greater or lesser degree, in a particular region.

Enterocytes: The cells that line the intestinal wall.

Enzootic: A disease that is constantly present in the animal population, to a greater or lesser degree, in a particular region.

Eosinophilia: An increase in the number of eosinophils, a type of white blood cell, in the blood. This can be a general indicator of infection with certain types of parasite.

Erythrocyte: Red blood cell.

Gram negative / Gram positive: A way of classifying bacteria according to their staining properties under the microscope; sometimes helpful in choosing the right antibiotic.

Haematocrit: Relative volume of the blood occupied by erythrocytes, usually around 45 per cent. Easy test to perform with limited laboratory facilities, so commonly used in the tropics.

Hepatocyte: Liver cell.

HIV: Human immunodeficiency virus — the virus that causes AIDS.

Host: Man or any animal that harbours a parasite.

Immunity: A state in which the individual is resistant to specific infections.

Immunoglobulin: A protein possessing antibody activity. Most immunoglobulins circulate in the bloodstream, and 'gamma-globulin' is a preparation of 'ready-made' antibodies from donated blood. 'Passive' immunization consists simply of injecting such ready-made antibody into someone who does not have it.

Incidence: The number of new cases of a disease in a given period.

Incubation period: The time between exposure to an infection and the first symptoms.

Intradermal; intramuscular; intravenous: These terms refer to the position of the tip of the needle during an injection. An intradermal injection is given as close to the skin surface as possible; an intramuscular injection is given deep into a muscle — often in the buttock; an intravenous injection is given into a vein, directly into the bloodstream.

Jaundice: Yellow discoloration of the skin and whites of the eyes, due to the presence in the blood of excess amounts of a substance called bilirubin, which is normally excreted by the liver into the bile. It occurs in hepatitis, other liver diseases, and sometimes malaria, and is a sign of reduced liver function. Lay people sometimes use this term to mean hepatitis.

Ketoacidosis: Acidosis (excesive blood acidity) arising from accumulation of ketones (acetone-like substances) in body tissues and fluids; this can be a complication of uncontrolled diabetes.

Lesion: Sore, wound, ulcer, or area of tissue damage.

Leukopenia: Reduction in the number of white blood cells.

Lymphocyte: A type of white blood cell.

Lumen: The cavity or channel within a tubular organ such as the intestine.

Lymph nodes (glands): Part of the immune system. Some can normally be felt as small lumps close to the skin in the neck, groin, and armpit. They may enlarge or become inflamed during an infection.

Maculo-papular: Term used to describe a spotty rash consisting of tiny circumscribed elevations of the skin.

Meningo-encephalitis: Inflammation of both the brain and meninges (its surrounding membranes).

Micro-organism: Any microscopic organism, including viruses, bacteria, funguses and yeasts, protozoa, and rickettsiae.

Muco-cutaneous: Affecting the mucous membranes and skin, commonly refers to a particular type of leishmaniasis common in Central and South America.

Myelitis: An inflammation of the spinal cord, often resulting in paralysis

Narcosis: Depression of the nervous system — by a drug or other agent such as an excess of dissolved nitrogen in the blood. (The latter is called nitrogen narcosis, which may occur in divers.)

Oedema (edema): Fluid in the tissues, causing swelling.

Oesophagus (esophagus): The gullet or food passage from mouth to stomach.

Papule: A small, circumscribed, solid elevation of the skin.

Parasite: An animal that lives within or upon man or any other animal (its host), and upon which it depends for nutrition and shelter — sometimes to the detriment of the host.

Pathogen; enteropathogen: Any disease-producing micro-organism. Enteropathogens produce intestinal disease.

PCR test (polymerase chain reaction): One of the most important advances in molecular biology, this is a very sensitive method for detecting tiny amounts of DNA.

Petechiae: Tiny, multiple haemorrhages, sometimes most easily seen in the skin, for example in the non-blanching rash of meningococcal meningitis.

Pharynx: Back of the throat.

Photophobia: Discomfort or pain from bright light.

Physiological: Normal or related to the way the body functions in health rather than in disease. Physiology is the science of the mechanisms of normal body function.

Pleural effusion: Fluid around the lung.

Prevalence: The total number of cases of a disease at a certain time in a given area.

Prophylaxis: A word that doctors use when they mean prevention!

Protozoa: The simplest organisms in the animal kingdom, consisting each of a single nucleated cell. Some of them cause disease. Malaria, amoebic dysentery, sleeping sickness, trichomoniasis, and giardiasis are all caused by protozoa.

Psychotropic: Mind- or mood-altering.

Purpura: Gross bleeding into the skin, resulting in large purple patches.

RAST test: Radioallergosorbent test — an allergy test done on a sample of blood.

Retro-orbital: Behind the eye.

Rickettsiae: A group of micro-organisms that have many similarities to bacteria. They include the micro-organisms that cause typhus.

Rigor: Shiver accompanying fever; may signify severe infection, or malaria.

Serology: A blood test that detects the presence of antibodies to a particular antigen (e.g. HIV test)

Serotype: The particular sub-type of bacteria or virus, as determined by antibody testing

Sputum: Phlegm; mucus secretions from the lung and respiratory passages.

Subcutaneous: Under all layers of the skin. Many immunizations are injected subcutaneously.

Sylvatic: Jungle or forest form, as in sylvatic yellow fever.

Systemic: Affecting the body as a whole. Systemic treatment is the opposite of local or topical treatment.

Thrombosis: Clotting of blood within a vein.

Thrombocytopenia: Reduction in the number of platelets in the blood may lead to bleeding.

Toxin: A specific chemical product produced by a living organism that damages or poisons another organism (e.g. man).

Trophozoite: The active, feeding, growing, disease-producing form of a protozoan parasite.

Ulcer: An inflamed defect following damage at the surface of the skin, the stomach lining, or any other tissue surface.

Vector: A carrier of infection or of a parasite from one host to the next.

Viruses: Tiny, particulate micro-organisms; much smaller than bacteria and too small to be seen without the aid of the electron microscope. They live inside our cells, multiplying within them, and it is this characteristic which protects them from antibodies and drugs, and makes viral infections so difficult to treat.

Visceral: Internal

Vitiligo: Patches of white, de-pigmented skin.

Index